Handbook of
PHARMACOLOGY of AGING
Second Edition

Handbook of PHARMACOLOGY of AGING

Second Edition

Edited by
Jay Roberts • David L. Snyder • Eitan Friedman

CRC Press
Boca Raton New York London Tokyo

Publisher/Life Sciences:	Robert B. Stern
Editorial Assistant:	Carol Messing
Project Editor:	Carrie L. Unger
Marketing Manager:	Susie Carlisle
Direct Marketing Manager:	Becky McEldowney
Cover design:	Shayna Murry
PrePress:	Kevin Luong
Manufacturing:	Sheri Schwartz

Library of Congress Cataloging-in-Publication Data

Handbook of pharmacology of aging / edited by David Snyder, Jay Roberts, Eitan Friedman. — 2nd ed.
p. cm. — (CRC Series on pharmacology and toxicology handbooks)
Rev. ed. of: CRC handbook of pharmacology of aging. 1983.
Includes bibliographical references and index.
ISBN 0-8493-8306-4 (alk. paper)
1. Geriatric pharmacology--Handbooks, manuals, etc. I. Snyder, David L. (David Leroy).
I. Roberts, Jay. III. CRC handbook of pharmacology on aging. IV. Series: Pharmacology and toxicology (Boca Raton, FL)
RC953.7.C73 1996
615.5′.8′0846—dc20

96-14773
CIP

International Standard Book Number 0-8493-8306-4
Library of Congress Card Number 96-14773
Printed in the United States of America 1 2 3 4 5 6 7 8 9 0
Printed on acid-free paper

Handbooks of

Pharmacology and Toxicology

A CRC Press Series

Mannfred A. Hollinger, Series Editor
University of California, Davis

Published Titles

Handbook of Pharmacokinetic and Pharmacodynamic Correlations with Computer Applications
Hartmut Derendorf

Handbook of Methods in Gastrointestinal Pharmacology
Timothy S. Gaginella

Handbook of Targeted Delivery of Imaging Agents
Vladimir P. Torchilin

Handbook of Pharmacology of Aging, Second Edition
Jay Roberts, David L. Snyder, and Eitan Friedman

Forthcoming Titles

Handbook of Theoretical Models in Biomedical Research
David B. Jack

Handbook of Mammalian Models in Biomedical Research
David B. Jack

Handbook of Plant and Fungal Toxicants
J. P. Felix D'Mello

Handbook of Opportunistic Infections
Vassil St. Georgiev

SERIES PREFACE

As the "graying" of America continues, the number of elderly people at risk from adverse drug reactions is also increasing. This is due to a number of factors including diminished physiological functions influencing both pharmacokinetic and pharmacodynamic aspects of drug effects. In addition, as people reach their sixth decade of life, the number of drugs that they concurrently use begins to increase in an almost linear fashion, thus raising the specter of drug interactions. This is particularly true for anticoagulant, anti-inflammatory, and oral hypoglycemic drugs which are routinely used by the geriatric population.

Since the publication of the first edition of this handbook in 1983, our knowledge of age-related factors influencing drug effects has increased significantly. It is timely, therefore, that this new information has been organized by the editors utilizing contributors of the highest stature. It is hoped that the material in this edition will contribute to an increased awareness of the special aspects of geriatric pharmacology and prevent needless toxic drug experiences in the elderly.

Mannfred Hollinger
Series Editor

PREFACE

In 1908 Elie Metchnikoff received the Nobel Prize for his many contributions to biology and the ***study of aging***. He introduced the concept that aging was caused by the continuous absorption of toxins from intestinal bacteria.

That singular event aside, little of significance to gerontology occurred during the next 40 years. Most authors regard the modern period of gerontology to have begun about 1950 when systematic studies that described the aging phenotype in terms of physiology, biochemistry, and cell morphology were carried out. The last 45 years might have led to better defined, experimentally testable hypotheses; however, that has not yet occurred.

The optimism that these studies would lead to well-developed, defined, experimentally testable hypotheses on the mechanisms of aging has not been fully realized. It is (arguably) probably fair to say that biological gerontology still lacks enough truly fundamental information to allow formulation of a central theme and of hypotheses which define the field. One theme, that aging is the result of the declining force of natural selection with age, has given us a kind of theoretical touchstone, but has done little to define experimental approaches.

The fact that there is no adequate theory of biological aging has done nothing to discourage the proliferation of theories. Historically, one of the major problems in gerontology is the ease and frequency with which new theories have appeared. Most researchers have viewed aging as "a thing" that happens rather than as a period of the life history of organisms that begins at maturity and lasts for the rest of the life span. Aging is not one thing and probably does not have a single cause. Furthermore, the changes that occur with age may be interdependent. Aging need not depend on a single mechanism. The major mechanisms regulating the aging rate in fixed postmitotic cells may be different from those operating in renewable tissues. Superimposed on all this is the fact that the combination of environmental damage and intrinsic processes further obscures the fundamental mechanisms operating. Our view of aging should be the same as our view of development. During both processes numerous primary and secondary changes occur. Some changes are caused by the environment; others seem to be programmed and directed within the body. Understanding aging and formulating coherent, testable hypotheses requires that these various aspects of aging be dissected from each other and examined critically. This has proven to be and undoubtedly is a complex task. No matter how complex, modern biology cannot realistically ignore a process that occurs with essentially the same scenario in the somatic cells of most eukaryotes. Nor can biologists avoid the challenge of exploring the differing trajectories of aging in different species. For example, the mouse and the human have similar physiologies and nearly identical quantities of DNA/cell and yet complete what we call their maximum life spans in a chronological period that differs by about 30-fold. Mice get cancer at about 30 times the rate of humans. This observation suggests that aging is regulated by a highly conserved mechanism that runs at a variable and species-specific rate. For the biologist, the compelling attraction of aging is the challenge of discovering how so fundamental and universal a biologic property works. To the geriatrician, the outcome of a better understanding of the process of aging means an improved armamentarium of treatments and strategies for improving the quality of life of elderly people.

To summarize briefly what we know about aging, it is clear that aging is characterized by an increasing vulnerability to environmental change. A consequence of this is that increasing chronological age brings with it an increasing probability of dying. Some biologists argue that the survivorship kinetics of biological aging may be an artifact of civilization, domestication, and zoos. In nature, populations of animals (including humans) only recently began to live long enough to show the characteristic kinetics of biological aging. Most species in the wild are killed by predators or die from accidents long before they have a chance to show the increasing vulnerability that characterizes biological aging.

In fact, we may ask why the biological aging process, characteristic of protected populations, should occur at all in nature. If we think of aging as a genetically programmed, purposeful process, in which vulnerability to the environment increases with time, then we must consider how evolution would have selected for such a process. Why should evolution select for a negative property? Perhaps the most attractive set of ideas has been proposed by Medawar (1952) and Williams (1957). Both argue that optimization of reproduction is what is selected for. Medawar pointed out that deleterious genes associated with senescence may be delayed until the postreproductive period. Williams (1957) introduced the idea of antagonistic pleiotropy, which states that genes expressed early in life and associated with optimization of fecundity have deleterious effects later in life. Thus, aging may be the price we pay for mechanisms that assure successful reproduction. Sacher (1968) and Cutler (1979) have argued that the important question is not why we grow old, but why we live as long as we do.

For the purpose of this volume and for placing the various chapters in perspective it might be helpful to the readers to review the various classes of theories of aging. I would emphasize that these theories, however classified, are not mutually exclusive and are global in nature.

The first class of theories can be described as stochastic theories. In this formulation, aging is caused by the accumulation of "insults" from the environment. The insults eventually reach a level incompatible with life. The most prominent specific example of this class of theories is the somatic mutation theory of aging. The theory states that mutations in somatic cells (genetic damage), presumably resulting from background radiation and perhaps radiomimetic agents, will accumulate and eventually produce functional failure and ultimately death. The major experimental support for this theory was derived from the well-documented observation that exposure to ionizing radiation shortens life span.

On logical grounds, life span shortening by radiation does not define whether the mechanism for this life span shortening bears any relationship to the normal mechanism of aging. One can envision numerous treatments that would shorten life span but are not related to normal aging. The pitfalls inherent in using death as an end point for aging are eminently obvious in this example.

The developmental-genetic theories consider the process of aging to be part of a continuum with development, genetically controlled, and programmed. Resistance to the idea of an aging process that is continuous with and probably operating through the same mechanisms as development derives from two sources. One has to do with the earlier discussed selection for aging mechanisms through evolution. The second results from an intuitive sense that the diverse scenarios and trajectories of aging are not likely to be controlled by a process whose mechanisms regulate the precise processes of development. I believe this negative view really derives from the notion that death is the relevant end point for aging, and that the regulation of aging depends on a single process.

We can consider three examples of developmental-genetic theories. The first group can be collected under the general heading of neuroendocrine theories of aging. This group of theories regard functional decrements in neurons and their associated hormones as central to the aging process. Given the major integrative role of the neuroendocrine system in physiology, this is an attractive approach. An important version of this theory proposes that the hypothalamic, pituitary, adrenal axis is the master timekeeper for the organism and the primary regulator of the aging process. Functional changes in this system are accompanied by or regulate functional decrements throughout the organism. The cascade effect of functional decrements in the hypothalamus, for example, and their potential sequelae are evident. The neuroendocrine system regulates early development, growth, puberty, the control of the reproductive system, metabolism and in part the activities of all the major organ systems in the body. Several lines of evidence have accumulated that support the neuroendocrine theory.

A second developmental-genetic theory is the immunological theory of aging. This theory, as proposed by Walford (1981), is based on two observations: (1) that the functional capacity of the immune system declines with age, as seen in reduced T-cell function (Walford, 1969) and in reduced resistance to infectious disease, and (2) that the fidelity of the immune system declines with age as evidenced by the striking age-associated increase in autoimmune disease. Walford (1979) has related these immune system changes to the genes of the major histocompatibility complex in rats and mice.

The third example of development-genetic theory has to de with free radicals. This theory proposes that most aging changes are due to damage caused by radicals. For example, autoxidation of lipids by free-radical pathways may lead to the formation of hydroperoxides, which then decompose to products such as ethane and pentane. Of course other molecules may be damaged by free radicals and reactive oxygen species may also operate to regulate gene expression directly.

This is an attractive theory because it provides a mechanism for aging that does not depend on tissue-specific action but is fundamental to all aerobic tissues.

Modern gerontologists emphasize that the failures of aging tissues probably result from both genetic changes and environmental insults. A view that I find appealing is that the genetic component of aging is really the component that maintains the regulatory fidelity of the organisms physiology for a period consistent with reproductive success. These putative *fidelity assurance mechanisms* have a limited life span after which they deteriorate, thus leaving the organism vulnerable to the random insults that result in dysregulation and ultimately death. Thus, the important issue may be why we live as long as we do and what mechanisms exist to assure that we do.

Sorting out these theoretical questions does not obviate studies on interventions which delay the deteriorative cascades we recognize as aging. Many, if not all, of them are amenable to pharmacological interventions. The collection of chapters in this volume will provide timely insights into these interventions as well as into the fundamental mechanisms of aging.

Vince Cristofalo, Ph.D.

REFERENCES

Cutler, R. G., Evolution of human longevity: a critical overview, *Mech. Ageing Dev.*, 9, 337, 1979.

Medawar, P. B., *An Unsolved Problem of Biology*, London, HK Lewis, 1952.

Sacher, G. A., Molecular versus systemic theories on the genesis of aging, *Exp. Gerontol.*, 3, 265, 1968.

Walford, R. L. et al., Immunopathology of aging, *Ann. Rev. Gerontol, Ger.*, Eisdorfer, C., Ed., New York, Springer-Verlag, 1981, 3.

Walford, R. L., Multigene families, histocompatibility system, transformation, meiosis, stem cells and DNA repair, *Mech. Ageing. Dev.*, 9, 19, 1979.

Walford, R., *The Immunologic Theory of Aging*, Copenhagen, Munksgaard, 1969.

Williams, G. C., Pleiotropy, natural selection and the evolution of senescence, *Evolution*, 11, 398, 1957.

INTRODUCTION

Since the *Handbook of the Pharmacology of Aging* was first published in 1983, several notable advances markedly accelerated research in this field and contributed to acquisition of important new information on pharmacogerontology, thereby necessitating an entirely new volume. First, the relevance of the whole field of pharmacogerontology to practical therapeutic issues became widely appreciated, often as a result of tragic consequences ensuing from inadvertent neglect of age-associated pharmacokinetic or pharmacodynamic changes while administering drugs to elderly patients.

Second, the pharmaceutical industry developed and successfully applied the principle of targeting specific, normally occurring enzymes, receptors and other proteins in the body as sites for inhibition or stimulation by new drugs. Such new agents were generally very potent, often with relatively low therapeutic indices, thereby necessitating a more rational use and more precise individualization of drug dosage.

Third, there has been expanded federal support by several NIH institutes, as well as other agencies, for research on several commonly occurring, highly debilitating diseases associated with aging, including neoplastic and cardiovascular disorders, osteoporosis, Parkinson's disease, and Alzheimer's disease. Many new drugs and novel therapeutic modalities have been developed for several of these diseases, and new lead compounds are in active development for neurodegenerative disorders. The recognition of specific problems associated with administering these agents to the elderly has lead to the development of pharmacogerontological principles. Elderly subjects have several special challenges compared to middle aged adults. Apparently normal elderly subjects must be carefully examined to exclude disease before assessing how drugs are handled in these subjects. Yet, the very changes that occur in drug action in the elderly take place largely because of degenerative alterations in the heart, liver, and kidneys (see Figure 1). For example, cardiac output declines approximately 1% per year from age 19 to 86 and a decreased proportion of cardiac output goes to the liver and kidney resulting in decreased drug elimination. Age-induced changes in the structure and function of critical organs and molecules probably occur at different rates in different individuals. Therefore individuals of the same chronological age can suffer different degrees of cardiovascular, hepatic, or renal degeneration with a corresponding variation in drug action. Exogenous environmental factors that can modify drug disposition also change with age. These include cigarette smoking, various dietary changes, alcohol, coffee and tea consumption, and exposure at home or at work to chemicals that can induce or inhibit hepatic drug metabolizing enzymes (Figure 1). In the elderly cumulative lifetime exposures to toxicants often become manifest as disease. With age, the following changes tend to occur, often concomitantly, thereby complicating analysis of drug disposition and response in the elderly: cigarette smoking decreases or stops, total caloric intake declines, the amount of exercise is reduced, retirement tends to make life more sedentary, alcohol, tea, and coffee consumption goes down, and exposure to chemicals at work and at home decreases. As a result of decreased caloric intake, the total body weight tends to decline. Relationships between total body fat, muscle, and extracellular fluids change; for example, body fat gradually increases with age at the expense of lean body mass (muscle) from 18 to 36% of the total body weight in men and from 33 to 48% in women. Each patient can often reveal a different mix of these factors and effects, thereby requiring individualization of drug selection and dosage. The elderly often receive multiple drugs simultaneously, magnifying enormously the problems described above for a single drug. Opportunities for interactions among drugs and host factors proliferate exponentially when many drugs are consumed by the same elderly patient.

The fourth notable advance to affect pharmacogerontology occurred in molecular biology. Basic advances in this field allowed definition at the molecular level of the specific enzymes, receptors and other proteins directly involved in pharmacokinetic and pharmacodynamic processes. Such new knowledge led to fresh insight into how aging at the molecular level affects these processes and alters drug response, Molecular biology has also revealed how some of the individual factors depicted in Figure 1 play a role in pharmacogerontology.

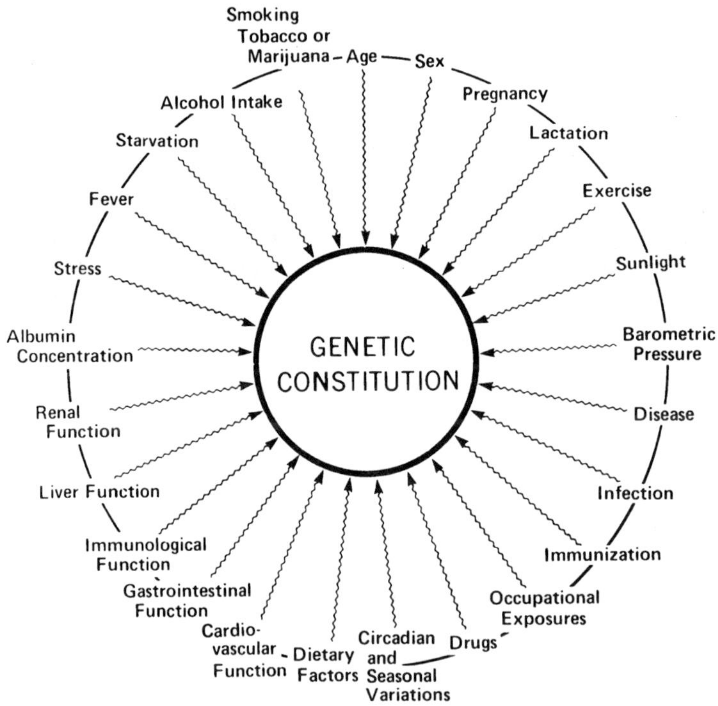

Figure 1. This circular design suggests the multiplicity of host factors that may influence drug response in humans. A line joins all such factors in the outer circle to indicate their close interrelationship. Arrows from each factor in the outer circle to genetic factors in the inner circle are wavy to indicate that effects of each host factor on genetically determined rates of drug response may occur at multiple sites and through different processes. These processes include drug absorption, distribution, metabolism, excretion, receptor action, and combinations thereof.

All authors of the individual chapters in this volume should be congratulated! Each has made an important contribution that will require this outstanding book to be widely read and quoted. The *Handbook* should stimulate even further advances in this exciting and rapidly developing field.

Ellito S. Vesell, MD., Sc.D.

THE EDITORS

Jay Roberts, Ph.D., is Professor and Chair of the Department of Pharmacology at the Medical College of Pennsylvania and Hahnemann University, Philadelphia, Pennsylvania.

Dr. Roberts received his B.S. degree from Long Island University, New York in 1949. He obtained his Ph.D. degree in 1953 from the Cornell University Graduate School of Medical Sciences. He was a member of the faculty of Cornell University Medical School from 1955 to 1966 and was appointed Associate Professor in 1962. He served as Professor of Pharmacology at the University of Pittsburgh in the Department of Pharmacology from 1966 through 1970. In 1970, he assumed the position as Professor and Chair of Pharmacology at the Medical College of Pennsylvania and became Professor and Chair in 1994 of the Department of Pharmacology of the Medical College of Pennsylvania and Hahnemann University when the two institutions merged.

Dr. Roberts is a member of American Society for Pharmacology and Experimental Therapeutics and is a Fellow of the American College of Clinical Pharmacology College of Physicians (Philadelphia) and the American College of Cardiology and the Gerontological Society of America. He has served on NIH study sections and review committees of the American Heart Association (Pennsylvania and South Eastern section). He has served as Chair and Member of the Revision of U.S. Pharmacopeia-Convention Geriatrics Division. He was a Reviewer for Technology Advisory Council on Advanced Medical and Biotechnologies for the Advanced Technology Center of Southeastern Pennsylvania. He is a member of the Gerontological Society of America and was the Chair of the Biological Sciences section in 1982.

Dr. Roberts has served on the Editorial Board of the *Journals of Geriatric Drug Therapy*; as *Ad hoc* reviewer for Veterans Administration merit award grants; and on the International Editorial Board of *Excerpta Medica* as Associate Editor. He became Assistant Editor of the *Journal of Pharmacology and Experimental Therapeutics* in 1991. He is also a member of the Society for Experimental Biology and Medicine, the Harvey Society, and American Association for the Advancement of Science.

He was an Associate Editor for the *Journal of Gerontology* — Biological Sciences, Pharmacology Section and became Editor in 1996. He has also served on the Editorial Board of the *Journal of Cardiovascular Pharmacology* and as a reviewer for *Experimental Aging Research*. Dr. Roberts was Chair of the American Heart Association Pennsylvania Affiliate Research Committee from 1976 through 1995. Dr. Roberts is presently on the Editorial Boards of the *Journal of Clinical Pharmacology* and the *Journal of Geriatric Drug Therapy*.

Dr. Roberts is author or co-author of more than 150 publications. His current major research interests include the effect of age, gender, and diet on the control of the heart by the adrenergic nervous system.

David Snyder, Ph.D., is an Assistant Professor in the Department of Pharmacology at the Medical College of Pennsylvania and Hahnemann University in Philadelphia.

Dr. Snyder received his B.S. and Ph.D. degrees from The Pennsylvania State University in 1975 and 1982, respectively. After doing postdoctoral work at the Lobund Institute at the University of Notre Dame, he was appointed Assistant Faculty Fellow with the Lobund Institute at the University of Notre Dame in 1985. Dr. Synder obtained a Postdoctoral Research Fellowship with the Department of Pharmacology and the Center for Gerontological Research at the Medical College of Pennsylvania, Philadelphia, Pennsylvania in 1990 and served as an Instructor in 1992. He became an Assistant Professor in 1994.

Dr. Snyder is a member of the Gerontological Society of America and the Association for Gnotobiotics. He was appointed to the Editorial Review Board of the *Journal of Gerontology* — Biological Sciences in 1996.

Dr. Snyder is the author of 29 peer-reviewed journal publications and in 1989 edited the book *Dietary Restriction and Aging*. His current research interests relate to aging of the sympathetic nervous system in the heart and spleen, dietary restriction's capacity to extend life span, and geriatric pharmacology.

Eitan Friedman, Ph.D., is Chief, Division of Molecular Pharmacology in the Department of Pharmacology at the Medical College of Pennsylvania and Hahnemann University in Philadelphia, Pennsylvania.

Dr. Friedman received his B.A. in Chemistry from Brooklyn College in 1966 and was awarded a Ph.D. from New York Medical College in 1971. Dr. Friedman did postdoctoral research in the Neuropsychopharmacology Research Unit at New York University School of Medicine in 1971–1972. In 1973, he was appointed Instructor in Experimental Psychiatry at New York University School of Medicine and moved up in rank at this institution and was appointed Associate Professor in 1979. Dr. Friedman was appointed Professor of Psychiatry and Pharmacology and Director of the Division of Neurochemistry at the Medical College of Pennsylvania, Philadelphia, Pennsylvania in 1986 and became Chief of the Division of Molecular Pharmacology at the Medical College of Pennsylvania and Hahnemann University in 1995.

Dr. Friedman is a member of American Association for the Advancement of Science, American College of Neuropsychopharmacology, New York Academy of Sciences, International Society for Neurochemistry, Society of Biological Psychiatry, European College of Neuropsychopharmacology, American Society for Neurochemistry, and the American Society of Pharmacological and Experimental Therapeutics.

Dr. Friedman has served on the Editorial Board of *Neurobiology of Aging* and is currently Deputy Editor of the *Journals of Gerontology* — Biological Science. He served as reviewer of research grants for the National Institutes of Health study section and a reviewer for numerous professional publications.

Dr. Friedman is author and co-author of more than 160 peer reviewed publications and numerous book chapters. His interests include the neurobiology of the aging brain, signal transduction in excitable tissue, and the neurobiology of Alzheimer's disease.

CONTRIBUTORS

James R. Docherty, Ph.D.
Department of Physiology
Royal College of Surgeons in Ireland
Green, Dublin, Ireland

Natalie D. Eddington, Ph.D.
Pharmacokinetic and Biopharmaceutical Laboratory
Department of Pharmaceutical Sciences
University of Maryland School of Pharmacy
Baltimore, Maryland

Lynn E. Fisher-Katz, Pharm.D.
Department of Pharmacy
Summa Health System
Akron, Ohio

Emil J Freireich, M.D.
University of Texas
M.D. Anderson Cancer Center
Houston, Texas

Walter Fried, M.D.
Department of Medicine
Division of Hematology and Oncology
Lutheran General Hospital
Park Ridge, Illinois

Eitan Friedman, Ph.D.
Department of Pharmacology
Medical College of Pennsylvania and Hahnemann University
Philadelphia, Pennsylvania

Samual Gershon, M.D.
Western Psychiatric Institute and Clinic
University of Pittsburgh Medical Center
Pittsburgh, Pennsylvania

Concetta Harakal, Ph.D.
Department of Pharmacology
Temple University School of Medicine
Philadelphia, Pennsylvania

Howard Hurtig, M.D.
Department of Neurology
Graduate Hospital
Philadelphia, Pennsylvania

Mark D. Johnson, Ph.D.
Department of Pharmacology
Medical College of Pennsylvania and Hahnemann University
Philadelphia, Pennsylvania

Richard A. Josephson, M.S., M.D
Department of Medicine
Northeastern Ohio Universities College of Medicine and
Department of Biomedical Engineering
University of Akron
Akron, Ohio and
Department of Medicine
Summa Health System
Akron, Ohio

Ti Li Loo, Ph.D.
Department of Pharmacology
The George Washington University Medical Center
Washington, D.C.

David R. Lynch , M.D., Ph.D.
Department of Neurology and Pediatrics
Children's Hospital of Philadelphia
The University of Pennsylvania and
Department of Neurology
Graduate Hospital
Philadelphia, Pennsylvania

H. George Mandel, Ph.D.
Department of Pharmacology
The George Washington University Medical Center
Washington, D.C.

Philip I. Markowitz, M.D.
Department of Psychiatry
Medical College of Pennsylvania and Hahnemann University
Philadelphia, Pennsylvania

J. Bruce Miller, M.D.
Department of Medicine
Division of Hematology and Oncology
Lutheran General Hospital
Park Ridge, Illinois

John M. Morgan
Departments of Medicine and Pharmacology
Medical College of Pennsylvania and Hahnemann University
Philadelphia, Pennsylvania

Njanoor Narayanan, Ph.D.
Department of Physiology
The University of Western Ontario
London, Ontario, Canada

Anthony J. Piraino
Departments of Medicine and Phamacology
Division of Clinical Pharmacology
The Medical College of Pennsylvania and
Hahnemann University
Philadelphia, Pennsylvania

Elliot Richelson, M.D.
Department of Research
Mayo Clinic Jacksonville
Jacksonville, Florida and
Departments of Pharmacology
Mayo Medical School
Rochester, Minnesota

Jay Roberts, Ph.D.
Department of Pharmacology
Medical College of Pennsylvania and
Hahnemann University
Philadelphia, Pennsylvania

Philip J. Scarpace, Ph.D.
Geriatric Research Education
and Clinical Center
Department of Veterans Affairs
Medical Center
Gainesville, Florida and
Department of Pharmacology
University of Florida
Gainesville, Florida

Jair C. Soares
Western Psychiatric Institute and Clinic
University of Pittsburgh Medical Center
Pittsburgh, Pennsylvania

David L. Snyder, Ph.D.
Department of Pharmacology
Medical College of Pennsylvania and
Hahnemann University
Philadelphia, Pennsylvania

Nihal Tümer, Ph.D.
Geriatric Research Education
and Clinical Center
Department of Veterans Affairs
Medical Center
Gainesville, Florida and
Department of Pharmacology
University of Florida
Gainesville, Florida

Ashiwel S. Undie, Ph.D.
Program in Pharmacology and Neuroscience
Department of Pharmaceutical Sciences
University of Maryland
School of Pharmacy
Baltimore, Maryland

Ellito S. Vesell, MD., Sc.D.
Department of Pharmacology
The Pennsylvania State University
College of Medicine
Hershey, Pennsylvania

James D. Winkler, Ph.D.
Department of Immunopharmacology
SmithKline Beecham Pharmaceuticals
King of Prussia, Pennsylvania

Mitsuhiko Yamada, M.D., Ph.D.
Department of Neuroscience Research
Mayo Clinic Jacksonville
Jacksonville, Florida

TABLE OF CONTENTS

Chapter 1

PHARMACOKINETICS

Natalie D. Eddington

CONTENTS

I. INTRODUCTION — DEMOGRAPHICS AND DRUG USAGE

The elderly population is one of the fastest growing segments of our society.[1] Today they comprise approximately 12% of the U.S. population. However, they consume more than 30% of the total prescription drugs purchased.[1] By the year 2030 the consumption of prescription drugs by the elderly may amount to more than 40%.[2] A large portion of this percentage will be used for the treatment of multiple chronic diseases in the elderly patient.[2] Due to the high incidence of polypharmacy in the elderly and more importantly the functional decline of various organ systems, this population is extremely sensitive to drug effects and is more susceptible to adverse drug reactions.

There is a rapidly accumulating literature that clearly documents pharmacokinetic differences due to aging.[3–7] Examining these alterations can provide insight on the degree to which those physiological processes responsible for drug biotransformation are altered in the aging patient. The physiological changes that accompany aging produce changes in pharmacokinetics, efficacy, and, of course, toxicity in the elderly population.

Advancing age produces physiological changes that have the potential of directly affecting the absorption, distribution, metabolism, and elimination of drugs. There are several age-related changes in gastrointestinal function that might alter the absorption of drugs. These include reductions in gastric acid secretion, gastrointestinal motility, and blood flow. Changes

0-8493-8306-4/96/$0.00+$.50

in body composition, such as reductions in the lean muscle mass, increase in the adipose tissue content, and decreases in total body water, can alter drug distribution. Age-related physiological changes in the P450 oxidative enzyme systems and diminished liver perfusion affect the metabolism of hepatically biotransformed agents. Diminished renal blood perfusion and reduction in the number of functioning nephrons lead to alterations in renal drug clearance in the elderly patient. For the most part the aging process results in alterations in the absorption, distribution, and elimination of various therapeutic agents. Circumspect examination of the age-related changes in pharmacokinetics allows for greater insight and understanding of the physiologic changes associated with the aging process.

II. ORAL ABSORPTION

A. PHYSIOLOGICAL AND PHYSIOCHEMICAL DETERMINANTS

The process of aging has a multifaceted effect on the physiological determinants of oral drug absorption. The age-related physiological changes, in turn, have a varied effect on the absorption of drugs along the gastrointestinal tract. In general, the physiological factors that control drug absorption are as follows: gastrointestinal pH, gastrointestinal enzymes, and gastrointestinal motility. Each of these operates in conjunction with the other factors to promote or hinder the absorption of drugs from the gastrointestinal tract. Because there are so many factors that can directly affect absorption, it is difficult to attribute a specific age-related pharmacokinetic change to a single age-related physiologic change. For example, if there is a reduction in the absorption rate constant (ka) in the elderly, is this reduction due to changes in motility or changes in the pH of the stomach? To further complicate this, the pharmacokinetics of oral absorption are also influenced by chronic disease states (e.g., congestive heart failure, hepatic and renal dysfunction) and the nutritional status of the geriatric patient. In addition to the age-associated changes in gastrointestinal physiology, the health status of the elderly patient also plays a significant role in drug absorption.

B. PHARMACOKINETICS OF DRUG ABSORPTION

Prior to discussing the consequence of aging on oral absorption, it is first important to review the pharmacokinetics of drug absorption. The rate and extent of absorption are represented by the following pharmacokinetic parameters: absorption rate constant (ka), maximal plasma concentration (C_{max}), time of maximal plasma concentration (T_{max}), area under the plasma concentration time curve, ($AUC_{0\text{-}\infty}$), and bioavailability (F).[8] The ka, C_{max}, and T_{max} provide an indication of the rate of absorption. The $AUC_{0\text{-}\infty}$ and F denote the extent of absorption. These absorption parameters represent the aggregate of the interplay between both the physiochemical drug properties (i.e., pKa, disintegration, solubility, dissolution) and the physiological factors associated with drug absorption (i.e., gastrointestinal pH, motility, blood flow). Since the parameters describe so many components, the difficulty of attributing an alteration in an absorption parameter to an age-related change in physiology is evident. If there is a reduction in ka for a particular drug in the elderly patient, it is difficult to definitively state that the decrease is solely due to a specific alteration in gastrointestinal physiology. This identifies one of the controversies in the gerontology literature. There are many investigators that state equivocally that there are no age-related changes in drug absorption, while other researchers report significant alterations due to aging.[3–7]

C. GASTROINTESTINAL TRACT AND ORAL ABSORPTION

The oral absorption of drugs is dependent on the physiological properties of the gastrointestinal tract and the physiochemical properties of the drug. Each factor plays an important role in drug absorption. Considering oral solid dosage forms, the stomach provides an environment for the disintegration, dissolution, and occasionally absorption of drugs. After the dosage form disintegrates in the stomach, dissolution is initiated. Dissolution is predicated on the physiochemical drug properties. Since most drugs are either weak acids or weak bases, the dictator of dissolution as well as absorption is the pKa of the drug and the pH of the environment. In general, the ionized form of the drug will have the fastest dissolution and the unionized form will be readily absorbed via passive processes. Absorption is highly dependent on the pH of the various segments of the gastrointestinal tract. The stomach with a pH of 1 to 2.5 provides an area for the absorption of most weak acids. On the other hand, weak bases, for the most part, are absorbed in the upper sections of the small intestine with a characteristic pH of 5 to 6. The aging process has numerous effects on the gastrointestinal tract that can potentially affect the drug absorption.

D. ACHLORHYDRIA AND ORAL DRUG ABSORPTION

One of the most pronounced and highly documented effects of aging on the gastrointestinal tract is a decrease in the production of hydrogen ions in the stomach.[9–11] Figure 1.1 illustrates the decrease in total and free acid as a function of age through the eighth decade of life in males and females. From 20 years of age, there is approximately a 30% decrease in the production of hydrogen ions in the gastric mucosa.[11] Basal and histamine-stimulated peak gastric secretion also declines with age.[10] Mojavereian and colleagues[9] reported similar findings by examining the gastric pH in a group of elderly subjects using telemetry. These investigators also reported higher postprandial gastric pH values in the older volunteers, and the mean duration in time to achieve a gastric pH of <4 was significantly longer in the elderly compared to the younger population. These results are most likely due to the reduced rate of gastric acid secretion in the older subjects.

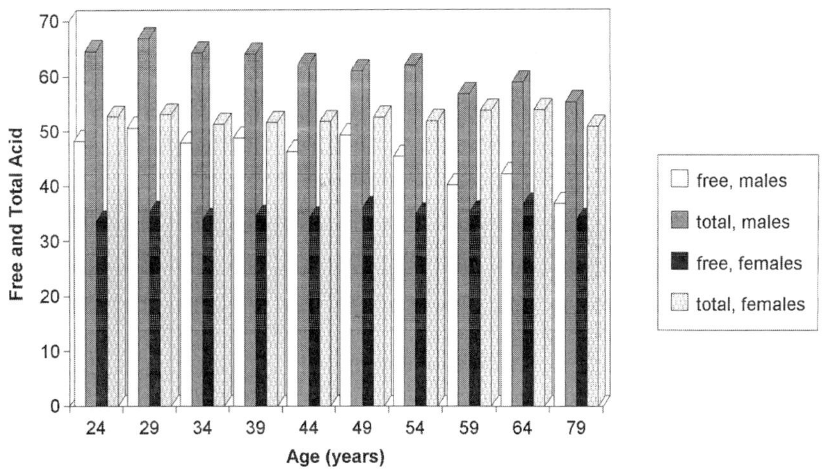

FIGURE 1.1. Total and free acid as a function of age in males and females. (Adapted from Vanzant, F. R. et al., *Arch. Intern. Med.*, 49, 345, 1932.)

The incidence of achlorhydria increases dramatically in males and females from age 29 (Figure 1.2). This change is more pronounced in females. Based on the degree of achlorhydria in the aged population, it is possible that the increase in gastric pH will modulate absorption from the gastrointestinal tract. The possible impact of this change is varied; however, the following might be expected: (1) an increase in pH would theoretically decrease the dissolution of those drugs which require a more acidic environment (i.e., weak bases); (2) an increase in pH would increase the dissolution of those agents which require a more basic environment; (3) the absorption of weak acids in the stomach would be reduced; (4) the absorption of weak bases would be promoted, or (5) those agents which usually degrade in the acidic media of the stomach would be more stable and display higher systemic availability after oral dosing.

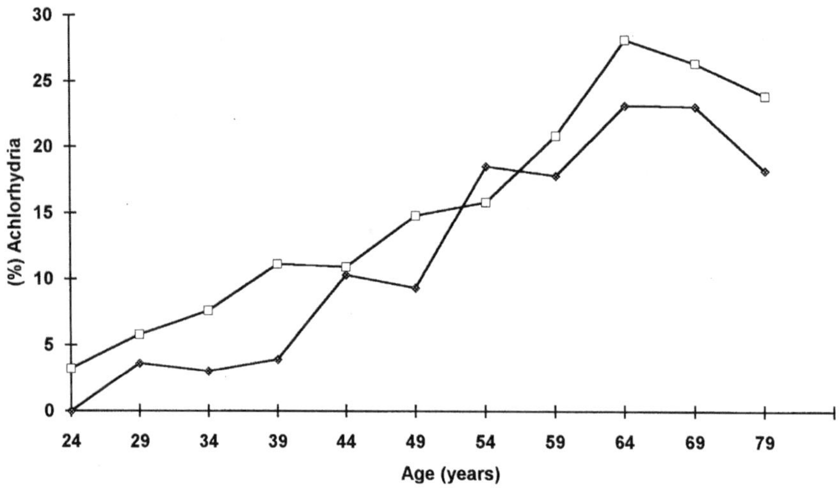

FIGURE 1.2. Percent of achlorhydria as a function of age in males (♦) and females (□). (Adapted from Vanzant, F. R. et al., *Arch. Intern. Med.*, 49, 345, 1932.)

There are no definitive studies in the literature that explicitly report a change in the absorption as a result of age-related alterations in the pH of the stomach. However, there are studies examining alterations in absorption due to achlorhydria. If achlorhydria is present, then the dissolution of weak bases would decrease. This reduction would subsequently diminish the extent of absorption into the systemic circulation in the elderly.

Clinical studies with tetracycline provide an informative example on the possible impact of achlorhydria on drug absorption. This agent requires the acidic pH of the stomach to promote dissolution.[12] The absorption of tetracycline was evaluated in a clinical study after administration to healthy young adults alone and concurrently with sodium bicarbonate.[12] The later treatment was used to mimic achlorhydria. The extent of absorption of tetracycline was markedly reduced when the drug was co-administered with sodium bicarbonate. Alkalinizing the gastric contents severely decreased the dissolution of the dosage form in the stomach. Another study conducted in achlorhydric elderly subjects did not find a decrease in the absorption of tetracycline.[13] There were differences in the formulation of tetracycline used in the two studies. The former study used a formulation with minimal bioavailability. Those differences found in the sodium bicarbonate leg of the study may reflect purely formulation differences and not the influence of simulated achlorhydria.

Glyburide, an oral hypoglycemic with limited solubility in the stomach, has a pKa of 5.3. An increase in gastric pH in the elderly may lead to reduced dissolution of this agent in the stomach. If dissolution is diminished, then the absorption of glyburide may be decreased or delayed. In a comparative study in young and old healthy subjects, the absorption of glyburide was found to be significantly slower in the geriatric group.[14] The T_{max} increased from 2.9 hr in the young to 3.7 hr in the old group. In addition to changes in T_{max}, both the AUC and C_{max} were also affected in the elderly. The AUC_{0-4hr} was reduced from 273 ng*hr/mL in the young to 186 ng*hr/mL in the old group, and the C_{max} was decreased from 138 ng/mL in the young to 95 ng/mL in the older group. The reason for the reduction in absorption is unknown. However, this change may be due to an age-related decrease in the dissolution of glyburide in the stomach, secondary to an increase in pH.

Drugs which degrade in the acidic contents of the stomach may display an increase in absorption due to the reduction of hydrogen ion production in the elderly. Since a lesser amount of the drug would be degraded in the stomach, a greater portion of the dose would reach the systemic circulation.

E. REDUCED GASTRIC EMPTYING AND ORAL DRUG ABSORPTION

Along with the high incidence of achlorhydria in the elderly population, there is an increase in the gastric residence time.[9,15,16] The gastric residence time is an indication of the time required for the contents of the stomach to empty into the small intestine. Table 1.1 summarizes the results from numerous investigations examining the gastric emptying half-time for both liquid and solid dosage forms in young and old volunteers. The gastric emptying half-time was significantly longer in the elderly for all dosage forms.[15,16] A more recent study evaluated gastric residence time with the nondisintegrating Heidleberg capsule.[9] These investigators found a significantly longer residence time in a group of twelve healthy elderly subjects compared to twelve young subjects. How these age-related changes in gastric emptying affect oral absorption is unclear. Depending on the absorption site, we might expect a prolonged absorption phase and an increase in the amount of drug reaching the systemic circulation in the elderly. Here, the slow trek along the gastrointestinal tract may increase the amount of time at the optimal site of absorption. The pharmacokinetic change that would be expected due to slower gastric emptying might be an increase in C_{max} along with a prolonged T_{max}. Evaluation of the absorption parameters without determining residence time will not determine if changes in parameters are due solely to age-related gastric emptying effects.

TABLE 1.1.
Mean Gastric Emptying Half-Times in Young and Elderly Subjects

Age (years)	n[a]	$t_{1/2}$[b] (min)	Ref.
22–31	7	46.7	15
72–86	11	123.3[c]	15
21–62	22	78.0	16
70–84	13	103.0[c]	16
28–39	9	145	9
65–79	12	187[c]	9

[a] n = number of subjects.
[b] $t_{1/2}$ = half-time for gastric emptying.
[c] $p < 0.05$.

The absorption of levodopa in the elderly provides insight on the possible age-related changes in gastric emptying as well as the status of extrahepatic enzymes in the geriatric subject. Levodopa, a high-clearance agent, undergoes presystemic metabolism by the enzyme decarboxylase located in gastrointestinal mucosa. In a study by Robertson et al.,[17] there was a statistically higher bioavailability (F) of levodopa in geriatric subjects compared with younger subjects (F = 63% [old] vs. 41% [young]). These investigators also reported a significantly higher C_{max} (1842 ng/mL [old] vs. 1077 ng/mL [young]) and significantly lower clearance (14.2 mL/min/kg [old] vs. 23.4 mL/min/kg [young]) in the elderly group. These results are also supported by Yeh et al.[18] and Broe et al.[19] who both reported increases in C_{max} and AUC after levodopa dosing in the elderly. The decarboxylase enzyme has been reported to be in high levels in the gastric mucosa[20] and the intestinal mucosa[21] with age-related decreases in activity. The age-related increase in the absorption for levodopa may be attributed to: (1) a decrease in the gastric emptying time, thus allowing more time at the optimal site of absorption and an increase in the amount of drug reaching the systemic circulation; or (2) a decrease in decarboxylase enzyme activity, thus reducing presystemic metabolism and increasing the amount of drug reaching the systemic circulation. The later seems more feasible. When the decarboxylase enzyme inhibitor, carbidopa, is given to young and old subjects the extent of absorption is relatively the same for both groups.[17]

Prolonged gastric residence time may also decrease the rate of absorption or delay the absorption process. This change may be manifested as a lag time in the plasma concentration time curve or an increase in the T_{max}. The antiarrhythmic agent, digoxin,[22] and the antiepileptic agent, vigabatrin,[23] both display an increase in T_{max} in the elderly. This prolonged absorption may be due to the age-related increase in gastric residence time.

F. REDUCED SPLANCHNIC BLOOD FLOW AND ORAL DRUG ABSORPTION

Even though it is difficult to determine the influence of aging on the physiological determinants of oral absorption, the impact of age-related changes in presystemic metabolism on absorption is somewhat clearer. Drugs that undergo a high degree of presystemic or first-pass metabolism are referred to as high-clearance or high-extraction drugs. Prior to reaching the systemic circulation, these agents are extracted or metabolized to a great extent by the liver. Since they are so highly hepatically metabolized, the rate at which they reach the liver via the hepatic blood flow determines the extent of metabolism. For this reason, both the systemic bioavailability and the clearance of these agents are dependent on hepatic blood flow.[24] Increases in hepatic blood flow will decrease the bioavailability and increase the clearance. Conversely, decreases in hepatic blood flow will increase bioavailability and decrease clearance. Both of these scenarios assume that there are no changes in protein binding, metabolizing capabilities of the liver, and volume of distribution.

Blood flow varies as a function of age. Figure 1.3 illustrates the cardiac output, cardiac index, and the splanchnic blood flow from the age of 30 to 79.[25–27] As a function of age, there is a consistent decrease in splanchnic and portal blood flow. By the seventh decade, the splanchnic blood flow has diminished by approximately 40%. High-clearance agents will be potentially sensitive to the changes observed in blood flow with age. Moreover, if these agents exhibit pronounced increases in bioavailability, this will further substantiate the age-related decrease in splanchnic blood flow.

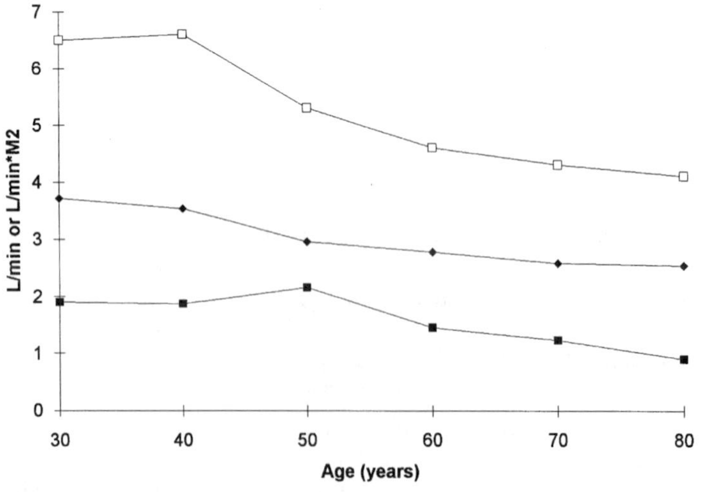

FIGURE 1.3. Decreases in splanchnic blood flow (■), cardiac output (□), and cardiac index (♦) as a function of age in males and females (cardiac index is expressed in L/minM²).[26,27]

An excellent example of a high-extraction drug which exhibits an increase in the extent of absorption is the calcium channel blocker, nifedipine. After a single oral dose of nifedipine the absolute bioavailability was found to be more than 30% higher in the elderly as compared to young adults (Table 1.2).[28] Associated with the increase in the bioavailability was a decrease in the clearance of nifedipine in the elderly (519 mL/min [young] vs. 348 ml/min [old]). The decrease in clearance was also reflected in the formation of the nitropyridine metabolite of nifedipine in the elderly. When comparing the ratio of the metabolite to the parent drug, a much lower ratio was found for the elderly subjects (0.3) as compared to the young volunteers (0.53).

Studies with verapamil, another high-clearance drug, support the findings observed with nifedipine. The clearance of verapamil is directly related to hepatic blood flow. Due to the decrease in splanchnic blood flow as a function of age, a decrease in clearance and an associated increase in bioavailability would be expected. The extent of absorption is increased for verapamil in the geriatric patients secondary to a reduction in the first-pass metabolism of this agent along with a decrease in hepatic blood flow (Table 1.2).[29] Other high-clearance agents that display increases in bioavailability are nalbuphine[30] (Table 1.2), propranolol,[31,32] and lidocaine.[32]

TABLE 1.2.
Bioavailability Differences for High-Clearance Agents in the Elderly

Drug	Young $AUC_{0-\infty}$ (ng·hr/mL)	Old $AUC_{0-\infty}$ (ng·hr/mL)	Young F (%)	Elderly F (%)	Ref.
Nifedipine	136 (56)	281 (64)	0.46 (0.2)	0.61 (0.07)	28
Nalbuphine	25.8 (6.3)	161 (61.2)	11.0 (0.035)	44.2 (0.279)	30
(*S*)-Verapamil	50.4 (36.5)	214 (123.0)	—	—	29

It should be reiterated that the changes noted in the bioavailability of high-clearance agents are due primarily to age-related alterations in liver blood flow. Some of the aforementioned increases in bioavailability may also be due to changes in the volume of distribution of the agent. It is important to keep this in mind when reviewing the pharmacokinetic gerontology literature. If no changes are observed in the volume of distribution after intravenous administration in young and old participants, then the increase in bioavailability may be due solely to reduction in liver blood flow.

III. DISTRIBUTION

A. PHYSIOLOGICAL AND PHYSIOCHEMICAL DETERMINANTS

Unlike absorption, there are specific age-related changes in the physiological determinants of drug distribution whose impact is appreciable and the degree of the change is quantifiable. There are three major physiological determinants of distribution: (1) body composition (i.e., adipose tissue content, muscle mass, and total body water); (2) plasma protein binding (i.e., affinity and capacity); and (3) blood perfusion or flow rate. The interdependency of these physiological factors on the physiochemical drug properties are critical in determining distributional behavior. A lipophilic agent will most likely bind to adipose tissue and its apparent volume of distribution may be rather large. Small volumes of distribution are characteristic of agents that are highly bound to plasma proteins with limited tissue binding. Age-related alterations in the physiological determinants of drug distribution will be apparent when the volume of distribution of various agents is compared between elderly and young subjects.

After drugs enter the systemic circulation they will distribute to various locations, depending on blood flow, protein binding, body composition, and, of course, their physiochemical properties. There are numerous studies in the literature which identify significant changes in those factors which affect drug distribution such as decreases in total body water content, decreases in circulating plasma albumin levels, and increases in adipose tissue content.[3,4,7] These factors play a significant role in the rate and extent of drug that reaches the receptor site.

B. BODY COMPOSITION AND DRUG DISTRIBUTION

Body compositional changes in adipose tissue content and lean muscle mass occur in the elderly. The lipid or adipose tissue content based on body weight increases markedly during the aging process, with a gender-related pattern.[34] Figure 1.4 presents the lean muscle mass and adipose tissue content as a function of age in males and females. Young adult males have a much lower percentage of total body fat (7 to 19%). Conversely, the body fat content of young females ranges from 27 to 33%. By the seventh decade of life, the body fat has risen to about 35% in males and up to as much as 50% of the total body weight of elderly women.

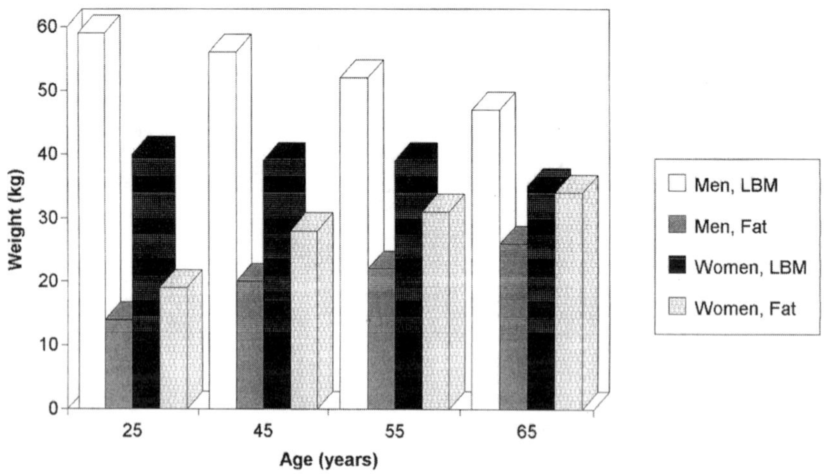

FIGURE 1.4. Age-related changes in lean body mass (LBM) and body fat in males and females. (Adapted from Forbes, G. B. and Reina, J. C., *Metabolism*, 19, 653, 1970.)

Pharmacokinetic evidence of increases in adipose tissue content would be enlargement of the distribution volume for drugs possessing strong lipophilic properties. The benzodiazepines provide an excellent illustration of distribution changes of nonpolar agents. The majority of these agents are very lipophilic, and increases in the volume of distribution have been found. The distribution volume of midazolam, a benzodiazepine used for anesthetic induction, increases in the elderly.[35] After a single intravenous dose the mean volume of distribution at steady state (Vd_{ss}) was found to be 1.22 L/kg in young males vs. 2.47 L/kg in elderly males. In young females the mean Vd_{ss} of midazolam was found to be 0.91 L/kg vs. 1.70 L/kg in older females. Diazepam, another lipophilic benzodiazepine, has also shown increases in the volume of distribution secondary to an age-related increase in body fat.[36] Similar findings have been reported for diazepam in nonelderly obese individuals whose total body fat is as high or higher than the adipose tissue content in the elderly.[37,38] The barbiturates, another class of lipophilic agents, exhibit increases in the volume of distribution associated with a decrease in the ratio of lean muscle to fat content in the elderly. The anesthetic agent, thiopental, tends to have a larger distributional pattern in elderly women compared to young women.[39] Each of these examples further accentuates the impact of increases in adipose tissue content on drug distribution in the geriatric subject.

Associated with the increase in body fat is a decrease in the lean muscle mass (see Figure 1.4). This decrease is more pronounced in females with a 25 to 30% decrease in muscle mass by the age of 70.[34] Reductions in muscle mass would be illustrated by decreases in the distribution volume for those agents with hydrophilic qualities that accumulate in lean tissue. Bromazepam,[40] oxaprozin,[41] and ethanol[42] each distribute to lean muscle and display a decrease in volume of distribution with age. It must be pointed out that the age-related changes noted for both bromazepam and oxaprozin may be due to changes in the bioavailability, since oral doses were administered in each study.

In addition to the body compositional changes in adipose tissue and muscle mass there is an age-related decline in total body water. Figure 1.5 displays the extracellular, intracellular, and total body water content from the third to the ninth decade. Studies by Schock and associates[43] clearly document a decrease in total body water as a function of age. A more recent study has also confirmed these findings.[44] The volume of distribution of agents that distribute into total body water will be influenced by this age-related change. Distribution is reduced for those drugs which are highly hydrophilic, such as ciprofloxacillin.[45] This change is primarily due to a decrease in total body water content as well as decreases in the lean muscle mass.

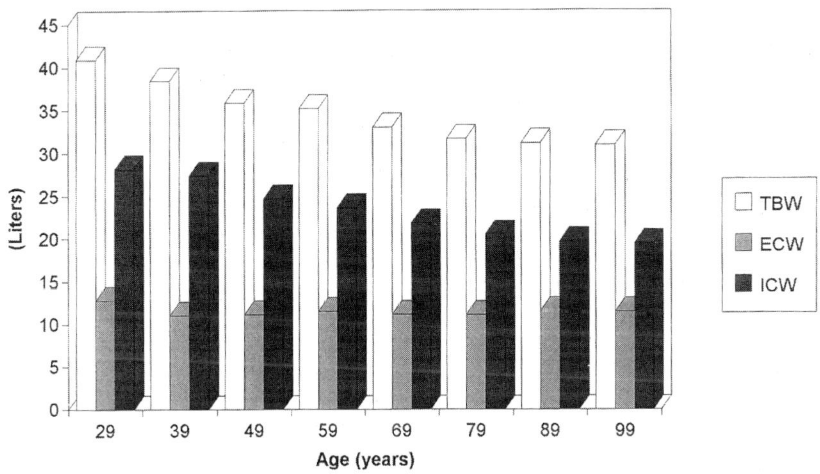

FIGURE 1.5. Changes in total body water (TBW), extracellular water (ECW), and intracellular water (ICW) as a function of age. (Adapted from Shock, N. W. et al., *J. Gerontol.*, 18, 1, 1963.)

The distributional characteristics of neuromuscular blocking agents have been extensively studied in the elderly. These investigations provide an excellent example of how age-related physiological alterations are manifested by changes in pharmacokinetic parameters. Neuromuscular blocking agents are large, polar compounds that tend to follow multicompartment characteristics, and hence their initial distribution is an important determinant of drug action.[46] If we assume a three-compartment model structure to characterize the pharmacokinetics of these agents, then the central compartment represents the blood and highly perfused tissues (i.e., liver, kidney). The second and third compartments represent those tissues that are more slowly perfused. The volume of the central compartment is referred to as the initial distribution volume (V_1) or volume of the central compartment (V_c). This volume represents the amount of drug in the body following intravenous injection and instantaneous mixing divided by the initial concentration of the drug in blood.

Due to the age-related reduction in total body water, decreases in the initial distribution volume would be expected for the hydrophilic neuromuscular blocking agents. After the administration of *d*-tubocurarine,[46] pancuronium,[47] and vecuronium[47] there was a significant decrease in the initial volume of distribution as compared to younger subjects (Table 1.3).

TABLE 1.3.
Age-Related Decreases in the Initial Distribution Volume (V_c) of Selected Agents

Drug	Young (years)	Old (years)	V_c, young (L/kg)	V_c, old (L/kg)	Ref.
Propofol	18–35	65–80	0.415 (0.055)	0.311 (0.080)	49
d-Tubocurarine	30–56	70–87	0.038 (0.007)	0.025[a] (0.006)	46
Metocurine	29–52	70–81	0.039 (0.009)	0.021[a] (0.008)	46
Etomidate	22–62	66–82	0.099 (0.024)	0.075 (0.026)	48

[a] $p < 0.05$.

The physiologic age-related mechanism for the decrease in V_1 of polar compounds is a reduction in total body water. However, this reduction in total body water should not affect the initial distribution of nonpolar, lipophilic compounds. Geriatric patients tend to have a higher initial concentration of most anesthetic agents as compared to younger patients. This is postulated to be due to a decrease in total body water for the polar agent and hence a smaller initial volume. However, these higher initial concentrations and smaller initial volumes have also been observed with lipophilic agents. The nonpolar anesthetic agents etomidate[48] and propofol[49] both show an age-related decrease in their initial distribution volume (Table 1.3). The reason for the smaller initial distribution volume is unclear. However, it may be due to inaccurate estimation of the initial distribution volume due to limited plasma samples at the earlier time points.

Thiopental is an interesting example of how an apparent change in dosing requirements can first be attributed to an age-induced alteration in one physiological process. However, with more accurate pharmacokinetic analysis, the actual physiological process was identified. Early studies with thiopental in the elderly reported significantly higher plasma concentrations after bolus dosing.[50] The increase in plasma concentration was proposed to be due to a shrinkage of the initial volume in the elderly. Recent studies with optimal sampling schemes have determined that the increase in thiopental levels was due to a decrease in the intercompartment clearance.[51–55] This clearance is dependent on blood flow to distribute drug from the central compartment to various peripheral compartments. Decreases in blood perfusion rate with age have been reported, and these changes may play an important role in the clearance of thiopental as opposed to a reduced initial volume. It is important to note that even though intercompartmental clearance of thiopental decreases with age, the volume of distribution at steady state increases as stated previously because of its lipophilic nature.

It appears from the previous example that blood perfusion is a critical determinant of drug distribution and the process of aging decreases blood flow to various tissues. Strum and associates[56] performed an elegant study examining the pharmacokinetics of several liophilic volatile anesthetic agents in the elderly. The agents investigated were isoflurane, enflurane, halothane, and methoxyflurane. Physiologically based compartment modeling was used to describe the distribution. The compartments of the model were as follows: compartment I represented the lungs and pulmonary capillary vasculature (volume of the compartment = V_1); compartment II represented the vessel-rich tissues such as liver, heart, kidneys, and brain (volume = V_2); compartment III represented the muscle tissue (volume = V_3); compartment

IV represented fat adjacent to well-perfused tissues (volume = V_4); and compartment V represented the remaining fat tissues (volume = V_5). Both V_4 and V_5 increased with age for each anesthetic agent. This corresponds to the increase in body fat observed in the elderly with lipophilic agents. Additionally, splanchnic perfusion also displayed an age-related decline in the model based on decreases in the rate constants to compartments II and V. The modulation of the distribution of these volatile anesthetic agents in the elderly highlights the interaction between adipose tissue content, blood perfusion, and the physical and chemical drug properties.

C. PROTEIN BINDING AND DRUG DISTRIBUTION

The volume of distribution is not only governed by blood perfusion and body composition, but protein binding also strongly influences drug distribution. Many drugs interact with plasma, serum, or tissue proteins to form a drug molecule-protein complex. This interaction is usually reversible, and the formation of this complex is dependent on the amount of protein, the physiochemical properties of the drug, and the affinity of the drug-protein complex. Albumin and α_1-acid glycoprotein (AAG) are the major proteins found in the plasma. Many weakly acidic drugs (anions) bind to albumin, whereas cations or basic drugs tend to bind to AAG. Displacement of drugs from protein binding sites will result in an increase in the free or unbound drug concentration and hence elicit a transient rise in the volume of distribution as well as an increase in the elimination of the drug.

Age-related changes in protein binding may be due to either changes in protein concentrations and/or changes in drug affinity for the protein molecule. Serum albumin decreases with age from 4.0% in young adults to 3.5% in elderly subjects.[57] The decrease in albumin is secondary to a decrease in protein synthesis in the liver as well as alterations in the elimination of these agents.[57] The decrease in available protein for drug binding purposes leads to an increase in unbound drug in the plasma. The unbound or free fraction of the drug is the entity that interacts with the receptor site, thus eliciting the pharmacological response.

Considering a drug highly protein bound to albumin, a decrease in plasma proteins will usually cause an increase in the free or unbound drug in the plasma. This free drug can either be transported to peripheral tissue sites for uptake or be eliminated by the excretory organs. If the former route is taken by the free drug, the volume of distribution increases as a function of age. Drugs which exhibit decreased binding (increased free fraction) in the elderly subjects are usually acidic and tend to bind to albumin. Accompanying this increase in the free fraction is usually an increase in the apparent volume of distribution at steady state. This relation is best illustrated by the following equation:

$$Vd_{ss} = Vp + fup / fut * VT \tag{1}$$

where Vp is volume of the plasma compartment, fup and fut are the fraction of drug unbound in plasma and tissue, and VT is the volume of the tissues. As can be seen from Equation 1, increases in fup will increase the Vd_{ss}.

Agents that are highly protein bound to albumin are sensitive to the age-related alteration in this serum protein. Protein binding as well as distributional changes have been reported for glyburide in the elderly.[14] Glyburide is a sulfonyl antidiabetic agent that is approximately 97% bound to albumin at physiological pH. In a study examining its pharmacokinetics in young (18 to 40 years) and elderly subjects (60 to 85 years), there was a significant increase in the volume of distribution secondary to a decrease in serum albumin. Associated with the increase in distribution was a 52% increase in the fraction of glyburide unbound in plasma in the elderly volunteers. This significant increase in free glyburide highlights the age-related decrease in available albumin.

The protein binding characteristics of the nonsteroidal anti-inflammatory drug (NSAID) naproxen has been extensively studied in the elderly and is summarized in Table 1.4.[58–62] Elderly patients tend to display an increased sensitivity to the effects of NSAIDs with a concomitant higher frequency of side effects.[58] Naproxen is usually highly protein bound to albumin with less than 2% of the total drug in the unbound form. In the elderly the fraction unbound is significantly higher, and in some instances almost doubled. This change is primarily due to a decrease in available albumin to bind free naproxen.

TABLE 1.4.
Effect of Age on the Protein Binding of Naproxen

Age range (years)	n[a]	Free naproxen (mg/L)	Albumin (g/dL)	Ref.
22–39	10	0.048 (0.025)	4.80 (0.15)	58
66–81	10	0.114[b] (0.070)	4.32 (0.16)	58
40–64	9	0.090 (0.088)	4.18 (4.6)	62
76–93	13	0.141[b] (0.089)	4.03 (3.5)	62
22–26	8	0.030 (0.01)	4.5 (2)	61
70–76	6	0.090[b] (0.02)	3.40 (2)	61

[a] n = number of subjects.
[b] $p < 0.05$.

Both valproic acid and theophylline display age-related changes in binding. The percent of valproic acid bound to albumin decreases as a function of age, with an associated increase in its free fraction.[63–65] In most instances, increases in the free fraction of drugs will elicit a concomitant increase in the Vd_{ss} if bioavailability remains constant. The relationship between aging and protein binding has also been examined with theophylline.[66–68] Unbound theophylline levels are significantly higher in the elderly and are highly correlated with the serum albumin level.

The change in protein binding with albumin may also be due to alterations in the binding capacity of the protein. Lesko and investigators[69] examined the protein binding of salicylate in healthy young and healthy elderly male volunteers. The fraction bound of salicylate was significantly lower in the elderly, but the decrease in binding was not due to an age-related decrease in serum albumin levels. This change was due to a lower binding affinity of salicyalte for albumin binding sites. Albumin has two classes of sites for the binding of salicylate, low- and high-affinity sites. The total binding capacity of the low affinity site was responsible for the age-related increase in the free fraction of salicylate. This study suggests that reductions in circulating albumin levels alone may not completely account for the age-related changes observed in protein binding of numerous agents. The affinity of the drug for the binding sites as well as the capacity for those sites are also important considerations in the geriatric patient.

Unlike acidic drugs which are usually bound to albumin, basic drugs tend to bind to AAG. Whereas there appears to be an age-related increase in the free fraction of drugs bound to albumin, the opposite has been observed with AAG.[57] The increase observed with this protein has been shown to decrease the free drug fraction and overall serves to decrease the Vd_{ss}.

Propranolol, a β-blocker, binds primarily to AAG.[70,71] This agent is administered as a racemic mixture with the *l*-isomer displaying the primary pharmacological properties. The effect of age on the stereoselective protein binding of propranolol has been recently examined (Table 1.5).[32,72] Significantly higher AAG levels were found along with a smaller free fraction of the *l*-propranolol in the elderly. There was a trend toward a smaller free fraction of *d*-isomer in the elderly, but this difference did not reach statistical significance. These investigators not only reported higher AAG levels in the elderly, they also pointed out differences in the affinity of the two isomers of propranolol for the binding sites on the AAG molecule. The change in protein binding does not only influence the Vd_{ss}, it also may alter the degree of metabolism or renal elimination.

TABLE 1.5.
Age-Related Stereoselective Differences in Propranolol Protein Binding

Age range (years)	Mean age (years)	n[a]	fu_d	fu_l	AAG (mg/dL)	Ref.
23–33	28.1	10	0.173 (0.031)	0.133 (0.025)	59 (13)	32
55–75	63.6	10	0.155 (0.023)	0.113[b] (0.014)	73[b] (15)	32

[a] n = number of subjects.
[b] $p < 0.05$.

IV. METABOLISM

The response of hepatic metabolism to the aging process is highly variable and unpredictable. Aging affects the three major factors responsible for biotransformation of drugs: liver hemodynamics, hepatic metabolic capacity, and protein binding. More specifically, the age-related physiological factors that affect biotransformation are (1) decreases in splanchnic blood flow; (2) decreases in the total number of functioning hepatocytes; (3) reduction in total liver mass; and (4) alterations in protein binding. Each of these changes can potentially alter the intrinsic metabolic capacity of the liver for various agents that are hepatically cleared. This will decrease hepatic clearance and increase elimination half-life if the volume of distribution remains constant.

The aging process does not affect biotransformation pathways in a uniform manner.[7,44,73,74] In general, drugs undergoing Phase I type reactions, such as hepatic microsomal oxidation, tend to display a slower clearance in the elderly. On the other hand, hydrolysis, reduction, and glucuronide conjugation, the Phase II-type reactions, are not significantly affected by the aging process. Not only does the liver succumb to these age-related alterations in drug metabolism, it also has to contend with a wide range of genetic, nutritional, and environmental factors (i.e., fluorocarbons, smoking).

To understand how the process of aging affects the physiological factors responsible for drug metabolism, it is first necessary to review hepatic drug clearance. There are three major determinants of hepatic clearance (Cl_H): liver blood flow (Q_H), intrinsic clearance of unbound drug (Cl_{uint}), and fraction of drug unbound (f_{ub}).[24] These parameters are related to hepatic drug clearance as shown in the following equation:

$$CL_H = Q_H \frac{f_{ub} * Cl_{uint}}{Q_H + f_{ub}Cl_{uint}} \tag{2}$$

The extraction ratio (ER) represents the ratio of drug eliminated when it traverses the liver and is represented by the following equation:

$$ER = \frac{f_{ub} * Cl_{uint}}{Q_H + f_{ub}Cl_{uint}} \tag{3}$$

Drugs are placed into three categories depending on their ER; high (ER >0.7), medium (ER 0.3 to 0.7), and low (ER <0.3). High-ER drugs are also known as flow-dependent agents and are sensitive to changes in Q_H. Age-related reductions in Q_H for high-ER agents will cause a decrease in Cl_H. Low-ER drugs, referred to as flow-independent agents, are most affected by changes in fraction of drug unbound (f_{ub}) and the intrinsic clearance of unbound drug (Cl_{uint}). Alterations in protein binding, as discussed previously, or decreases in P450 microsomal enzyme content in the aged will affect the clearance of these agents.

A. HEPATIC BLOOD FLOW AND METABOLISM

There is approximately a 1% decline after the age of 30 in the cardiac output.[25–27,75] This translates into a 0.5 to 1.0% reduction in hepatic blood flow. Liver blood flow is usually determined by idocyanine green (ICG), an agent that is highly extracted from the liver and is not protein bound. Studies by Wood et al.[76] have reported a reduction in the clearance of ICG in the elderly. This decrease in liver clearance is a direct reflection of the age-related reduction in liver blood flow. There is also a 1% decrease in liver mass annually.[74] Figure 1.6 illustrates the reduction in liver weight and the reduction in the number of liver cells with age. Decreases in liver blood flow and the reduction in liver mass may partially account for the diminished metabolism in the elderly.

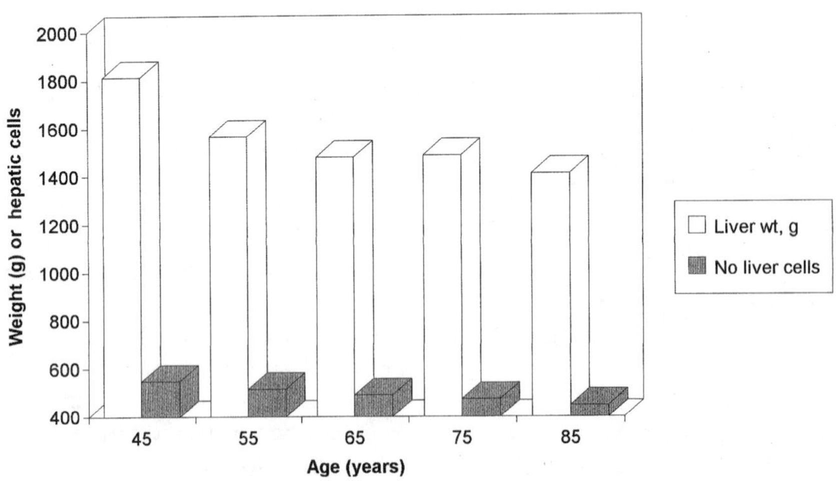

FIGURE 1.6. Changes in liver weight and number of hepatic cells as a function of age. Adapted from Sato, T. Miwa, T., and Tauchi, H., *Gerontologia*, 16, 368, 1970.)

Unlike renal function, there are no routine laboratory tests to determine liver metabolizing capabilities. However, antipyrene is metabolized exclusively by microsomal oxidation and is used to assess this pathway. The hepatic clearance of this agent, which is not protein bound, is significantly reduced in the elderly.[76]

To evaluate how the aging process affects microsomal oxidation as well as other metabolic pathways, the benzodiazepines provide an informative example. These agents have been extensively studied in the elderly and display selective reductions in certain metabolic pathways with age, while other pathways remain intact (Table 1.6). As a group, the benzodiazepines demonstrate an age-related reduction in hepatic metabolism for those agents that undergo hepatic oxidation such as diazepam,[77] desalkylflurazepam,[78] desmethlydiazepam,[78] bromazepam,[78] triazolam,[79] adinazolam,[80] and lorazepam.[81] Conversely, no significant changes in metabolic clearance have been reported for benzodiazepines biotransformed by phase II-type reactions, such as reduction (nitrazepam)[83] or glucuronide conjugation (oxazepam,[82] temazepam).[78]

Alprazolam, metabolized by microsomal oxidation, exhibits a decrease in clearance in the elderly.[84,85] When the clearance of this agent was compared to the disposition of antipyrene, the elimination of these two agents was highly correlated. There is an indication that the metabolism of this agent is also altered in a gender-related manner.[85] After a single oral dose, no significant differences in clearance were found between elderly women and young women. However, clearance and half-life were reduced in elderly men when compared to younger men.[85] Both parameters were significantly changed with a longer half-life and lower clearance in the elderly males.

Similar gender-related results have been found with the hepatically oxidized benzodiazepine, midazolam.[86] After a single intramuscular dose, a decrease in the rate of midazolam elimination was found in elderly males compared to young men. Conversely, there were no age-related decreases in clearance for older women. Another study reported a slight reduction in midazolam clearance in geriatric subjects after administration to young and old women.[87] In a previous study, where only male subjects were enrolled, midazolam displayed a significant increase in the elimination half-life, although the age-related differences in clearance did not reach significance.[88] Nonetheless, these findings suggest a gender-related and age-related decrease in the microsomal pathway for oxidative metabolism. Furthermore, it appears that this pathway is more sensitive to age-related changes in males as compared to females.

TABLE 1.6.
Elimination Parameters (CL, $t_{1/2}$) for Selected Benzodiazepine in Young and Elderly Subjects

Benzodiazepine	Metabolism	Young mean CL (min/mL/kg)	Old mean CL (min/mL/kg)	Young mean $t_{1/2}$ (hr)	Old mean $t_{1/2}$ (hr)	Ref.
Lorazepam	Oxidation	0.99	0.77[a]	14.1	15.9	81
Alprazolam	Oxidation	1.33	0.64[a]	11.1	19.0[a]	85
Midazolam	Oxidation	7.26	6.95	2.7	3.2	86
Nitrazepam	Reduced	0.95	0.85	20	28.0[a]	83
Diazepam	Oxidation	0.39	0.24[a]	36	97.5[a]	77

[a] $p < 0.05$.

As a group, most tricyclic antidepressants are eliminated by the liver. The metabolism of these agents displays a high degree of interindividual variability stemming from numerous metabolic phenotypes. Due to the presence of slow and fast metabolizers in the population, it is difficult to establish a clear difference in drug metabolism between young and old patients. For the most part the demethylation pathways for the metabolism of imipramine, amitriptyline, trazodone, and clomipramine are reduced in the elderly.[89] Hepatic hydroxylation for trazodone and clomipramine metabolism demonstrates reduced clearance in the elderly. On the other hand, desimipramine, which is also hydroxylated, does not display a significant reduction in clearance in the elderly.[89]

B. STEREOISOMERS AND METABOLISM

It is apparent from reviewing the gerontology literature on drug metabolism that the hepatic isozymes are affected to a different extent by the aging process. This premise is even more apparent when the metabolism of racemic mixtures is evaluated in the elderly. Recent studies have highlighted the stereoselective reduction in the hepatic metabolism of various enantiomeric compounds. With the development of analytical methods to separate chiral compounds, investigators have begun to examine the effect of aging on the biotransformation of racemic mixtures.

Recent studies have examined the metabolism of verapamil, the calcium channel inhibitor in young and old volunteers (Table 1.7). After the administration of racemic verapamil, the clearance of both the (*S*)- and (*R*)-verapamil was prolonged in the elderly.[29] The clearance of the (*S*)-isomer was reduced more than the (*R*)-isomer. This suggests that the pathway for (*S*)-verapamil is more sensitive to age-related changes in hepatic metabolism, such as reduction in hepatic blood flow, as compared to (*R*)-verapamil. Schwartz et al.[90] also reported similar findings with the (*S*)-verapamil. After separate intravenous administrations of the (*R*)- and (*S*)-enantiomers, there were significant reductions in the clearance of the (*S*)-isomer in older subjects, but no age-related change in (*R*)-verapamil clearance.

TABLE 1.7.
Age-Related Stereoselective Differences in Verapamil Metabolism

Age range (years)	n[a]	Cl_o, R-isomer (L/hr/kg)	Cl_o, S-isomer (L/hr/kg)	AAG (mg/dL)	Ref.
20–25	12	1.30 (0.67)	22.5 (21.3)	59 13	29
60–79	12	0.53[b] (0.20)	4.8[b] (3.0)	73[b] (15)	29

[a] n = number of subjects.
[b] $p < 0.05$.

Stereoisomeric changes have also been found for the metabolism of the barbiturate, mephobarbital, in the elderly.[91] After administration of a single oral dose of racemic (400 mg) mephobarbital to young and old subjects, the apparent total body clearance of the (*R*)-enantiomer was much slower and the elimination half-life was much longer in the older group. Another barbiturate, hexobarbital, displays stereoselective metabolism in the elderly. In a study by Chandler et al.,[92] the disposition of *d*- and *l*-hexobarbital was examined. The mean oral clearance of the *d*-isomer was unaffected by the aging process; however, the *l*-isomer was cleared to a significantly slower extent in the elderly.

In addition to hexobarbital, propranolol has also exhibited a decrease in the intrinsic hepatic clearance of (*S*)-propranolol in the elderly.[93] This stereoselective behavior in drug metabolism strongly supports an age-related alteration in metabolism that discriminates based on the expression of certain hepatic isozymes.

C. RENAL ELIMINATION

As with liver function, there is a reduction in renal function with age that has been well documented.[94–98] A progressive reduction in renal blood flow after the age of 20 has been reported, with approximately a 1 to 2% decline in renal blood flow per year after the second decade.[96,97] In addition, the renal mass declines appreciably due to the aging process with an associated reduction in the number of functioning nephrons.[96,99,100]

The renal processes glomerular filtration, tubular secretion, and tubular reabsorption are also affected by aging. The glomerular filtration rate (GFR) has been shown to decline at a rate of less than 1% per year after the second decade of life.[94] Tubular secretion as determined by the maximal reabsorption capacity of glucose decreases by approximately 0.5% per year.[95] Additionally, there is a 1% decrease in the total renal plasma flow, based on para-aminohippuric acid clearance measurements.[94] Figure 1.7 presents the inulin clearance (GFR), diodrast clearance (renal plasma flow), and renal blood flow as a function of age.[94] The decrease in renal function in the elderly has been studied extensively, and drugs eliminated solely or to a significant extent by the kidney display a reduced rate of clearance in the elderly.

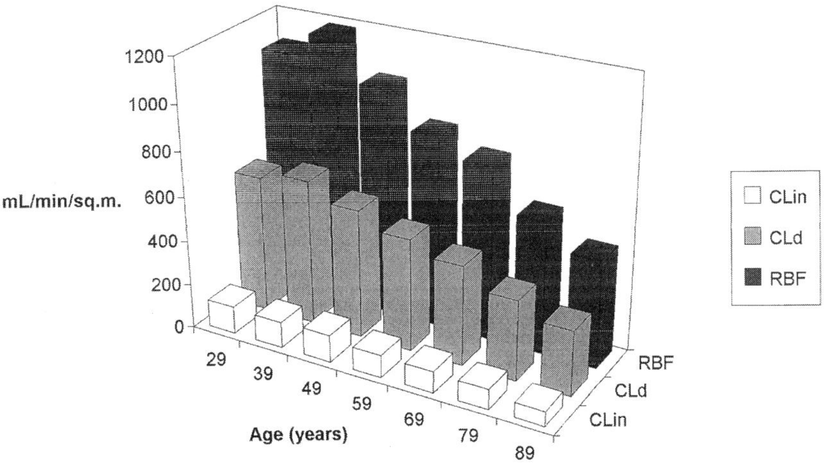

FIGURE 1.7. Changes in inulin clearance (CLin), diodrast clearance (CLd), and renal blood flow (RBF) as a function of age. (Adapted from Davies, D. F. and Shock, N. W., *J. Clin. Invest.*, 29, 496, 1950.)

Serum creatinine levels are used routinely to determine creatinine clearance and hence the GFR. Creatinine levels are based on the catabolism of muscle. The sole use of serum creatinine levels to determine the GFR may provide false measurements in the elderly population. As was noted in the section on distribution, there is a significant decrease in skeletal muscle mass in the elderly. Furthermore, there is a decrease in the renal elimination of creatinine. Estimation of creatinine clearance based on serum creatinine levels yields an inaccurate measurement and should not be used as a measure of GFR.

The progressive structural changes and reduction of the functional capabilities of the kidney with age leads to significant decreases in the renal clearance of various agents. Quinolone antibiotics are excreted to a large extent by the kidney. Elderly patients with reduced GFR tend to eliminate these compounds at a much slower rate. Quinolone antibiotics that show an age-related reduction in renal clearance are ofloxacin,[101] temafloxacin,[102] amifloxacin,[103] and lomefloxacin.[104] The cephalosporin and aminoglycoside antibiotics also display a reduced renal clearance. The cephalosporins, cefmetazole[105] and ceftriaxone,[106] and the aminoglycosides, kanamycin[107] and vancomycin,[108] each display a significant decrease in renal clearance in the elderly. Clarithromycin, a macrolide antibiotic, has been reported to display diminished elimination in geriatric patients.[109] Each of these antibiotics is excreted by the kidney and exhibit an age-related decrease in renal clearance. Selected antibiotics are presented in Table 1.8.

Acebutolol and vigabatrin are both chiral compounds eliminated by the kidney and also display reduced renal clearance in the elderly. Acebutolol is a chiral β-blocker that is metabolized to an equipotent chiral metabolite, diacetolol.[110] After single-dose administration of acebutolol as a racemate, a significant reduction in the renal clearance and urinary excretion of both parent drug and metabolite has been reported.[110] This reduction in the renal clearance was displayed in a stereoselective manner with a decrease in the ratio of (*S*)-enantiomer to (*R*)-enantiomer in plasma and urine for both the parent drug and metabolite. This age-related

TABLE 1.8.
Age-Related Changes in Renal Clearance and Creatinine Clearance

Drug	Young CL_{Cr} (mL/min)	Elderly CL_{Cr} (mL/min)	Young CL_R (mL/min)	Elderly CL_R (mL/min)	Ref.
Vancomycin	129.6 (7.7)	97.7 (8.3)	70 (5)	56.7 (3.3)	108
Ceftriaxone	114 (26)	92 (14)	6.9 (1.2)[a]	5.3 (1.1)[a]	106
Clarithromycin	116.3 (17.9)	67.2 ± 15.3	168 ± 35[a]	84 ± 31[a]	109

[a] $p < 0.05$.

reduction in the renal clearance suggests that the renal processes (i.e., filtration and possibly secretion) are affected in a stereoselective manner.

Vigabatrin displays a stereoselective decrease in the elimination of one enantiomer.[111] After a single oral dose of vigabatrin to healthy young subjects and elderly subjects with compromised renal function, there was a significant reduction in the urinary excretion of both the (*S*)- and (*R*)-enantiomers. Further examination of the results displayed a trend toward a reduction in the enantiomer ratio (S/R) for the pharmacokinetic parameters AUC, renal clearance (Cl_{R}) and amount of drug excreted in the urine (A_e) between the young and the renally compromised group. These enantiomeric differences in the renal clearance of vigabatrin imply that the changes in the kidney are isomer specific, meaning that the clearance of one pathway of renal elimination is more sensitive to age-related changes in filtration, secretion, and reabsorption than another pathway.

The effect of age-related physiologic changes in renal clearance on the renal elimination pathways of metabolites is exhibited by the asthmatic agent, theophylline. The renal elimination of theophylline and its metabolites was compared in a group of young and old volunteers.[112] A significant decrease in the renal clearance of theophylline was found in the elderly. However, the urinary excretion patterns were completely different between the young and old groups. The elderly were found to have excreted a significantly higher amount of the metabolite, 1-methyluric acid, and a lower amount of the parent drug in the urine as compared to the younger subjects. These differences in renal elimination may be due to both the age-related changes in hepatic intrinsic clearance as well as the effect of physiological changes in kidney function on renal clearance.

Further advances in assessing gastrointestinal changes in the elderly, and the evidence of stereospecific changes in not only drug metabolism, but also in renal elimination, provide further understanding about the specific sensitivity of some physiological processes to aging.

D. SUMMARY

Aging has a variable effect on the pharmacokinetics of drugs. The alterations in drug disposition observed in the geriatric patient are primarily due to age-related changes in those physiological processes that are responsible for the absorption, distribution, and elimination of therapeutic agents. Examination of altered pharmacokinetic parameters provides indirect evidence of the physiological functions (i.e., diminished tubular absorption, diminished production of gastric hydrogen ions) affected by aging. There are numerous informative examples that elucidate age-related changes in physiological function by displaying alterations in pharmacokinetic parameters. Some of these changes have a minimal impact, such as the decrease in hydrogen ion production on the absorption of drugs in the elderly. On the other hand, age-related reduction in blood flow has direct consequences on drug absorption, distribution, and metabolism, as well as the renal elimination of drugs.

The next emphasis in geriatric pharmacokinetics should be additional research in the area of metabolism and disposition of stereoisomers. Studies in the literature have provided significant evidence on the specificity of the aging process as it relates to the elimination enantiomers. It is apparent that the process of aging selectively alters the absorption, distribution, metabolism and elimination of one isomer while minimally affecting another. Research should be conducted to examine why the process of aging selectively alters the pharmacokinetics of certain enantiomers. This will further enhance our understanding of the influence of the aging process on those physiologic processes responsible for drug disposition in the geriatric patient.

REFERENCES

1. **Sloan, R. W.,** Principles of drug therapy in geriatric patients, *Am. Fam. Physician*, 45, 2709, 1992.
2. **Butler R. N.,** Introduction, in Hayne, S. G., Feinleib, M., Eds.: Second Conference on the Epidemiology of Aging. USDHHS, Public Health Service, NIH Publication. No. 80–969, Washington, D.C., 1980, p. 4.
3. **Cutler N. R. and Narang P. K., Eds.,** *Drug Studies in the Elderly*, Williams & Wilkins, Baltimore, 1988.
4. **Lamy, P. P.,** Comparative pharmacokinetic changes and drug therapy in an older population, *J. Am. Geriatr. Soc.*, Suppl. 30, S11, 1982.
5. **Lamy, P. P.,** The elderly, undernutrition and pharmacokinetics, *J. Am. Geriatr. Soc.*, 31, 560, 1983.
6. **Cohen, J. L.,** Pharmacokinetic changes in aging, *Am. J. Med.*, 80 (Suppl. 5A), 31, 1980.
7. **Mayerson, M.,** Special Pharmacokinetic Considerations in the Elderly, in Evans, W. E., Schentag, J. J., and Juslo, W. J., *Applied Pharmacokinetics: Principles of Therapeutic Drug Monitoring,* 3rd ed., Applied Therapeutics, Vancouver, WA, 1992, chap. 9.
8. **Gibaldi, M. and Perrier, D.,** *Pharmacokinetics*, 2nd ed., Marcel Dekker, New York, 1982, chap 4.
9. **Mojaverian, P., Vlassws, P. H., Kellner, P. E., and Rocci, M. L.,** Effects of gender, posture and age on gastric residence time of an indigestible solid: pharmaceutical considerations, *Pharm. Res.*, 5, 639, 1988.
10. **Baron, J. H.,** Studies of basal and peak acid output with an augmented histamine test, *Gut,* 4, 136, 1963.
11. **Vanzant, F. R., Alvarez, W. C., Eusterman, G. B., Dunn, H. L., and Berkson, J.,** The normal range of gastric acidity from youth to old age, *Arch. Intern. Med.*, 49, 345, 1932.
12. **Barr, W. H., Adir, J., and Garrettson, L.,** Decrease of tetracycline absorption in man by sodium bicarbonate, *Clin. Pharmacol. Ther.,* 12, 779, 1971.
13. **Kramer, P. A., Chapron, D. J., Benson, J., and Mercik, S. A.,** Tetracycline absorption in elderly patients with achlorhydria, *Clin. Pharmacol. Ther.,* 23, 467, 1978.
14. **Schwinghammer, T. L., Antal, E. J., Kubacka, R. T., Hackimer, M. E., and Johnston, J. M.,** Pharmacokinetics and pharmacodynamics of glyburide in young and elderly nondiabetic adults, *Clin. Pharm.,* 10, 532, 1991.
15. **Evans, M. A., Triggs, E. J., Cheung, M., Broe, G. A., and Creasey, H.,** Gastric emptying rate in the elderly: implications for drug therapy, *J. Am. Geriatr. Soc.*, 29, 201, 1981.
16. **Horowitz, M., Maddern, G. J., Chatterton, B. E., Collins, P. J., Harding, P. E., and Shearman, D. J.,** Changes in gastric emptying with age, *Clin. Sci.*, 67, 213–218, 1984.
17. **Robertson, D. R., Wood, N. D., Everest, H., Monks, K., Waller, D. G., Renwick, A. G., and George, C. F.,** The effect of age on the pharmacokinetics of levodopa administered alone and in the presence of carbidopa, *Br. J. Clin. Pharmacol.*, 28, 61, 1989.
18. **Yeh, K. C., August, T. F., Bush, D. F., Lasseter, K. C., Musson, D. G., Schwartz, S., Smith, M. E., and Titus, D. C.,** Pharmacokinetics and bioavailability of Sinemet CR: a summary of human studies, *Neurology,* 39, 25, 1989.
19. **Broe, G. A., Evans, M. A., and Triggs, E. J.,** Senile Parkinsonism and dopa pharmacokinetics, *Clin. Exp. Neurol.,* 18, 174, 1981.
20. **Rivera-Calimlim, L., et al.,** Absorption and metabolism of L-dopa by the human stomach, *Eur. J. Clin. Invest.,* 1, 1313, 1971.
21. **Iwamoto, K., Wantanabe, J., and Atsumi, F.,** Age dependence in capacity limited jejunal decarboxylation of levodopa in rats, *Biochem. Pharmacol.,* 36, 2151, 1987.
22. **Cusack, B., Kelly, J., O'Malley, K. O., Noel, J., Lavan, J., and Horgan, J.,** Digoxin in the elderly: pharmacokinetic consequences of old age, *Clin. Pharmacol. Ther.,* 25, 772, 1978.
23. **Rey, E., Pons, G., and Vigabatrin, O. G.,** Clinical pharmacokinetics, *Clin. Pharmacokin.,* 23, 267, 1992.
24. **Wilkinson, E. R. and Shand, D. G.,** A physiological approach to hepatic drug clearance, *Clin. Pharmacol. Ther.,* 18, 377, 1975.
25. **Bender, A. D.,** The effect of increasing age on the distribution of the peripheral blood flow in man, *J. Am. Geriatr. Soc.,* 13, 192, 1965.

26. **Sherlock, S., et al.,** Splanchnic blood flow in man by the bromsulfalein method: the relation of peripheral plasma by bromsulfalein level to calculated flow, *J. Lab. Clin. Med.*, 35, 923, 1950.
27. **Brandfonbrener, M., Landowne, M., and Shock, N.,** Changes in cardiac output with age, *Circulation,* 12, 557, 1955.
28. **Robertson, D. R., Waller, D. G., Renwick, A. G., and George, C. F.,** Age-related changes in the pharmacokinetics and pharmacodynamics of nifedipine, *Br. J. Clin. Pharmacol.,* 25, 297, 1988.
29. **Sasaki, M., Tateishi, T., and Ebihara, A.,** The effects of age and gender on the stereoselective pharmacokinetics of verapamil, *Clin. Pharmacol. Ther.*, 54, 278, 1993.
30. **Jaillon, P., Gardin, M. E., Lecocq, B., Richard, M. O., Meignan, S., Blondel, Y., Grippat, J. C., Bernieres, J., and Vergnoux, O.,** Pharmacokinetics of nalbuphine in infacts, young healthy volunteers and elderly patients, *Clin. Pharmacol. Ther.*, 46, 226, 1989.
31. **Castleden, C. M. and George, C. F.,** The effect of aging on the hepatic clearance of propranolol, *Br. J. Clin. Pharmacol.,* 7, 49, 1979.
32. **Lalonde, R. L., Tenero, D. M., Burlew, B. S., Herring, V. L., and Bottorff, M. B.,** Effects of age on the protein binding and disposition of propranolol stereoisomers. *Clin. Pharmacol. Ther.*, 4, 447, 1990.
33. **Cusack, B.,** Protein binding of lignocaine in the elderly, *Eur. J. Clin. Pharmacol.,* 29, 323, 1985.
34. **Forbes, G. B. and Reina, J. C.,** Adult lean body mass declines with age: some longitudinal observations, *Metabolism,* 19, 653, 1970.
35. **Servin, F., Enriquez, I., Fournet, M., Failler, J. M., Farinotti, R., and Desmonts, J. M.,** Pharmacokinetics of midazolam used as an intravenous induction agent for patients over 80 years of age, *Eur. J. Anaesthesiol.,* 4, 1, 1987.
36. **Wills, R. J.,** Pharmacokinetics of diazepam from a controlled release capsule in healthy elderly volunteers, *Biopharm. Drug Dispos.,* 5, 241, 1984.
37. **Abernathy, D., et al.,** Alterations in drug distribution and clearance due to obesity, *J. Pharmacol. Exp. Ther.,* 217, 681, 1981.
38. **Abernathy, D., et al.,** Prolonged accumulation of diazepam in obesity, *J. Clin. Pharmacol.,* 23, 369, 1983.
39. **Jung, D., et al.,** Thiopental disposition as a function of age in female patients undergoing surgery, *Anesthesiology,* 56, 2633, 1982.
40. **Ochs, H. R., Greenblatt, D. J., Friedman, H., Burstein, E. S., Locniskar, A., Harmatz, J. S., and Shader, R. I.,** Bromazepam pharmacokinetics: influence of age, gender, oral contraceptives, cimetidine, and propranolol, *Clin. Pharmacol. Ther.,* 41, 562, 1987.
41. **Greenblatt, D. J., Matlis, R., Scavone, J. M., Blyden, G. T., Harmatz, J. S., and Shader, R. I.,** Oxaprozin pharmacokinetics in the elderly, *Br. J. Clin. Pharmacol.,* 19, 373, 1985.
42. **Vestal, R. E., et al.,** Aging and ethanol metabolism, *Clin. Pharmacol. Ther.,* 21, 343, 1977.
43. **Shock, N. W., Watkin, D. M., Yiengst, M. J., Norris, A. H., Gaffney, G. W., Gregerman, R. I., and Falzone, J. A.,** Age differences in water content of the body as related to basal oxygen consumption in males, *J. Gerontol.,* 18, 1, 1963.
44. **Greenblatt, D. G., Sellers, E. M., and Shader, R. I.,** Drug disposition in old age, *N. Engl. J. Med.,* 306, 1081, 1982.
45. **Lebel, M. and Bergeron, M. G.,** Pharmacokinetics in the elderly. Studies on ciprofloxacin, *Am. J. Med.,* 82, 108, 1987.
46. **Matteo, R. S., Backus, W. W., McDaniel, D. D., Brotherton, W. P., Abraham, R., and Diaz, J.,** Pharmacokinetics and pharmacodynamics of d-tubocurarine and metocurine in the elderly, *Anesth. Analg.*, 64, 23, 1985.
47. **Rupp, S. M., Castagnoli, K. P., Fisher, D. M., and Miller, R. D.,** Pancuronium and vecuronium pharmacokinetics and pharmacodynamics in younger and elderly adults, *Anesthesiology,* 67, 45, 1987.
48. **Arden, J. R., Holley, F. O., and Stanski, D. R.,** Increased sensitivity to etomidate in the elderly: initial distribution versus altered brain response, *Anesthesiology,* 65, 19, 1986.
49. **Kirkpatrick, T., Cockshott, I. D., Douglas, E. J., and Nimmo, W. S.,** Pharmacokinetics of propofol (diprivan) in elderly patients, *Br. J. Anaesth.*, 60, 146, 1988.
50. **Homer, T. D. and Stanski, D. R.,** The effect of increasing age on thiopental disposition and anesthetic requirement, *Anesthesiology*, 62, 714, 1985.
51. **Shock, N. W., Watkin, D. M., Yiengst, M. J., Norris, A. H., Gaffney, G. W., Gregerman, R. I., and Falzone, J. A.,** Age differences in water content of the body as related to basal oxygen consumption in males, *J. Gerontol.,*18, 1,1963.
52. **Christensen, J. H., Andreasen, F., and Jansen, J. A.,** Influence of age and sex on the pharmacokinetics of thiopentone, *Br. J. Anaesth.*, 53, 1189, 1981.
53. **Christensen, J. H., Andreasen, F., and Jansen, J. A.,** Pharmacokinetics and pharmacodynamics of thiopentone, a comparison between young and elderly patients, *Anaesthesia*, 37, 398, 1982.
54. **Avram, M. J., Krejcie, T. C., and Henthorn, T. K.,** The relationship of age to the pharmacokinetics of early drug distribution: the concurrent disposition of thiopental and indocyanine green, *Anesthesiology,* 72, 403, 1990.

55. **Stanski, D. R. and Maitre, P. O.,** Population pharmacokinetics and pharmacodynamics of thiopental: the effect of age revisited, *Anesthesiology*, 72, 412, 1990.
56. **Strum, D. P., Eger, E. I., II, Unadkat, J. D., Johnson, B. H., and Carpenter, R. L.,** Age affects the pharmacokinetics of inhaled anesthetics in humans, *Anesth. Analg.*, 73, 310, 1991.
57. **Wallace, S. M. and Verbeeck, R. K.,** Plasma protein binding of drugs in the elderly, *Clin. Pharmacokin.*, 12, 41, 1987.
58. **Upton, R. A., Williams, R. L., Kelly, J., and Jones, R. M.,** Naproxen pharmacokinetics in the elderly, *Br. J. Clin. Pharmacol.*, 18, 207, 1984.
59. **Gotzsche, P. C., Andreasen, F., Egsmose, C., and Lund, B.,** Steady state pharmacokinetics of naproxen in elderly rheumatics compared with young volunteers, *Scand. J. Rheumatol.*, 17, 11, 1988.
60. **Schmitt, M. and Guentert, T. W.,** Effect of age on the pharmacokinetics of tenoxicam in comparison to other non-steroidal anti-inflammatory drugs (NSAIDs), *Scand. J. Rheumatol.*, Suppl. 80, 86, 1989.
61. **Van den Ouweland, F. A., Jansen, P. A., Tan, Y., Van de Putte, L. B., Van Ginneken, C. A., and Gribnau, F. W.,** Pharmacokinetics of high-dosage naproxen in elderly patients, *Int. J. Clin. Pharmacol. Ther. Toxicol.*, 26, 143, 1988.
62. **McVerry, R. M., Lethbridge, J., Martin, N., Mukerjee, S. K., Littler, T., Tallis, R., Sibeon, R., and Orme, M. L.,** Pharmacokinetics of naproxen in elderly patients, *Eur. J. Clin. Pharmacol.*, 31, 463, 1986.
63. **Perucca, E., Grimaldi, R., Gatti, G., Pirracchio, S., Crema, F., and Frigo, G. M.,** Pharmacokinetics of valproic acid in the elderly, *Br. J. Clin. Pharmacol.*, 17, 665, 1984.
64. **Bryson, S. M., Verma, N., Scott, P. J., and Rubin, P. C.,** Pharmacokinetics of valproic acid in young and elderly subjects, *Br. J. Clin. Pharmacol.*, 16, 104, 1983.
65. **Bauer, L. A., Davis, R., Wilensky, A., Raisys, V., and Levy, R. H.,** Valproic acid clearance: unbound fraction and diurnal variation in young and elderly adults, *Clin. Pharmacol. Ther.*, 37, 697, 1985.
66. **Antal, E. J., Kramer, P. A., Mercik, S. A., Chapron, D. J., and Lawson, I. R.,** Theophylline pharmacokinetics in advanced age, *Br. J. Clin. Pharmacol.*, 12, 637, 1981.
67. **Rammohan, M.,** Theophylline pharmacokinetics in normal elderly subjects, *Clin. Pharmacol. Ther.*, 44, 522, 1988.
68. **Lesko, L. J., Tabor, K. J., and Johnson, B. F.,** Theophylline serum protein binding in obstructive airway disease, *Clin. Pharmacol. Ther.*, 29, 776, 1981.
69. **Lesko, L. J., Narang, P. K., Yeager, L., and Cutler, N. R.,** Salicylate protein binding in serum from young and elderly subjects as measured by diafiltration, *Eur. J. Clin. Pharmacol.*, 28, 339, 1985.
70. **Walle, U. K., Walle, T., Bai, S., and Olanoff, S.,** Stereoselective binding of propranolol to human plasma, alpha-1-acid glycoprotein and albumin, *Clin. Pharmacol. Ther.*, 34, 718, 1983.
71. **Bendayan, R., Pieper, J. A., Stewart, R. B., and Caranasos, G. J.,** Influence of age on serum protein binding of propranolol, *Eur. J. Clin. Pharmacol.*, 26, 251, 1984.
72. **Tenero, D. M., Bottorff, M. B., Burlew, B. S., Williams, J. B., and Lalonde, R. L.,** Altered beta-adrenergic sensitivity and protein binding to 1-propranolol in the elderly, *J. Cardiovasc. Pharmacol.*, 16, 702, 1990.
73. **Greenblatt, D. J., et al.,** Antipyrene kinetics in the elderly: prediction of age-related changes in benzodiazepin oxidizing capacity, *J. Pharmacol. Exp. Ther.*, 220, 120, 1982.
74. **Sato, T., Miwa, T., and Tauchi, H.,** Age changes in the human liver of the different races, *Gerontol.*, 16, 368, 1970.
75. **Bach, B., Hansen, J. M., Kampmann, J. P., et al.,** Disposition of antipyrine and phenytoin correlated with age and liver volume in man, *Clin. Pharmacokinet.*, 6, 396, 1981.
76. **Wood, A. J., Vestal, R. E., Wilkinson, G., Branch, R. A., and Shard, D. G.,** Effect of aging and cigarette smoking on antipyrine and indocyanine green elimination, *Clin. Pharmacol. Ther.*, 26, 16, 1979.
77. **Greenblatt, D. J., Abernathy, D. R., Locniskar, A., Ochs, H. R., Harmatz, J. S., and Shader, R. I.,** Diazepam disposition determinants, *Clin. Pharmacol. Ther.*, 27, 301, 1980.
78. **Greenblatt, D. J., Harmatz, J. S., and Shader, R. I.,** Clinical pharmacokinetics of anxiolytics and hypnotics in the elderly. Therapeutic considerations (Part I), *Clin. Pharmacokin.*, 21, 165, 1991.
79. **Greenblatt, D. J., Harmatz, J. S., Shapiro, L., Engelhardt, N., and Gouthro, T. A.,** Shader Sensitivity to triazolam in the elderly, *N. Engl. J. Med.*, 324, 1691, 1991.
80. **Fleishaker, J. C., Hulst, L. K., Ekernas, S. A., and Grahnen, A.,** Pharmacokinetics and pharmacodynamics of adinazolam and N-desmethyladinazolam after oral and intravenous dosing in healthy young and elderly volunteers, *J. Clin. Psychopharmacol.*, 12, 403, 1992.
81. **Greenblatt, D. J., Allen, M. D., Locniskar, A., Harmatz, J. S., and Shader, R. I.,** Lorazepam kinetics in the elderly, *Clin. Pharmacol. Ther.*, 26, 103, 1979.
82. **Sonne, J., Loft, S., Dossing, M., Boesgaard, S., and Andreasen, F.,** Single dose pharmacokinetics and pharmacodynamics of oral oxazepam in very elderly institutionalised subjects, *Br. J. Clin. Pharmacol.*, 31, 719, 1991.
83. **Greenblatt, D. J., Abernethy, D. R., Locniskar, A., Ochs, H. R., Harmatz, J. S., and Shader, R. I.,** Age, sex and nitrazepam kinetics: relation to antipyrene disposition, *Clin. Pharmacol. Ther.*, 38, 697, 1985.

84. **Greenblatt, D. J. and Wright, C. E.,** Clinical pharmacokinetics of alprazolam. Therapeutic implications, *Clin. Pharmacokin.*, 24, 453, 1993.
85. **Greenblatt, D. J., Allen, M. D., Abernethy, D. R., Moschitto, L. J., Smith, R. B., and Shader, R. I.,** Alprazolam kinetics in the elderly. Relation to antipyrine disposition, *Arch. Gen. Psychiatry*, 40, 287, 1983.
86. **Holazo, A. A., Winkler, M. B., and Patel, I. H.,** Effects of age, gender and oral contraceptives on intramuscular midazolam pharmacokinetics, *J. Clin. Pharmacol.*, 28, 1040, 1988.
87. **Avram, M. J., Fragen R. J., and Caldwell N. J.,** Midazolam kinetics in women of two age groups, *Clin. Pharmacol. Ther.*, 34, 505, 1983.
88. **Smith, M. T., Heazlewood, V., Eadie, M. J., Brophy, T. O., and Tyrer, J. H.,** Pharmacokinetics of midazolam in the aged, *Eur. J. Clin. Pharmacol.*, 26, 381, 1984.
89. **Von Moltke, L. L., Greenblatt, D. J., and Shader, R. I.,** Clinical pharmacokinetics of antidepressants in the elderly. Therapeutic implications, *Clin. Pharmacokin.*, 24, 141, 1993.
90. **Schwartz, J. B., Troconiz, I. F., Verotta, D., Liu, S., and Capili, H.,** Aging effects on stereoselective pharmacokinetics and pharmacodynamics of verapamil, *J. Pharmacol. Exp. Ther.*, 265, 690, 1993.
91. **Hooper, W. D. and Qing, M. S.,** The influence of age and gender on the stereoselective metabolism and pharmacokinetics of mephobarbital in humans, *Clin. Pharmacol. Ther.*, 48, 633, 1990.
92. **Chandler, M. H., Scott, S. R., and Blouin, R. A.,** Age associated stereoselective alterations in hexobarbital metabolism, *Clin. Pharmacol. Ther.*, 43, 436, 1988.
93. **Gilmore, D. A., Gal, J., Gerber, J. G., and Nies, A. S.,** Age and gender influence the stereoselective pharmacokinetics of propranolol, *J. Pharmacol. Exp. Ther.*, 261, 1181, 1992.
94. **Davies, D. F. and Shock, N. W.,** Age changes in glomerular filtration rate, effective renal plasma flow and tubular excretory capacity in adult males, *J. Clin. Invest.*, 29, 496, 1950.
95. **Miller, J. H., McDonald, R. K., and Shock, N. W.,** Age changes in the maximal rate of renal tubular reabsorption of glucose, *J. Gerontol.*, 7, 196, 1952.
96. **Hollenberg, N. K., Adams, D. F., Solomon, H. S., Rashid, A., Abrams, H. L., and Merrill, J. P.,** Senescence and the renal vasculature in normal man, *Circ. Res.*, 15, 31, 1976.
97. **Papper, S.,** Effects of age in reducing renal function, *Geriatrics*, 2* 83, 1973.
98. **Hansen, J., Kampmann, J., and Laursen, H. M.,** Renal excretion of drugs in the elderly, *Lancet*, 1, 1170, 1970.
99. **Tauchi, H., Tsuboi, K., and Okutomi, J.,** Age changes in the human kidney of different races, *Gerontologia*, 17, 87, 1971.
100. **Moore, R. A.,** Total number of glomeruli in the normal kidney, *Anat. Rec.*, 48, 153, 1931.
101. **Nilsson-Ehle, I., and Ljungberg, B.,** Quinolone disposition in the elderly. Practical implications, *Drugs Aging*, 1, 279, 1991.
102. **Granneman, G. R. and Guay, D. R.,** The influence of age on the pharmacokinetics of temafloxacin, *Am. J. Med.*, 91, 71S, 1991.
103. **Stroshane, R. M., Silverman, M. H., Sauerschell, R., Brown, R. R., Boddy, A. W., and Cook, J. A.,** Preliminary study of the pharmacokinetics of oral amifloxacin in elderly subjects, *Antimicrob. Agent Chemother.*, 34, 751, 1990.
104. **Kovarik, J. M., Hoepelman, A. I., Smit, J. M., Sips, P. A., Rozenberg-Arska, M., Glerum, J. H., and Verhoef, J.,** Steady-state pharmacokinetics and sputum penetration of lomefloxacin in patients with chronic obstructive pulmonary disease and acute respiratory tract infections, *Antimicrob. Agents Chemother.*, 36, 2458, 1992.
105. **Borin, M. T., Peters, G. R., and Smith, T. C.,** Pharmacokinetics and dose proportionality of cefmetazole in healthy young and elderly volunteers, *Antimicrob. Agents Chemother.*, 34, 1944, 1990.
106. **Luderer, J. R., Patel, I. H., Durkin, J., and Schneck, D. W.,** Age and ceftriaxone kinetics, *Clin. Pharmacol. Ther.*, 35, 19, 1983.
107. **Lumholtz, B., et al.,** Dose regimen of kanamycin and gentamycin, *Acta Med. Scand.*, 196, 521, 1974.
108. **Cutler, N. R., Narang, P. K., Lesko, L. J., Ninos, M., and Power, M.,** Vancomycin disposition: the importance of age, *Clin. Pharmacol. Ther.*, 36, 803, 1984.
109. **Chu, S., Wilson, D. S., Guay, D. R., and Craft, C.,** Clarithromycin pharmacokinetics in healthy young and elderly volunteers, *Clin. Pharmacol.*, 32, 1045, 1992.
110. **Piquette-Miller, M., Foster, R. T., Kappagoda, C. T., and Jamali, F.,** Effect of aging on the pharmacokinetics of acebutolol enantiomers, *J. Clin. Pharmacol.*, 32, 148, 1992.
111. **Haegele, K. D., Huebert, N. D., Ebel, M., Tell, G. P., and Schechter, P. J.,** Pharmacokinetics of vigabatrin: implications of creatinine clearance, *Clin. Pharmacol. Ther.*, 44, 558, 1988.
112. **Antal, E. J., Kramer, P. A., Mercik, S. A., Chapron, D. J., and Lawson, I. R.,** Theophylline pharmacokinetics in advanced age, *Br. J. Clin. Pharmacol.*, 12, 637, 1981.

Chapter 2

ADRENERGIC FUNCTION IN AGING: FOCUS ON THE CARDIOVASCULAR SYSTEM

Nihal Tümer and Philip J. Scarpace

CONTENTS

I. ABSTRACT

Catecholamines (CA) have an important endocrine and neuroendocrine role in mediating a variety of autonomic functions. One consequence of normal aging, in particular in the cardiovascular system, is a decline in β-adrenergic function associated with an alteration in responsiveness to β-adrenergic therapy. The intrinsic ability for muscle contractility or relaxation is maintained with age, and there appears to be an alteration in the process linking the receptor with the contractile or relaxation mechanisms.

0-8493-8306-4/96/$0.00+$.50

Plasma norepinephrine (NE) concentration increases with age, as does the biosynthesis of CA in the adrenal gland. The latter appears to be a consequence of the increased expression of tyrosine hydroxylase (TH), the key enzyme in the CA biosynthetic pathway. Despite the increased synthesis and circulating NE concentrations, adrenergic neurotransmission is diminished in heart and vasculature with age. The number of β-adrenergic receptors for the most part does not decline with age, but postreceptor signal transduction, in particular the amount of adenylyl cyclase activity, decreases with age. There is some indication that homeostatic and adaptive regulation of β-adrenergic signal transduction is impaired in the aged and may contribute to underlying pathology and therapeutic responsiveness.

II. INTRODUCTION

Catecholamines (CAs) have an important endocrine and neuroendocrine role in mediating a variety of autonomic functions in the periphery and have a profound influence over central neurologic processes. Considering their broad distribution and diverse influence on physiology, normal CA function is critical for maintaining homeostasis. Pathologic alterations in peripheral and central catecholaminergic mechanisms, in particular β-adrenergic mechanisms, have been implicated in many diseases.

One consequence of normal aging is a decline in β-adrenergic function.[1,2] This is associated with an increase in autonomic dysfunction with age and an alteration in responsiveness to β-adrenergic therapy in the elderly. Understanding the basic pharmacologic consequences of aging is critical to safe and effective therapy in the elderly.

For a drug to exert a therapeutic effect on a specific end organ, both the concentration of the drug as well as the sensitivity and efficacy of the drug must be considered. The processes that determine the end organ concentration of the drug are pharmacokinetic and those that govern the end organ responses are pharmacodynamic.

Pharmacokinetic considerations include absorption, distribution, metabolism, and excretion of drugs. Often, changes in the sum total of these processes with aging result in a higher concentration of drug delivered to the end organ for a given dose. For example, with propranolol, a β-adrenergic blocker used widely as an antihypertensive agent, the volume of distribution decreases with age and the rate of elimination is reduced with age due to diminished hepatic metabolism.[3] The end result is that for a given dose, the plasma concentration may be up to 16-fold higher in the elderly.[3]

Pharmacodynamic considerations include receptor number and affinity, signal transduction mechanisms, cellular responses, and homeostatic regulation. Whereas for a given dose, pharmacokinetic changes in senescence often result in a higher concentration of a drug delivered to the end organ, pharmacodynamic changes often result in a reduced cellular response for the same concentration of a drug. In the example given above, a given dose of propranolol results in a 16-fold higher plasma concentration in the elderly than in the young. However, this same dose in the elderly has a diminished ability to antagonize the stimulatory response of the β-agonist, isoproterenol, on heart rate as compared to the young.[4] However, this is not universally true. Some responses do not change in old age, but may be altered earlier in life, and there are a few in which responsiveness actually increases. In the great majority, however, responsiveness declines either over the entire life span or during the postmaturational phase. The variations may be explained by the different rates at which individual cells, tissues, and organs age.[1]

There are only a few receptor systems that have been examined in sufficient detail to allow us to begin to understand the contribution of pharmacokinetic and pharmacodynamic changes with age to the end organ responsiveness with senescence. Among those best studied are the α- and β-adrenergic signal transduction systems. Despite the dramatic changes in the pharmacokinetics of adrenergic drugs that result in elevated plasma concentrations, particularly with the β-adrenergic antagonists, it is the decrease in pharmacodynamic parameters that, for the most part, governs the overall responsiveness of adrenergic drugs with age. In this chapter we will consider the changes in CA function with senescence and, as an example, we will discuss how these changes alter the responsiveness of the cardiovascular system, in particular the regulation of blood pressure.

We will consider the age-related changes in CA synthesis, adrenergic neurotransmission, plasma CA levels, α-adrenergic responsiveness, and β-adrenergic responsiveness. In addition, we will consider alterations in the homeostatic regulation of these pathways with age and the adaptive regulation by exercise. The former may be contributing to the altered CA action with age, whereas the latter may improve functional responsiveness.

III. ADRENERGIC REGULATION OF BLOOD PRESSURE

The role of the adrenergic function in the regulation of blood pressure is complex.[5] We will limit our brief discussion to the cardiovascular system and sympathetic nerves (Table 2.1). β-Adrenergic receptors mediate increases in both the rate and force of contraction in the heart, both of which in turn elevate blood pressure. In vascular tissue, β-adrenergic receptors mediate relaxation, and thus decrease blood pressure. An acute infusion of the β-adrenergic agonist, isoproterenol, results in widening of the pulse pressure due to both increased cardiac output and increased vasodilation. The net result is a decrease in the mean blood pressure. Paradoxically, β-adrenergic blockers also decrease blood pressure. The mechanism involves the inhibition of the release of adrenergic transmitters at neuroeffector junctions (Table 2.1). The α_2-adrenergic receptors mediate vasoconstriction, which increases blood pressure, and in addition these receptors facilitate presynaptic inhibition of NE release (discussed below), leading to a net decrease in blood pressure (Table 2.1). The α_1-adrenergic receptors mediate myocardial contraction and vasoconstriction with a profound positive effect on blood pressure (Table 2.1).

TABLE 2.1.
Adrenergic Regulation of Blood Pressure

	Heart		**Vascular**		**Sympathetic nerves**		**Net effect**	
βAR	↑ Rate	↑ BP	↑ Relaxation	↓ BP	↑ Facilitate NE release		Agonist	↓ BP
	↑ Contraction						Blockers	↓ BP
α_2AR			↑ Constriction	↑ BP	↑ Sympathetic Drive	↓↓ BP		↓ BP
α_1AR	↑ Contraction	↑ BP	↑↑Constriction	↑↑BP				↑↑ BP

Note: βAR, β-adrenergic receptors; α_2AR, α_2-adrenergic receptors; α_1AR, α_1-adrenergic receptors; BP, blood pressure. Arrows indicate increase (↑), large increase (↑↑), decrease (↓), or large decrease (↓↓).

IV. CATECHOLAMINE BIOSYNTHESIS

The CAs, including dopamine, NE, and epinephrine, are formed from their amino acid precursor tyrosine in the brain, in the chromaffin cells of the adrenal medulla, and in the sympathetic nerves (Figure 2.1). TH is the key enzyme involved in this pathway.[6] TH is generally regarded as the rate-limiting step in the biosynthesis of CA, and its activity is the important regulatory step in the biosynthesis pathway.[6]

TH facilitates the hydroxylation of tyrosine-producing dopamine. Among the mechanisms that control the rate of this reaction, two types of changes in TH activity are particularly important. First, rapid (within minutes) changes in TH activity are modulated by phosphorylation/ dephosphorylation, in particular, cAMP-dependent protein kinase A phosphorylation of serine 40, which increases the affinity for the biopterin cofactor.[7,8] TH activity is also

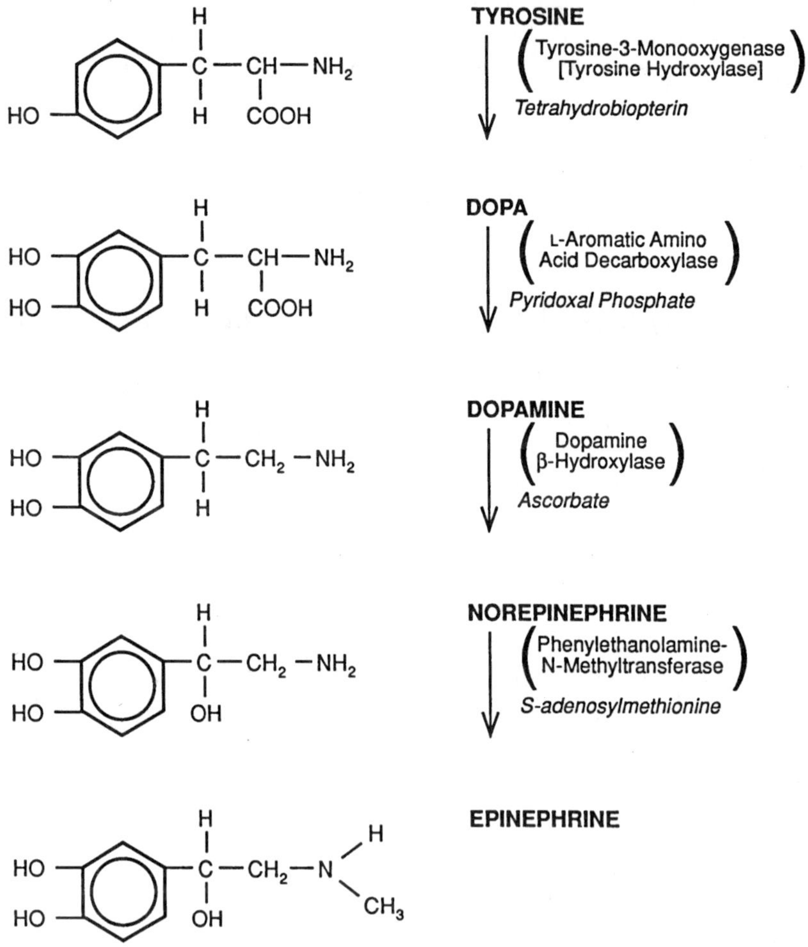

FIGURE 2.1. The enzymatic steps in the synthesis of norepinephrine and epinephrine from tyrosine. The rate-limiting step is the conversion of tyrosine to dopa by tyrosine hydroxylase.

regulated by competitive inhibition by CAs. The CA-bound enzyme is particularly sensitive to modulation by protein kinase A, which increases the V_{max} value tenfold.[8] Second, prolonged activation of catecholaminergic cells leads to a gradual increase in TH activity, caused by the apparent formation of new TH molecules as the result of increases in TH mRNA levels.[7,9] For example, cold stimulus and chemical sympathectomy are known to increase the synthesis and release of CAs in the brain, adrenal medulla, and heart.[9–11]

The effect of age on the biosynthesis of CAs has been studied in the adrenal medulla, heart, brain, and sympathetic ganglia. In the heart, dopa decarboxylase and dopamine-β-hydroxylase activities are reduced with age. However, there was no significant difference in CA synthesis with age in the heart using ^{14}C-tyrosine as an indicator of synthesis rate of CAs.[12] In contrast to the heart, there is a dramatic 50 to 75% increase in TH activity and TH mRNA with age in rat adrenal medulla.[13–15] Parallel to these changes, there is an equal increase in CA content with age in adrenal medulla. TH mRNA levels do not change in the superior cervical ganglion between 10 and 24 months of age,[14] and TH activity is diminished in the hypothalamus with age.[16]

A. BIOSYNTHESIS FOLLOWING ENVIRONMENTAL STIMULI

One of the most serious consequences of the aging process is an inability to respond to environmental stimuli. Older rats do not maintain their body temperature as well as young rats when exposed to the cold.[17] However, in response to acute cold, plasma epinephrine increases equally in young and old rats.[18] This represents release of stored adrenal medullary epinephrine and indicates the adrenal gland is receiving an adequate signal to respond to the cold stress. Despite the similar release of epinephrine between age groups, TH activity, TH immunoreactivity, and TH gene expression do not change following cold exposure in old F-344 rats, although there was a significant increase in all these parameters in adrenals from young animals.[19] This suggests that induction of TH activity is impaired in senescent rats following cold exposure; this inability to increase TH activity in cold-exposed senescent rats could be a failure in TH gene regulation or due to an inability to further stimulate the overactive TH synthesis in the adrenal medulla of old rats. One interpretation of this latter observation is that the maximum capacity for synthesis of TH in the old rats has been reached and that they simply cannot respond to additional stimulation.

Partanen et al.[20] have studied the recovery of reserpine-depleted CA stores and CA loss following inhibition of synthesis and intraneuronal degradation in sympathetic ganglia. TH activities were 37% higher in the superior cervical ganglia and 156% higher in adrenal glands of aged compared with young rats. More importantly, recoveries of reserpine-depleted CA stores in the superior cervical and hypogastric ganglia of aged rats were slower than in young rats. Further supporting this loss of plasticity with age is another study by Strong et al.[13] in which TH mRNA and TH activity in the adrenal medulla were assessed after reserpine treatment. TH mRNA increased after reserpine treatment in all ages (1.5-fold in the 2-month-old, 3-fold in the 12-month-old, and 1.75-fold in the 27-month-old rats); however, TH activity increased only in the 2-month-old animals. These results suggest impaired post-transcriptional or post-translational regulation with age.

V. ADRENERGIC NEUROTRANSMISSION

The adrenergic neurotransmission of the cardiovascular system is mediated by NE release at neuroeffector junctions. There is only limited knowledge concerning the release of adrenergic neurotransmitters with age. The NE content of rat arteries and veins either decreases or does not change with age.[21] In isolated heart preparations, following equal sympathetic nerve stimulation, the amount of NE released is greater in hearts from young compared with senescent male rats.[22] This is not the case with female F-344 rats, who demonstrated a decrease in NE release with age up to 12 months and then an increase between 12 and 24 months to a value equal to young rats.[23] The reduction in NE release with age in male rats appears to be a result of a defect in Ca^{2+} channels.[24] This is further supported by studies in cardiac synaptosomes.[25,26] An age-related decline in NE release due to a defect in Ca^{2+} channels was demonstrated in cardiac synaptosomes prepared from senescent male F-344 rats.[25] Again, this was not the case in female senescent F-344 rats, who demonstrated no age-related defect in Ca^{2+} channel function.[26]

In addition, it has been reported that NE content in both the atria and ventricles decreases with increasing age.[2] Furthermore, the disappearance of CA histofluorescence with age in the nerve cell bodies of human and rat sympathetic ganglia indicated decreased storage of NE[20] and is consistent with a decrease in CA content in the heart with age. It is important to note that the decrease in CA content in the rat heart appears to be associated with decreased capacity of the storage granules in the adrenergic nerve terminals to retain the transmitter.[12] The density of adrenergic nerves innervating arteries and veins of older rats, guinea pigs, and rabbits also is diminished with age.[21] These findings are in contrast to the adrenal medulla, in which CA content and release increase with age.[27] The majority of the released NE from nerve terminals does not find its way to its intended targets, the postsynaptic α- and β-adrenergic receptors. Most of the NE is either cleared by the circulation, undergoes reuptake into the nerve terminal, or undergoes uptake into extraneuronal storage sites. The effects of age on the latter uptake processes are controversial. In the rat heart and vasculature, the uptake processes have either been reported to decrease or increase with age.[28]

VI. PLASMA CATECHOLAMINES WITH AGE

It is well established that circulating levels of NE increase with age in man, whereas circulating epinephrine levels are unchanged.[2] In rats, both circulating levels of epinephrine and NE increase with age. This may be due to the increase with age in adrenomedullary synthesis and secretion of CAs. For the most part, epinephrine in the circulation originates in the adrenal medulla and represents adrenal medullary activity. Although the adrenal medulla contains considerable amounts of NE, the majority of NE found in the circulation originates in the nerve terminals and represents adrenergic neural activity. As indicated above, the CA content of the rat adrenal medulla increases with age. There is a progressive increase in the synthesis of both epinephrine and NE content with age in adrenal medulla of old rats.[27]

Secretion rates of epinephrine from the adrenal gland under resting conditions are two to four times greater in old rats. The stimulus for adrenal medulla to synthesize new epinephrine originates in the sympathetic ganglia of the hypothalamus. These sympathetic efferent pathways innervate the adrenal medulla, and this neural activity increases with age. The increase in neural activity parallels the increase in TH mRNA and TH activity in the adrenal medulla, resulting in an increase in epinephrine synthesis as described above. With aging there is a 50 to 75% increase in CA content and increased CA secretion from the medulla. In addition to the increased secretion of CA from the adrenal medulla, the clearance of NE decreases and the rate of appearance of NE is increased with age.[28] All of these factors are contributing to the increase in plasma NE levels with age.

A. ADRENAL MEDULLARY INFLUENCES ON ADRENERGIC NEUROTRANSMISSION

Changes in adrenal medullary secretion with age may be contributing to the alterations in adrenergic nervous system activity. The adrenal medulla is known to play a major role in maintaining homeostasis.[29] Many investigators[30,31] have reported that the role of the adrenal medulla in cardiac regulation becomes more important when adrenergic neural influence in the heart is decreased. Because adrenergic nervous input to the heart decreases with age,[22] it would be expected that the influence of adrenal medullary CAs on adrenergic neurochemical transmission at the cardiac neuroeffector junction would increase. For instance, Mueller et al.[31] have shown that after the destruction of cardiac postganglionic sympathetic nerve endings by the selective neurotoxin, 6-hydroxydopamine, an increase in TH activity occurs in the rat adrenal medulla. It was suggested that this increased activity was the result of a reflex increase in sympathoadrenal activity. Conversely, when the heart is exposed to increased CAs from a hyperactive adrenal medulla, there is a desensitization of cardiac β-adrenergic receptors.[32] Thus, it is important to consider both adrenergic neural input and adrenomedullary input when evaluating chemical transmission processes at the adrenergic neuroeffector junctions as a function of age.

VII. PERIPHERAL ADRENERGIC FUNCTION WITH AGE

From the above discussion, we know that senescence results in increased plasma NE, unchanged epinephrine, and decreased adrenergic nervous system activity in the heart and the vascular system. Both the α- and β-adrenergic receptors located in numerous organs in the body are responsive to both adrenergic innervation and circulating CAs. For the most part, the physiological responsiveness declines with age (Table 2.2). The end organ adrenergic responsiveness in the cardiovascular system will now be considered.[1]

The increase in heart rate after β-adrenergic agonist infusion is a common method of evaluating the cardiovascular response to β-adrenergic stimulation. However, the genesis of tachycardia after β-adrenergic stimulation is complex. There are direct chronotropic effects mediated by β_1-stimulation, reflex tachycardia mediated by β_2-vasodilation, reflex withdrawal

TABLE 2.2.
β-Adrenergic Responsiveness with Age

Species and tissue	Receptor	Physiological role	Physiological responsiveness with age	Receptor density with age	Signal transduction with age	Ref.
Rat myocardium	β,β1,β2	Rate and contractility	↓	↔	↓	1
Rat salivary glands	β1	Secretion	↓	↓	↓	110, 111
Cerebral microvessels	β			↓	↓	112
Rat brain	β,β2	Neurotransmission	↓ ↔	↓	↔	113
Rat vasculature	β2	Relaxation	↓	↔	↓ ↔	38, 50
Rat liver	β2	Glycolysis	↑	↑	↑	114, 115
Rat lung	β2	Relaxation	↔	↔ ↑	↓	55, 72, 116
Rat white fat	β3	Lipolysis	↓	↓	↓	49, 68
Rat brown fat	β3	Heat generation	↓	↓	↓	69
Human heart	β1	Rate and contractility	↓			4
Human vasculature	β2	Relaxation	↓			40
Human lymphocyte	β2	Inhibition of immune function		↔	↑ ↔ ↓	60, 85, 117
Human pancreas	β2	Insulin release	↔			118

Note: Arrows indicate increase (↑), decrease (↓), or no change (↔). When more than three references exist a review article is cited.

of vagal tone, as well as the negative modulation by adenosine. Nonetheless, in humans the dose of isoproterenol required to increase the resting heart rate by 25 bpm increases with age, indicating a decreased sensitivity to this drug.[4,33] The chronotropic and inotropic responses to isoproterenol are diminished with aging, not only in humans, but in rats, dogs, and isolated rat cardiac muscle strips.[34–36] However, the chronotropic response to electrical pacing and the positive inotropic response to calcium are unaltered with age, suggesting the β-adrenergic signal transduction pathway is deficient with age rather than the intrinsic function of the cardiac muscle (Table 2.2).[2]

The loss of β-adrenergic receptor-mediated responsiveness with age extends to arterial smooth muscles.[37,38] Isolated aortas from rats, rabbits, and guinea pigs are less responsive to the relaxing effects of isoproterenol at older ages. In contrast, the maximum relaxation in the presence of sodium nitrite is unchanged with age, again implicating the β-receptor-mediated pathway.[2] In the case of veins, there are conflicting results between rats and humans. One report indicated no change in β-adrenergic relaxation with age in rat veins[39], and another indicated reduced relaxation with age in the human dorsal hand vein[40] (see Table 2.2 and Reference 28).

In addition to the smooth muscle of the vascular, the tracheal smooth muscle from rats also demonstrates a reduced responsiveness to isoproterenol with age.[41] Moreover, other smooth muscle including the vas deferens, ileum, colon, and uterus demonstrate decreased sensitivity to NE with age.[2]

In summary, β-adrenergic responsiveness declines with age in cardiac and most smooth muscles. The intrinsic ability for muscle contractility or relaxation is maintained with age, and there appears to be an alteration in the process linking the receptor with the contractile or relaxation mechanisms. Although the latter is an attractive hypothesis, it would be naive to conclude that deficient adrenergic signal transduction is solely responsible for the reduced physiological responsiveness. For example, a recent study in isolated hearts from Sprague-Dawley rats demonstrated that the hearts from the presenescent (22-month-old) rats had both reduced inotropic response and generated more adenosine than young rats. When the adenosine receptor was blocked with theophylline, the difference in contractile response to isoproterenol was eliminated, suggesting the reduced adrenergic responsiveness with age may in part be due to increased inhibition by adenosine.[42] Similarly, a study in young and elderly humans demonstrated that the age-related increase in the isoproterenol dose required to increase heart rate by 25 bpm was obliterated by a 30-min infusion of theophylline.[43] Thus, the age-related modulation of adrenergic signal transduction may be as important as impaired signal transduction in explaining the loss of responsiveness in the cardiovascular system. Having recognized that multiple signal transduction systems and their interactions play an important role in the final physiological responsiveness, the remainder of the chapter will focus on adrenergic signal transduction.

VIII. ADRENERGIC SIGNAL TRANSDUCTION

The α_2- and β-adrenergic receptors are linked to the adenylyl cyclase signal transduction pathway, whereas the α_1-adrenergic receptor is a linked phospholipase C signal transduction pathway. We will first consider the adenylyl cyclase-linked receptors. The α_2- and β-adrenergic signal transduction system consists of three major components (Figure 2.2). The first components are the β-adrenergic or α_2-adrenergic receptors, which have a specific recognition site oriented towards the external cell surface for the binding of epinephrine, NE, and adrenergic drugs. The second component is a guanine nucleotide-binding regulatory protein, a heterotrimer that links receptor occupancy by agonist to adenylyl cyclase activation. The third component is the catalytic unit, which is the site of the conversion of adenosine triphosphate (ATP) to cAMP.

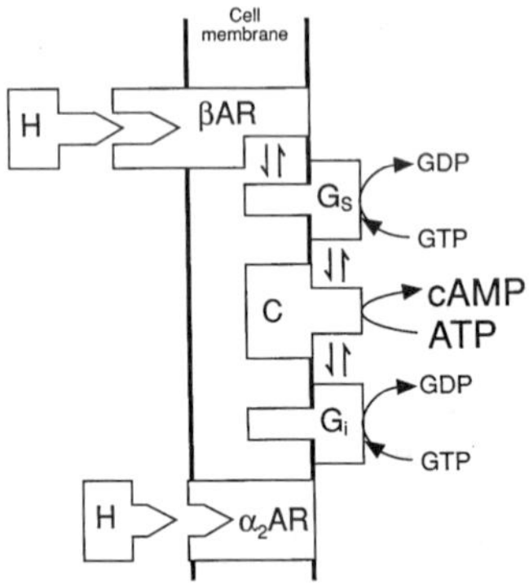

FIGURE 2.2. Schematic model of the hormone-sensitive adenylate cyclase system. ATP = adenosine triphosphate; C = catalytic unit; cAMP = cyclic adenosine monophosphate (adenosine 3′,5′-cyclic phosphate); GDP = guanosine 5′-diphosphate; GTP = guanosine 5′-triphosphate; H = hormone; G_s = stimulatory guanine nucleotide regulatory component; G_i = inhibitory guanine nucleotide regulatory component; βAR = β-adrenergic receptor; α_2AR = α-adrenergic receptor.

The α- and β-adrenergic receptors are part of the ever-growing family of receptors that are characterized by seven membrane-spanning domains with the amino terminus extracellular and the carboxyl terminus intracellular.[44] The β-adrenergic receptors are subdivided into the β_1, β_2, and β_3 subtypes. These receptors share structural homology with the α-adrenergic receptors that include the α_1- and α_2-adrenergic subtypes as well as the dopamine, the five muscarinic-cholinergic, two serotonin, substance K, rhodopsin receptors, and many others.[45] The transmembrane domains of these receptors are most important for ligand binding, including distinguishing between antagonists and agonists. For example, the substitution of a single amino acid (aspartate[113]) with glutamic acid in the third transmembrane domain of the hamster

β_2-adrenergic receptor results in the recognition of the β-antagonists, alprenolol and pindolol, as partial agonists.[46]

The β-adrenergic receptors are coupled to the activation of adenylyl cyclase, whereas the α_2-adrenergic receptor is linked to the inhibition of adenylyl cyclase. Signal transduction between these receptors and adenylyl cyclase is mediated by guanosine 5′-triphosphate (GTP)-binding proteins (G proteins). These G proteins are part of a larger family of G proteins that provide signal transduction to a variety of specific effector enzymes and ion channels, including adenylyl cyclase, phospholipase C, cyclic GMP, phosphodiesterase, Ca^{2+} channels, and K^+ channels.[45,47] Two of these proteins, termed G_s and G_i, are involved in both the stimulation and inhibition of adenylyl cyclase activity by β- and α-adrenergic receptors, respectively. They are thought to exist as heterotrimers, with G_s and G_i apparently having similar β and γ subunits and a unique α subunit. The G proteins appear to oscillate between two activity forms, an inactive guanosine 5′-diphosphate (GDP)-bound form and an active GTP-bound form. The binding of ligand to the stimulatory receptor activates the G proteins by promoting the replacement of bound GDP by GTP in the G protein α subunit. The GTP-α subunit interacts with the third component of the enzyme complex, the catalytic unit, to form an active enzyme that is the site of the conversion of ATP to cAMP. Similarly, activation of the inhibitory receptor, α_2, promotes formation of the GTP-α subunit of the G_i protein, which may inhibit adenylyl cyclase directly. In addition, the dissociated βγ subunits from G_i protein can either inhibit or activate the enzyme, depending on the adenylyl cyclase isoform, or can reassociate with the α subunit from G_s, preventing the activation of adenylyl cyclase.[48]

A. β-ADRENERGIC RECEPTORS

The number of β-adrenergic receptors can be directly assessed by the use of radiolabeled antagonists. There have been numerous investigations detailing the changes in receptors with age. Numerous reports, with one exception, have determined that the number of β-adrenergic receptors is unaltered with age in humans (Table 2.2). These findings are also true in rats whose β-adrenergic receptor number is unchanged with age in the heart, lung, and lymphocytes (Table 2.2). In addition, both the β_1 and β_2 subtypes do not change with age in the rat heart. There are isolated reports of decreases in the receptor number in the rat heart and increases in the rat lungs, but the predominance of evidence suggests the receptor number is unchanged with age in these tissues (Table 2.2).[1]

This is not the case from all organs, as receptor density increases in the rat liver and decreases with age in brown and white adipocytes of rats (Table 2.2). In the latter, the mRNA levels for β_1- and β_3-adrenergic receptors also decrease with age.[49] Also, in the rat the predominance of evidence suggests β-adrenergic receptors diminish in most areas of the brain with age (Table 2.2). Numerous reports indicate that in the cerebellum, striatum, pineal, brain stem, forebrain, and hindbrain there is a decrease in receptor density with age. Only in the cortex is there conflicting evidence as to whether or not β-adrenergic receptor density is unchanged or decreased with age. In contrast to rats, in humans there is no change in β-adrenergic receptor density in brains sampled at autopsy.[1]

In summary, in the aged rats, β-adrenergic receptors decrease in adipose tissues and all brain areas investigated except the cortex. Receptors are unchanged in most peripheral organs, including lymphocytes, heart, and lung; however, receptors increase in the liver. In humans, there are no changes with age in either lymphocytes or brain, the only organs investigated.

B. POSTRECEPTOR SIGNAL TRANSDUCTION

Three aspects of β-adrenergic signal transduction have been investigated with respect to aging: the coupling of agonist-occupied receptors to G proteins, the levels of G proteins, and the intrinsic activity of the catalytic unit of adenylyl cyclase. The binding of agonists to the β-adrenergic receptor promotes the formation of an agonist high-affinity binding complex. This process is referred to as receptor coupling, and those receptors that form the high-affinity complex are referred to as coupled receptors. The formation of this high-affinity binding complex is rate limiting in the activation of adenylyl cyclase. It was previously believed that the G_s protein was necessary for the formulation of this agonist high-affinity complex; however, recent evidence indicates the high-affinity complex may form prior to association with the G protein.[51] The number of high-affinity receptors (or coupled receptors) can be assessed by binding competition between radiolabeled antagonists and unlabeled agonists. In contrast to assessment of total receptor density, the number of high-affinity receptors decreases with age in most tissues that have been investigated, including rat heart, lung, and lymphocytes.[52–56] In particular, this decrease in coupled receptors with age may be contributing to the well-documented loss of sensitivity of β-agonists with age.[1]

Despite the critical role of G protein function in signal transduction of the β-adrenergic receptor, there have been few studies that assessed G protein function with age in the heart. Experiments using antibodies directed towards the α subunits of G_s and G_i proteins have indicated the amount of these proteins are unchanged with age in the F-344 rats.[57] In contrast, in the Wistar rat, the amount of G_{sa} immunoreactivity and G_{sa} mRNA decrease with age with no change in G_{ia} immunoreactivity.[58] This is supported by functional studies in the F-344 rat that assessed reconstitution of solubilized myocardial G protein with S49 cyc^- cells and found that G protein function is decreased with age.[59] Similarly, in the rat aorta, β-adrenergic receptor-G-protein coupling is decreased with age as evidenced by a decrease in both isoproterenol affinity for the receptor and the amount of β-adrenergic receptors that coprecipitates with G protein-directed antisera.[50] In contrast, in human lymphocytes, G protein function is unaltered with age.[60]

The predominance of evidence for changes in signal transduction with age is derived from studies of membrane adenylyl cyclase activity or cellular production of cAMP. With those studies, the overwhelming majority of the evidence suggests a decrease with age. Agonist-stimulated adenylyl cyclase activity or cAMP production is decreased with age in human lymphocytes,[60–63] rat heart,[56,59,64–67] rat lung,[55] and rat adipocytes.[68,69] There are two studies indicating no change in cAMP production in human lymphocytes[70,71] and one study indicating no change in the isoproterenol-stimulated adenylyl cyclase activity in rat lung.[72]

Whereas β-agonists activate adenylyl cyclase through the β-adrenergic receptor by the mechanism described earlier, forskolin, a cardioactive diterpene, activates adenylyl cyclase by a direct interaction with the catalytic unit. By using this compound, this laboratory determined that the loss of adenylyl cyclase activity can specifically be attributed to the diminished activity of the catalytic unit of adenylyl cyclase.[57,59,60,67] First, the decrease in adenylyl cyclase activity maximally stimulated by both isoproterenol (receptor mediated) and by forskolin (catalytic unit mediated) is approximately the same. These pharmacological data suggest that the loss of adenylyl cyclase function can account for the diminished receptor and postreceptor activation of adenylyl cyclase with age.[67] In addition, the number of forskolin binding sites as assessed by [^{3}H] forskolin binding is decreased by 41% in hearts from senescent rats compared with young rats.[57] Furthermore, this loss of binding sites is paralleled by a decrease in the capacity of forskolin to activate adenylyl cyclase.[57] In some preparations, the ability of forskolin to stimulate adenylyl cyclase is dependent upon the association of adenylyl cyclase with the GTP-bound α subunit of the G_s protein.[73] That is, in the presence of this complex, forskolin binds with high affinity and fully activates, whereas in the absence of Gs_a, forskolin binds with low affinity and partially activates adenylyl cyclase. However, this is not the case with myocardial preparations from F-344 rats. The efficacy and sensitivity of forskolin activation is equivalent in the absence or presence of the GDP analog, GDP-βS.[67] This compound blocks the activation of G_s protein by preventing the binding of GTP to the α subunit, and thus no association with the catalytic unit occurs. In addition, the forskolin binding assay is unaffected by preactivating G_s protein with isoproterenol or $Gpp(NH)_p$ or by deactivating with GDP. Collectively, these data suggest that the amount of adenylyl cyclase catalytic units diminishes with age and that this decrease correlates with the diminished capacity to activate adenylyl cyclase with age. It may also account for the reduced β-adrenergic signal transduction observed in senescent rat hearts. In addition, our laboratory recently demonstrated that steady-state mRNA levels for type V and VI adenylyl cyclase are altered at 12 months of age, but are unchanged between 6 and 24 months of age, and thus do not correlate with the age-related loss of adenylyl cyclase activity.[74]

C. α-ADRENERGIC RECEPTORS

Studies on changes in α-adrenergic receptors and responsiveness are sparse and conflicting. The α_2 subtype is linked to the inhibition of adenylyl cyclase, and α_2-receptor density is either reduced, increased, or not changed in human platelets (Table 2.3). However, responsiveness to a_2-adrenergic-mediated vasoconstriction in most rat tissues is markedly reduced by aging.[28] The a_1 subtype activates phospholipase C, and the density of this receptor subtype is reduced in the rat heart and the liver, but not in the smooth muscle (Table 2.3). Stimulation of phospholipase C activity through the α_1 receptor is reduced in the rat heart, but not in the liver (Table 2.3). More importantly, α-adrenergic response in the human vasculature is probably unchanged with age (Table 2.3).

In summary, β-adrenergic responsiveness is decreased with age, including the rate and force of contractility on the heart as well as vascular relaxation. The mechanism for the most part involves impaired postreceptor signal transduction with unchanged receptor density. In contrast, at least in humans, α-adrenergic responsiveness is unchanged with age, thus in the elderly there is a shift toward dominance by α-adrenergic processes and a vasoconstrictive state.

TABLE 2.3.
α-Adrenergic Responsiveness with Age

Species and tissue	Receptor	Physiological role	Physiological responsiveness with age	Receptor density with age	Signal transduction with age	Ref.
Rat heart	α_1	Rate and contractility	↓	↓	↔ ↓	119–122
Rat liver	α_1	Glycolysis		↓	↔	123, 124
Rat vas deferens	α_1	Contraction	↔			125
Rat aorta	α_1	Contraction	↓		↓ ↔	28, 126
Rat parotid gland	α_1	Metabolism/ secretion	↓	↔	↓	127, 128
Rat vasculature	α_2	Contractility	↓			28
Human vasculature	α_1	Contractility	↔ ↓			129–132
Human veins	α_2	Contractility	↓			133, 134
Human platelet	α_2	Aggregation	↔ ↑	↑ ↓ ↔		28, 135

Note: Arrows indicate increase (↑), decrease (↓), or no change (↔). When more than three references exist a review article is cited.

IX. HOMEOSTATIC AND PHYSIOLOGICAL REGULATION

A. DESENSITIZATION

One of the most important manifestations of aging is a decrease in the ability to adapt to changes in the environment. Adrenergic receptors self-regulate their own responsiveness and are regulated by a number of hormones and drugs. An important aspect of this self-regulation is desensitization of the β-adrenergic receptor. Following agonist binding to the receptor and activation of adenylate cyclase, the receptor is left in the uncoupled state. This event is associated with phosphorylation of the receptor by a specific kinase. Functionally, the receptor expresses low-affinity binding for the agonist, and there is a decrease in the ability of agonists to further stimulate adenylate cyclase.[75] A portion of the cell surface receptors are internalized during the desensitization process (receptor down-regulation). These internalized receptors are sequestered in membrane vesicles that are distinct from the plasma membrane, containing the other components of the adenylate cyclase complex.[76] The up- and down-regulation of the β-adrenergic receptor with age has been investigated in a variety of organ systems, including the rat heart,[1,77] the rat brain,[78] rat salivary glands,[79] and human lymphocytes.[52,71] For the most part, we will limit our discussion to the heart.[78] Though the density of β-adrenergic receptors does not decrease with age in the rat heart, it has been suggested that homeostatic regulation of this receptor may be impaired with age. Treatment with β-adrenergic antagonists induces supersensitivity, whereas treatment with β-adrenergic agonists leads to CA refractoriness. It was determined that up-regulation of β-adrenergic receptors occurs in older rat hearts[80] and that both subtypes of cardiac β-adrenergic receptors participate in the up-regulation response to chemical denervation by 6-hydroxydopamine regardless of age.[81] Similarly, the up-regulation of β-adrenergic receptors in the rat heart in response to thyroid hormone administration is also unchanged with age. Receptor density increased twofold in hearts from 3-, 12-, and 24-month-old rats.[82] The down-regulation of cardiac β-adrenergic receptors also occurs equally in younger and older rats exposed to the receptor agonist metaproterenol.[56,77] Moreover, the recovery from receptor-down regulation was faster in senescent rats.[77] In this latter study, β-adrenergic receptor mRNA levels did correlate with receptor down regulation.[77] In another study, Tümer et al.[83] investigated the effect of decreased adrenal medullary CAs due to adrenal demedullation on the regulation of cardiac β-adrenergic receptors with age. Surprisingly, adrenal demedullation down-regulated cardiac β-receptor numbers; however, this down-regulation of β-receptors was unaffected by age. In contrast, the rate of β-adrenergic receptor regeneration after irreversible blockade is slower in senescent rats compared with young rats.[84] However, the rate of up-regulation and recovery from down-regulation with age has not been studied in the rat heart. A slower rate of response might compromise the capacity of the heart to respond to homeostatic challenges. In both the rat cortex and the salivary glands the rate of β-adrenergic receptor recovery after desipramine desensitization was slower in aged rats[78,79] and, additionally, in rat submandibular glands the rate of recovery of postreceptor-mediated adenylyl cyclase activity was impaired with senescence.[79]

In human lymphocytes, there are no changes in β-adrenergic receptors with age.[85] In addition, the β-adrenergic receptor-induced down-regulation by the β_2-agonist, terbutaline, occurred equally in young and elderly subjects.[86] However, upright posture induces an acute increase in receptor density in young subjects that does not occur in older subjects.[71] Moreover, following thyroidectomy the number of lymphocyte β-adrenergic receptors decreases equally in young and elderly subjects, but recovery of the receptor number is delayed in the aged patients.[87] Thus, in the human lymphocyte, down-regulation is normal, but up-regulation is impaired with age. This is in contrast to the rat heart where up-regulation is normal, but similar to the rat brain and salivary glands, where up-regulation is impaired with age.

The endogenous concentration of CAs increases with age (see section on Plasma Catecholamines with Age). Some of the changes in receptors and post-receptor mechanisms with age may be a result of homeostatic regulation by increasing CA concentrations with age.[75] There is some similarity between the changes in β-adrenergic receptors and signal transduction with age and the changes in response to homologous desensitization to CAs. More receptors from aged animals and humans appear to be in the desensitized state compared with their young counterparts.[52,75] Especially significant is an age-related increase in the number of receptors sequestered in light membrane (or internalized) vesicles, suggesting that there is a receptor down-regulation occurring in older rats.[88] More compelling is a study in which a β-adrenergic agonist was administered to both young and senescent rats.[56] The number of high-affinity (coupled receptors) receptors and the amount of isoproterenol-stimulated adenylate cyclase decreased in the untreated animals with age. These parameters were further reduced by β-adrenergic agonist treatment, but to a lesser extent in the older animals. Thus, the effects of age and agonist desensitization are not additive and suggest that aged animals may already be partially desensitized. In this same study, NaF-stimulated adenylate cyclase activity was less in the older untreated rats, but was unaffected by β-adrenergic treatment in either age group. This suggests that there is an additional postreceptor deficit independent of CA desensitization.

The reduced receptor number in some tissues (down-regulation), the reduced high-affinity receptors (coupled receptors), and the reduced hormone-stimulated adenylate cyclase activity with age suggests receptor desensitization to increased plasma NE concentrations with age (Table 2.3). The inability of older animals to desensitize to β-adrenergic agonists further supports this hypothesis. However, there is an additional postreceptor reduction in catalytic unit activity with age independent of desensitization. These data suggest that desensitization of the β-adrenergic receptor may be contributing, but does not totally account for the reduced hormonal responsiveness in senescence.

B. EXERCISE ADAPTATIONS

Exercise is known to help control hypertension and emotional stress, to reduce risk factors for coronary artery disease, and to help prevent cardiovascular disease.[89] Endurance exercise training lowers blood pressure in hypertensive subjects, producing an approximate 10-mmHg reduction in systolic and diastolic pressures in subjects with either systolic or diastolic hypertension.[90] This effect is independent of any weight loss and is seen in both old and young individuals. Interestingly, long-term training at 40 to 70% of maximal oxygen uptake appears to elicit the same or greater reductions in blood pressure than higher-intensity training in both human and animal studies.[91]

Whether the training-related reduction in blood pressure is a result of reduced peripheral vascular resistance, cardiac output, or both is unclear. Results of studies measuring the effects of endurance training on cardiac output in hypertensive subjects have been inconsistent. Though peripheral resistance correlates strongly with blood pressure reduction in some studies, in others the relationship is weak.

There has been great interest in determining the mechanism of lowered resting blood pressure after endurance training. As the sympathetic nervous system is affected by exercise and is also involved in blood pressure regulation, investigators have tried to prove whether or not changes in plasma CAs with training are causally related to blood pressure changes. Though most studies of non-elderly hypertensive subjects find significant decreases in plasma NE levels with training, with the magnitude of blood pressure reduction correlated to the decrease in NE, other studies have found no reduction in plasma NE in older hypertensive individuals who undergo training.[92] In the nonhypertensive elderly there are conflicting data as to whether fit, active older men have higher[93] or lower[90] resting plasma NE levels than their sedentary counterparts.

Studies in rats have provided insight as to how exercise influences the sympathetic nervous system with age. In young animals, exercise training reduces blood pressure, resting heart rate, and plasma CAs. The reduction in plasma CAs may account for the decrease in both heart rate and blood pressure.

Exercise training decreases the heart rate at rest and in response to submaximal exercise. Withdrawal of vagal tone contributes to this bradycardia as it may diminish responsiveness to CAs, and several investigators have suggested that the latter is a result of decreased β-adrenergic receptors in the sinoatrial node.[94,95] However, it is controversial as to whether or not training alters β-adrenergic receptor numbers. Several laboratories have reported no change in receptor numbers with training, whereas others have found a decrease in receptor numbers after training. The latter studies were in young rats. In senescent rats there was no effect of age or exercise on β-adrenergic receptor density and affinity.[96] This suggests that bradycardia following training is not due to changes in density of β-receptors, but possibly may be due to changes in the release of CAs or in postreceptor signal transduction mechanisms. There is evidence to support both of these hypotheses. Exercise training decreases the synthesis of TH and thus the available CA.[97] Exercise training also diminished the maximum stimulation of adenylyl cyclase by isoproterenol, Gpp(NH)p, and forskolin with no change in G_sa protein immunoreactivity in the ventricles of young rats.[98] This latter observation suggests that exercise training decreases the capacity for β-adrenergic signal transduction, and if this generalized decrease in postreceptor signal transduction in the ventricle extends to the sinoatrial node, then this may help explain the bradycardia observed following physical training.

In contrast to the decrease in β-adrenergic signal transduction observed in the young rats, the senescent rats demonstrated an increase in signal transduction following training, partially offsetting the age-related decline in signal transduction. The combination of the decrease in the young rats and the increase in old rats results in a level of signal transduction that is no longer significantly different with age.[98]

Older animals have a higher NE turnover rate in the heart and the adrenal medulla in response to exercise (reflecting elevated sympathetic activity). Resting cardiac CA content declines significantly with age. Moreover, in response to an acute exercise bout, epinephrine levels in the heart are further reduced with age. Similarly, the NE content in the heart in response to acute exercise was also markedly reduced with advanced age. In summary, turnover and circulating levels of peripheral CAs measured both at rest and in response to exercise are reduced by chronic exercise in both hypertensive humans and rodents.[99]

It has been proposed that the decrease in NE turnover and plasma CAs following exercise training may be a result of decreased CA synthesis. This has been investigated by assessing the amount of TH hydroxylase expression and activity in the adrenal medulla in young and senescent rats following exercise training. TH is the key enzyme in the CA biosynthetic pathway (see Catecholamine Biosynthesis). Exercise training decreases both the expression and activity of TH in the adrenal medulla of young, but not old rats. This suggests that the diminution of CAs following exercise training may be a result of diminished CA biosynthesis. However, the older rats do not demonstrate this adaptive change, suggesting the effects of exercise are blunted with senescence.[99]

In summary, sympathetic nervous system activity diminishes in the heart, as does the responsiveness to β-adrenergic agonists. In contrast, CA biosynthesis increases with age in the adrenal medulla with a concomitant elevation of plasma CA levels. The combination of these factors may be contributing to the increased incidence of hypertension in the elderly. Exercise training reduces both systolic and diastolic blood pressure in young and elderly hypertensive subjects. The reduction in CA synthesis following training may be linked to the beneficial effects of exercise in hypertensive individuals.[99]

X. PATHOPHYSIOLOGY

A review of age-associated changes in the anatomy and physiology of systems that may alter blood pressure regulation is provided in Table 2.4. Arterial compliance decreases secondary to atherosclerosis, fibrosis, and smooth muscle hypertrophy, which makes blood pressure more sensitive to changes in cardiac output and blood volume. In the same fashion, the venous system increases in tortuosity with age, thus enhancing venous pooling. Age and disease-associated cardiac hypertrophy impair the diastolic filling phase of the cardiac cycle. Renal sodium conservation is impaired in the aging kidney and may partly explain the age-related decrease in plasma volume. Neurohypophyseal release of vasopressin is blunted in response to volume stress. Renin, angiotensin, and aldosterone levels are lower in elderly subjects and do not rise after standing to the same degree as in younger individuals. Plasma NE levels increase with age under both basal and stress conditions such as standing, isometric exercise, or cold stimulation.[2,100]

TABLE 2.4.
Risk Factors for Disordered Blood Pressure Regulation

Factors that predispose to postural hypotension	Factors that predispose to hypertension
Blunted baroreceptor response	Impaired β-adrenergic-mediated vasodilation
Decreased renin, angiotensin, and aldosterone levels	Normal α-adrenergic-mediated vasoconstriction
Decreased arterial compliance	Elevated plasma norepinephrine levels
Increased venous tortuosity	Increased prevalence of atherosclerosis
Decreased cardiac compliance	Decreased aortic compliance
Decreased renal sodium conservation	Increased vascular resistance
Decreased plasma volume	
Blunted vasopressin release to volume decrease	

A. POSTURAL HYPOTENSION

If the changes described above are combined with the data from the previous section on peripheral adrenergic function, it is apparent that there are age-related changes that may impair the maintenance of blood pressure (changes in heart rate response, cardiac and vascular compliance, vasopressin, renin, angiotensin, and renal concentrating ability). In addition, because cerebral blood flow declines with age, any decline in blood pressure may precipitate symptomatic cerebral hypoperfusion. Conversely, the increased plasma NE levels seen with standing, diminished β-adrenergic vasodilation, and unaltered α-adrenergic sensitivity would suggest that aging should be associated with a predominant vascular α-adrenergic activity and enhanced vasoconstriction and therefore resistance to hypotension (Table 2.4).[101]

In the undisturbed state the elderly appear to be resistant to hypotension. The key phase in this statement is the "undisturbed state." If we examine Table 2.4, the factors that protect against hypotension are all dependent on adrenergic function, whereas the factors that predispose to hypotension, except for the first two, are dependent on nonadrenergic mechanisms. If the homeostasis is disturbed or if a drug is present that disrupts adrenergic function, then the factors in Table 2.4 that protect will be affected more so than the factors that predispose, and the balance will tip toward an increase in the susceptibility for hypotension. For example, diuretic-induced volume depletion causes significant postural hypotension in a group of elderly subjects who previously had a normal blood pressure response to upright tilt.[102] This did not occur in the younger controls. Elderly subjects also have a decline in both supine and sitting blood pressure after meals, which does not occur in younger subjects.[103,104] Therefore, it appears that the sum effect of adrenergic and nonadrenergic changes leads to impaired blood pressure regulation, which may increase the likelihood of postural hypotension.[101]

B. HYPERTENSION

A number of the factors that predispose the elderly to postural hypotension also contribute to hypertension. The factors that cause the development of hypertension in the elderly are unknown, but those that contribute to the increased peripheral resistance are considered likely candidates. As discussed in the previous section, the diminished β-adrenergic vasodilation with age coupled with unchanged α-adrenergic vasoconstriction and elevated CAs suggest a predominant vasoconstrictive state in the elderly. This, coupled with a decrease in connective tissue elasticity and increased atherosclerosis, contributes to increased vascular resistance. Collectively, these factors lead to impaired blood pressure regulation, which contributes to the prevalence of hypertension in the elderly.[100]

C. HEART FAILURE

The β-adrenergic signal transduction pathway plays an important role in the pathophysiology of heart failure. An increase in the sympathetic tone is one of the major responses to reduced cardiac output. The decline in cardiac function results in a decrease in blood pressure, triggering the baroreceptor reflex system to increase sympathetic tone. If the heart cannot respond to this increased sympathetic stimulation, baroreceptor function may continue unchecked, leading to further neurohormonal activation and a hyperadrenergic state. This escalating, spiraling cycle of increasing adrenergic tone reflects the downwardly spiraling myocardial function of heart failure. This inverse relationship between cardiac function and sympathetic tone is well documented in patients with heart failure. It is controversial whether the increased sympathetic activity simply reflects the deterioration of cardiac failure or directly contributes to the decline in cardiac performance.[105]

The increases in epinephrine and NE plasma concentrations with heart failure are also associated with a decline in inotropic responsiveness to β-adrenergic agonists. It is unclear whether this abnormality is contributory to the heart failure or a consequence of the increased sympathetic tone. There is a decrease in the density of the β_1-adrenergic receptor subtype that is proportional to the severity of the heart disease.[106,107] However, the decrease in receptor number is also proportional to the increase in CAs observed with heart failure, suggesting that the receptor loss may be a consequence of desensitization to CAs. Receptor-mediated as well as postreceptor activation of adenylyl cyclase are diminished.[108] This may be a result of both increased amounts of G_i protein and decreased amounts of G_s protein.[109] Since CAs can regulate the gene expression of G proteins and CAs increase with heart failure, it is also difficult to determine whether the changes in G protein with heart failure are a cause or consequence of the disease. Postreceptor stimulation of adenylyl cyclase activity is also diminished with heart failure, suggesting a loss of catalytic unit enzyme activity. In summary, decreases in β-adrenergic receptor number, G protein, and catalytic unit activity with heart failure may contribute to the development of the disease. However, because cardiac failure is associated with elevated plasma CAs, the possibility exists that the altered signal transduction is a result of these elevated concentrations.[106]

In conclusion, pharmacodynamic changes with age include selected receptor alterations, impaired signal transduction, and decreased homeostatic regulation. From these theoretical considerations, it is difficult to predict the therapeutic effect of a given drug in senescence. However, thorough examination of the principles discussed above contributes to our understanding of clinical therapeutics in the elderly.

REFERENCES

1. **Scarpace, P. J., Tümer, N., and Mader, S. L.,** Beta-adrenergic function in aging: basic mechanisms and clinical applications, *Drugs Aging*, 1, 116, 1991.
2. **Roberts, J. and Tümer, N.,** Age-related changes in autonomic function of catecholamines, in *Review of Biological Research in Aging*, Vol. 3, Rothstein, M., Ed., Alan R. Liss, New York, 1987, 257.
3. **Platt, D.,** Pharmacotherapy and old age, *Triangle (Sandoz J. Med. Sci.)*, 25, 43, 1986.
4. **Vestal, R. E., Wood, A. J. J., and Shand, D. G.,** Reduced β-adrenergic sensitivity in the elderly, *Clin. Pharmacol. Ther.*, 26, 181, 1979.
5. **Hoffman, B. B. and Lefkowitz, R. J.,** Catecholamines and sympathomimetic drugs, in *Goodman and Gilman's the Pharmacological Basis of Therapeutics*, Gilman, A. G., Rall, T. W., Nies, A. S., and Taylor, P., Eds., Pergamon Press, New York, 1990, 220.
6. **Nagatsu, T., Levitt, M., and Udenfriend, S.,** Tyrosine hydroxylase: the initial step in norepinephrine biosynthesis, *J. Biol. Chem.*, 238, 2910, 1964.
7. **Acheson, A. L. and Zigmond, M. J.,** Short and long term changes in tyrosine hydroxylase activity in rat brain after subtotal destruction of central noradrenergic neurons, *J. Neurosci.*, 1, 493, 1981.
8. **Daubner, S. C., Lauriano, C., Haycock, J. W., and Fitzpatrick, P. F.,** Site-directed mutagenesis of serine 40 of rat tyrosine hydroxylase, *J. Biol. Chem.*, 267, 12639, 1992.
9. **Chuang, D. M. and Costa, E.,** Biosynthesis of tyrosine hydroxylase in rat adrenal medulla after exposure to cold, *Proc. Natl. Acad. Sci. U.S.A.*, 71, 4570, 1974.
10. **Fluharty, S. J., Rabow, L. E., Zigmond, M. J., and Stricker, E. M.,** Tyrosine hydroxylase activity in the sympathoadrenal system under basal and stressful conditions: effect of 6-hydroxydopamine, *J. Pharmacol. Exp. Ther.*, 235, 354, 1985.

11. **Stachowiak, M. K., Fluharty, S. J., Stricker, E. M., Zigmond, M. J., and Kaplan, B. B.,** Molecular adaptations in catecholamine biosynthesis induced by cold stress and sympathectomy, *J. Neurosci. Res.*, 16, 13, 1986.
12. **Limas, C. J.,** Comparison of the handling of norepinephrine in the myocardium of adult and old rats, *Cardiovasc. Res.*, 9, 664, 1975.
13. **Strong, R., Moore, M. A., Hale, C., Wessels-Reiker, M., Armbrecht, H. J., and Richardson, A.,** Modulation of tyrosine hydroxylase gene expression in the rat adrenal gland by age and reserpine, *Brain Res.*, 525, 126, 1990.
14. **Kedzierski, W. and Porter, J. C.,** Quantitative study of tyrosine hydroxylase mRNA in catecholaminergic neurons and adrenals during development and aging, *Mol. Br. Res.*, 7, 45, 1990.
15. **Voogt, J. L., Arbogast, L. A., Quadri, S. K., and Andrews, G.,** Tyrosine hydroxylase messenger RNA in the hypothalamus, substantia nigra and adrenal medulla of old female rats, *Br. Res. Mol. Brain Res.*, 8, 55, 1990.
16. **Reymond, M. J., Arita, J., Dudley, C. A., Moss, R. L., and Porter, J. C.,** Dopaminergic neurons in the mediobasal hypothalamus of old rats: evidence for decreased affinity of tyrosine hydroxylase for substrate and cofactor, *Brain Res.*, 304, 215, 1984.
17. **Scarpace, P. J., Matheny, M., Borst, S. E., and Tümer, N.,** Thermoregulation with age: role of thermogenesis and uncoupling protein expression in brown adipose tissue, *Proc. Soc. Exp. Biol. Med.*, 205, 154, 1994.
18. **Avakian, E. V., Horvath, S. M., and Colburn, R. W.,** Influence of age and cold stress on plasma catecholamine levels in rats, *J. Auton. Nerv. Syst.*, 10, 127, 1984.
19. **Tümer, N., LaRochelle, J., Yenice, S., and Yürekli, M.,** Effect of mild cold exposure and age on tyrosine hydroxylase gene expression, *Endocrinology*, 131 (Suppl.) 77, 1993.
20. **Partanen, M., Waller, S., London, E., and Hervonen, A.,** Indices of neurotransmitter synthesis and release in aging sympathetic nervous system, *Neurobiol. Aging*, 6, 227, 1985.
21. **Handa, R. K. and Duckles, S. P.,** Influence of age on norepinephrine content in arteries and veins of Fischer 344 rats, *Neurobiol. Aging*, 8, 511, 1987.
22. **Daly, R. N., Goldberg, P. B., and Roberts, J.,** The effect of age on presynaptic $alpha_2$ adrenoceptor autoregulation of norepinephrine release, *J. Gerontol.*, 44, B59, 1989.
23. **Tümer, N., Mortimer, M. L., and Roberts, J.,** Gender differences in the effect of age on adrenergic neurotransmission in the heart, *Exp. Gerontol.*, 27, 301, 1992.
24. **Roberts, J., Mortimer, M. L., Ryan, P. J., Johnson, M. D., and Tümer, N.,** The role of calcium in adrenergic neurochemical transmission in the aging heart, *J. Pharmacol. Exp. Ther.*, 253, 957, 1990.
25. **Snyder, D. L., Johnson, M. D., Aloyo, V., Eskin, B., and Roberts, J.,** Age-related changes in cardiac norepinephrine release: role of calcium movement. *J. Gerontol. Biol. Sci.*, 50A, B358, 1995.
26. **Snyder, D. L., Johnson, M. D., Eskin, B. A., Wang, W., and Roberts, J.,** Effect of age on cardiac norepinephrine release in the female rat, *Aging Clin. Exp. Res.* 7, 210, 1995.
27. **Ito, K., Sato, A., Sato, Y., and Suzuki, H.,** Increases in adrenal catecholamine secretion and adrenal sympathetic nerve unitary activities with aging in rats, *Neurosci. Lett.*, 69, 263, 1986.
28. **Docherty, J. R.,** Effect of age on the response of target organs to autonomic neurotransmitters, in *Aging of the Autonomic Nervous System*, Amenta, F., Ed., CRC Press, Boca Raton, FL, 1993, 109.
29. **Axelrod, J. and Reisine, T. D.,** Stress hormones: their interaction and regulation, *Science*, 244, 452, 1984.
30. **Gauthier, P., Nadeau, R., and de Champlain, J.,** Acute and chronic cardiovascular effects of 6-hydroxydopamine in dogs, *Circ. Res.*, 31, 207, 1972.
31. **Mueller, R. A., Thoene, H., and Axelrod, J.,** Adrenal tyrosine hydroxylase: compensatory increase in activity after chemical sympathectomy, *Science*, 163, 468, 1969.
32. **Torda, T., Yamaguchi, I., Hirata, F., Kopin, I. J., and Axelrod, J.,** Quinacrine-blocked desensitization of adrenoceptors after immobilization stress or repeated injection of isoproterenol in rats, *J. Pharmacol. Exp. Ther.*, 216, 334, 1981.
33. **Bertel, O., Buhler, F. R., Kiowski, W., and Lutold, B. E.,** Decreased beta-adrenoceptor responsiveness as related to age, blood pressure and plasma catecholamines in patients with essential hypertension, *Hypertension*, 2, 130, 1980.
34. **Abrass, I. B., Davis, J. L., and Scarpace, P. J.,** Isoproterenol responsiveness and myocardial beta adrenergic receptors in young and old rats, *J. Gerontol.*, 37, 156, 1982.
35. **Yin, F., Spurgeon, H., Green, H., Lakatta, E., and Weisfeldt, M. L.,** Age associated decrease in heart rate response to isoproterenol in dogs, *Mech. Ageing Dev.*, 10, 17, 1979.
36. **Lakatta, E. G., Gerstenblith, G., Angell, C. S., Shock, N. W., and Weisfeldt, M. L.,** Diminished inotropic response of aged myocardium to catecholamines, *Circ. Res.*, 36, 262, 1975.
37. **Crass, M. F., Borst, S. E., and Scarpace, P. J.,** β-Adrenergic responsiveness in cultured aorta smooth muscle cells: effects of subculture and aging, *Biochem. Pharmacol.*, 43, 1811, 1992.
38. **Chin, J. H. and Hoffman, B. B.,** Age-related deficit in beta receptor stimulation of cAMP binding in blood vessels, *Mech. Ageing Dev.*, 53, 111, 1990.

39. **Duckles, S. P. and Hurlbert, J. S.,** Effect of age on beta adrenergic relaxation of the rat jugular vein, *J. Pharmacol. Exp. Ther.*, 236, 71, 1986.
40. **Pan, H. Y.-M., Hoffman, B. B., Pershe, R. A., and Blaschke, T. F.,** Decline in beta adrenergic receptor-mediated vascular relaxation with aging in man, *J. Pharmacol. Exp. Ther.*, 239, 802, 1986
41. **Fleisch, J. H., Maling, H. M., and Brodie, B. B.,** Beta-receptor activity in aorta, *Circ. Res.*, 26, 151, 1970.
42. **Dobson, J. G., Jr., Fenton, R. A., and Romano, F. D.,** Increased myocardial adenosine production and reduction of β-adrenergic contractile response in aged hearts, *Cir. Res.*, 66, 1381, 1990.
43. **Suteparuk, S., Nies., A. S., Andros, E., and Gerber, J. G.,** The role of adenosine in promoting cardiac β-adrenergic subsensitivity in aging humans, *J. Gerontol.*, 50A, 128, 1993.
44. **Collins, S., Caron, M. G., and Lefkowitz, R. J.,** Regulation of adrenergic receptor responsiveness through modulation of receptor gene expression, *Annu. Rev. Physiol.*, 53, 497, 1991.
45. **Martens, G. J. M.,** Molecular biology of G-protein-coupled receptors, *Prog. Brain Res.*, 92, 17, 201, 1992.
46. **Strader, C. D., Candelore, M. R., Hill, W. S., Dixon, R. A. F., and Sigal, I. S.,** A single amino acid substitution in the β-adrenergic receptor promotes partial agonist activity from antagonists, *J. Biol. Chem.*, 264, 16470, 1989.
47. **Spiegel, A. M., Shenker, A., and Weinstein, L. S.,** Receptor-effector coupling by G-proteins: implications for normal and abnormal signal transduction, *Endocrin. Rev.*, 1303, 536, 1992.
48. **Birnbaumer, L., Abramowitz, J., and Brown, A. M.,** Receptor-effector coupling by G proteins, *Biochem. Biophys. Acta*, 1031, 163, 1990.
49. **Gettys, T. W., Rohlfs, E. M., Prpic, V., Daniel, K. W., Taylor, I. L., and Collins, S.,** Age-dependent changes in β-adrenergic receptor subtypes and adenylyl cyclase activation in adipocytes from Fischer 344 rats, *Endocrinology*, 136, 2022, 1995.
50. **Gurdal, H., Friedman, E., and Johnson, M. D.,** β-Adrenoceptor-G_{as} coupling decreases with age in rat aorta, *Mol. Pharmacol.*, 47, 772, 1995.
51. **Lefkowitz, R. J., Cotecchia, S., Samama, P., and Costa, T.,** Constitutive activity of receptors coupled to guanine nucleotide regulatory proteins, *Trends Pharmacol. Sci.*, 14, 303, 1993.
52. **Feldman, R. D., Limbird, L. E., Nadeau, J., Robertson, D., and Wood, A. J. J.,** Alterations in leukocyte β-receptor affinity with aging. A potential explanation for altered β-adrenergic sensitivity in the elderly, *N. Engl. J. Med.*, 310, 815, 1984.
53. **Montamat, S. C. and Davies, A. O.,** Physiological response to isoproterenol and coupling of beta-adrenergic receptors in young and elderly human subjects, *J. Gerontol.*, 44, M100, 1989
54. **Narayanan, N. and Derby, J. A.,** Alterations in the properties of beta-adrenergic receptors of myocardial membranes in aging: impairments in agonist-receptor interactions and guanine nucleotide regulation accompany diminished catecholamine-responsiveness of adenylate cyclase, *Mech. Ageing Dev.*, 19, 127, 1982.
55. **Scarpace, P. J. and Abrass, I. B.,** Decreased beta-adrenergic agonist affinity and adenylate cyclase activity in senescent rat lung, *J. Gerontol.*, 38, 143, 1983.
56. **Scarpace, P. J. and Abrass, I. B.,** Beta-adrenergic agonist-mediated desensitization in senescent rats, *Mech. Ageing Dev.*, 35, 255, 1986.
57. **Shu, Y. and Scarpace, P. J.,** Forskolin binding sites and G-protein immunoreactivity in rat hearts during aging, *J. Cardiovasc. Pharmacol.*, 23, 188, 1994.
58. **Miyamoto, A., Kawanam, S., Kimura, H., and Oshsika, H.,** Impaired expression of G_{sa} protein mRNA in rat ventricular myocardium with aging, *Eur. J. Pharmacol.*, 266, 147, 1994.
59. **O'Connor, S. W., Scarpace, P. J., and Abrass, I. B.,** Age-associated decrease in the catalytic unit activity of rat myocardial adenylate cyclase, *Mech. Ageing Dev.*, 21, 357, 1983.
60. **Abrass, I. B. and Scarpace, P. J.,** Catalytic unit of adenylate cyclase: reduced activity in aged-human lymphocytes, *J. Clin. Endocrinol. Metab.*, 55, 1026, 1982.
61. **Krall, J. F., Connelly, M., Weisbart, R., and Tuck, M. L.,** Age-related elevation of plasma catecholamine concentration and reduced responsiveness of lymphocyte adenylate cyclase, *J. Clin. Endocrinol. Metab.*, 52, 863, 1981.
62. **Stressman, J., Eliakim, R., Cahan, C., and Ebstein, R. P.,** Deterioration of beta-receptor-adenylate cyclase function in elderly, hospitalized patients, *J. Gerontol.*, 39, 667, 1984.
63. **O'Hara, N., Daul, A. E., Fesel, R., Siekmann, U., and Brodde, O. E.,** Different mechanisms underlying reduced β_2-adrenoceptor responsiveness in lymphocytes from neonates and old subjects, *Mech. Ageing Dev.*, 31, 115, 1985.
64. **O'Connor, S. W., Scarpace, P. J., and Abrass, I. B.,** Age-associated decrease of adenylate cyclase activity in rat myocardium, *Mech. Ageing Dev.*, 16, 91, 1981.
65. **Kusiak, J. W. and Pitha, J.,** Decreased response with age of the cardiac catecholamine sensitive adenylate cyclase system, *Life Sci.*, 33, 1679, 1983.
66. **Fan, T.-H. M. and Banerjee, S. P.,** Age-related reduction of beta-adrenoceptor sensitivity in rat heart occurs by multiple mechanisms, *Gerontology*, 31, 373, 1985.
67. **Scarpace, P. J.,** Forskolin activation of adenylate cyclase in rat myocardium with age: effects of guanine nucleotide analogs, *Mech. Ageing Dev.*, 52, 169, 1990.

68. **Giudicelli, V. and Pecquery, R.,** Beta adrenergic receptors and catecholamine sensitive adenylate cyclase in rat fat cell membranes. Influence of growth, cell size and aging, *Eur. J. Biochem.*, 90, 413, 1978.
69. **Scarpace, P. J., Mooradian, A. D., and Morley, J. E.,** Age-associated decrease in beta-adrenergic receptors and adenylate cyclase activity in rat brown adipose tissue, *J. Gerontol.*, 43, B65, 1988.
70. **Zahniser, N. R., Parker, D. C., Bier-Laning, C. M., Miller, J. A., Gerber, J. G., and Nies, A. S.,** Comparison between the effects of aging on antagonist and agonist interactions with beta-adrenergic receptors on human mononuclear and polymorphonuclear leukocyte membranes, *J. Gerontol.*, 43, M151, 1988.
71. **Mader, S. L. and Davis, P. B.,** Effect of age on acute regulation of beta-adrenergic responses in mononuclear leukocytes, *J. Gerontol.*, 44, M-168, 1989.
72. **Vanscheeuwijck, P., Van de Velde, E., and Fraeyman, N.,** Effect of aging on properties and function of β-adrenoceptors in rat lung, *Eur. J. Pharmacol.*, 172, 373, 1989.
73. **Seamon, K. B. and Daly, J. W.,** Forskolin: its biological and chemical properties, in *Advances in Cyclic Nucleotide and Protein Phosphorylation Research*, Greengard, P. and Robison, G. A., Eds., Raven Press, New York, 1986, 150.
74. **Scarpace, P. J., Mathey, M. K., and Tümer, N.,** Myocardial adenylyl cyclase: correlation between activity and type V and VI mRNA with age, *ASBMB*, 9, A1373, 1995.
75. **Scarpace, P. J.,** Decreased receptor activation with age. Can it be explained by desensitization?, *J. Am. Geriatr. Soc.*, S 36, 1067, 1988.
76. **Collins, S.,** Recent perspectives on the molecular structure and regulation of the β_2-adrenoceptor, *Life Sci.*, 52, 2083, 1993.
77. **Raitt, M. H., Tamblyn, C., Allen, J. M., and Abrass, I. B.,** Beta-adrenergic receptor downregulation and recovery in heart and lung in the Fischer 344 rat: effects of aging and correlation with mRNA levels, *J. Gerontol.*, 4, 213, 1995.
78. **Weiss, B., Clark, M. B., and Greenberg, L. H.,** Modulation of catecholaminergic receptors during development and aging, in *Handbook of Neurochemistry*, Vol. 6, Lajtha, A., Ed., Plenum Press, New York, 1984, 595.
79. **Scarpace, P. J., Koller, M. M., and Rajakumar, G.,** Desipramine desensitizes β-adrenergic signal transduction in salivary glands: differential regulation with age, *Eur. J. Pharmacol.*, 247, 65, 1993.
80. **Tümer, N., Houck, W. T., and Roberts, J.,** Effect of age on upregulation of the cardiac adrenergic beta receptors, *J. Gerontol.*, 45, B48, 1990.
81. **Tümer, N., Houck, W. T., and Roberts, J.,** Upregulation of adrenergic beta receptor subtypes in the senescent rat heart, *Mech. Ageing Dev.*, 49, 235, 1989.
82. **Scarpace, P. J. and Abrass, I. B.,** Thyroid hormone regulation of beta-adrenergic receptor number in aging rats, *Endocrinology*, 108, 1276, 1981.
83. **Tümer, N., Houck, W. T., Boehm, C., and Roberts, J.,** Cardiac adrenergic beta receptor binding characteristics with age following adrenal demedullation, *Br. J. Pharmacol.*, 99, 87, 1990.
84. **Pitha, J., Hughes, B. A., Kusiak, J. W., Dax, E. M., and Baker, S. P.,** Regeneration of β-adrenergic receptors in senescent rats: a study using an irreversible binding antagonist, *Proc. Natl. Acad. Sci. U.S.A.*, 79, 4424, 1982.
85. **Abrass, I. B. and Scarpace, P. J.,** Human lymphocyte beta-adrenergic receptors are unaltered with age, *J. Gerontol.*, 26, 298, 1981.
86. **Zahniser, N. R., Wiser, A., Cass, W. A., Curella, P., Gerber, J. G., and Nies, A. S.,** Terbutaline-induced desensitization of polymorphonuclear leukocyte β_2-adrenergic receptors in young and elderly subjects, *Clin. Pharmacol. Ther.*, 51, 432, 1992.
87. **Basso, A., Veccia, V., Masera, N., and Piantanelli, L.,** Delayed recovery of lymphocyte β-adrenoceptors in thyroidectomized aging patients, *Gerontology*, 39, 327, 1993.
88. **Scarpace, P. J. and Baresi, L. A.,** Increased beta-adrenergic receptors in the light-density membrane fraction in lungs from senescent rats, *J. Gerontol.*, 43, B163, 1988.
89. **McHenry, P. L., Ellestad, M. H., Fletcher, G. F., Froelicher, V., Hartley, H., Mitchell, J. H., and Froelicher, E. S. S.,** A position for health professionals by the committee on exercise and cardiac rehabilitation of the council on clinical cardiology, American Heart Association, Special Report, *Circulation*, 81, 396, 1990.
90. **Hagberg, J. M., Seals, D. R., Yerg, J. E., Gavin, J., Gingerich, R., Premachandra, B., Holloszy, J. O., et al.,** Metabolic responses to exercise in young and older athletes and sedentary men, *J. Appl. Physiol.*, 65, 900, 1988.
91. **Tipton, C. M.,** Exercise, training and hypertension, in *Exercise and Sports Sciences Reviews*, Holloszy, J. O., Ed., Williams & Wilkins, Baltimore, 1991, 505.
92. **Hagberg, J. M.,** Exercise, fitness and hypertension, in *Exercise, Fitness and Health*, Bouchard, C., Shephard, R. J., Stephens, T., Sutton, J. R., and McPherson, B. D., Eds., Human Kinetics, Champaign, IL, 1990, 466.
93. **Poehlman, E. T., McAuliffe, T., and Danforth, E., Jr.,** Effects of age and level of physical activity on plasma norepinephrine kinetics, *Am. J. Physiol.*, 258, E256, 1990.

94. **Hammond, H. K., White, F. C., Brunton, L. L., and Longhurst, J. C.,** Association of decreased myocardial β-receptors and chronotropic response to isoproterenol and exercise in pigs following chronic dynamic exercise, *Circ. Res.*, 60, 720, 1987.
95. **Williams, R. S.,** Role of receptor mechanisms in the adaptive response to habitual exercise, *Am. J. Cardiol.*, 55, 68D, 1985.
96. **Scarpace, P. J., Lowenthal, D. T., and Tümer, N.,** Influence of age and exercise on myocardial β-adrenergic receptor properties, *Exp. Gerontol.*, 27, 169, 1992.
97. **Tümer, N., Hale, C., Lawler, J., and Strong, R.,** Modulation of tyrosine hydroxylase gene expression in the rat adrenal gland by exercise: effects of age, *Brain Res. Mol. Brain Res.*, 14, 51, 1992.
98. **Scarpace, P. J., Shu, Y., and Tümer, N.,** Influence of exercise training on myocardial β-adrenergic signal transduction: differential regulation with age, *J. Appl. Physiol.*, 77, 737, 1994.
99. **Tümer, N. and Lowenthal, D. T.,** Sympathetic nervous system: aging and exercise, *South. Med. J.*, 205, S42, 1994.
100. **Applegate, W. B. and Rutan, G. H.,** Advances in management of hypertension in older persons, *J. Am. Geriatr. Soc.*, 40, 1162, 1992.
101. **Scarpace, P. J., Mader, S. L., and Tümer, N.,** Adrenergic receptors: implications for falls, in *Aging and Musculoskeletal Disorders*, Perry, H. M., III, Morley, J. E., and Coe, R. M., Eds., Springer-Verlag, New York, 1993, 166.
102. **Shannon, R. P., Wei, J. Y., Rosa, R. M., Epstein, F. H., and Rowe, J. W.,** The effect of age and sodium depletion on cardiovascular responses to orthostasis, *Hypertension*, 8, 438, 1986.
103. **Lipsitz, L. A. and Fullerton, K. J.,** Postprandial blood pressure reduction in healthy elderly, *J. Am. Geriatr. Soc.*, 34, 267, 1986.
104. **Mader, S. L.,** Effects of meals and time of day on postural blood pressure responses in healthy young and elderly subjects, *Arch. Int. Med.*, 149, 2757, 1989.
105. **Sloman, G.,** Angiotensin-converting enzyme inhibition, the sympathetic nervous system, and congestive heart failure, *Am. J. Cardiol.*, 70, 113C, 1992.
106. **Horn, E. M. and Bilezikian, J. P.,** Mechanisms of abnormal transmembrane signaling of the β-adrenergic receptor in congestive heart failure, *Circulation*, 82, I26, 1990.
107. **Bristow, M. R., Hershberger, R. E., Port, J. D., Gilbert, E. M., Sandoval, A., Rasmussen, R., Cates, A. E., and Feldman, A. M.,** β-Adrenergic pathways in nonfailing and failing human ventricular myocardium, *Circulation*, 82 (Suppl. I), I12, 1990.
108. **Hammond, H. K., Roth, D. A., Insel, P. A., Ford, C. E., White, F. C., Maisel, A. S., Ziegler, M. G., and Bloor, C. M.,** Myocardial β-adrenergic receptor expression and signal transduction after chronic volume-overload hypertrophy and circulatory congestion, *Circulation*, 85, 269, 1992.
109. **Feldman, A. M.,** Modulation of adrenergic receptors and G-transduction proteins in failing human ventricular myocardium, *Circulation*, 87 (Suppl. IV), IV27, 1993.
110. **Rajakumar, G. and Scarpace, P. J.,** β-Adrenergic signal transduction in aging parotid and submandibular glands, *J. Gerontol.*, 46, B249, 1991.
111. **Rajakumar, G., Koller, M. M., and Scarpace, P. J.,** β-Adrenergic receptors and salivary gland secretion with aging, *Growth Dev. Aging*, 56, 215, 1992.
112. **Mooradian, A. D. and Scarpace, P. J.,** β-Adrenergic receptor activity of cerebral microvessels is reduced in aged rats, *Neurochem. Res.*, 16, 447, 1991.
113. **Scarpace, P. J. and Abrass, I. B.,** Alpha- and beta-adrenergic receptor function in the brain during senescence, *Neurobiol. Aging*, 9, 53, 1988.
114. **Katz, M. S., Dax, E. M., and Gregerman, R. I.,** Beta adrenergic regulation of rat liver glycogenolysis during aging, *Exp. Gerontol.*, 28, 329, 1993.
115. **Dax, E. M., Partilla, J. S., Pineyro, M. A., and Gregerman, R. I.,** β-Adrenergic receptors, glucagon receptors, and their relationship to adenylate cyclase in rat liver during aging, *Endocrinology*, 120, 1534, 1987.
116. **Scarpace, P. J. and Yu, P.,** Effect of diet restriction on rat lung beta-adrenergic receptors and adenylate cyclase activity, *J. Gerontol.*, 42, 442, 1987.
117. **Feldman, R. D.,** Physiological and molecular correlates of age-related changes in the human beta-adrenergic receptor system, *Fed. Proc., Fed. Am. Soc. Exp. Biol.*, 45(1), 48, 1986.
118. **Morrow, L. A., Rosen, S. G., and Halter, J. B.,** Beta-adrenergic regulation of insulin secretion: evidence of tissue heterogeneity of beta-adrenergic responsiveness in the elderly, *J. Gerontol. Med. Sci.*, 46, M108, 1991.
119. **Miyamoto, A. and Ohsha, H.,** Age-related changes in [^{3}H]-prazosin binding and phosphoinositide hydrolysis in rat ventricular alpha-adrenoceptors during aging, *Life Sci.*, 31, 2507, 1982.
120. **Borst, S. E., Narang, N., Crews, F. T., and Scarpace, P. J.,** Reduced alpha$_1$-adrenergic receptor-mediated inositide hydrolysis in cardiac atria of senescent rats, *J. Cardiovasc. Pharmacol.*, 16, 444, 1990.
121. **Partilla, J. S., Hoopes, M. T., Ito, H., Dax, E. M., and Roth, G. S.,** Loss of rat ventricular alpha-1 adrenergic receptors during aging, *Life Sci.*, 31, 2507, 1982.

122. **Kimball, K. A., Cornett, L. E., Seifen, E., and Kennedy, R. H.,** Aging: changes in cardiac a-1 adrenoceptor responsiveness and expression, *Eur. J. Pharmacol.*, 208, 231, 1991.
123. **Borst, S. E. and Scarpace, P. J.,** Alpha$_1$-adrenergic stimulation of inositide hydrolysis in liver of senescent rats, *Mech. Aging Dev.*, 56, 275, 1990.
124. **Borst, S. E. and Scarpace, P. J.,** Reduced high affinity alpha$_1$-adrenoceptors in liver of senescent rats: implication of assessment at various temperatures, *Br. J. Pharmacol.*, 101, 650, 1990.
125. **Pagenkopf, C. W., Bourreau, J.-P., and Challice, C. E.,** Changes in prejunctional potency of B-HT 933 during aging in the rat vas deferens, *Clin. Exp. Pharmacol. Physiol.*, 17, 557, 1990.
126. **Gurdal, H., Friedman, E., and Johnson, M. D.,** Effects of dietary restriction on the change in aortic a1-adrenoceptor mediated responses during aging in Fischer 344 rats, *J. Gerontol.*, 50A, B67, 1995.
127. **Gee, M. V., Ishikawa, Y., Baum, B. J., and Roth, G. S.,** Impaired adrenergic stimulation of rat parotid cell glucose oxidation during aging: the role of calcium, *J. Gerontol.*, 41, 331, 1986.
128. **Ishikawa, Y., Gee, M. V., Baum, B. J., and Roth, G. S.,** Decreased signal transduction in rat parotid cell aggregates during aging is not due to loss of alpha-1 adrenergic receptors, *Exp. Gerontol.*, 24, 25, 1989.
129. **Scott, P. J. W. and Reid, J. L.,** The effect of age on the response of human isolated arteries to noradrenaline, *Br. J. Clin. Pharmacol.*, 13, 237, 1982.
130. **Stevens, M. J., Lipe, S., and Moulds, R. F. W.,** The effects of age on the response of human isolated arteries and veins to noradrenaline, *Br. J. Clin. Pharmacol.*, 14, 750, 1982.
131. **Supiano, M. A., Hogikyan, R. V., Stolz, A. M., Orstan, N., and Halter, J. B.,** Regulation of venous α-adrenergic responses in older humans, *Am. J. Physiol.*, 260, E599, 1991.
132. **McDonald, A., MacDonald, E., Fulton, J. D., Wadsworth, R. M., Scott, P. J. W., and Howie, K. A.,** No evidence for a general change in contractile responsiveness of the mesenteric artery with aging, *J. Gerontol.*, 50A, B20, 1995.
133. **Docherty, J. R.,** Effects of ageing on contractions to noradrenaline and 5-HT in human saphenous vein, *Br. J. Pharmacol.*, 105, 305P, 1992.
134. **Miyamoto, A., Villalobos-Molina, R., Kowatch, M. A., and Roth, G. S.,** Altered coupling of alpha 1-adrenergic receptor-G protein in rat parotid during aging, *Am. J. Physiol.*, 262, C1181, 1992.
135. **Supiano, M. A. and Hogikyan, R. V.,** High affinity platelet a$_2$-adrenergic receptor density is decreased in older humans, *J. Gerontol. Biol. Sci.*, 48, B173, 1993.

Chapter 3

CHOLINERGIC REGULATION OF HEART FUNCTION IN AGING

Njanoor Narayanan

CONTENTS

I. ABSTRACT

Cardiac performance is determined by the integrated function of multiple interdependent variables including heart rate, contractility, coronary flow, preload, and afterload, all of which are subject to regulation by the adrenergic and cholinergic divisions of the autonomic nervous system. There exists an impressive body of evidence showing that the adrenergic control of heart function declines with aging in humans and animals due, in part, to impaired β-adrenergic signal transduction at the postsynaptic level. On the other hand, information about the impact of aging on cholinergic control of heart function is scanty, and limited *in vivo* studies have produced conflicting results. Interestingly, recent studies utilizing isolated perfused whole heart, ventricular myocardium, and atrial tissue preparations from rats have demonstrated a striking enhancement of the negative chronotropic, negative inotropic, and coronary vasoconstriction responses of the aging heart to postsynaptic cholinergic stimulation. The mechanisms underlying the age-associated exaggeration of myocardial cholinergic

0-8493-8306-4/96/$0.00+$.50

responses are only beginning to be explored. Available evidence suggests that an age-associated decrease in acetylcholinesterase activity in atria and ventricles as well as age-related alterations in muscarinic receptor-linked signal transduction processes may underlie the cholinergic hyper-responsiveness of the aging heart. Data from electrophysiological studies have shown that muscarinic receptor activation results in greater hyperpolarization of the membrane potential in atria from aged animals, presumably due to greater muscarinic activation of K^+ channels (I_{KACh}). If such an age-related difference involves the sinoatrial node, this would result in depression of pacemaker activity, leading to enhanced bradycardic response to cholinergic stimulus with aging. Muscarinic receptor stimulation also results in greater shortening of action potential duration (APD_{50}) in aged heart ventricle; this may compromise trans-sarcolemmal Ca^{2+} influx and, consequently, intracellular Ca^{2+} mobilization for myofilament activation, thus contributing to the greater negative inotropic response to cholinergic stimulation in aging. The mechanisms underlying the age-associated increase in coronary vasoconstriction response to cholinergic stimulus are not known, but it does not appear to be due to age-related decrement in the rate of synthesis of endothelium-derived relaxing factor (EDRF) or diminished responsiveness of the coronary vascular smooth muscle to EDRF. Whether or not the hyper-responses of the myocardium to cholinergic agonists observed in the aging rat model is applicable to humans is uncertain. However, these observations suggest need for caution in the therapeutic use of cholinomimetics in the elderly so as to guard against the occurrence of exaggerated bradycardia and coronary spasm.

The ability of cholinergic agonists to attenuate β-adrenergic stimulation of adenylate cyclase activity decreases with aging in the rat model, suggesting an age-associated diminution in adrenergic-cholinergic interactions in the heart. This may be a protective adaptation occurring in the face of diminished adrenergic control of the aging heart.

II. INTRODUCTION

The autonomic nervous system exerts profound control on heart function. The sympathetic nerves innervating the heart release norepinephrine, which in turn produces increases in heart rate, contractile force, and cardiac output through activation of adrenergic (mainly β-adrenergic and to some extent α-adrenergic) receptor-linked pathways.[1–8] On the other hand, the parasympathetic nerves innervating the heart release acetylcholine, which in turn produces decrements in heart rate, contractile force, and cardiac output through activation of muscarinic receptor-linked pathways.[1–4,7–9] Additionally, muscarinic receptor activation leads to attenuation of the β-adrenergic responses of the heart.[2,7,10] Thus, the integrated and coordinated control of heart function by both the adrenergic and cholinergic divisions of the autonomic nervous system is central to the maintenance of circulatory homeostasis.

A large body of evidence from studies in intact organisms and in cardiovascular tissues, cells, and subcellular organelles isolated from animals indicates that β-adrenergic modulation of cardiovascular function diminishes with postmaturational aging in humans and animals.[11–15] To a considerable extent, this age-associated change appears to be due to a reduction in the cardiovascular target organ response to the β-adrenergic stimulation. The cellular mechanisms underlying the age-associated deficit in cardiac response to β-adrenergic stimulation may include diminished agonist binding affinity of β-adrenergic receptors,[11,12,16,17] decreased activity of G_s protein[11,12,16,17] and adenylate cyclase catalytic subunit,[18,19] as well as selective changes in the phosphorylation of target proteins by cAMP-dependent protein kinase and their dephosphorylation by protein phosphatases.[11–17,20–22] Studies on the impact of aging on α-adrenergic and cholinergic modulation of cardiovascular function have been much less extensive. The effects of age on α-adrenergic receptors and responsiveness may vary, depending on the receptor subtype (α_1 or α_2) and target tissue (artery, vein, cardiac muscle) involved.[14,15,23] The current general view appears to be that in contrast to the age-related decline in β-adrenergic responses of the heart and vasculature, the α-adrenergic-mediated vasoconstriction is not compromised with aging, at least in humans.[14,15,23] On the other hand, age-related decrease in α-receptor density[24,25] and reduced contractile response to α-adrenergic stimulation[26] have been observed in rat cardiac tissue. In this chapter I will review the evidence suggesting changes in cholinergic regulation of cardiovascular function with aging. The review will be confined to alterations during postmaturational aging (as opposed to developmental changes) and will focus primarily on age-related changes in the responses of the heart and coronary vasculature to cholinergic agonists as well as the mechanisms underlying the age-related changes. The latter will take into account the influence of aging on acetylcholine biosynthesis and degradation, cholinergic signal transduction mechanisms, and adrenergic-cholinergic interactions in the heart, and the pathophysiological implications of age-associated changes will be indicated.

III. AGE-RELATED CHANGES IN CARDIOVASCULAR RESPONSES TO CHOLINERGIC STIMULATION IN INTACT ORGANISMS

In vivo studies have indicated alterations in cholinergic control of cardiovascular function with aging, but the evidence is conflicting. One study reported that the negative chronotropic responses of the heart to vagal stimulation and administration of cholinergic agonists are reduced in aged rats compared to adult rats.[27] The positive chronotropic response which normally follows vagotomy or blockade of muscarinic receptors with atropine has been reported to be minimal or absent in aged rats, also suggesting age-associated reduction in cholinergic control.[27] In contrast, another study reported markedly larger bradycardia in the aged compared with young rats in response to vagal stimulation and intravenous injections of acetylcholine.[28] In another *in vivo* study using rats and rabbits, the age-related change in hemodynamic responses to acetylcholine was found to be dose dependent. Thus, a low dose (0.05 μg/kg) of acetylcholine was found to produce a greater decline in cardiac output and blood pressure in the aged compared with adult animals, but, at a higher dose (2 μg/kg), the magnitude of hemodynamic responses was lower in the aged compared with adult animals.[29] Data obtained in human studies have shown that aging is accompanied by an attenuation of the tachycardia induced by muscarinic receptor blockade with atropine,[30] of the bradycardia induced by baroreceptor stimulation,[31] and of spontaneous heart rate variability.[32] These observations are consistent with the possibility that a reduction in parasympathetic tone with aging may contribute, in part, to a decrease in heart rate variability at rest or in response to a postural stress in older humans.

The reasons for the conflicting evidence from *in vivo* studies regarding cholinergic modulation of cardiovascular function are not clear. Assessment of age-related changes in cardiovascular responses to experimental interventions in intact organisms is complicated by the interplay of multiple interdependent factors controlling cardiovascular performance *in vivo*. The various factors (e.g., heart rate, intrinsic myocardial contractility, preload, afterload, coronary flow, and properties of the arterial and venous vasculature) influencing cardiovascular performance *in vivo* are in turn subject to modulation by the autonomic nervous system.[13,14] With aging, nonuniform changes may occur in the various factors governing cardiovascular performance, and the direction and magnitude of age-related changes may differ at the level of the nervous system components (afferent, efferent, and central) of the cholinergic regulatory pathway and the target organs, namely, the heart and vascular tissues. While a number of studies have described age-related changes in the biosynthesis and degradation of acetylcholine (implying age-related changes at the presynaptic level), only recently have some efforts been made to delineate age-related changes in the postsynaptic components of the cholinergic control system. The following sections of this review will address the current state of knowledge regarding age-related changes in the cholinergic responses of the heart and coronary vasculature and the cellular mechanisms underlying the age-related changes.

IV. POSTSYNAPTIC CHOLINERGIC RESPONSES OF THE HEART IN AGING

The impact of aging on the responsiveness of the heart to cholinergic stimulation was assessed in a recent study which utilized isolated perfused heart preparations from adult (6 to 8 months) and aged (28 to 30 months) Fischer 344 rats.[33] The results of this study demonstrated that in isolated perfused spontaneously beating hearts, the negative chronotropic response to acetylcholine (10^{-9} to 10^{-5} M) was up to fourfold greater in the aged compared with adult hearts; this age-related difference was less marked (twofold), but not abolished in the presence of a maximally effective concentration of the cholinesterase inhibitor, eserine. The cholinesterase-resistant agonist carbachol (10^{-9} to 2.5×10^{-6} *M*) also elicited a two- to threefold greater negative chronotropic response in the aged compared with adult hearts (Figure 3.1). Taken together, these findings suggest that the age-related increase in cholinergic responsiveness cannot be attributed exclusively to an age-related decline in acetylcholinesterase activity in the myocardium (see Section V below). An age-related increase in negative chronotropic response to acetylcholine has also been observed in another study which utilized isolated right atrial preparations from adult and aged rats.[34] In this case, however, the age-related difference was abolished upon pretreatment of the tissue with an irreversible inhibitor of acetylcholinesterase.[34]

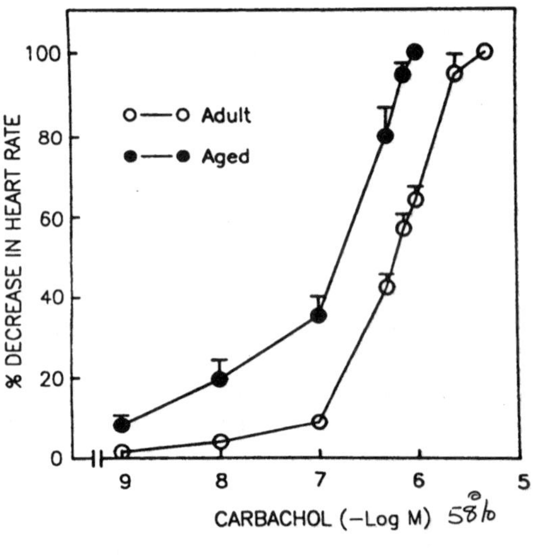

FIGURE 3.1. Negative chronotropic response of isolated perfused spontaneously beating adult (6 to 8 months) and aged (28 to 30 months) rat hearts to carbachol. (From Su, N. and Narayanan, N., *Can. J. Physiol. Pharmacol.*, 70, 1618, 1992. With permission.)

The effect of aging on the inotropic response of the heart to cholinergic stimulation has been determined in isolated heart preparations.[33] In isolated perfused hearts paced electrically (4 Hz), carbachol (10^{-9} to 10^{-5}) elicited a concentration-dependent negative inotropic response, which was twofold greater in the aged compared with adult; both maximal response and sensitivity to carbachol were greater in the aged (Figure 3.2). Thus, the data from studies utilizing isolated perfused beating hearts[33] and atrial tissue preparations[34] have provided direct evidence of a striking age-associated enhancement in the chronotropic and inotropic responses of the heart to cholinergic agonists. This age-associated exaggeration of the cholinergic responses of the heart at the postsynaptic level contrasts with the well-recognized decline in the β-adrenergic responses of the heart in aging.

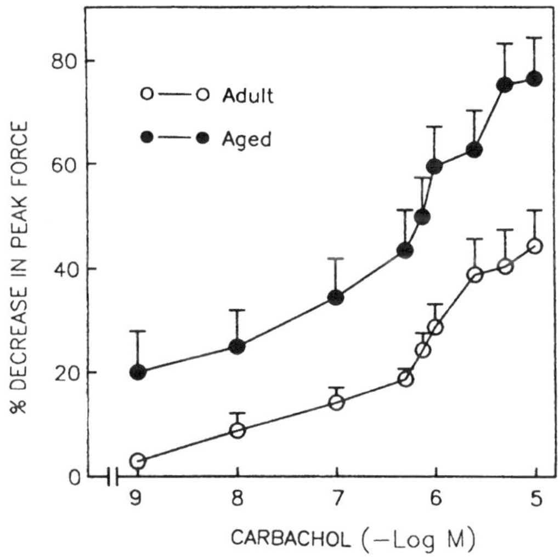

FIGURE 3.2. Negative inotropic response of isolated perfused, electrically paced (240 beats per minute) adult (6 to 8 months) and aged (28 to 30 months) rat hearts to carbachol. (From Su, N. and Narayanan, N., *Can. J. Physiol. Pharmacol.*, 70, 1618, 1992. With permission.).

V. BIOSYNTHESIS AND DEGRADATION OF ACETYLCHOLINE WITH AGING

Age-related changes in the synthesis of acetylcholine in cholinergic neurons as well as in the degradation of acetylcholine upon its release into the synaptic junction can contribute to age-related alterations in target organ responses to this neurotransmitter. The activity of choline acetyltransferase, the enzyme which catalyzes the synthesis of acetylcholine from acetyl-CoA and choline, has been found to be reduced in hearts from aged rats (24 to 26 months) when compared with that from young (1 month) or adult (8 to 10 months) rats.[35,36] This age-related decline in enzyme activity was more pronounced in the atrial compared to the ventricular tissue. In the rat, age-related decrease in the activity of choline acetyltransferase has also been described in neural tissues, including various areas of the brain (striatum, hippocampus, and cerebral cortex) and in the peripheral nervous system.[36,37] Overall, these data suggest that acetylcholine biosynthesis in the central and peripheral synapses may become less intense in old age. Such an age-related change can be expected to result in attenuation or exhaustion of the neurotransmitter release during prolonged cholinergic stimulation.

The effect of acetylcholine released into the synaptic cleft is terminated mainly by the action of the enzyme acetylcholinesterase, which hydrolyzes acetylcholine into choline and acetate. The enzyme is localized on the presynaptic membrane as well as the postsynaptic membrane. Several studies have reported substantial decline in the activity of acetylcholinesterase in atria and ventricles of aged compared with adult rats.[26,36,38–40] Decreased activity of this enzyme would increase the effective synaptic concentration of acetylcholine (released by cholinergic nerves or administered exogenously in experiments performed *in vivo*); this may explain, in part, the enhanced bradycardic response to acetylcholine observed in experiments performed *in vivo*[28] and *in vitro*.[33,34] Certain observations made in studies using isolated perfused heart preparations also suggest that the enhanced negative chronotropic and inotropic responses of the aging heart to cholinergic agonists cannot be attributed exclusively to age-associated decline in acetylcholinesterase activity. For example, (1) at a maximally effective concentration of the cholinesterase inhibitor eserine, significant age-related differences in the chronotropic response to acetylcholine persisted and (2) marked age-related differences could be observed in the chronotropic and inotropic responses to carbachol, a cholinesterase-resistant cholinergic agonist.[33] Thus, it is likely that age-associated alterations at the level of postsynaptic effectors for cholinergic agonists also contribute to the cholinergic hyper-responses of the aging heart.

VI. CHOLINERGIC SIGNAL TRANSDUCTION IN THE AGING HEART

Cholinergic effects on the heart are mediated through muscarinic-cholinergic receptors. As is generally the case with hormone and neurotransmitter receptors, muscarinic receptors are coupled to guanosine 5′-triphosphate (GTP)-binding proteins (G proteins) which, in turn, interact with cellular effectors to produce physiological responses.[1–4,41] In the heart, muscarinic receptors are known to be coupled to multiple cellular effectors. Thus, binding of acetylcholine (or other cholinergic agonists) to the cardiac muscarinic receptors and consequent activation of receptor-G protein-linked pathways (Figure 3.3) lead to (a) increase in K^+ conductance (I_{KACh}) and efflux of K^+ and resultant hyperpolarization,[1–4, 7, 42–45] (b) inhibition of slow L-type Ca^{2+} current ($I_{Ca}L$) limiting trans-sarcolemmal Ca^{2+} influx,[46–50] (c) inhibition of hyperpolarization-activated pacemaker current (I_f, slowly activating inward current carried by Na^+ and K^+ ions),[51–53] (d) inhibition of β-adrenergic-mediated increase in cellular cAMP level,[2,3,54–56] (e) increase in cellular cGMP level,[2,3,57] and (f) increase in the hydrolysis of phosphoinositide.[2,3,58] The precise relationships of all of these pathways to negative chronotropic and inotropic responses of the heart to muscarinic receptor activation are not yet clearly understood. Also, important differences exist in the functional responsiveness of atrial and ventricular myocardium to muscarinic-cholinergic stimulation[2,3] and, therefore, it is likely that some, but not all, of these signal transduction pathways are shared by atrial and ventricular tissues.[2,3] It is generally thought that muscarinic activation of I_{KACh} and inhibition of I_f and $I_{Ca(L)}$ at the level of pacemaker cells of the sinoatrial node contribute to the inhibition of heart rate. The inhibition of contractile force may involve inhibition of the rise in cytosolic Ca^{2+} upon excitation either due to direct effect on ion channels (e.g., inhibition of $I_{Ca(L)}$) or through second messenger-mediated processes (e.g., inhibition of $I_{Ca(L)}$ through cGMP-mediated phosphorylation of Ca^{2+} channel compare References 59 and 60). Conceivably, age-related changes at the level of muscarinic receptors, G proteins, and their effectors as well as alterations in the functional interactions between these macromolecular components can contribute to the cholinergic hyper-responses of the aging heart. To date, only a few studies have examined the effect of postmaturational aging on the postsynaptic cholinergic signal transduction processes in the heart. The available data from biochemical and electrophysiological studies in this regard are reviewed in the following sections.

A. MUSCARINIC RECEPTORS

Pharmacological and molecular cloning studies have demonstrated that muscarinic-cholinergic receptors comprise at least five genetically distinct subtypes (M_1 to M_5) that are characterized by different structure, tissue distribution, and functional properties.[41,61–63] Major responses to muscarinic receptor agonists in cardiac muscle appear to be mediated by a well-characterized M_2 muscarinic receptor that may couple to different signal transduction pathways.[2–4,41,45] The possibility that altered cholinergic responses of the heart in aging may be associated with age-related changes in the number of myocardial muscarinic receptors and (or) their functional properties has been investigated in some studies. In a study using Sprague-Dawley rats, a significant (24%) increase in muscarinic receptor density was observed in aged (24 to 25 months) atria compared with adult (7 to 8 months) atria, while no age-related change was seen in receptor density in the ventricles or in agonist or antagonist binding affinities of atrial and ventricular receptors.[64] Another study using Fischer 344 (F-344) rats reported no age-related difference in muscarinic receptor density in atria and ventricles, but

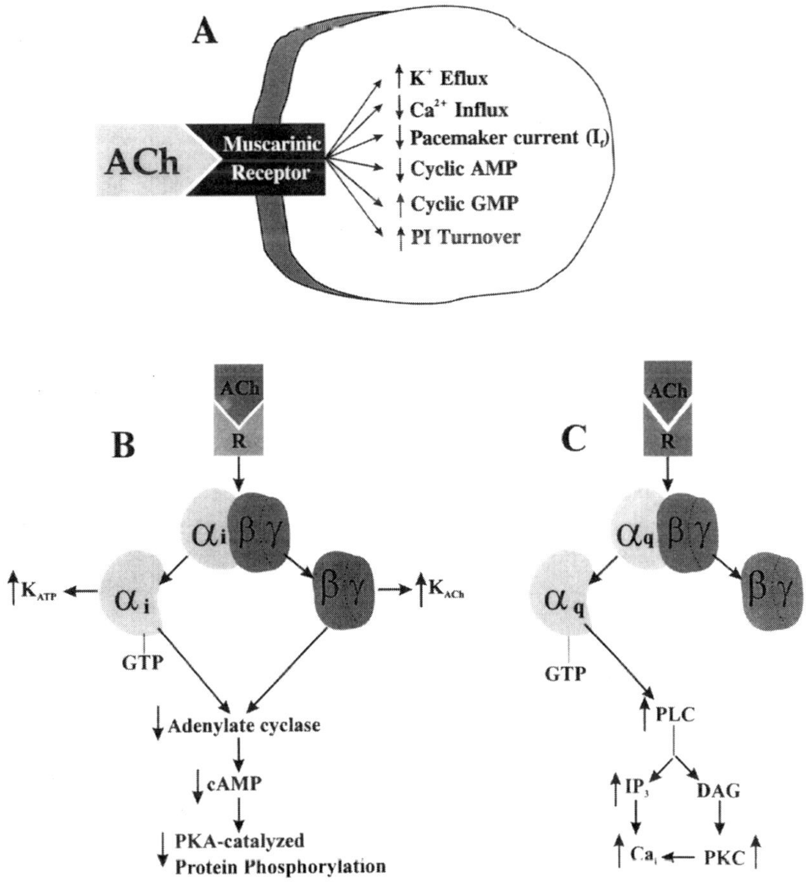

FIGURE 3.3. Schematic representation of the cellular responses to cholinergic stimulation of cardiac muscarinic receptors. Acetylcholine (ACh) released from parasympathetic nerve endings stimulates postjunctional muscarinic receptors to elicit multiple cellular responses which include enhancement of potassium efflux, cGMP production, and phosphatidylinositol (PI) breakdown as well as inhibition of calcium influx, pacemaker current (I_f), and cAMP production (A). The muscarinic receptor (R) is coupled to multiple effector pathways through heterotrimeric G proteins composed of α, β, and γ subunits which dissociate into the GTP-bound form of the α subunit (α_{GTP}) and $\beta\gamma$ upon receptor activation. Either of these subunits of the G protein may regulate effectors. Muscarinic activation of K^+ channels and inhibition of adenylate cyclase are mediated through a pertussis toxin-sensitive G protein, G_i (B). There has been controversy regarding the G protein subunit (α or $\beta\gamma$) mediating muscarinic activation of the K_{ACh} channel, but it now appears that the $\beta\gamma$ subunit is the physiological effector of K_{ACh}, whereas the α subunit may serve to stimulate another type of K^+ channel, the ATP-sensitive K^+ (K_{ATP}) channel.[3] Both α and $\beta\gamma$ subunits have been implicated in the muscarinic inhibition of adenylate cyclase[3,138] which results in decreased cAMP production and consequently diminished phosphorylation of cellular proteins by protein kinase A (PKA). A pertussis toxin-insensitive G protein (G_q) couples the muscarinic receptor to phospholipase C (PLC). Muscarinic stimulation of this pathway results in the formation of second messengers inositol 1,4,5-triphosphate (IP_3) and diacylglycerol (DAG), which enhance intracellular Ca^{2+} (Ca_i) levels. IP_3 releases Ca^{2+} from sarcoplasmic reticulum and DAG stimulates protein kinase (PKC) which may also serve to enhance Ca_i through protein phosphorylation.[3] Stimulation of muscarinic receptor is also associated with activation of guanylate cyclase and increase in cGMP production; the mechanisms underlying this pathway and its physiological implications are not yet clear.

noted an age-associated enhancement in the agonist (carbachol) binding affinity of atrial (but not ventricular) muscarinic receptors.[33] Other studies using ventricular tissue from Wistar rats have reported conflicting findings, and these include no age-related changes in receptor density,[65] decrease in receptor density,[66] and decrease in agonist binding affinity of the receptor;[65] these studies[65,66] did not examine the effect of aging on atrial muscarinic receptors. The reasons for the above disparate observations are not clear, and at present no definitive conclusions regarding age-related changes at the level of myocardial muscarinic receptors and their contribution to altered cholinergic responses of the heart can be made. Nevertheless, the age-associated enhancement in muscarinic receptor density in atria[64] and agonist binding affinity of atrial muscarinic receptors[33] observed in some studies seems to correlate with the enhanced negative chronotropic response of the aging heart to cholinergic agonists.[28,33,34]

B. POSTRECEPTOR SIGNAL TRANSDUCTION MECHANISMS

In the heart, the muscarinic receptors are coupled to multiple effectors via guanine nucleotide binding proteins (G proteins) which serve as signal transducers to bring about cellular physiological responses to muscarinic receptor stimulation.[2–4,41,67,68] There exists considerable heterogeneity among G proteins,[41,68,69] and at least four types of G proteins have been identified in cardiac tissue.[70] These include (i) G_s which mediates β-adrenergic-stimulated cAMP production and modulates the activity of voltage-dependent ion channels;[2,3,41,70] (ii) G_i, which mediates muscarinic activation of K^+ (I_{KACh}) channels[2–4,67,68] and inhibition of β-adrenergic-stimulated adenylate cyclase activity (and hence decrease in cAMP production) by muscarinic cholinergic, α-adrenergic, and adenosine A_1-receptor agonists;[2,3,71] (iii) G_o, the function of which is not yet clear, but may be involved in muscarinic inhibition of adenylate cyclase and pacemaker current;[3,4] and (iv) G_q, which is involved in muscarinic and α-adrenergic stimulation of phospholipase C[72] and phospholipase A_2.[73] Each G protein is a heterotrimer composed of G_α, G_β, and G_γ subunits.[69] The G_α subunit contains the binding site for guanine nucleotides and a specific GTP-hydrolyzing enzyme (GTPase). G_α interacts reversibly with its respective receptor and confers specificity to the holoprotein by virtue of α-subunit structural heterogeneity relative to the more homogeneous structures of β- and γ-subunits.[69] Another characteristic of the G_α subunit is its ability to undergo nicotinamide adenine dinucleotide-dependent ADP-ribosylation by bacterial toxins. Thus, $G_{s\alpha}$ undergoes ADP-ribosylation by choleratoxin, whereas $G_{i\alpha}$ and $G_{o\alpha}$ are ADP-ribosylated by pertussis toxin; G_q appears not to be ADP-ribosylated by either toxin. ADP-ribosylation of $G_{s\alpha}$ inhibits GTPase activity, thus irreversibly activating the subunit to stimulate adenylate cyclase and ion channels.[74] ADP-ribosylation of $G_{i\alpha}$ and $G_{o\alpha}$ inhibits the interaction between subunits and receptors.[74] These functional modifications make ADP-ribosylation a means for detecting, quantifying, and localizing G proteins. The G_i, G_o, and G_q proteins appear to be the major G proteins involved in muscarinic signal transduction in the heart.

In the process of signal transduction, the G proteins undergo a regulatory cycle triggered by agonist occupation of the receptor.[69] The agonist-receptor complex interacts with the guanosine 5′-diphosphate (GDP)-bound form of the G protein which in turn binds GTP through a GDP-GTP exchange reaction to form $G_{\alpha\text{-GTP}.\beta\gamma}$. The binding of GTP to the heterotrimeric G protein results in dissociation of its subunits (G_α-GTP and $G_{\beta\gamma}$) as well as the agonist-receptor complex. Either of the dissociated G protein subunits ($G_{\alpha\text{-GTP}}$ and $G_{\beta\gamma}$) may regulate effectors through generation of second messengers (e.g., cAMP, cGMP, inositol 1,4,5-triphosphate [IP_3], diacylglycerol) or through direct interaction with effectors (e.g., ion channels)[2–4,41,67,68,70] (see Figure 3.3). Termination of the cycle occurs with the hydrolysis of GTP to GDP and reassociation of $G_{\alpha\text{-GDP}}$ with $G_{\beta\gamma}$ to form the inactive complex.

In addition to changes at the level of muscarinic receptors, age-related alterations in the signal transduction process due to changes in the amount and/or function of G proteins and their effectors can result in altered physiological responses. To date, only a few studies have examined the effects of aging on postreceptor muscarinic signal transduction processes in the heart. One study compared the expression of $G_{i\alpha}$ subunits in atria and ventricles of adult (6 to 8 months) and aged (28 to 30 months) Fischer 344 rats using Western immunoblotting and ADP-ribosylation techniques. It was found that the steady-state levels of $G_{i\alpha}$ were ~two-fold greater in total particulate fractions (40,000 × *g* pellets) of both atria and ventricles from the aged compared to adult rats.[75a] Another study in Fischer 344 rats, aged 6 and 24 months, showed no age-related differences in the amounts of $G_{s\alpha}$ and $G_{i\alpha}$ proteins in ventricular particulate fractions (27,000 × g pellet) as determined by Western immunoblotting analysis.[76] The latter study did not examine the effect of aging on atrial G proteins. The difference in the nature of particulate membrane fractions (total vs. heavy particulate fractions) used in the two studies may have contributed to the disparate observations regarding the effect of aging on $G_{i\alpha}$ content in the ventricle. It is worth noting here that increased expression of $G_{i\alpha}$ has been documented in hypothyroid rat heart[77] and failing human[78–80] and hamster[81] hearts. Further, in some studies, increased expression of $G_{i\alpha}$ has been correlated with enhanced negative inotropic response of the heart to cholinergic agonists.[82–84] Such findings strengthen the possibility that increased amounts of $G_{i\alpha}$ protein in aged atria and ventricles may contribute to age-related enhancement in the negative chronotropic and inotropic responses of the heart to cholinergic agonists.

As noted earlier, in the process of signal transduction, the binding of GTP to the G_α subunit of the G protein not only leads to dissociation of the G protein subunits, but also dissociation of the agonist-receptor complex; the latter event is apparently due to a decrease in receptor affinity for agonist, induced by the binding of GTP to G_α. Therefore, the functional interactions between agonist-receptor complexes and G proteins can be monitored experimentally by determining the ability of guanine nucleotides to induce a decrement in receptor affinity for agonists. In experiments performed using atrial and ventricular membranes from adult and aged rat hearts, guanine nucleotides [GTP and its hydrolysis-resistant analogue, Gpp(NH)p] were found to produce pronounced decrements in muscarinic receptor affinity for the agonist carbachol.[75a] No age-related difference was seen in the magnitude of guanine nucleotide-mediated shift in receptor affinity for agonist, showing that this signal transduction step is not altered with aging.

Biochemical studies examining age-related changes in cellular effectors for muscarinic signal transduction in the heart are very few. Significantly greater increases in cGMP in response to submaximal doses of acetylcholine have been observed in aged (24 to 26 months) compared to adult (6 to 8 months) rat hearts.[85] This difference persisted in the presence of acetylcholinesterase blockade, suggesting that the mechanisms of the age-associated difference were at or distal to the muscarinic receptor. It remains to be determined whether aging is accompanied by alterations in the content and/or activities of guanylate cyclase, or cGMP-phosphodiesterases in the heart. Decreased activity of the catalytic unit of adenylate cyclase has been observed in studies using ventricular membranes from aged rat hearts compared to adult rat hearts,[18,19,76] and decrements in both G_s protein activity as well as adenylate cyclase activity have been implicated in the age-related decline in β-adrenergic signal transduction in the heart.[11–15] Also, the ability of the muscarinic agonist, carbachol, to inhibit β-adrenergic-mediated activation of adenylate cyclase was found to be significantly reduced with aging in the rat heart suggesting that, postsynaptically, the antiadrenergic action of cholinergic stimulus (mediated via G_i protein) declines with aging.[86] As yet, no information is available regarding the effect of postmaturational aging on the muscarinic receptor-G_q protein-linked phosphoinositide pathway. Muscarinic effects directed through this pathway appear to be positively inotropic,[2,3,70,72] which is in contrast to the predominant negative inotropic effect that usually results from muscarinic receptor stimulation. The physiological significance of the muscarinic-phosphoinositide pathway is not yet clear.[2,3,70]

C. ELECTROPHYSIOLOGICAL RESPONSES

Insights into the likely mechanisms underlying the postsynaptic cholinergic hyper-responses of the heart have also been provided by a recent study which examined the electrophysiological basis of this phenomenon. This study[75] determined the effects of muscarinic receptor stimulation by carbachol on transmembrane action potential parameters in right atrial tissue and right ventricular free wall preparations from adult (6 to 8 months) and aged (26 to 28 months) F-344 rats. In addition, the effect of carbachol on atrioventricular conduction time (AVT) was assessed in isolated perfused beating hearts from both age groups. The results showed that, under basal conditions (i.e., in the absence of carbachol), myocardial aging is associated with (a) partial depolarization of the maximum diastolic potential (MDP) in the atrium, but not ventricle; (b) increase in AVT; and (c) prolongation of APD in the ventricle.[75] An age-associated prolongation of ventricular APD in the absence of age-related change in MDP has also been observed in other studies using rat cardiac muscle preparations including right ventricle,[87] left ventricle,[88] papillary muscle, and left ventricular myocytes.[89] Also, an age-associated increase in AVT has been observed in humans.[90] The mechanisms underlying these age-related electrophysiological alterations (seen under basal conditions) are not well understood at present. Presumably, significant alterations occur in ionic homeostasis of the myocardial fibers with aging contributing to changes in electrophysiological properties. Evidence from recent studies suggests that decrements in (a) the rate of inactivation of Ca^{2+} current[89] and the magnitude of outward directed K^+ current (I_{to})[89] contribute to the prolonged APD in the ventricle. Cytosolic Ca^{2+} (Ca^{2+}_i) transient has been shown to modulate action potential in rat ventricular myocytes[91] and Ca_i transient is prolonged with aging in the rat heart.[92] Therefore, the prolongation of ventricular APD with aging may also relate to a prolonged Ca_i transient. In both adult and aged hearts, the major electrophysiological responses to muscarinic receptor stimulation included (1) hyperpolarization of MDP (in atria), (2) shortening of APD, and (3) increase in AVT.[75] Interestingly, certain of these electrophysiological responses to muscarinic receptor stimulation were found to be selectively and significantly modified with aging. Thus, the results revealed that in the rat model studied, aging is accompanied by (1) enhancement in carbachol-induced hyperpolarization of MDP in atria (Figure 3.4), (2) more pronounced carbachol-induced shortening of APD (particularly APD_{50}) in the ventricle (Figure 3.5), and (3) unaltered negative dromotropic response to carbachol (Figure 3.6). The age-associated enhancement in carbachol-induced hyperpolarization in atria may be due to a greater increase in I_{KACh} in the aged atria, since the key mechanism for hyperpolarization of MDP is the activation of I_{KACh} through stimulation of muscarinic receptors in the atria.[7,42,47,93,94] This action of muscarinic agonists may result in depression of excitability and pacemaker activity at the sinoatrial node. Therefore, the greater bradycardic response of the aged compared to adult heart to carbachol appears to be linked to an aged-associated difference in muscarinic modulation of I_{KACh}.

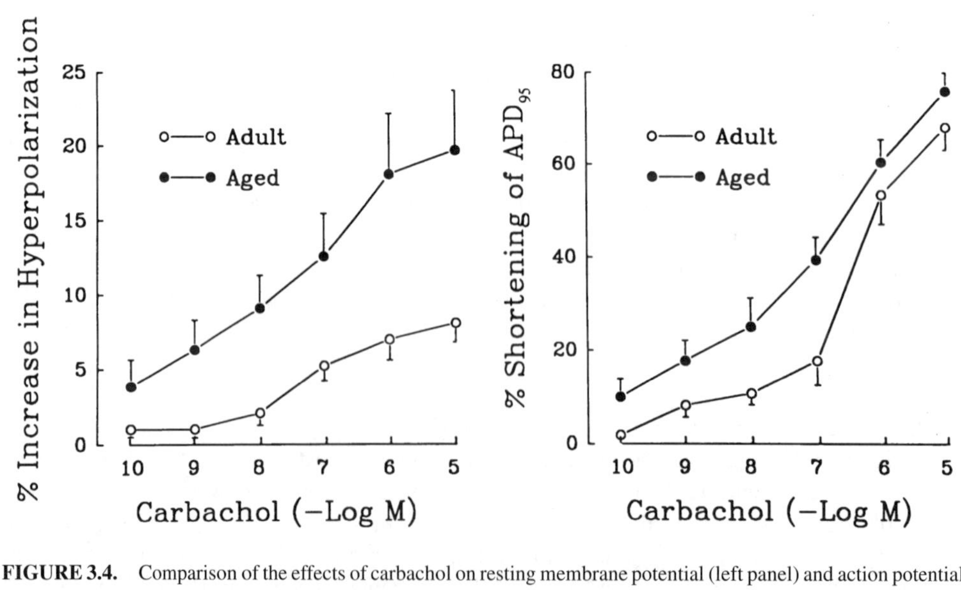

FIGURE 3.4. Comparison of the effects of carbachol on resting membrane potential (left panel) and action potential duration (right panel) in atria from adult (6 to 8 months) and aged (28 to 30 months) rats. The age-related difference in membrane hyperpolarization (but not APD_{95}) is significant at all carbachol concentrations. (From Su, N., Duan, J., Moffat, M. P., and Narayanan, N., *Can. J. Physiol. Pharmacol.*, 73, 1430, 1995. With permission.)

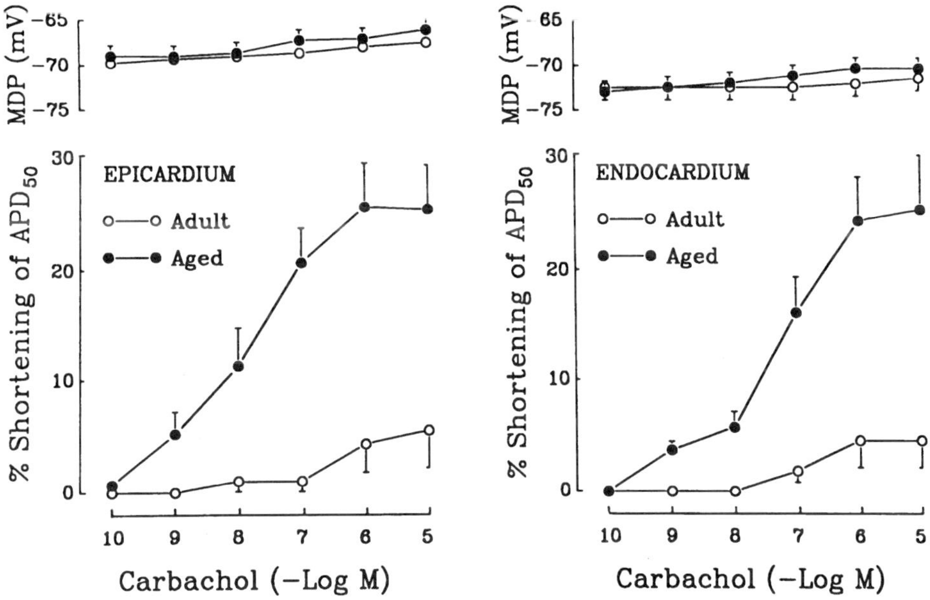

FIGURE 3.5. Comparison of the effects of carbachol on maximum diastolic potential (MDP) and action potential duration measured at 50% repolarization (APD_{50}) in ventricular epicardium (left panel) and endocardium (right panel) from adult (6 to 8 months) and aged (28 to 30 months) rats. Carbachol had no significant effect on MDP in epicardium or endocardium. The carbachol-induced shortening of APD_{50} differed significantly with age in epicardium and endocardium. (From Su, N., Duan, J., Moffat, M. P., and Narayanan, N., *Can. J. Physiol. Pharmacol.*, 73, 1430, 1995. With permission.)

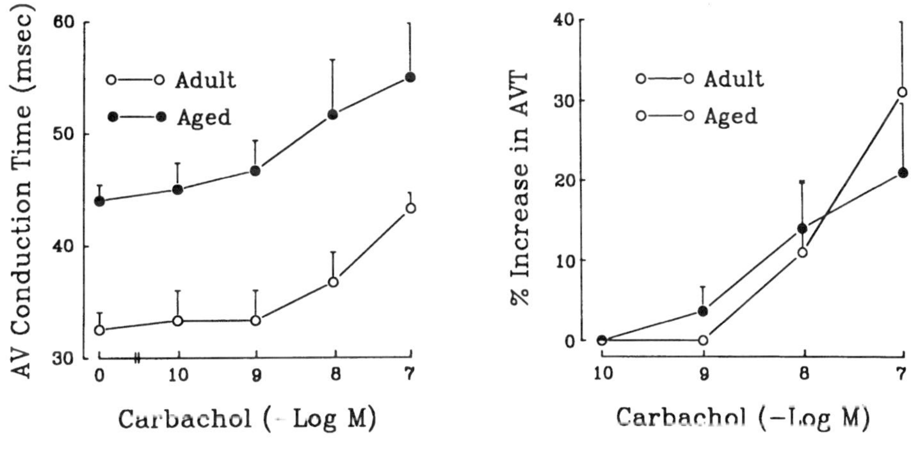

FIGURE 3.6. Comparison of the effect of carbachol on atrioventricular conduction time (AVT) in isolated perfused atrial-paced (240 beats per minute) hearts from adult (6 to 8 months) and aged (24 to 30 months) rats. Aging is associated with a significant increase in AVT (left panel). However, the magnitude of carbachol-induced increase in AVT does not differ significantly with aging. (From Su, N., Duan, J., Moffat, M. P., and Narayanan, N., *Can. J. Physiol. Pharmacol.*, 73, 1430, 1995. With permission.)

The observation that aging is associated with a more pronounced effect of carbachol on the shortening of APD_{50} in the ventricle has mechanistic relevance to the age-associated enhancement in the negative inotropic response of the heart to muscarinic receptor stimulation. The ionic basis of the shortening of APD_{50} by muscarinic agonists likely involves a reduction in $I_{Ca(L)}$[46–52] and, perhaps, activation of I_{KACh} as well.[95] Reduction in $I_{Ca(L)}$ and/or activation of I_{KACh} will shorten APD_{50}, thus shortening the plateau phase and diminishing Ca^{2+} influx during the action potential. This effect has been suggested to be responsible for the negative inotropic response of the heart to muscarinic-cholinergic stimulation.[46–50] Thus, age-related enhancement in carbachol-induced shortening of APD_{50} may have resulted from a more potent inhibition of $I_{Ca(L)}$ in the aged compared to adult ventricle, and this would contribute to the enhanced negative inotropic response of the aged heart to carbachol.[33] However, the precise ionic mechanisms for the age-related alterations in carbachol-induced hyperpolarization of MDP and shortening of APD need to be verified in further studies using voltage or patch clamp techniques.

VII. CORONARY VASCULAR RESPONSE TO CHOLINERGIC STIMULATION WITH AGING

Considerable evidence suggests that blood vessels are affected by the aging process, but the age-related changes may vary with specific vascular bed, type of vessel, and species.[96–100] Although age-related pathological changes have been reported to occur in coronary arteries in humans and experimental animals, a consistent pattern indicative of physiological aging has not been established. In the rat model, an age-related deficit in coronary vascular function has been suggested from structural studies showing decreased capillary density due to inadequate capillary growth in the face of excessive hypertrophic enlargement of myocyte compartment of the ventricle; there is also indirect evidence of subendocardial ischemia under stressful conditions.[101–104] While *in vitro* measurements did not show age-related changes in resting coronary blood flow,[104,105] recent evidence from *in vivo* measurements has revealed decrements in coronary blood flow as well as coronary vascular reserve and increments in coronary vascular resistance in aging rats.[106] Whether or not age-related changes in autonomic tone in coronary vasculature contribute to alterations in coronary vascular function parameters measured *in vivo* remains unclear.

Most of the published work on the impact of aging on vascular responses to autonomic stimulation has focused on age-related changes in responsiveness to adrenergic drugs in blood vessels isolated from various vascular beds and perfused organs. The data from these studies suggest that β-adrenergic-mediated vasodilation decreases with aging in various vascular beds, including coronary arteries.[14,99] The impact of aging on α-adrenergic-mediated vasoconstriction, however, is controversial, with studies showing an increase[107,108] a decrease,[109,110] or no change.[111,112] In isolated perfused rat hearts, no age-related difference was observed in α-receptor-mediated vasoconstriction in coronary vasculature.[112] In contrast, enhanced contractile response to α-receptor stimulation was observed in coronary arteries isolated from senescent compared to young beagles.[108] Very little is known about the influence of aging on vascular responses to cholinergic stimulation. Results from a recent study[112] showed (a) that the cholinergic agonist, carbachol, causes coronary vasoconstriction in isolated constant flow perfused rat heart and (b) that the maximum response and the sensitivity of coronary vasculature to carbachol are strikingly enhanced with aging (Figure 3.7). Based mainly on evidence from experiments performed on dogs,[113–117] it has long been assumed that cholinergic agonists are vasodilators of coronary arteries and that parasympathetic innervation of coronary vessels mediates vasodilation.[9,118] However, in recent years it has become clear that the dog is an exception, and in most species cholinergic stimulation in fact produces coronary vasoconstriction. Thus, isolated coronary arteries from most species, including human, sheep, pig, rabbit, and rat, contract in response to acetylcholine and other cholinergic agonists.[8,119] Furthermore, in isolated rat heart preparations perfused at constant pressure, electrical stimulation of the vagus nerve leads to decrease in coronary flow (due to coronary vasoconstriction), suggesting a functional parasympathetic innervation of the coronary arteries in this species.[120] The pressor response to carbachol observed in isolated, constant-flow perfused rat hearts[112] provides further confirmation of the vasoconstrictor action of cholinergic agonists in the coronary vasculature. Coronary vasodilation due to EDRF (which has been identified as nitric oxide)[121] has been reported in some studies.[122–124] In isolated perfused rat hearts, no significant age-related difference was observed in the degree of coronary vasoconstriction induced by the inhibition of EDRF synthesis, whereas the age-associated enhancement in carbachol-induced coronary vasoconstriction prevailed after blockade of EDRF synthesis.[112] Therefore, it is unlikely that impaired generation of EDRF by coronary endothelial cells or reduced sensitivity of vascular smooth muscle to EDRF contributes to the enhanced coronary vasoconstrictor effect of cholinergic stimulus in the aged rat heart.

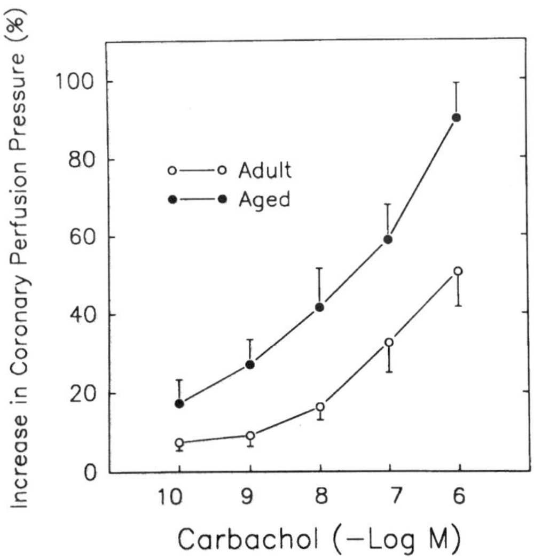

FIGURE 3.7. Comparison of the effects of carbachol on coronary perfusion pressure in isolated, constant flow perfused, electrically paced (250 beats per minute) hearts from adult (6 to 8 months) and aged (28 to 30 months) rats. Since the hearts were perfused in the constant flow mode, changes in coronary perfusion pressure reflect changes in coronary vascular resistance. The results show striking enhancement in carbachol-induced coronary vasoconstriction with aging. (From Su, N. and Narayanan, N., *Cardiovasc. Res.*, 27, 284, 1993. With permission.)

In isolated coronary arteries[8,119,125–128] and other blood vessels,[8,119,128–130] cholinergic agonists induce vasoconstriction by direct activation of muscarinic receptors (M_3 subtype), which are distinct from muscarinic receptors in cardiomyocytes (M_2 subtype). However, it has been suggested that in the intact beating heart cholinergic coronary vasoconstriction may also result indirectly from decrease in cardiac work owing to activation of the M_2 muscarinic receptors in cardiomyocytes.[125] The carbachol-induced coronary vasoconstriction in adult and aged rat hearts appears to result mainly, if not exclusively, from the activation of vascular muscarinic receptors, since the nonsubtype-selective muscarinic receptor antagonist atropine, but not the cardioselective muscarinic receptor antagonist AFDX-116, blocked this response.[112] Minimal involvement of carbachol-induced decrease in cardiac metabolism in the coronary vascular response to carbachol is also suggested by the observations that (a) carbachol-induced coronary vasoconstriction in spontaneously beating and electrically paced hearts was similar to that in potassium-arrested hearts, and (b) despite the greater negative chronotropic and inotropic effects of carbachol on aged compared to adult hearts, the age-related difference in coronary vascular response to carbachol could be observed in beating and nonbeating heart preparations.[112]

The postreceptor mechanisms governing cholinergic coronary vasoconstriction are not yet clearly understood. In earlier studies, vasoconstriction of coronary arteries by cholinergic agonists was reported to occur with membrane depolarization,[131] hyperpolarization,[132] or constant membrane potential.[133] This inconsistency of results has been attributed, in part, to the presence of endothelium in the multicellular tissue and it has been shown recently that in isolated coronary smooth muscle cells, acetylcholine induces hyperpolarization through stimulation of Ca^{2+}-activated potassium channels.[134] In any case, muscarinic receptor-mediated increase in intracellular Ca^{2+} is considered essential for the vasoconstrictor action and the hyperpolarizing effect of cholinergic agonists.[125,134] In isolated perfused rat hearts, the carbachol-induced coronary vasoconstriction was markedly attenuated by verapamil, a sarcolemmal Ca^{2+} channel antagonist, suggesting that a large component of the contractile Ca^{2+} mobilized by muscarinic receptor activation is derived via influx of extracellular Ca^{2+}.[112] However, since verapamil did not abolish the vasoconstrictor response to carbachol,[112] it is likely that muscarinic receptor activation also leads to Ca^{2+} mobilization from intracellular sources. Such a possibility is supported by the recent observation that in isolated coronary smooth muscle cells, acetylcholine augments Ca^{2+} release from sarcoplasmic reticulum,[134] apparently through activation of muscarinic receptor-linked phospholipase C and production of IP_3.[135] The mechanisms underlying the age-associated enhancement in coronary vasoconstriction in response to muscarinic receptor activation remain to be determined. In this regard, it is noteworthy that in rat hearts, attenuation of carbachol-induced coronary vasoconstriction by verapamil resulted in abolition of the age-related difference in pressor response.[112] This observation suggests that a relatively greater influx of extracellular Ca^{2+} upon muscarinic receptor activation in the aged compared to adult heart may be a factor contributing to the age-related enhancement in coronary vascular response to cholinergic stimulus.

VIII. ADRENERGIC-CHOLINERGIC INTERACTIONS IN THE AGING HEART

Pronounced interactions among the adrenergic and cholinergic limbs of the autonomic nervous system, occurring both peripherally and centrally, play an important role in the integration of the autonomic control of heart function.[10,136,137] In the periphery, acetylcholine released from the parasympathetic nerve endings produces antiadrenergic effects on the heart in addition to direct negative chronotropic and inotropic effects. The antiadrenergic action of acetylcholine involves both prejunctional and postjunctional mechanisms. Prejunctionally, interaction of acetylcholine with muscarinic receptors on postganglionic sympathetic terminals causes inhibition of norepinephrine release; postjunctionally, interaction of acetylcholine with cardiac muscarinic receptors causes inhibition of β-adrenergic activation of adenylate cyclase.[2,3,10] Conceivably, age-associated exaggeration of the antiadrenergic effects of cholinergic stimulus can contribute to the decline in adrenergic responses of the aging heart. This possibility was addressed in one study which examined the postjunctional antiadrenergic action of cholinergic stimulus on the heart by determining the effect of a cholinergic agonist (carbachol) on β-adrenergic activation of adenylate cyclase in myocardial membranes from adult and aged rats. Interestingly, the results from this study showed that the ability of carbachol to inhibit β-adrenergic activation of adenylate cyclase is significantly reduced in the aged heart, suggesting an age-associated diminution in adrenergic-cholinergic interaction in the heart.[86] Thus, postsynaptically, exaggerated cholinergic antagonism of adrenergic stimulation does not appear to contribute to the decline in adrenergic control of the heart in aging. On the other hand, the age-dependent decline in the antiadrenergic action of cholinergic stimulation may be construed as a protective adaptation occurring in the face of diminished adrenergic control of the aging heart.

As noted earlier (Section VI), muscarinic cholinergic inhibition of adenylate cyclase and β-adrenergic activation of adenylate cyclase are mediated through G_i and G_s proteins, respectively. The mechanism by which G_i attenuates adenylate cyclase activity has not been clearly established. Inhibition of adenylate cyclase has been proposed to occur by at least two mechanisms: directly by $G_{i\alpha}$ GTP inhibition of adenylate cyclase and/or indirectly via inactivation of $G_{s\alpha}$ GTP by $G_{\beta r}$ released from G_i and possibly G_o.[2,3,138] The mechanistic basis of the age-associated decline in muscarinic inhibition of β-adrenergic-stimulated adenylate cyclase activity is yet to be determined. It has been suggested that in the adult rat heart, about 50% of the total cardiac β-receptor-G_s-linked adenylate cyclase units in cardiac membranes are coupled to the muscarinic receptor-G_i-linked inhibitory pathway, and that with aging a much lesser fraction of the cyclase units may be coupled to the inhibitory pathway.[86]

IX. PATHOPHYSIOLOGICAL IMPLICATIONS OF CHOLINERGIC HYPER-RESPONSES OF THE AGING HEART

The enhanced responsiveness of the heart and coronary vasculature to cholinergic agonists with aging may have pathophysiological and clinical implications. In the pathophysiological setting, the enhanced cholinergic responsiveness of the heart implies that age-related decline in baroreceptor control of heart rate,[31,139,140] a function largely mediated by the vagus,[141] is not due to effector organ hyporesponsiveness. Consequently, the defect is likely located elsewhere in the reflex arc. In the clinical setting, cholinergic hypersensitivity of the heart may contribute to inordinate sinus node depression and carotid sinus syndrome prevalent in the elderly.[142] At the level of the coronary vasculature, cholinergic hypersensitivity may result in greater coronary vasoconstriction at any level of cholinergic tone, thus compromising coronary blood flow, energy metabolism, and contractility in the aging heart. Thus, age-related decrease in coronary blood flow and increase in coronary vascular resistance encountered *in vivo*,[106] but not *in vitro*,[104] can be explained in part on the basis of age-associated change in vasoregulatory response to endogenously released acetylcholine. In the clinical setting, cholinergic constriction is recognized to be an underlying factor in the pathogenesis of coronary spasm.[119,143] Hence, cholinergic hypersensitivity of the coronary vasculature in aging may contribute to higher incidence of coronary spasm in the elderly. Whether or not the hyper-responses to cholinergic agonists observed in the aging rat model are applicable to humans is uncertain. However, these observations suggest need for caution in the therapeutic use of cholinomimetics in the elderly so as to guard against the occurrence of exaggerated bradycardia and coronary vasospasm.

X. ACKNOWLEDGMENTS

Studies from the author's laboratory cited in this review were supported by the Heart and Stroke Foundations of Ontario and Saskatchewan. I thank Dr. Na Su, who did her Ph.D. research in my laboratory, for her contributions to studies in this field. I also thank Ande Xu for preparing some of the illustrations, and Susan Hunt for secretarial assistance.

REFERENCES

1. **Wikberg, J. E. S. and Lefkowitz, R. J.,** Adrenergic receptors in the heart: pre and postsynaptic mechanisms, in *Nervous Control of Cardiovascular Function*, Randall, W. C., Ed., Oxford University Press, New York, 1984, 95.
2. **Lindeman, J. P. and Watanabe, A. M.,** Mechanisms of adrenergic and cholinergic regulation of myocardial contractility, in *Physiology and Pathophysiology of the Heart*, Sperelakis, N., Ed., Kluwer Academic Publishers, Boston, 1994, 467.
3. **Fleming, J. W., Wisler, P. L., and Watanabe, A. M.,** Signal transduction by G proteins in cardiac tissues, *Circulation*, 85, 420, 1992.
4. **Brown, A. M.,** Regulation of heartbeat by G protein-coupled ion channels, *Am. J. Physiol.*, 259, H1621, 1990.

5. **Scholz, H.,** Effects of β- and α-adrenoceptor activators and adrenergic transmitter releasing agents on the mechanical activity of the heart, in *Handbook of Experimental Pharmacology*, Vol. 54, part 1, Szekeres, L., Ed., Springer-Verlag, 1980, 651.
6. **Benfey, B. G.,** Function of myocardial α-adrenoceptors, *Life Sci.*, 46, 743, 1990.
7. **Loffelholz, K. and Pappano, A. J.,** The parasympathetic neuroeffector junction of the heart, *Pharmacol. Rev.*, 37, 1, 1985.
8. **Doods, H. N., Dammgen, N., Mayer, N., Rinner, I., and Trach, V.,** Muscarinic receptors in heart and vascular system, in *Progress in Pharmacology and Clinical Pharmacology*, Vol. 7, part 1, Van Zwieten, P. A. and Schonban, E., Eds., Gustav Fischer Verlag, Stuttgart, 1989, 47.
9. **Higgins, C. B., Vatner, S. F., and Braunwald, E.,** Parasympathetic control of the heart, *Pharmacol. Rev.*, 25, 119, 1973.
10. **Levy, M. N.,** Cardiac sympathetic-parasympathetic interactions, *Fed. Proc., Fed. Am. Soc. Exp. Biol.*, 43, 2598, 1984.
11. **Narayanan, N. and Derby, J. A.,** Alterations in the properties of β-adrenergic receptors of myocardial membranes in aging: impairments in agonist-receptor interactions and guanine nucleotide regulation accompany diminished catecholamine responsiveness of adenylate cyclase, *Mech. Ageing Dev.*, 19, 127, 1982.
12. **Scarpace, P. J.,** Decreased beta adrenergic responsiveness during senescence, *Fed. Proc., Fed. Am. Soc. Exp. Biol.*, 45, 51, 1986.
13. **Lakatta, E. G.,** Cardiac muscle changes in senescence, *Annu. Rev. Physiol.*, 49, 519, 1987.
14. **Lakatta, E. G.,** Cardiovascular regulatory mechanisms in advanced age, *Physiol. Rev.*, 73, 413, 1993.
15. **Tumer, N. and Scarpace, P. J.,** Adrenergic function in aging: focus on the cardiovascular system, in *Handbook of Pharmacology of Aging*, 2nd ed., Roberts, J., Snyder, D. L., and Friedman, E., Eds., CRC Press, Boca Raton, FL, 1995, p 23.
16. **Scarpace, P. J.,** Decreased receptor activation with age. Can it be explained by desensitization?, *J. Am. Geriatr. Soc.*, 36, 1067, 1988.
17. **Scarpace, P. J.,** Forskolin activation of adenylate cyclase in rat myocardium with age: effects of guanine nucleotide analogs, *Mech. Ageing Dev.*, 52, 169, 1990.
18. **Kusiak, J. W. and Pitha, J.,** Decreased response with age of the cardiac catecholamine sensitive adenylate cyclase system, *Life Sci.*, 33, 1679, 1983.
19. **O'Connor, S. W., Scarpace, P. J., and Abrass, I. B.,** Age-associated decrease in the catalytic unit activity of rat myocardial adenylate cyclase, *Mech. Ageing Dev.*, 21, 357, 1983.
20. **Guarnieri, T., Filburn, C. R., Zitnik, G., Roth, G. S., and Lakatta, E. G.,** Contractile and biochemical correlates of β-adrenergic stimulation of the aged heart, *Am. J. Physiol.*, 239, H501, 1980.
21. **Sakai, M., Danziger, R. S., Staddon, J. M., Lakatta, E. G., and Hansford, R. G.,** Decrease with senescence in the norepinephrine-induced phosphorylation of myofilament proteins in isolated cardiomyocytes, *J. Mol. Cell. Cardiol.*, 21, 1327, 1989.
22. **Jiang, M. T., Moffat, M. P., and Narayanan, N.,** Age-related alterations in phosphorylation of sarcoplasmic reticulum and myofibrillar proteins and diminished contractile response to isoproterenol in intact rat ventricle, *Circ. Res.* 72, 102, 1993.
23. **Docherty, J. R.,** Effect of age on the response of target organs to autonomic neurotransmitters, in *Aging of the Autonomic Nervous System*, Amenta, F., Ed., CRC Press, Boca Raton, FL, 1993, 109.
24. **Patrilla, J. S., Hoopes, M. T., Ito, H., Dax, E. M., and Roth, G. S.,** Loss of rat ventricular α-adrenergic receptors during aging, *Life Sci.*, 31, 2507, 1982.
25. **Gascon, S., Dierssen, M., Marmol, F., Vivas, N. M., and Badia, A.,** Effect of age on αl-adrenoceptor subtypes in the heart ventricular muscle of the rat, *J. Pharm. Pharmacol.*, 45, 907, 1993.
26. **Kimball, K. A., Cornett, L. E., Seifen, E., and Kennedy, R. H.,** Aging: changes in cardiac α-l adrenoceptor responsiveness and expression, *Eur. J. Pharmacol.*, 208, 231, 1991.
27. **Kelliher, G. J. and Conahan, S. T.,** Changes in vagal activity and response to muscarinic receptor agonists with age. *J. Gerontol.*, 35, 842, 1980.
28. **Ferrari, A. U., Daffonchio, A., Gerosa, S., and Mancia, G.,** Alterations in cardiac parasympathetic function in aged rats, *Am. J. Physiol.*, 260, H647, 1991.
29. **Frolkis, V. V., Bezrukov, V. V., Duplenko, Y. K., Stachegoleua, I. V., Sheutchuk, V. G., and Verkhratsky, N. S.,** Acetylcholine metabolism and cholinergic regulation of functions in ageing, *Gerontologia* (Basel), 19, 45, 1973.
30. **Nafelski, L. A. and Brown, C. F. G.,** Action of atropine on the cardiovascular system in normal persons, *Arch. Int. Med.*, 86, 898, 1950.
31. **Gribben, B., Pickering, T. G., Sleight, P., and Peto, R.,** Effect of age and high blood pressure on baroreflex sensitivity in man, *Circ. Res.*, 29, 421, 1971.
32. **Mancia, G., Ferrari, A., Gregorini, L., Parati, G., Pomidossi, G., Bertinieri, G., Grassi, G., Di Rienzo, M., Pedotti, A., and Zanchetti, A.,** Blood pressure and heart rate variabilities in normotensive and hypertensive human beings, *Circ. Res.*, 53, 96, 1983.

33. **Su, N. and Narayanan, N.,** Enhanced chronotropic and inotropic responses of rat myocardium to cholinergic stimulus with aging, *Can. J. Physiol. Pharmacol.*, 70, 1618, 1992.
34. **Kennedy, G. J. and Seifen, E.,** Aging: effects on chronotropic actions of muscarinic agonists in isolated rat atria, *Mech. Ageing Dev.*, 51, 81, 1990.
35. **Vekhratsky, N. S.,** Acetylcholine metabolism peculiarities in aging, *Exp. Gerontol.*, 5, 49, 1970.
36. **Frolkis, V. V.,** *Aging and Life-Prolonging Processes*, translated from the Russian by Bobrov, N., Springer-Verlag Wien, New York, 1982, 124.
37. **Morgan, D. G. and May, P. C.,** Age-related changes in synaptic neurochemistry, in *Handbook of the Biology of Aging*, 3rd ed., Schneider, E. L. and Rowe, J. W., Eds., Academic Press, San Diego, CA, 1990, 219.
38. **Frolkis, V. V., Shevtchuk, V. G., Verkhratsky, N. S., Stupina, A. S., Karpova, S. M., and Lakiza, T. Y.,** Mechanisms of neurohumoral regulation of heart function in aging, *Exp. Aging Res.*, 5, 441, 1979.
39. **Mayer, E. M., Momol, A. E., and Baker, S. P.,** Age-related reductions in rat atrial high affinity choline uptake, ACh synthesis and ACh release. A brief note, *Mech. Ageing Dev.*, 30, 221, 1985.
40. **Sket, D. and Brzin, M.,** Activity of cholinergic enzymes in the rat heart as a function of age, *Period. Biol.*, 87, 383, 1985.
41. **Birnbaumer, L., Abramowitz, J., Yatani, A., Okabe, K., Mattera, R., Graf, R., Sanford, J., Codina, J., and Brown, A. M.,** Roles of G proteins in coupling of receptors to ionic channels and other effector systems, *Crit. Rev. Biochem. Mol. Biol.*, 25, 225, 1990.
42. **Pfaffinger, P. J., Martin, J. M., Hunter, D. D., Nathanson, N. M., and Hille, B.,** GTP-binding proteins couple cardiac muscarinic receptors to a K channel, *Nature*, 317, 536, 1985.
43. **Sakman, B., Noma, A., and Trautwein, W.,** Acetylcholine activation of single muscarinic K^+ channels in isolated pacemaker cells of the mammalian heart, *Nature*, 303, 250, 1983.
44. **Soejima, M. and Noma, A.,** Mode of regulation of ACh-sensitive K-channel by the muscarinic receptor in rabbit atrial cells, *Pflugers Arch.*, 400, 424, 1984.
45. **Schimerlik, M. I.,** Structure and regulation of muscarinic receptors, *Annu. Rev. Physiol.*, 51, 217, 1989.
46. **Ten Eick, R., Nawrath, H., McDonald, T. F., and Trautwein, W.,** On the mechanism of the negative inotropic effect of acetylcholine, *Pflugers Arch.*, 361, 207, 1976.
47. **Giles, W. R. and Noble, S. J.,** Changes in membrane currents in bullfrog atrium produced by acetylcholine, *J. Physiol. (London)*, 261, 103, 1976.
48. **Hino, N. and Ochi, R.,** Effect of acetylcholine on membrane currents in guinea pig papillary muscle, *J. Physiol. (London)*, 307, 183, 1980.
49. **Hartzell, H. C.,** Regulation of cardiac ion channels by catecholamines, acetylcholine and second messenger systems, *Prog. Biophys. Mol. Biol.*, 52, 165, 1988.
50. **Petit-Jacques, J., Bois, P., Bescond, J., and Lenfant, J.,** Mechanism of muscarinic control of the high threshold calcium current in rabbit sino-atrial node myocytes, *Pflugers Arch.*, 423, 21, 1993.
51. **DiFrancesco, D. and Tromba, C.,** Acetylcholine inhibits activation of the cardiac hyperpolarization-activated current, I_f, *Pflugers Arch.*, 410, 139, 1987.
52. **DiFrancesco, D. and Tromba, C.,** Inhibition of the hyperpolarization-activated current induced by acetylcholine in rabbit sino-atrial node myocytes, *J. Physiol. (London)*, 405, 477, 1988.
53. **DiFrancesco, D. and Tromba, C.,** Muscarinic control of the hyperpolarization-activated current (I_f) in rabbit sino-atrial node myocytes, *J. Physiol. (London)*, 405, 493, 1988.
54. **George, W. J., Wilkerson, R. D., and Kadowitz, P. J.,** Influence of acetylcholine on contractile force and cyclic nucleotide levels in the isolated perfused rat heart, *J. Pharmacol. Exp. Ther.*, 184, 228, 1973.
55. **Hazeki, O. and Ui, M.,** Modification by islet-activating protein of receptor mediated regulation of cyclic AMP accumulation in isolated rat heart cells, *J. Biol. Chem.*, 256, 2856, 1981.
56. **Brown, B. S., Polson, J. B., Krzanowski, J. J., and Wiggins, J. R.,** Influence of isoproterenol and methylisobutylxanthine on the contractile and cyclic nucleotide effects of methacholine in isolated rat atria, *J. Pharmacol. Exp. Ther.*, 212, 325, 1980.
57. **Goldberg, N. D. and Haddox, M. K.,** Cyclic GMP metabolism and involvement in biological regulation, *Annu. Rev. Biochem.*, 46, 823, 1977.
58. **Brown, J. H. and Jones, L. G.,** Phosphoinositide metabolism in the heart, in *Phosphoinositides and Receptor Mechanisms*, 7th ed., Venter, J. C. and Harrison, L. C., Eds., Alan R. Liss, New York, 1986, 245.
59. **Sperelakis, N.,** Regulation of calcium slow channels of cardiac muscle by cyclic nucleotides and phosphorylation, *J. Mol. Cell. Cardiol.* 20, 75, 1988.
60. **Sperelakis, N.,** Cyclic GMP regulation of calcium slow channels in cardiac muscle and vascular smooth muscle cells, *Adv. Pharmacol.*, 26, 217, 1994.
61. **Nathanson, N. M.,** Molecular properties of the muscarinic acetylcholine receptor, *Annu. Rev. Neurosci.*, 10, 195, 1987.
62. **Bonner, T. I.,** New subtypes of muscarinic acetylcholine receptors, *Trends Pharmacol.*, Suppl. IV, 11, 1989.
63. **Ehlert, F. J., Delen, F. M., Yun, S. H., Friedman, D. J., and Self, D. W.,** Coupling of subtypes of the muscarinic receptor to adenylate cyclase in the corpus striatum and heart, *J. Pharmacol. Exp. Ther.*, 254, 660, 1989.

64. **Narayanan, N. and Derby, J. A.,** Effects of age on muscarinic cholinergic receptors in rat myocardium, *Can. J. Physiol. Pharmacol.*, 61, 822, 1983.
65. **Baker, S. P., Marchand, S., O'Neil, E., Nelson, C. A., and Posner, P.,** Age-related changes in cardiac muscarinic receptors: decreased ability of the receptor to form a high affinity agonist binding state, *J. Gerontol.*, 40, 141, 1985.
66. **Chevalier, B., Mansier, P., Teiger, E., Callens-El Amrani, F., and Swynghedauw, B.,** Alterations in β adrenergic and muscarinic receptors in aged rat heart. Effects of chronic administration of propranolol and atropine, *Mech. Ageing Dev.*, 60, 215, 1991.
67. **Brown, A. M. and Birnbaumer, L.,** Ionic channels and their regulation by G protein subunits, *Annu. Rev. Physiol.*, 52, 197, 1990.
68. **Kurachi, Y.,** G-Protein control of cardiac potassium channels, *Trends. Cardiovasc. Med.*, 4, 64, 1994.
69. **Gilman, A. G.,** G Proteins: transducers of receptor-generated signals, *Annu. Rev. Biochem.*, 56, 615, 1987.
70. **Robishaw, J. D. and Foster, K. A.,** Role of G proteins in the regulation of the cardiovascular system, *Annu. Rev. Physiol.*, 51, 229, 1989.
71. **Neumann, J., Schmitz, W., Scholz, H., and Stein, B.,** Effects of adenosine analogues on contractile response and cAMP content in isolated guinea pig ventricular myocytes, *Naunyn-Schmiedeberg's Arch. Pharmacol.*, 332, 403, 1989.
72. **Pappano, A. J., Matsumoto, K., Tagima, T., Agnarsson, U., and Webb, W.,** Pertussis toxin-insensitive mechanism for carbachol-induced depolarization and positive inotropic effect in heart muscle, *Trends. Pharmacol. Sci.*, 9 (Suppl.), 35, 1988.
73. **Kim, D., Lewis, D. L., Graziadei, L., Neer, E. J., Bar-Sagi, D., and Clapham, D. E.,** G-Protein βγ-subunits activate the cardiac K^+ channel via phospholipase A_2, *Nature*, 337, 557, 1989.
74. **Milligan, G.,** Techniques used in the identification and analysis of function of pertussis toxin-sensitive G proteins, *Biochem. J.*, 235, 1, 1988.
75. **Su, N., Duan, J., Moffat, M. P., and Narayanan, N.,** Age-related changes in electrophysiological responses to muscarinic receptor stimulation in rat myocardian, *Can. J. Physiol. Pharmacol.*, 73, 1430, 1995.

75a. **Su, N. and Narayanan, N.,** Unpublished data.

76. **Shu, Y. and Scarpace, P. J.,** Forskolin binding sites and G-protein immunoreactivity in rat hearts during aging, *J. Cardiovasc. Pharmacol.*, 23, 188, 1994.
77. **Levine, M. A., Feldman, A. M., Robishaw, J. D., Ladenson, P. W., Ahn, J. G., Moroney, J. F., and Smallwood, P. M.,** Influence of thyroid hormone status on expression of genes encoding G protein subunits in the rat heart, *J. Biol. Chem.*, 265, 3553, 1990.
78. **Feldman, A. M., Cates, A. E., Veazey, W. B., Hershberger, R. E., Bristow, M. R., Baughman, K. I., Baumgartner, W. A., and VanDop, C.,** Increase of the 40,000 mol wt pertussis toxin substrate (G protein) in the failing human heart, *J. Clin. Invest.*, 82, 189, 1988.
79. **Neumann, J., Scholz, H., Doring, V., Schmitz, W., Von Meyerinck, L., and Kalmar, P.,** Increase in myocardial G_i-proteins in heart failure, *Lancet*, 2, 936, 1988.
80. **Feldman, A. M., Cates, A. E., Bristow, M. R., and Van Dop, C.,** Altered expression of α-subunits of G proteins in failing human hearts, *J. Mol. Cell. Cardiol.*, 21, 359, 1989.
81. **Sen, L., Liang, B. T., and Smith, T. W.,** Enhanced α_1-adrenergic responsiveness via a pertussis toxin (PT)-sensitive pathway in myocytes from cardiomyopathic hearts (abstract), *Circulation*, 78 (Suppl. II), 111, 1988.
82. **Bristow, M. R. and Feldman, A. M.,** Changes in the receptor-G protein-adenylate cyclase system in heart failure from various types of heart muscle disease, *Basic Res. Cardiol.*, 87 (Suppl. I), 15, 1992.
83. **Urasawa, K., Sato, K., Igarashi, Y., Kawaguchi, H., and Yasuda, H.,** A mechanism of catecholamine tolerance in congestive heart failure — alterations in the hormone-sensitive adenylate cyclase system of the heart, *Jpn. Circ. J.*, 56, 456, 1992.
84. **Eschenhagen, T., Mende, U., Nose, M., Schmitz, W., Scholz, H., Schulte, A. E. J., Sempell, R., Warnholtz, A., and Wustel, J. M.,** Regulation and possible functional implications of G-protein mRNA expression in non failing and failing ventricular myocardium, *Basic Res. Cardiol.*, 87 (Suppl. I) 51, 1992.
85. **Kulchitskii, O. K.,** Effect of acetylcholine on the cyclic GMP level in the rat heart at different ages, *Bull. Exp. Biol. Med.*, 90, 1237, 1980.
86. **Narayanan, N. and Tucker, L.,** Autonomic interactions in the aging heart: age-associated decrease in muscarinic cholinergic receptor mediated inhibition of β-adrenergic activation of adenylate cyclase, *Mech. Ageing Dev.*, 34, 249, 1986.
87. **Wey, J. Y., Spurgeon, H. A., and Lakatta, E. G.,** Excitation-contraction in rat myocardium: alterations with adult aging, *Am. J. Physiol.*, 246, H784, 1993.
88. **Capasso, J. M., Malhotra, A., Remily, R. M., Scheuer, J., and Sonnenblick, E. H.,** Effect of age on mechanical and electrical performance of rat myocardium, *Am. J. Physiol.*, 245, H72, 1983.
89. **Walker, K. E., Lakatta, E. G., and Houser, S. R.,** Age-associated changes in membrane currents in rat ventricular myocytes, *Cardiovasc. Res.*, 27, 1968, 1993.
90. **Bachman, S., Sparrow, D., and Smith, L. K.,** Effect of aging on the electrocardiogram, *Am. J. Cardiol.*, 48, 513, 1981.

91. **Dubell, W. H., Boyett, M. R., Spurgeon, H. A., Talo, A., Stern, M. D., and Lakatta, E. G.,** The cytosolic calcium transient modulates the action potential of rat ventricular myocytes, *J. Physiol. (London)*, 436, 347, 1991.
92. **Orchard, J. and Lakatta, E. G.,** Intracellular calcium transients and developed tensions in rat heart muscle. A mechanism for the negative interval-strength relationship, *J. Gen. Physiol.*, 86, 637, 1985.
93. **Noma, A. and Trautwein, W.,** Relaxation of ACh-induced potassium current in the rabbit sino-atrial node, *Pflugers Arch.*, 377, 193, 1978.
94. **DiFrancesco, D., Ducouret, P., and Robinson, R. B.,** Muscarinic modulation of cardiac rate at low acetylcholine concentrations, *Science*, 243, 669, 1989.
95. **Ochi, R.,** Decrease in calcium conductance by acetylcholine in mammalian ventricular muscle, in *The Mechanism of Gated Calcium Transport Across Biological Membranes*, Ohnishi, S. T. and Endo, M., Eds., Academic Press, New York, 1981, 79.
96. **Tomanek, R. J.,** Coronary vasculature of the aging heart, in *The Aging Heart*, Weisfeldt, M. L., Ed., Raven Press, New York, 1980, 115.
97. **Yin, F. C.,** The aging vasculature and its effects on the heart, in *The Aging Heart*, Weisfeldt, M. L., Ed., Raven Press, New York, 1980, 137.
98. **Lakatta, E. G.,** Hemodynamic adaptation to stress with advancing age, *Acta Med. Scand.* (Suppl.), 711, 39, 1986.
99. **Vanhoutte, P. M.,** Aging and vascular responsiveness, *J. Cardiovasc. Pharmacol.*, 12 (Suppl. 8), S11, 1988.
100. **Tomanek, R. J., Aydelotte, M. R., and Torry, R. J.,** Remodelling of coronary vessels during aging in purebred beagles, *Circ. Res.*, 69, 1068, 1991.
101. **Anversa, P., Hiler, B., Ricci, R., Guideri, G., and Olivetti, G.,** Myocyte cell loss and myocyte hypertrophy in aging rat heart, *J. Am. Coll. Cardiol.*, 8, 1441, 1986.
102. **Guideri, G., Olivetti, G., Hiler, B., Ricci, R., and Anversa, P.,** Increased incidence of isoproterenol-induced ventricular fibrillation in aging rats, *Can. J. Physiol. Pharmacol.*, 65, 504, 1987.
103. **Tomanek, R. J.,** Effect of age and exercise on the extent of the myocardial capillary bed, *Anat. Rec.*, 167, 55, 1970.
104. **Weisfeldt, M. L., Wright, J. R., Shreiner, D. P., Lakatta, E. G., and Shock, N. W.,** Coronary flow and oxygen extraction in the perfused heart of senescent male rats, *J. Appl. Physiol.*, 30, 44, 1971.
105. **Friberg, P., Nordlander, M., Lundin, S., and Folkow, B.,** Effects of aging on cardiac performance and coronary flow in spontaneously hypertensive and normotensive rats, *Acta Physiol. Scand.*, 125, 1, 1985.
106. **Hachamovitch, R., Wicker, P., Capasso, J. M., and Anversa, P.,** Alterations in coronary blood flow and reserve with aging in Fischer 344 rats, *Am. J. Physiol.*, 256, H66, 1989.
107. **Olah, M. E. and Rahwan, R. G.,** Age-related changes in responsiveness of the rat aorta to depolarizing and receptor-mediated contractile stimuli and to calcium antagonism, *Pharmacology*, 35, 163, 1987.
108. **Toda, N. and Miyazaki, M.,** Senescent beagle coronary arteries in response to catecholamines and adrenergic nerve stimulation, *J. Gerontol.*, 42, 210, 1987.
109. **Hamilton, C. A., Dalrymple, H. W., Jones, C. R., and Reid, J. L.,** The effect of aging on alpha-adrenoceptors and their responses in rabbits, *Clin. Exp. Pharmacol. Physiol.*, 12, 535, 1985.
110. **Nielsen, H., Hasenkam, J. M., Pilegaard, H. K., Aalkjaer, C., and Mortensen, F. V.,** Age-dependent changes in α-adrenoceptor-mediated contractility of isolated human resistance arteries, *Am. J. Physiol.*, 263, H1190, 1992.
111. **Stevens, M. J., Lipe, S., and Moulds, R. F. W.,** The effect of age on the responses of human isolated arteries and veins to noradrenaline, *Br. J. Clin. Pharmacol.*, 14, 750, 1982.
112. **Su, N. and Narayanan, N.,** Age-related alteration in cholinergic but not α adrenergic response of rat coronary vasculature, *Cardiovasc. Res.*, 27, 284, 1993.
113. **Hashimoto, K., Shiegei, T., and Imai, S.,** Oxygen consumption and coronary vascular tone in isolated fibrillated dog heart, *Am. J. Physiol.*, 198, 965, 1960.
114. **Blesav, M. I. and Ross, G.,** Cholinergic mechanisms on the heart and coronary circulation, *Br. J. Pharmacol.*, 38, 93, 1970.
115. **Glaviano, V. V., Goldberg, J. M., Pindok, M., Wallick, D., and Aravanis, C.,** Cholinergic intervention on myocardial dynamics and metabolism in the non-working dog heart, *Circ. Res.*, 41, 508, 1977.
116. **Gross, G. J., Buck, J. D., and Waltier, D. C.,** Transmural distribution of blood flow during activity of coronary muscarinic receptors, *Am. J. Physiol.*, 240, H941, 1981.
117. **Cox, D. A., Hintzo, T. H., and Vatner, S. F.,** Effects of acetylcholine on large and small arteries in conscious dogs, *J. Pharmacol. Exp. Ther.*, 225, 704, 1983.
118. **Feigl, E. O.,** Coronary physiology, *Physiol. Rev.*, 63, 1, 1983.
119. **Kalsner, S.,** Cholinergic constriction in the general circulation and its role in coronary artery spasm, *Circ. Res.*, 65, 237, 1989.
120. **Van Charldrop, K. J., De Jonge, A., Davidesko, D., Rinner, I., Doods, H. N., and Van Zwieten, P. A.,** Coronary constriction induced by vagal stimulation in the isolated rat heart, *Eur. J. Pharmacol.*, 136, 135, 1987.

121. **Palmer, R. M. J., Ferridge, A. G., and Moncada, S.,** Nitric oxide release accounts for the biological activity of endothelium-derived relaxing factor, *Nature*, 327, 524, 1987.
122. **Stewart, D. J., Munzel, T., and Bassenge, E.,** Reversal of acetylcholine-induced coronary resistance vessel dilation by hemoglobin, *Eur. J. Pharmacol.*, 136, 239, 1987.
123. **Amezcua, J. L., Palmer, R. M. J., de Souza, B. M., and Moncada, S.,** Nitric oxide synthesized from L-arginine regulates vascular tone in the coronary circulation of the rabbit, *Br. J. Pharmacol.*, 97, 1119, 1989.
124. **Klem, M. and Schrader, J.,** Control of coronary vascular tone by nitric oxide, *Circ. Res.*, 66, 1561, 1990.
125. **Nuutinen, E. M., Wilson, D. F., and Erecinska, M.,** The effects of cholinergic agonists on coronary flow rate and oxygen consumption in isolated perfused rat heart, *J. Mol. Cell. Cardiol.*, 17, 31, 1985.
126. **Van Charldrop, K. J. and Van Zwieten, P. A.,** Comparison of the muscarinic receptors in coronary artery, cerebral artery and atrium of the pig, *Naunyn-Schmiedebergs Arch. Pharmacol.*, 339, 403, 1989.
127. **Entzeroth, M., Doods, H. N., and Mayer, N.,** Characterization of porcine coronary muscarinic receptors, *Naunyn-Schmiedebergs Arch. Pharmacol.*, 341, 432, 1990.
128. **Duckles, S. P. and Garcia-Villalon, A. G.,** Characterization of vascular muscarinic receptors. Rabbit ear artery and bovine coronary artery, *J. Pharmacol. Exp. Ther.*, 253, 608, 1990.
129. **Kuriyama, H. and Suzuki, H.,** The effects of acetylcholine on the membrane and contractile properties of smooth muscle cells of the rabbit superior mesenteric artery, *Br. J. Pharmacol.*, 64, 493, 1978.
130. **Vanhoutte, P. M.,** Inhibition by acetylcholine of adrenergic neurotransmission in vascular smooth muscle, *Circ. Res.*, 34, 317, 1974.
131. **Suyama, A. and Kuriyama, H.,** Mechanisms of the ergonovine-induced vasoconstriction in the rabbit main coronary artery, *Naunyn-Schmiedebergs Arch. Pharmacol.*, 326, 357, 1984.
132. **Kitamura, K. and Kuriyama, H.,** Effects of acetylcholine on the smooth muscle cells of isolated main coronary artery of the guinea pig, *J. Physiol.* (London), 293, 357, 1979.
133. **Ito, T., Kajiwana, M., Kitamura, K., and Kuriyama, H.,** Roles of stored calcium on the mechanical response evoked in smooth muscle cells of the porcine coronary artery, *J. Physiol.* (*London*), 322, 107, 1982.
134. **Gamitkevich, V. and Isenberg, G.,** Isolated guinea pig coronary smooth muscle cells. Acetylcholine induces hyperpolarization due to sarcoplasmic reticulum calcium release activating potassium channels, *Circ. Res.*, 67, 525, 1990.
135. **Berridge, M. J. and Irvine, R. F.,** Inositol phosphates and cell signalling, *Nature*, 341, 197, 1989.
136. **Muscholl, E.,** Peripheral muscarinic control of norepinephrine release in cardiovascular system, *Am. J. Physiol.*, 239, H713, 1980.
137. **Wurster, R. D.,** Central nervous system regulation of the heart: an overview, in *Nervous Control of Cardiovascular Function*, Randall, W. C., Ed., Oxford University Press, New York, 1984, 307.
138. **Gilman, A. G.,** G Proteins and dual control of adenylate cyclase, *Cell*, 36, 377, 1984.
139. **Lowenthal, D. T., Kim, K. E., Affrine, B., and Falkner, B.,** Overview of physiology in senescence, *Chest*, 83, 408, 1983.
140. **Pfeifer, M. A., Weinberg, C. R., Cook, D., Best, J. D., Rennan, A., and Halter, J. B.,** Differential changes of autonomic nervous system function with age in man, *Am. J. Med.*, 75, 249, 1983.
141. **Mancia, G. and Marks, A. I.,** Arterial baroreflex in humans, *Handbook Physiol.*, Sect. 2, Cardiovasc. Syst. III (2), 755, 1983.
142. **Thomas, J. E.,** Hyperactive carotid sinus reflex and carotid sinus syncope, *Mayo Clin. Proc.*, 44, 127, 1969.
143. **Yasue, H., Horio, Y., Nakamura, N., Fujii, H., Imoto, N., Sonada, R., Kugiyama, K., Obata, K., Morikami, Y., and Kimura, T.,** Induction of coronary artery spasm by acetylcholine in patients with variant angina: possible role of the parasympathetic nervous system in the pathogenesis of coronary artery spasm, *Circulation*, 74, 955, 1986.

Chapter 4

ANTIHYPERTENSIVE AND VASODILATOR DRUGS IN AGING

James R. Docherty

CONTENTS

0-8493-8306-4/96/$0.00+$.50

I. INTRODUCTION

The purpose of this article is to review the cardiovascular effects of antihypertensive and vasodilator drugs and how these effects are altered by the aging process. A wide range of antihypertensive and vasodilator agents are available for the treatment of cardiovascular disorders, and it is crucial to know how the response to these agents is altered by aging given the increasing proportion of the population in the aged group and the increased level of prescribing for the elderly.

Aging is associated with a variety of alterations in cardiovascular function, yet, despite these changes, the cardiovascular system continues to function reasonably well in supplying the needs of tissues (see Reference 1). However, aging is also associated with an increased incidence of cardiovascular disorders including coronary artery disease, heart failure, hypertension, and postural hypotension, and it is difficult to separate purely age-related changes from underlying pathological changes, or from the effects of prescribed drugs, in humans. The object of this chapter is to document age-related changes in the response to antihypertensives and vasodilator agents, whether due to normal aging or pathology, and to interpret the mechanisms underlying these changes. The use of animal models of aging in which cardiovascular disease is less prevalent can give insights into the normal aging process. Hence, it is necessary both to discuss human aging and how far similar effects are seen in animal models. Diuretic agents will be discussed in a separate chapter.

II. THE MODE OF ACTION OF ANTIHYPERTENSIVE AND VASODILATOR AGENTS

The major factors determining blood pressure are the cardiac output and peripheral resistance, related by the following equation:

$$\textit{Blood pressure} = \textit{cardiac output} \times \textit{total peripheral resistance}$$

i.e., blood pressure is produced by the pumping action of the heart (and so is dependent on cardiac output), but the actual level of blood pressure is affected by the resistance to pumping caused by the arteries (the total peripheral resistance): a decreased peripheral resistance results in lower blood pressure, as the heart has to pump less strongly against this decreased resistance to flow. Vasodilator agents, by reducing peripheral resistance, decrease blood pressure (useful in the treatment of hypertension) and reduce the work load on the heart (useful in angina). Agents which have a cardioinhibitory action can also act to lower blood pressure by decreasing cardiac output.

Left ventricular hypertrophy occurs in the majority of hypertensive patents, and a further beneficial effect of some antihypertensive and vasodilator drugs is reduction of this hypertrophy. Centrally acting agents such as α-methyl-dopa, as well as calcium entry blockers and agents like captopril, are reported to reduce left ventricular mass.[2]

In considering the effects of drugs on the cardiovascular system in aging, it is also necessary to consider whether or not the resting parameters of the cardiovascular system are altered by aging: heart rate, cardiac output, blood pressure, and whether or not cardiovascular reflex function is altered. Alterations in basal parameters may influence the response to drugs. Let us first of all consider basal cardiovascular parameters.

III. AGE-RELATED CHANGES IN CARDIOVASCULAR PARAMETERS

A. CARDIAC OUTPUT

It has often been reported that there is a gradual decrease in cardiac output with increasing age, falling by approximately one third by the age of 70,[3] but this may be due to a decreased skeletal muscle mass and decreased metabolic rate so that the resting cardiac output still meets the demands of the tissues. Certainly, many studies find a relatively small reduction in cardiac output with age in healthy subjects (e.g., a 10% reduction).[4] Resting supine heart rate is widely reported to be unchanged by aging, although there are reports of differences on standing (see Reference 1).

In the rat, there is no consistent evidence for an age-related alteration in resting heart rate, whether in conscious or anesthetized animals (see Reference 1).

B. RESTING BLOOD PRESSURE

Since cardiac output is only slightly altered by age in the healthy elderly and reduced by age in the average elderly population, blood pressure increases with age are likely to reflect mainly diminished aortic compliance and alterations in total peripheral resistance. Blood pressure increases with age in Western societies, although this may not be a purely age-related phenomenon, since blood pressure does not necessarily increase with age in some, usually small isolated "primitive" communities.[5,6] However, in most large studies of Western societies, systolic blood pressure tends to increase with age throughout life, whereas diastolic pressure tends to increase to the age of about 60 years and then stabilize or even fall[5] (see Figure 4.1). Hence, the prevalence of isolated systolic hypertension increases with age.[7] Systolic hypertension, i.e., where the systolic pressure and thus the pulse pressure is higher than could be predicted from diastolic pressure, can be due to a large stroke volume or decreased arterial compliance. However, decreased arterial compliance is the main cause of systolic hypertension in the elderly as the compliance of the aorta falls by a factor of 3 to 4 over the age range 20 to 80 years (see Reference 8).

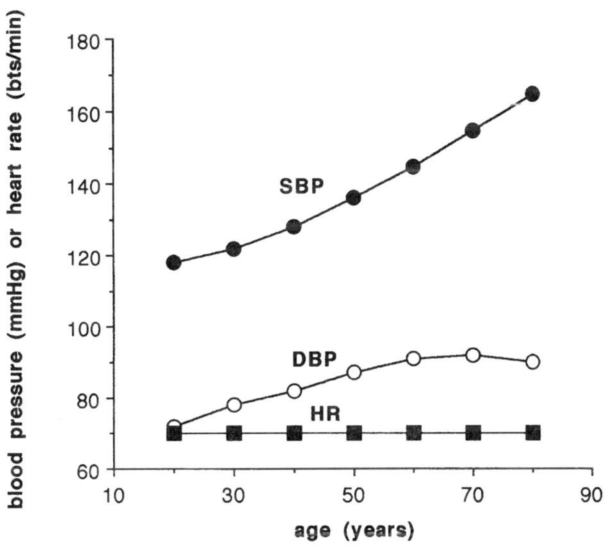

FIGURE 4.1. Schematic representation of the effects of increasing age on blood pressure and heart rate. Symbols: systolic blood pressure (SBP, ●); diastolic blood pressure (DBP, ○); resting heart rate (HR, ■).[5,6,23]

Blood pressure shows a circadian rhythm, and the majority of subjects show a nocturnal dip in blood pressure. However, there appears to be no age-related difference in the magnitude of this nocturnal dip.[9]

In the rat there are various reports of no change or altered resting blood pressure with aging (see Reference 1), suggesting that blood pressure is generally little altered by aging in the rat.

Hence, aging in humans is associated with a slightly diminished cardiac output and increased blood pressure, particularly systolic, so that these differences must be considered when comparing effects of drugs in young and old. However, antihypertensive and vasodilator therapy, by their nature, are normally only given to those with some degree of cardiovascular disease. Even so, elderly and young hypertensives differ in the prevalence of isolated systolic hypertension. Many of the studies discussed in this manuscript refer to laboratory animals where aging changes in cardiovascular parameters tend to be less marked.

IV. CLASSES OF ANTIHYPERTENSIVE AND VASODILATOR DRUGS

Antihypertensive and vasodilator agents can be subdivided into a number of groups, based on their modes of action (see Table 4.1 and Figure 4.2).

TABLE 4.1.
Major Classes of Antihypertensive and Vasodilator Drugs

1. Cardioinhibitory actions
   - β-Adrenoceptor antagonists: propranolol (calcium entry blockers)
2. Sympathoinhibitory actions
   - α_2-Adrenoceptor agonists: α-methyl-dopa, clonidine, guanabenz reserpine
3. Peripheral vasodilator actions
   - (a) Inhibition of actions of endogenous vasoconstrictor
     - α_1-Adrenoceptor antagonists: prazosin, doxazosin
     - ACE inhibitors: captopril
     - 5-HT_2 receptor antagonists: ketanserin
     - Other potential agents
   - (b) Mimic endogenous vasodilator
     - Nitrates, sodium nitroprusside, NO donors, hydralazine
   - (c) Interaction with ion channels
     - Calcium entry blockers: verapamil, nifedipine, diltiazem
     - Potassium channel openers: cromakalin, minoxidil
   - (d) Interfere with second messenger levels
     - PDE inhibition: milrinone, enoximone

A. DRUGS WITH CARDIOINHIBITORY ACTIONS

1. β-Adrenoceptor Antagonist Drugs

The level of noradrenergic cardioaccelerator nerve activity can be gauged by the effects of β-adrenoceptor antagonists, which act by blocking the ongoing actions of the neurotransmitter. At first sight, given the numerous reports of decreased β-adrenoceptor function with aging both in humans and in experimental animals (see Table 4.2) and the decreased cardiac output found in the elderly, it might be expected that β-adrenoceptor antagonists would be less suitable in the elderly. Although there are some reports that β-adrenoceptor antagonists are less effective at lowering blood pressure in elderly hypertensives as compared to younger hypertensives,[19,20] other studies have reported that β-adrenoceptor antagonists are effective at lowering blood pressure in the elderly.[21] Certainly, useful reductions in blood pressure have been reported in elderly hypertensive patients treated with β-blockers,[22] and early studies showed that the β-adrenoceptor antagonist propranolol was as effective in older subjects at reducing cardiac output and heart rate during exercise.[23]

2. Cardiovascular β-Adrenoceptors and G Proteins

One of the most studied G protein-linked receptor systems is the β-adrenoceptor-G protein (Gs)-adenylate cyclase system (see Reference 24), so that there is a great deal of information on how aging affects not just the β-adrenoceptor, but also steps beyond the receptor. Most studies report no change with age in the number of β-adrenoceptor binding sites of rat heart

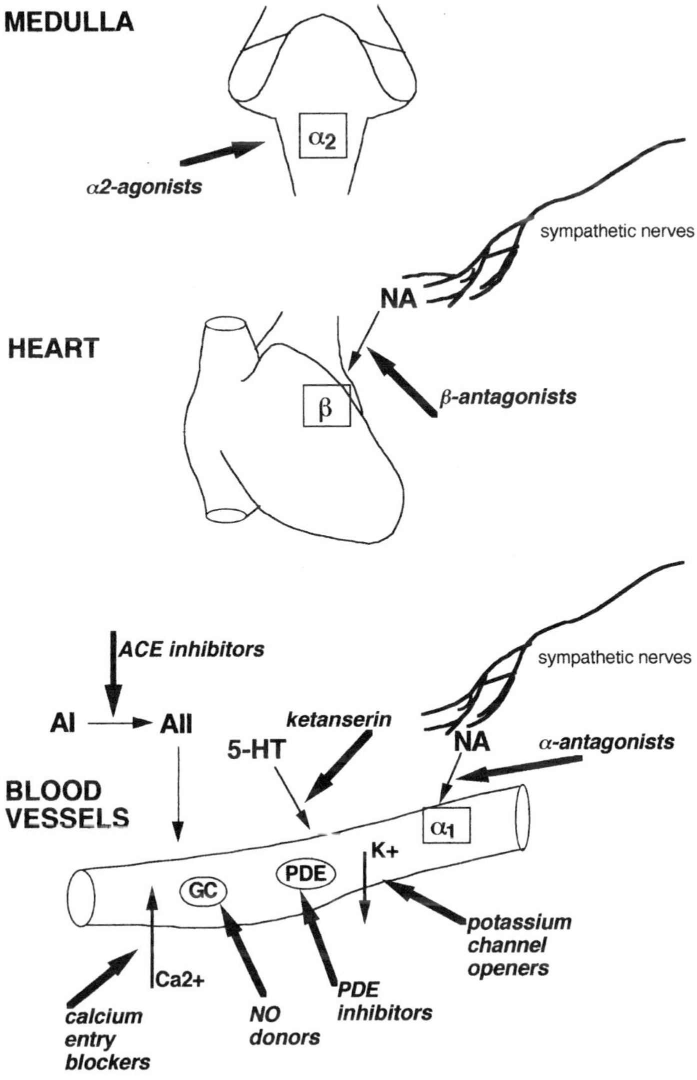

FIGURE 4.2. Schematic representation of the sites of action of antihypertensive and vasodilator drugs. Abbreviations: angiotension I and II (AI and AII), angiotension converting enzyme (ACE), noradrenaline (NA), phosphodiesterase (PDE), guanylate cyclase (GC).

(Table 4.2), and since responses to forskolin (activates adenylate cyclase), sodium fluoride (NaF) (activates the G_s G protein), glucagon (acts on glucagon receptors to stimulate adenylate cyclase), and dibutyryl cyclic AMP (mimicks cyclic AMP) are also reduced by aging in rat myocardium and human lymphocyte, it seems likely that the age-related alteration is not at the β-adrenoceptor level, but at some step beyond this in the activation of the enzyme via the G protein or even after formation of cAMP.[17,24,25] In agreement with this, there are reports of a decreased affinity of β-adrenoceptor binding sites for the β-adrenoceptor agonist isoprenaline with aging due to a decreased coupling to the G protein (the receptor-G protein complex has high affinity for the agonist, whereas the receptor dissociated from the G protein has low affinity for the agonist) (see Reference 24). A diminished production of cAMP by a β-agonist, NaF or forskolin, could be the result of increased activity of the enzyme phosphodiesterase (PDE), and there is a report of an age-related increase in the activity of this enzyme in rat aorta.[26] An age-related reduction in the protein kinase A response to β-adrenoceptor stimulation

TABLE 4.2.
Effects of Aging on Cardiac β-Adrenoceptor-Mediated Responses

Species and tissue	Response	Effect of aging	Ref.
Human systemic	Tachycardia to isop	Decrease	10
Dog systemic	Tachycardia to isop	Decrease	11
Rat systemic	Tachycardia to isop	Decrease	12, 13
	Tachycardia to NA	No change	13
Rat heart	Ligand binding	No change	14, 15
		Decrease	16
		Increase	17
Rat heart	$G_{s\alpha}$	Decrease	18

Note: Abbreviations: isoprenaline (isop), noradrenaline (NA), α subunit of G protein G_s ($G_{s\alpha}$).

and cAMP has also been reported in vascular smooth muscle.[27] There is evidence of an age-related decline in the expression of $G_{s\alpha}$ in rat ventricle by about 25%,[18] which might explain, at least in part, the decreased response to β-stimulation.

3. Calcium Entry Blockers

In addition to vascular actions, cardiac negative inotropic actions of certain calcium entry blockers, especially verapamil, may contribute to their therapeutic actions, particularly in angina. Calcium entry blockers will be discussed in detail later.

B. CENTRAL AND PERIPHERAL SYMPATHOINHIBITORY ACTIONS

Little is known about how central control of the sympathetic nervous system is altered in aging, but many studies have examined the catecholamine content of peripheral tissues as an indication of how the noradrenergic innervation is changed, with conflicting results, some studies showing a decline with age in content, others showing no change. Several studies have reported a decreased release of neurotransmitter with aging in response to electrical stimulation in isolated cardiovascular tissues, and this fits in with evidence for decreased adrenergic innervation of tissues with age (see Reference 1).

1. Prejunctional α_2-Adrenoceptors

Central antihypertensive drugs such as clonidine and guanabenz (α-methyl-dopa acts via a metabolite) mediate their effects by action at neuronal inhibitory α_2-adrenoceptors in the brain and periphery to inhibit sympathetic transmission to the heart and blood vessels, resulting in vasodilatation and cardioinhibition (see Reference 28). The effects of aging on prejunctional α_2-adrenergic receptors have been studied in detail, and most studies report a decreased responsiveness in aging (see Table 4.3). In the rat vas deferens, there is an age-related decline in both prejunctional α_2- and 5-hydroxytryptamine (5-HT_1)-receptor responsiveness,[13,31] suggesting that the decline in response occurs at a postreceptor level, either at the level of the G protein or beyond (these two receptors may couple to the same G protein, as yet unidentified, employing the same intracellular mechanism: possibly opening of K^+ channels or inhibition of Ca^{2+} channels). In aged rats, the centrally mediated depressor response to injection of clonidine into the nucleus tractus solitarius was absent despite depressor responses in younger animals.[33] However, clonidine produces at least part of its antihypertensive actions by a peripheral action at prejunctional α_2-adrenoceptors, effects not examined in the latter study.

In terms of antihypertensive drugs, a decreased function of prejunctional α_2-adrenoceptors might be expected to result in a decreased effectiveness of antihypertensive agents acting via prejunctional α_2-adrenoceptors. However, there is no clear evidence to support this premise,

TABLE 4.3.
Effects of Aging on the Responsiveness of Prejunctional Inhibitory α_2-Adrenoceptors

Species and tissue	Response	Effects of aging	Ref.
Rat heart	Inhibit tachycardia	Decrease	29
Rat vas deferens	Inhibit twitch	Decrease	31
Rat heart	Inhibit overflow	Decrease	30
Rat vas deferens	Inhibit overflow	No change	31
Human saphenous vein	Inhibit overflow	No change	32
Rat brain	Sympathoinhibitory	Decrease	33
Rat brain	Inhibit overflow	No change	34

and agents such as α-methyl-dopa have been widely used in the elderly (e.g., in a survey of prescribing in Ireland, α-methyl-dopa represented 13% of the cardiovascular drugs prescribed to those over 65).[35] Indeed, it has been shown that the depressor response to clonidine in healthy humans is unaffected by aging.[36] It is difficult to explain this difference between clinical findings and animal studies, unless pharmacokinetic factors or differences in cardiovascular control balance out a reduced response to clonidine at a receptor level.

Other agents which have central or peripheral sympathoinhibitory actions include reserpine, which has been widely used as an antihypertensive agent in the elderly. Little is known of alterations in its effects on the cardiovascular system in aging.

C. VASODILATORS

1. Block Actions of Endogenous Vasoconstrictors

a. α-Adrenoceptor Antagonists

α-Adrenoceptor antagonists lower blood pressure by blocking the vasoconstrictor actions of the catecholamines noradrenaline and adrenaline.

i. α_1-Adrenoceptors

α_1-Adrenoceptors are the predominant subtype of adrenoceptor involved in vasoconstriction, and this is mediated by a G protein-coupled stimulation of phospholipase C, leading to phosphoinositol (PI) hydrolysis. Responsiveness of vascular α_1-adrenergic receptors has been widely studied in relation to aging (Table 4.4); however, most studies have failed to find any change with age in contractile responses of isolated blood vessels or in pressor responses to agonists. Studies of the rat aorta, widely used in aging research, have generally reported a reduced responsiveness during maturation and aging (Table 4.4) or a reduced receptor reserve in tissues from aged rats.[42] The rat aorta may not be the most suitable tissue for the study of age-related changes specifically in α-adrenoceptor function, because the response to a variety of vasoconstrictors including 5-HT and angiotensin are reduced by maturation and aging.[1,42,47] This may suggest that the change occurring in rat aorta is at a postreceptor level, and may make the tissue suitable for investigation of changes in intracellular signaling with age. In rat heart there is some evidence for a decrease in α_1-adrenoceptor ligand binding sites with age, which may be linked to a decrease in PI response.[48,49]

α-Adrenoceptor antagonists, which like all antagonists can only have effects by blocking the actions of endogenous neurotransmitter (thus indirectly demonstrating the ongoing level of nervous control of tissues), can be used to examine changes with age in noradrenergic control of blood pressure. Agents used clinically include older compounds like phentolamine and phenoxybenzamine, and newer compounds such as prazosin and doxazosin. The hypotensive actions of the selective α_1-adrenoceptor antagonist prazosin[45] and the nonselective α_1- and α_2-adrenoceptor antagonist phentolamine[50] are reported to be unchanged by aging in humans, and the hypotensive actions of prazosin are unchanged in the rat[1] and rabbit.[46]

TABLE 4.4.
Effects of Aging on α_1- and α_2-Adrenoceptors

Species and tissue	Response	Effect of aging	Ref.
	α_1-Adrenoceptors		
Human arteries	Contraction to NA	No change	37
Dog arteries	Contraction	No change	38
Rat aorta	Contraction	No change	39
		Decrease	40–42
Rat blood vessels	Contraction	No change	43
		Decrease	44
Human systemic	Pressor	Decrease	45
Rabbit systemic	Pressor	No change	46
Rat systemic	Pressor	No change	47
	α_2-Adrenoceptors		
Human saphenous vein	Contraction	Decrease	32
Rat systemic	Pressor	Decrease	47

ii. α_2-Adrenoceptors

α_2-Adrenoceptors, as well as being present on nerve terminals (see above), are also present postjunctionally on smooth muscle, where like α_1-adrenoceptors they mediate a contraction. Selective α_2-adrenoceptor antagonists have not yet been shown to be useful antihypertensive agents, presumably due to prejunctional actions, although nonselective antagonists such as phentolamine also act on α_2-adrenoceptors. Studies of the effects of aging on α_2-adrenoceptors mediating contractions of smooth muscle have been hindered by the lack of suitable isolated tissues containing α_2- adrenergic receptors. However, the human saphenous vein is an example of a tissue in which contractions to norepinephrine are mediated predominantly, if not exclusively, by α_2-adrenoceptors. In a study of vessels obtained from varicose vein surgery of both male and female (predominantly female) patients, a significant age-related correlation between noradrenaline potency and age has been reported,[51] suggesting that the ability of these veins to respond to sympathetic stimulation is decreased by age and that this may contribute to postural hypotension in the elderly (as discussed later).

Vascular α_2-adrenergic receptors mediating contraction can be relatively easily identified *in vivo*, and the pressor potency of the α_2-adrenoceptor agonist xylazine is reduced by aging in the rat.[47] However, this age-related difference in xylazine pressor potency is abolished by the angiotensin converting enzyme inhibitor captopril, suggesting that an age-related decline in angiotensin levels (or responsiveness) causes the change in α_2-adrenoceptor responsiveness. It is well known that the demonstration of an α_2-adrenoceptor-mediated contraction *in vitro* can be dependent on an on-going contraction to other vasoconstrictors such as angiotensin, and so alterations in levels of angiotensin *in vivo* may also have implications for α_2-responsiveness.

b. 5-Hydroxytryptamine Antagonists

5-Hydroxytryptamine (5-HT), although present as a neurotransmitter in some peripheral nerves, is located mainly in platelets and chromaffin cells in the periphery. 5-HT content of platelets is reported to be decreased by aging in humans,[52] but this decreased content is not due to diminished uptake, since uptake of 5-HT into platelets is reported to increase with age,[53] but is perhaps due to enhanced release.

Most studies looking at the effects of aging on smooth muscle contractions mediated by 5-HT have failed to examine which subtype of 5-HT was involved. However, since the predominant 5-HT receptor mediating contractions in many tissues is the 5-HT$_2$ receptor, it can be assumed, except if noted otherwise, that 5-HT_2 receptors are being examined (these receptors, like α_1-adrenoceptors, are linked to phospholipase C). During aging, most studies report no change in the contractile potency of 5-HT, e.g., there is no change in the constrictor potency to 5-HT (but a large increase in maximum response) with age in dog coronary artery,[54] but a decreased or even increased potency has been reported in the rat aorta (see Reference 1). Increased maximum responses to 5-HT during maturation and aging have also been reported in rat mesenteric artery.[55] In a study of the cerebral circulation, it was found that aging augmented the constrictor response to 5-HT so that cerebral blood flow was decreased by 5-HT only in aged rats.[56] In the human saphenous vein, the potency of 5-HT declined with age in veins obtained from a group of predominantly female patients undergoing varicose vein surgery, and this decline in response involved both 5-HT_1 and 5-HT_2 receptors.[51]

Ketanserin is an antagonist acting at 5-HT_2 receptors, which also has actions as an α_1-adrenoceptor antagonist. The ability of ketanserin to decrease blood pressure is reported to increase with age in humans,[57–59] although this is not true of the selective 5-HT_2 antagonist ritanserin.[60] This may suggest that the actions of ketanserin seen also involve α_1-adrenoceptors or that the pharmacokinetics of ketanserin differ in the elderly. However, other authors have reported that although diastolic pressure was reduced with ketanserin in the elderly, blood pressure control was less effective in ambulatory recordings.[61]

c. *Inhibition of Angiotensin*

Angiotensin, or, more correctly, the renin-angiotensin-aldosterone system, is of importance both in the short-term control of blood pressure and in the long-term control of blood pressure and blood volume. In the short-term control, angiotensin acts both as a direct vasoconstrictor and to facilitate vascular contractions, particularly those involving vascular α_2-adrenoceptors. Pressor responses to α_2-adrenoceptor agonists can be critically dependent on angiotensin: block of angiotensin formation with the converting enzyme inhibitor captopril markedly reduces the pressor response to the α_2-agonist xylazine.[47] Interestingly, while this is true of young rats, in old rats the pressor response to xylazine is much reduced as compared with young rats, and captopril has no effect.[47] Hence, the difference between young and old rats appears to be due to a decreased responsiveness to angiotensin in old rats. Indeed, there are several reports of an age-related decline in the renin-angiotensin-aldosterone system in terms of plasma renin activity, and plasma renin and plasma aldosterone levels (see Reference 62). The precise mechanism of the age-related decline in renin is uncertain, but may be due to altered synthesis due to changes in the aging kidney, high blood pressure, decreased β-adrenoceptor-mediated stimulation of renin release, or perhaps due to the high levels of atrial natriuretic peptide in the elderly, since this peptide exerts an inhibitory effect on renin secretion (see Reference 62). Decreased plasma levels of aldosterone may be due to diminished renin activity, resulting in decreased angiotensin and thus decreased stimulation of aldosterone secretion.

In rat aorta, although responses to angiotensin II, like responses to α_1-adrenoceptor agonists and 5-HT, decrease with increasing age, this change occurs mainly in maturation (see Reference 1). Hence, the rat aorta may not be the most useful model of the effects of aging on blood vessel function. The vasoconstrictor response to angiotensin is reported to be unchanged by aging in the human vasculature,[63] but the number of binding sites on human platelet for angiotensin is reported to increase with age,[64] perhaps due to receptor up-regulation in response to diminished plasma levels of angiotensin II.

Despite the decline in plasma renin activity, angiotensin-converting enzyme inhibitors such as captopril (which prevent the formation of angiotensin II from angiotensin I) still lower blood pressure in elderly hypertensives.[61,65] However, captopril may have more than one mechanism of action in lowering blood pressure since it also prolongs the actions of bradykinin, which causes endothelium-dependent relaxations (see Section IV.C.2). In particular, it has been suggested that angiotensin-converting enzyme inhibitors may be particularly useful for elderly hypertensive patients with congestive heart failure,[61] and have been shown to be useful in the treatment of heart failure in the very old.[66]

d. *Endothelin Antagonist*

Endothelin is a potent vasoconstrictor peptide released from the endothelium. In studies of the rat aorta, it has been reported that the contractile response decreases during maturation with no further change in aging,[67] although contractile responses to a variety of agents including norepinephrine and 5-HT decline with maturation in this vessel (see above). The potency of endothelin is reported to decrease with age in rat perfused blood vessels,[68] and the vasoconstrictor response to endothelin increased with age in rat coronary artery, although this latter effect appears to be due to diminished endothelial function with age.[69] Antagonism of the actions of endothelin may represent a future strategy for antihypertensive therapy in the elderly.[70]

e. *Blockade of Vasoconstriction Involving Other Autonomic Neurotransmitters*

In recent years, it has become clear that the peripheral nervous system contains, in addition to NA and acetylcholine (ACh), many amine neurotransmitters such as 5-HT and dopamine, as well as peptides such as neuropeptide Y, vasoactive intestinal polypeptide, calcitonin gene-related peptide, and substance P, which may be involved in the innervation of certain blood vessels. Additionally, the hormone vasopressin has a major role in the control of blood pressure, and its secretion in response to increased blood osmolality is increased with age.[71,72] However, little or nothing is known about the effects of aging on responses to these other neurotransmitters, and little is known of the therapeutic potential of blocking the actions of any of these agents.

2. MIMIC ENDOGENOUS VASODILATORS

a. *NO Donors*

The endothelium is the main barrier to the passage of substances from the blood to the tissues, but also functions as an endocrine gland to modulate vascular resistance. Whereas some vasodilators such as adrenaline and ANP produce vasodilatation by action at receptors on vascular smooth muscle, various physiological and pharmacological stimuli cause release of a substance from the endothelium, endothelium-dependent relaxant factor (EDRF), thought to be nitric oxide (NO),[73] which acts on vascular smooth muscle to stimulate the enzyme guanylate cyclase, and so cause vascular relaxation (see Figure 4.3). The nitrovasodilators such as glyceryl trinitrite and sodium nitroprusside act in the same way as EDRF by releasing NO, stimulating guanylate cyclase to produce relaxation by increasing cGMP levels.

In isolated tissues, nitrovasodilators such as nitroglycerine, nitrite, or nitroprusside produce powerful relaxations of a magnitude sufficient to abolish the precontraction, whereas the relaxation to other relaxants may be submaximal. Hence, one problem in investigating age-related changes in responses to nitrovasodilators is to ensure that the response is not supramaximal to allow age-related changes to be seen. This is illustrated by Figure 4.4, which shows altered relaxations during maturation in the rat aorta. There was a diminished relaxation to isoprenaline during maturation whether tissues were precontracted with KCl 20 or 40 m*M*, but diminished response to nitroprusside was only seen with KCl 40 m*M*. Responses to nitrovasodilators are also reported to decline during maturation and aging in rabbit aorta.[74] Responses were unaltered by aging in rat mesenteric artery[55] and in rabbit portal vein.[74]

The nitrovasodilator sodium nitroprusside is more effective at decreasing blood pressure in old than in young humans[75,76] and conscious rats,[77] presumably due to a diminished baroreflex compensation (see later), since the depressor response to sodium nitroprusside was little affected by age in pentobarbitone-anesthetized rats in which the baroreflex is markedly attenuated.[1] Indeed, in the latter study, the calcium entry blocker nifedipine proved to be more effective in the elderly than sodium nitroprusside.

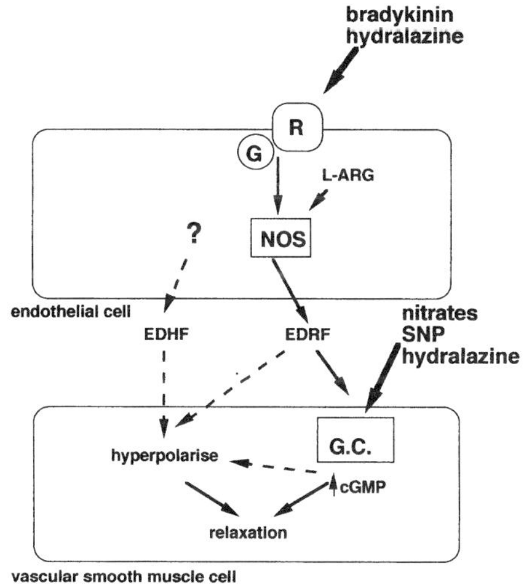

FIGURE 4.3. Schematic representation of endothelium-dependent or NO donor actions of vasodilator drugs. Agents such as bradykinin (actions potentiated by ACE inhibitors) and possibly hydralazine act to stimulate nitric oxide synthase (NOS) to produce nitric oxide (NO) from L-arginine (L-ARG), which acts on vascular smooth muscle cells to stimulate guanylate cyclase (GC), and the resultant increase in cGMP produces relaxation. Endothelium-dependent relaxation can also be produced by membrane hyperpolarization, due probably to NO, or possibly another relaxant factor termed endothelium-dependent hyperpolarizing factor (EDHF). Agents such as nitrites, sodium nitroprusside (SNP), and hydralazine are thought to produce relaxation by stimulation of GC as NO donors. Note: R, receptor; G, G protein.

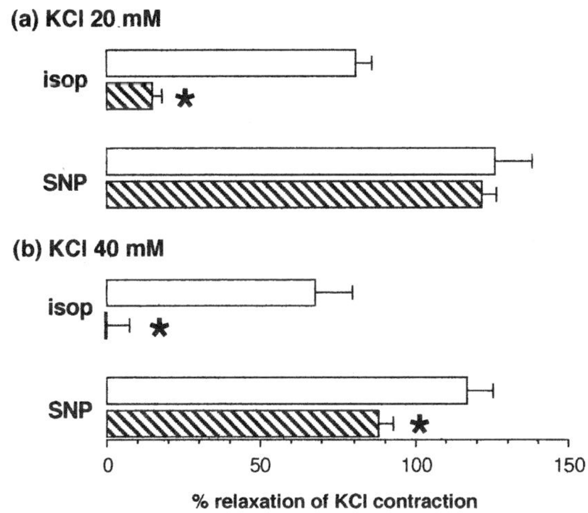

FIGURE 4.4. Relaxations to the β-adrenoceptor agonist isoprenaline (isop) and the NO donor sodium nitroprusside (SNP) in aorta from immature (6-week-old: open columns) and adult (6-month-old: hatched columns) rats, contracted with (a) KCl 20 m*M* or (b) 40 m*M*. Asterisks denote significant age-related changes. Note that responses to isop are significantly reduced in tissues from adult animals whether contracted with KCl 20 or 40 m*M*, whereas responses to SNP were only significantly reduced in tissues from adult animals contracted with KCl 40 m*M*.[1,41,91]

Endothelium-dependent relaxations (EDR) to histamine and ACh are reported to be unchanged by aging in rat basilar artery,[78] whereas EDR to ACh or bradykinin are significantly reduced in rat cerebral arteries, without change in the relaxation to nitroglycerine.[79] In systemic arteries, relaxations to ACh are generally reported to be unchanged or decreased in maturation and aging.[1] It has been reported for the rat coronary artery that a diminished endothelial function, as demonstrated by an age-related decrease in the relaxation to ACh, results in an age-related increase in the contractile response to endothelin (since endothelin presumably acts directly to contract the artery and indirectly via release of NO to relax the artery).[69] Similarly, in rat cerebral arterioles, the relaxation to ADP was decreased in aging and the response to 5-HT was changed from a small relaxation to a small contraction.[79] In rat mesenteric artery, EDR and hyperpolarizations to ACh were impaired by aging in SHR and Wistar-Kyoto rats,[80] and EDR to histamine were impaired in normotensive Wistar rats.[81] There is a decrease with age in the EDR to ACh in dog coronary artery[54] and dog mesenteric artery.[82] An increase in sensitivity to methacholine has been reported during maturation in rat aorta and tail artery with no change in the response to the calcium ionophore A23187, suggesting an alteration in the ability of muscarinic agonists to release EDRF.[39]

Many of these studies have looked at the effects of aging on vascular relaxations mediated by EDRF in terms of the ability of a substance like histamine to cause vascular relaxation; age-related changes may occur not only in the effects of EDRF, but also in the ability of the substance to release EDRF, loss of endothelial cells, or in the tissue response to activation of guanylate cyclase. Hydralazine, which has been widely used in elderly hypertensives, may, for convenience, be included in this section, as its arterial vasodilator actions are thought to be due, at least in part, to release of and formation of NO. There is a report that the fall in peripheral resistance per milligram of hydralazine is greater in patients over 70 years,[83] although this may reflect diminished baroreflex function.

b. *Other Potential Agents*

At physiological concentrations, atriopeptin increases sodium excretion with little effect on blood pressure in humans, although it will decrease blood pressure in higher concentrations. Despite increased resting plasma levels of atriopeptin,[84] the elderly have a reduced ability to excrete a saline load, at least partly due to the up to 50% decrease in renal blood flow which occurs during aging (see References 72, 85). The higher plasma levels of atriopeptin found in the elderly may be caused by a decreased clearance,[86] a decreased renal responsiveness to atriopeptin, or to the increased atrial pressure (increased preload resulting in increased ventricular volumes) found in the elderly. In humans, there is a report of an age-related increase in skin blood flow to atriopeptin,[87] although vascular actions of atriopeptin are less important physiologically than the renal actions. Whether or not a mimetic of the actions of atriopeptin will be a useful antihypertensive agent remains to be seen.

3. BLOCK OR OPEN ION CHANNELS

a. *Calcium Entry Blockers*

In humans, there has been speculation as to whether or not certain types of antihypertensive therapy may be especially effective in lowering blood pressure in the elderly, with reports that calcium entry blockers such as nifedipine[19] are more effective at lowering blood pressure in the elderly. However, results in these clinical studies are complicated by hypertension and by baroreflex function.

In a study in anesthetized rats, in which baroreflex function is considerably dampened, the NO donor sodium nitroprusside was less effective than the calcium entry blocker nifedipine and the β-adrenoceptor agonist isoprenaline at lowering blood pressure in old rats.[88] This study was complicated by the fact that diastolic blood pressure was significantly lower in the aged anesthetized rats, so that sodium nitroprusside was more effective at lowering blood pressure in the young than the old (in terms of absolute falls in blood pressure), but this difference may have been due to differences in resting diastolic blood pressure, since the minimum diastolic blood pressure reached during sodium nitroprusside infusion was similar in young and old rats. However, in contrast, nifedipine and isoprenaline were as effective in absolute terms at lowering blood pressure in young and old rats so that these agents were relatively more effective than sodium nitroprusside at lowering blood pressure in aged rats.[88]

Hence, nifedipine is at least as effective in old as in young rats in terms of absolute fall in blood pressure, but more effective in old in terms of percentage falls in pressure.

At the isolated tissue level, there are reports that diltiazem has increased effectiveness against noradrenaline (NA), but unchanged effectiveness against 5-HT or KCl, in rat aorta, although the potency of diltiazem against Ca^{2+} decreased with age.[42] No change in the response to diltiazem was found with age in rat pulmonary artery.[42] Other authors report no age-related change in the response to verapamil,[89] but a small age-related increase in the potency of nifedipine[90] in rat aorta.

Calcium channel blockers like nimodipine can reduce the decline in motor and cognitive function in aged rats, at least partly by altering microvascular structure,[91] so that the decline may be due to a dominance of vasoconstrictor over vasodilator influences. At the cardiac level, verapamil produced greater depression of spontaneous pacemaker activity in right atria from senescent than adult rats.[92]

b. Potassium Channel Openers

Potassium channel openers cause K^+ to leave cells, resulting in hyperpolarization and thus vascular relaxation. Relatively few studies have examined the effects of aging on responses to these agents. In rat mesenteric artery, hyperpolarizations and relaxations to the potassium channel opener cromakalin were relatively unaffected by aging,[80] with small increases in SHR with age and small decreases in Wistar rats with age.

4. Interfere with Second Messengers

Inhibitors of PDE act to increase cellular levels of cAMP and cGMP. Increased cAMP and cGMP have similar actions in vascular smooth muscle to cause relaxation, but opposing actions in cardiac muscle, causing cardiac stimulation and inhibition, respectively. Agents used clinically include milrinone and enoximone, which selectively inhibit PDE III which hydrolyzes only cAMP, producing vasodilatation and increasing cardiac contractility, making them useful in the treatment of heart failure.

Many studies of isolated blood vessels have looked at how aging affects the response to PDE inhibition. In rat aorta, some authors report a significant decrease in the relaxation to the nonselective PDE inhibitor isobutyl-methylxanthine (IBMX) during maturation, with similar change occurring in the relaxation to β-adrenoceptor agonists, forskolin (which activates adenylate cyclase), and to sodium nitroprusside (see Figure 4.5). This may suggest that during maturation in rat aorta, there is a decreased responsiveness to the intracellular signals cAMP and cGMP (see Reference 1), perhaps due to an increased activity of PDE in maturation.[26] Other authors report that responses to β-adrenoceptor agonists and adenosine decrease with aging in rat aorta with no change in responses to forskolin, IBMX, or in EDR to ACh,[93,94] suggesting that the age-related alteration is at the level of the G protein.[93] A decline in response to forskolin and PDE inhibitors has been reported in rat mesenteric artery[55] during maturation. Despite many reports of reduced vasodilator responses to β-adrenoceptor agonists in isolated tissues, particularly arteries (e.g., Reference 74; see Reference 1), no change in potency or maximum depressor response to β-adrenoceptor agonists was found during aging in the human vasculature *in vivo* (terbutaline).[95] Hence, differences found in isolated tissues are not always reflected in changes in overall cardiovascular responsiveness, especially when other factors such as reflexes come into play.

V. AUTONOMIC REFLEX FUNCTION

The aging cardiovascular system is likely to have an altered responsiveness to a whole range of antihypertensive and vasodilator agents due to altered cardiovascular reflex function. Cardiovascular homeostatic reflexes have evolved particularly to maintain blood flow to vital organs in hypotensive situations, and hence come into play when drugs alter blood pressure.

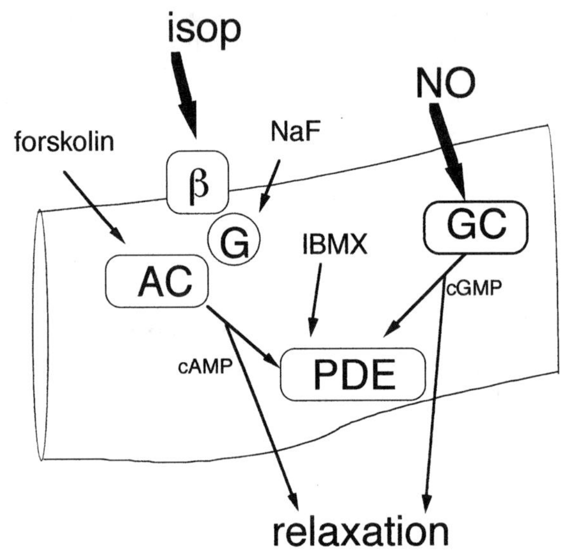

FIGURE 4.5. Schematic representation of the mode of action of vasodilator drugs. Isoprenaline (isop) binds to β-adrenoceptors (β_2) to activate adenylate cyclase (AC) via the G protein G_s. Increased production of cAMP produces vascular relaxation, the cAMP being metabolized by phosphodiesterase (PDE). Nitric oxide (NO) or NO donors act to stimulate guanylate cyclase (GC), and increased production of cGMP results in relaxation, the cGMP being metabolized by PDE. Sodium fluoride (NaF) stimulates G_s, forskolin stimulates AC, and IBMX inhibits PDE.

The most important short-term autonomic cardiovascular reflex is the baroreflex mediated by the baroreceptors in the aortic arch and carotid sinus, which respond to stretch of the blood vessel wall produced by changes in blood pressure.

Baroreflex function is measured in terms of the tachycardia to falls in blood pressure produced by a vasodilator, or in terms of the bradycardia to rises in blood pressure produced by a vasoconstrictor, and so may involve both sympathetic and vagal function. A fall in blood pressure is detected by the baroreceptors, which act via the medulla to cause sympathetic activation to produce vasoconstriction, and cardiac chronotropic (heart rate) and inotropic (force of contraction) effects in an attempt to counteract the fall in pressure. Baroreflex sensitivity is reported to be reduced by aging in humans[96] and rats.[77,97] Increased arterial stiffness occurs with aging (see Reference 8), and such could explain diminished baroreflexes, but the baroreflex could equally well be altered due to diminished central integration, diminished efferent nerve activity, or diminished target organ response to transmitter. Agents with direct vasodilator actions might be expected to be more effective at lowering blood pressure in the elderly, due to diminished reflex compensation.

A. POSTURAL HYPOTENSION

On assuming the upright position, the effects of gravity result in a shifting of about 10 to 15% of the total blood volume to the lower limbs, and most of this shift occurs in the first 2 to 3 min after standing.[98] This shift in blood results in a fall in systemic blood pressure which results in baroreflex compensation. The immediate compensation is a tachycardia to increase cardiac output. Smith et al.[4] examined the effects of graded tilting from the supine to upright position and found similar increases in leg volume (as a measure of pooling of blood in the legs) in young and old, but diminished increases in heart rate and diastolic pressure in the elderly group.

The incidence of postural hypotension is reported to increase in the elderly so that postural hypotension becomes common with an overall incidence of as high as 24%,[99] or as low as 6.4% in a group of elderly in which other risk factors for postural hypotension were excluded.[100] Various factors can explain differences between studies in the incidence of postural hypotension in the elderly, including drug therapy. Vasodilators of differing classes do not have similar propensities to cause postural hypotension. In theory, agents which cause direct or indirect vasodilatation while allowing sympathetic reflexes to counteract postural change should not cause a major incidence of postural hypotension, but may be more likely to cause reflex tachycardia. Some drugs in particular may predispose to postural hypotension such as those which interfere with the baroreflex at the vascular level — α-adrenoceptor antagonists, calcium entry blockers. Diminished baroreflex function, diminished venous tone, reduced function of the skeletal muscle pump which squeezes blood back to the heart, failing venous valves, or drug therapy may contribute to susceptibility to postural hypotension (see Table 4.5). There is evidence that with increasing age, the human saphenous vein responds less well to norepinephrine or noradrenergic nerve stimulation so that its ability to contract in response to noradrenergic nerve activation is diminished.[31,51] This failure to contract sufficiently may result in decreased ability to mobilize blood from the veins during postural change.

TABLE 4.5.
Possible Causes of Age-Related Increase in Incidence of Postural Hypotension

Factor	Effects of aging
Baroreflex	Decreased function
Tachycardia	Decreased
Vasoconstriction	Decreased
Veniconstriction	Decreased
Cardiac function	Decreased β-adrenoceptor function
	Increased cardiac work
Vasculature	Large increase systolic pressure
	Increased diastolic pressure
	Decline of renin-angiotensin system
	Blood volume decrease
Venous function	Skeletal muscle pump decreased?
	Decreased response to norepinephrine
	Venous valves: decreased function?
Postprandial hypotension	Increased incidence
Vasodilator drug therapy	Increased prescribing
	Increased effectiveness?
	Cardiovascular side effects of other therapy
Underlying disease	Increased incidence

VI. SUMMARY

Our knowledge of the effects of aging on the cardiovascular system and how it affects the responses to vasodilators and antihypertensive agents is clearly incomplete. One must also consider whether changes reported are due to aging, per se, or to a combination of aging and underlying pathology. Calcium entry blockers and the 5-HT_2 receptor antagonist ketanserin, but not β-adrenoceptor antagonists, are claimed to be especially effective in the elderly. However, it is perhaps less important to find antihypertensive agents that are more effective at lowering pressure in the elderly as compared to young hypertensives than to find useful antihypertensive agents effective in the elderly with few side effects, whether or not they are more or less effective in the young. Angiotension converting enzyme inhibitors (despite the reported decline in the renin-angiotension system with age: see above), α-methyldopa, and verapamil have all been shown to be beneficial in the treatment of hypertension and/or heart failure in the elderly. Because left ventricular hypertrophy is linked to morbidity in the elderly, treatments have been sought that can regress myocardial hypertrophy.

Side effects may make effective antihypertensive agents less useful in the elderly: postural hypotension may make vasodilators less useful; cardiodepressant actions may make β-blockers and some calcium entry blockers unsuitable in those with congestive heart failure; and centrally acting agents may be less useful due to sedation. Glomerular filtration rate decreases with age, and this decline is accompanied by a decrease in renal clearance of drugs, resulting in the need to prescribe lower doses in the elderly.

Studies at the tissue, cellular, and molecular level are leading to an increased understanding of the cardiovascular system and how it is altered in aging: the crucial protective role of the vascular endothelium in preventing cardiovascular disease has only recently been elucidated.

ACKNOWLEDGMENTS

Work carried out in the author's laboratory was supported by the Health Research Board (Ireland), the Royal College of Surgeons in Ireland, and the Irish Heart Foundation.

REFERENCES

1. **Docherty, J. R.,** Cardiovascular responses in aging: a review, *Pharmacol. Rev.*, 42, 103, 1990.
2. **Lakatta, E. G., Cohen, J. D., Fleg, J. L., Frohlich, E. D., and Gradman, A. H.,** Hypertension in the elderly: age- and disease-related complications and therapeutic implications, *Cardiovasc. Drugs Ther.*, 7, 643, 1993.
3. **Guyton, A. C.,** *Cardiac Output and Its Regulation*, W. B. Saunders, Philadelphia, 1963.
4. **Smith, J. J., Hughes, C. V., Ptacin, M. J., Barney, J. A., Tristani, F. E., and Ebert, T. J.,** The effect of age on hemodynamic response to graded postural stress in normal men, *J. Gerontol.*, 42, 406, 1987.
5. **Kotchen, J. M., McKean, H. E., and Kotchen, T. A.,** Blood pressure trends with aging, *Hypertension*, 4 (Suppl. III), III–128, 1982.
6. **Ikeme, A. C.,** Hypertension studies in developing countries, *Clin. Exp. Hypertension*, A11, 825, 1989.
7. **Probstfield, J. L., Applegate, W. B., Borhani, N. O., Curb, J. D., Cutler, J. A., Davis, B. R., Furberg, C. D., Hawkins, C. M., Lakatos, E., Page, L. B., Perry, H. M., Schron, E., and Smith, W. M.,** The systolic hypertension in the elderly program (SHEP): an intervention trial on isolated systolic hypertension, *Clin. Exp. Hypertension*, A11, 973, 1989.
8. **De Meersman, R. E.,** Aging as a modulator of respiratory sinus arrhythmia, *J. Gerontol.*, 48, B74, 1993.
9. **Imai, Y., Abe, K., Minami, N., Nihei, M., Munakata, M., Sakuma, H., Hashimoto, J., Imai, K., Sekino, H., and Yoshinaga, K.,** Influence of age on the nocturnal fall of blood pressure and its modulation by long-acting calcium antagonists, *Clin. Exp. Hypertension*, A12, 1077, 1990.
10. **Vestal, R. E., Wood, A. J. J., and Shand, D. G.,** Reduced beta-adrenoceptor sensitivity in the elderly, *Clin. Pharmacol. Ther.*, 26, 181, 1979.
11. **Yin, F. C. P., Spurgeon, H. A., Greene, H. L., Lakatta, E. G., and Weisfeldt, M. L.,** Age-associated decrease in heart rate response to isoproterenol in dogs, *Mech. Ageing Dev.*, 10, 17, 1978.
12. **Simpkins, J. W., Field, F. P., and Ress, R. J.,** Age-related decline in adrenergic responsiveness of the kidney, heart and aorta of male rats, *Neurobiol. Aging*, 4, 233, 1983.
13. **Borton, M. and Docherty, J. R.,** The effects of aging on neuronal uptake of noradrenaline in the rat, *Naunyn-Schmiedeberg's Arch. Pharmacol.*, 340, 139, 1989.
14. **Narayanan, N. and Derby, J. A.,** Alterations in the properties of beta-adrenergic receptors of myocardial membranes in aging: impairments in agonist-receptor interactions and guanine nucleotide regulation accompany diminished catecholamine responsiveness of adenylate cyclase, *Mech. Ageing Dev.*, 19, 127, 1982.
15. **Tumer, N., Houck, W. T., and Roberts, J.,** Upregulation of adrenergic beta-receptor subtypes in the senescent rat heart, *Mech. Ageing Dev.*, 49, 235, 1989.
16. **Fan, T. H.-M. and Banerjee, S. P.,** Age-related reduction of beta-adrenoceptor sensitivity in rat heart occurs by multiple mechanisms, *Gerontology*, 31, 373, 1985.
17. **Kusiak, J. W. and Pitha, J.,** Decreased response with age of the cardiac catecholamine sensitive adenylate cyclase system, *Life Sci.*, 33, 1679, 1983.

18. **Miyamoto, A., Kawana, S., Kimura, H., and Ohshika, H.,** Impaired expression of $G_{s\alpha}$ protein mRNA in rat ventricular myocardium with aging, *Eur. J. Pharmacol.,* 266, 147, 1994.
19. **Buhler, F. R.,** Age and cardiovascular response adaptation. Determinants of an antihypertensive treatment concept primarily based on beta-blockers and calcium entry blockers, *Hypertension,* 5 (Suppl. III), III-94, 1983.
20. **Greenberg, G., Brennan, P. J., and Miall, W. E.,** Effects of diuretic and beta-blocker therapy in the Medical Research Council Trial, *Am. J. Med.,* 76, 45, 1984.
21. **Klein, C., Gerber, J. G., Gal, J., and Nies, A. S.,** Beta-adrenergic receptors in the elderly are not less sensitive to timolol, *Clin. Pharmacol. Ther.,* 40, 161, 1986.
22. **Coope, J. and Warrender, T. S.,** Randomised treatment of hypertension in primary care, *Br. Med. J.,* 291, 1145, 1985.
23. **Conway, J., Wheeler, R., and Sannerstedt, R.,** Sympathetic nervous activity during exercise in relation to age, *Cardiovasc. Res.,* 5, 577, 1971.
24. **Xiao, R.-P. and Lakatta, E. G.,** Mechanisms of altered β-adrenergic modulation of the cardiovascular system with aging, *Rev. Clin. Gerontol.,* 1, 309, 1991.
25. **Robberecht, P., Gillard, M., Waelbroeck, M., Camus, J.-C., De Neef, P., and Christophe, J.,** Alterations of rat cardiac adenylate cyclase activity with age, *Eur. J. Pharmacol.,* 126, 91, 1986.
26. **Schoffter, P. and Stoclet, J.-C.,** Age-related differences in cyclic AMP metabolism and their consequences on relaxation induced by isoproterenol and phosphodiesterase inhibitors in rat isolated aorta, *Mech. Ageing Dev.,* 54, 197, 1990.
27. **Deisher, T. A., Mankani, S., and Hoffman, B. B.,** Role of cyclic AMP-dependent protein kinase in the diminished BBBB-adrenergic responsiveness of vascular smooth muscle with increasing age, *J. Pharmacol. Exp. Ther.,* 249, 812, 1989.
28. **Starke, K.,** Regulation of noradrenaline release by presynaptic systems, *Rev. Physiol. Biochem. Pharmacol.,* 77, 1, 1977.
29. **Docherty, J. R. and Hyland, L.,** Alpha-adrenoceptor responsiveness in the aged rat, *Eur. J. Pharmacol.,* 126, 75, 1986.
30. **Daly, R. N., Goldberg, P. B., and Roberts, J.,** The effect of age on presynaptic $alpha_2$ adrenoceptor autoregulation of norepinephrine release, *J. Gerontol.,* 44, 859, 1989.
31. **Hyland, L. and Docherty, J. R.,** Further examination of the effects of aging on the adrenoceptor responsiveness of the rat vas deferens, *Eur. J. Pharmacol.,* 110, 241, 1986
32. **Hyland, L. and Docherty, J. R.,** An investigation of age-related changes in pre- and postjunctional α-adrenergic receptors in human saphenous vein, *Eur. J. Pharmacol.,* 110, 241, 1985.
33. **Nistico, G., De Sarro, G. B., Bagetta, G., and Mollace, V.,** Altered sensitivity of alpha 2-adrenoceptors in the brain during aging in rats, *Ann. N.Y. Acad. Sci.,* 673, 206, 1992.
34. **Schlicker, E., Betz, R., and Gothert, M.,** Investigation into the age-dependence of release of serotonin and noradrenaline in the rat brain cortex and of autoreceptor-mediated modulation of release, *Neuropharmacology,* 28, 811, 1989.
35. **Nolan, L. and O'Malley, K.,** Age-related prescribing patterns in general practice, *Comp. Gerontol. A,* 1, 97, 1987.
36. **Klein, C. E., Gerber, J. G. and Nies, A. S.,** Lack of an effect of age on the response to clonidine, *Clin. Pharmacol. Ther.,* 47, 61, 1990.
37. **Scott, P. J. W. and Reid, J. L.,** The effect of age on the response of human isolated arteries to noradrenaline, *Br. J. Clin. Pharmacol.,* 13, 237, 1982.
38. **Toda, N. and Shimizu, I.,** Neuroeffector function in mesenteric arteries isolated from beagles of different ages, *J. Pharmacol. Exp. Ther.,* 240, 223, 1987.
39. **Hynes, M. R. and Duckles, S. P.,** Effect of increasing age on the endothelium-mediated relaxation of rat blood vessels in vitro, *J. Pharmacol. Exp. Ther.,* 241, 387, 1987.
40. **Tuttle, R. S.,** Age related changes in the sensitivity of rat aortic strips to norepinephrine and associated chemical and structural alterations, *J. Gerontol.,* 21, 510, 1966.
41. **Hyland, L., Warnock, P., and Docherty, J. R.,** Age-related alterations in α_1- and β-adrenoceptor mediated responsiveness of rat aorta, *Naunyn-Schmiedeberg's Arch. Pharmacol.,* 335, 50, 1987.
42. **Wanstall, J. C. and O'Donnell, S. R.,** Inhibition of norepinephrine contractions by diltiazem on aorta and pulmonary artery from young and aged rats: influence of alpha-adrenoceptor reserve, *J. Pharmacol. Exp. Ther.,* 245, 1016, 1988.
43. **Duckles, S. P., Carter, B. J., and Williams, C. L.,** Vascular adrenergic neuroeffector function does not decline in aged rats, *Circ. Res.,* 56, 109, 1985.
44. **Fouda, A.-K. and Atkinson, J.,** Sensitivity to noradrenaline and electrical stimulation decreases with age in the rat tail artery, *Naunyn-Schmiedeberg's Arch. Pharmacol.,* 334, 37, 1986.
45. **Elliott, H. L., Sumner, D. J., McLean, K., and Reid, J. L.,** Effect of age on the responsiveness of vascular alpha-adrenoceptors in man, *J. Cardiovasc. Pharmacol.,* 4, 388, 1982.

46. **Dalrymple, H. W., Hamilton, C. A., and Reid, J. L.,** The effect of age on peripheral alpha-adrenoceptors in vivo and in vitro in the rabbit, *Br. J. Pharmacol.*, 77, 322P, 1982.
47. **Docherty, J. R.,** The effects of ageing on vascular alpha-adrenoceptors in pithed rat and rat aorta, *Eur. J. Pharmacol.*, 146, 1, 1988.
48. **Miyamoto, A. and Ohshika, H.,** Age-related changes in [^{3}H]prazosin binding and phosphoinositide hydrolysis in rat ventricular myocardium, *Gen. Pharmacol.*, 20, 647, 1989.
49. **Borst, S. E., Narang, N., Crews, F. T., and Scarpace, P. J.,** Reduced alpha-1 adrenergic receptor-mediated inositide hydrolysis in cardiac atria of senescent rats, *J. Cardiovasc. Pharmacol.*, 16, 444, 1990.
50. **Buhler, F. R., Kiowski, W., Van Brummelen, P., Amann, F. W., Bertal, O., Landemann, R., Lutold, B.-E., and Bolli, P.,** Plasma catecholamines and cardiac, renal and peripheral vascular adrenoceptor mediated responses in different age groups in normal and hypertensive subjects, *Clin. Exp. Hypertension*, 2, 409, 1980.
51. **Docherty, J. R.,** Effects of aging on the vasoconstrictor responses to norepinephrine and 5-hydroxytryptamine in the human saphenous vein, *Cardiol. Elderly*, 1, 327, 1993.
52. **Shuttleworth, R. D. and O'Brien, J. R.,** Intraplatelet serotonin and plasma 5-hydroxyindoles in health and disease, *Blood*, 57, 505, 1981.
53. **Marazziti, D., Falcone, M., Rotondo, A., and Castrogiovanni, P.,** Age-related differences in human platelet 5-HT uptake, *Naunyn-Schmiedeberg's Arch. Pharmacol.*, 340, 593, 1989.
54. **Toda, N., Bian, K., and Inoue, S.,** Age-related changes in the response to vasoconstrictor and dilator agents in isolated beagle coronary arteries, *Naunyn-Schmiedeberg's Arch. Pharmacol.*, 336, 359, 1987.
55. **Tsujimoto, G., Lee, C.-H., and Hoffman, B. B.,** Age-related decrease in beta-adrenergic receptor-mediated vascular smooth muscle relaxation, *J. Pharmacol. Exp. Ther.*, 239, 411, 1986.
56. **Hajdu, M. A., McElmurry, R. T., Heistad, D. D., and Baumbach, G. L.,** Effects of aging on cerebral vascular responses to serotonin in rats, *Am. J. Physiol.*, 264, H2136, 1993.
57. **De Cree, J., Hoing, M., de Ryck, M., and Symoems, J.,** The acute antihypertensive effect of ketanserin increases with age, *J. Cardiovasc. Pharmacol.*, 7, S126, 1985.
58. **Rosendorff, C. and Murray, G. D.,** Ketanserin versus metoprolol and hydrochlorothiazide in essential hypertension: only ketanserin's hypotensive effect is age-related, *J. Hypertension*, 4, S109, 1988.
59. **Duggan, J., Kilfeather, S., Lightman, S., and O'Malley, K.,** The effect of age on platelet angiotensin II and ANP receptor density, *Br. J. Clin. Pharmacol.*, 26, 629P, 1988.
60. **Blauw, G. J., Van Brummelen, P., Chang, P. C., Vermrij, P., and Van Zwieten, P. A.,** Arterial dilatation and venous constriction induced by serotonin in the elderly, *Drugs*, 36 (Suppl. 1), 74, 1988.
61. **O'Malley, K., Cox, J. P., and O'Brien, E.,** Choice of drug treatment for elderly hypertensive patients, *Am. J. Med.*, 90 (Suppl. 3A), 27S, 1991.
62. **Bauer, J. H.,** Age-related changes in the renin-aldosterone system, *Drugs Aging*, 3, 238, 1993.
63. **Rosendorff, C., Kalliatakis, B., Radford, H. M., and Patton, J.,** Age-dependence of the pressor sensitivity to noradrenaline and angiotensin II during calcium channel blockade in hypertensive patients, *J. Cardiovasc. Pharmacol.*, 12, S69, 1988.
64. **Breckenridge, A.,** Aging, serotonin and ketanserin, *Drugs*, 36 (Suppl. 1), 44, 1988.
65. **Breckenridge, A.,** Age-related effects of angiotensin converting enzyme inhibitors, *J. Cardiovasc. Pharmacol.*, 12 (Suppl. 8), S100, 1988.
66. **De Bock, V., Mets, T., Romagnoli, M., and Derde, M. P.,** Captopril treatment of chronic heart failure in the very old, *J. Gerontol.*, 49, M148, 1994.
67. **Ishihata, A., Katano, Y., Morinobu, S., and Endoh, M.,** Influence of aging on the contractile response to endothelin of rat thoracic aorta, *Eur. J. Pharmacol.*, 200, 199, 1991.
68. **Dohi, Y. and Luscher, T. F.,** Aging differentially affects direct and indirect actions of endothelin-1 in perfused mesenteric resistance arteries of the rat, *Br. J. Pharmacol.*, 100, 889, 1990.
69. **Katano, Y., Ishihata, A., Morinobu, S., and Endoh, M.,** Modulation by aging of the coronary vascular response to endothelin-1 in the rat isolated perfused heart, *Naunyn-Schmiedeberg's Arch. Pharmacol.*, 348, 82, 1993.
70. **Levesque, H., Moore, N., Cailleux, N., Richard, V., Thuillez, C., and Courtois, H.,** Endothelins. A potential target for pharmacological intervention in diseases of the elderly, *Drugs Aging*, 4, 221, 1994.
71. **Vargas, E., Lye, M., Fargher, E. B., Goddard, C., Moser, B., and Davies, I.,** Cardiovascular haemodynamics and the response of vasopressin, aldosterone, plasma renin activity and plasma catecholamines to head-up tilt in young and old healthy subject, *Age Aging*, 15, 17, 1986.
72. **Davis, P. J. and Davis, F. B.,** Water excretion in the elderly, *Endocrinol. Aging*, 16, 867, 1987.
73. **Furchgott, R. F.,** Studies on endothelium-dependent vasodilation and the endothelium-derived relaxing factor, *Acta Physiol. Scand.*, 139, 257, 1990.
74. **Fleisch, J. H. and Hooker, C. S.,** The relationship between age and relaxation of vascular smooth muscle in the rabbit and rat, *Circ. Res.*, 38, 243, 1976.
75. **McGarry, K., Laher, M., Fitzgerald, D., Horgan, J., O'Brien, E., and O'Malley, K.,** Baroreflex function in elderly hypertensives, *Hypertension*, 5, 765, 1983.

76. **Irvine, N. A. and Shepherd, A. M. M.,** Age and blood pressure determine vasodepressor response to sodium nitroprusside, *J. Cardiovasc. Pharmacol.,* 6, 816, 1984.
77. **Docherty, J. R., Fitzgerald, D., and O'Malley, K.,** Age-related reduction of baroreflex tachycardia without loss of β-adrenoceptor-mediated tachycardia in Sprague-Dawley rats, *J. Cardiovasc. Pharmacol.,* 8, 376, 1986.
78. **Hamel, E., Assumel-Lurden, C., Bouloy, M., and MacKenzie, E. T.,** Selective age-related changes in neuronal markers and smooth muscle reactivity in cerebrovascular beads of Fischer F344 rats, *Neurobiol. Aging,* 11, 631, 1990.
79. **Mayhan, W. G., Faraci, F. M., Baumbach, G. L., and Heistad, D. D.,** Effects of aging on responses of cerebral arteries, *Am. J. Physiol.,* 258, H1138, 1990.
80. **Fujii, K., Ohmori, S., Tominaga, M., Abe, I., Takata, Y., Ohya, Y., Kobayashi, K., and Fujishima, M.,** Age-related changes in endothelium-dependent hyperpolarization in the rat mesenteric artery, *Am. J. Physiol.,* 265, H509, 1993.
81. **Moritoki, H., Hosoki, E., and Ishida, Y.,** Age-related decrease in endothelium-dependent dilator response to histamine in rat mesenteric artery, *Eur. J. Pharmacol.,* 126, 61, 1986.
82. **Shimizu, I. and Toda, N.,** Alterations with age of the response to vasodilator agents in isolated mesenteric arteries of the beagle, *Br. J. Pharmacol.,* 89, 769, 1986.
83. **Rowell, N. P. and Clark, K.,** The effects of oral hydralazine on blood pressure, cardiac output and peripheral resistance with respect to dose, age and acetylator status, *Radiother. Oncol.,* 18, 293, 1990.
84. **Haller, B. G. D., Zust, H., Shaw, S., Gnadinger, M. P., Uehlinger, D. E., and Weidmann, P.,** Effects of posture and aging on circulating atrial natriuretic peptide levels in man, *J. Hypertension,* 5, 551, 1987.
85. **Schmucker, D. L.,** Aging and drug disposition: an update, *Pharmacol. Rev.,* 37, 133, 1985.
86. **Legault, L., van Nguyen, P., Holliwell, D. L., and Leenen, F. H. H.,** Hemodynamic and plasma atrial natriuretic factor responses to cardiac volume loading in young versus older normotensive humans, *Can. J. Physiol. Pharmacol.,* 70, 1549, 1992.
87. **Jansen, T. L. Th. A., Tan, A. C. I. T. L., Wollersheim, H., Benraad, Th., and Thien, Th.,** Age-dependent vasodilatation of the skin microcirculation by atrial natriuretic factor, *J. Cardiovasc. Pharmacol.,* 18, 622, 1991.
88. **Docherty, J. R.,** Age-related differences in the depressor responses to sodium nitroprusside and nifedipine in anaesthetized rats, *J. Auton. Pharmacol.,* 10, 49, 1990.
89. **Olah, M. E. and Rahwan, R. G.,** Age-related changes in responsiveness of rat aorta to depolarizing and receptor-mediated contractile stimuli and to calcium antagonists, *Pharmacology,* 35, 163, 1987.
90. **Carvajal, A., Shafii, M., and Docherty, J. R.,** Effects of maturation and aging on the response to vasodilators in the rat aorta, *Br. J. Pharmacol.,* 96, 190P, 1989
91. **de Jonge, G. I., Jansen, A. S. P., Horvath, E., Gispen, W. H. and Luiten, P. G. M.,** Nimodipine effects on cerebral microvessels and sciatic nerve in aging rats, *Neurobiol. Aging,* 13, 73, 1991.
92. **Schwartz, J. B.,** The effects of aging on responses to verapamil in isolated right atria, *J. Gerontol.,* 44, M201, 1989.
93. **Kazanietz, M. G. and Enero, M. A.,** Decreased beta-adrenoceptor-mediated vasodilation in aorta from aged rats: possible involvement of a stimulatory GTP-binding protein, *Eur. J. Pharmacol.,* 198, 177, 1991.
94. **O'Donnell, S. R. and Wanstall, J. C.,** Thyroxine treatment of aged or young rats demonstrates that vascular responses mediated by β-adrenoceptor subtypes can be differentially regulated, *Br. J. Pharmacol.,* 88, 41, 1986.
95. **Kendall, M. J., Woods, K. L., Wilkins, M. R., and Worthington, D. J.,** Responsiveness to beta-adrenergic receptor stimulation: the effects of age are cardioselective, *Br. J. Clin. Pharmacol.,* 14, 821 1982,.
96. **Collins, K. J., Exton-Smith, A. N., James, M. H., and Oliver, D. J.,** Functional changes in autonomic nervous responses with aging, *Age Aging,* 9, 17, 1980.
97. **Rothbaum, D. A., Shaw, D. G., Angell, C. S., and Shock, N. W.,** Age differences in the baroreceptor response of rats, *J. Gerontol.,* 29, 488, 1974.
98. **Smith, J. J. and Porth, C. J. M.,** Posture and the circulation: the age effect, *Exp. Gerontol.,* 26, 141, 1991.
99. **Caird, F. I., Andrews, G. R., and Kennedy, R. D.,** Effect of posture on blood pressure in the elderly, *Br. Heart J.,* 35, 527, 1973.
100. **Mader, S. L., Josephson, K. R., and Rubenstein, L. Z.,** Low prevalence of postural hypotension among community-dwelling elderly, *J. Am. Med. Soc.,* 258, 1511, 1987.

Chapter 5

ANTIARRHYTHMIC DRUGS — AGENTS AFFECTING MYOCARDIAL EXCITABILITY

Richard A. Josephson and Lynn E. Fisher-Katz

CONTENTS

I. INTRODUCTION

There are numerous factors influencing the genesis, propagation, maintenance, termination, and prophylaxis of cardiac arrhythmias. This section will focus on those agents that directly affect neuronal excitability. Cardiac arrhythmias are often influenced by alterations in autonomic tone. Agents that directly affect the autonomic nervous system (e.g., β-blockers, anticholinergics) may have a profound effect on cardiac rhythm; however, the reader is referred to other sections of this text for information on these agents. Similarly, calcium

0-8493-8306-4/96/$0.00+$.50

channel blockers have widespread effects in addition to affecting cardiac arrhythmias. Other sections of this text provide important information on these agents.

The alteration of the effects of antiarrhythmic agents with increasing age are often the net result of multiple interacting forces. Readers of this text are likely most familiar with alterations in the ***pharmacokinetic*** parameters as a function of advancing age. Alterations in the absorption, distribution, and elimination phases of many antiarrhythmic drugs are known to vary with aging. In addition, there may be alterations in the ***pharmacodynamic*** effects of a given agent with advancing age (i.e., despite similar plasma concentrations an agent may have enhanced toxicity or efficacy in the elderly). A third factor, which may be difficult to distinguish from direct pharmacodynamic effects, is the notion that the underlying cardiovascular substrate varies with age, either because of changes that may be properly ascribed to aging effects per se, or perhaps secondary to co-existent illnesses/dysfunctions which increase in prevalence with advancing age. The interplay of these three important facets of drug action is at present incompletely elucidated for many antiarrhythmic agents.

II. IMPLICATIONS OF CURRENT DATA FOR FUTURE DRUG TRIALS IN THE ELDERLY

Analysis of past as well as design of future clinical studies of antiarrhythmic drugs in the elderly is fraught with numerous limitations. Considerable prior work may be hampered by unintentional "ageism", where drug dosages or therapeutic blood levels determined in young and middle-aged adults are then assumed to be applicable in the elderly. To the extent that changes in drug effects with aging are due to altered pharmacokinetics, frequent measurement of drug levels may minimize this problem. Measuring a pharmacodynamic alteration is more complex. Given that the underlying cardiovascular (as well as other) substrate is known to change with advancing age, it may be predicted that the efficacy, as well as the therapeutic/toxic ratio, will be altered in the elderly. It is well known that the prevalence of coronary artery disease (both symptomatic, as well as clinically occult) increases with advancing age. Similarly, it has been documented that there is decreased β-adrenergic responsiveness of the aging myocardium. To the extent that the spectrum of action of a drug is dependent on one or both of these factors, for example, the overall therapeutic profile of the drug is likely to be different in the elderly than in the non-elderly. Careful, and perhaps large studies will be required so that apparent age-related effects may be more precisely dissected into those actions which are related to aging, per se, vs. those which are secondary to increasing prevalence of diseases with advancing age. Only then will true age effects be discernible and quantifiable.

III. CLASSIFICATION OF ANTIARRHYTHMIC AGENTS

For the past 20 years, classification of cardiac antiarrhythmic agents has been based on a scheme described by Vaughn Williams. This scheme is described in Figure 5.1, with agents in Class I and Class III being the ones primarily thought to affect myocardial excitability. Though considerable use has been made of this classification scheme, it has serious limitations which have become more evident as our knowledge of basic pharmacologic and physiologic processes increases. The limitations of this classification were brought to the fore by the Task Force of the Working Group on Arrhythmias of the European Society of Cardiology. This group met in Sicily and produced a document justifying a new approach for the classification of antiarrhythmic agents based on fundamental mechanisms of arrhythmogenesis and antiarrhythmic drug action; it is called the Sicilian gambit (Figure 5.2).[1,2] There is much to recommend the use of this classification by serious students of cardiac pharmacology. It is argued that the Vaughan Williams classification should be supplanted because of several serious limitations:

1. The classification principles are multiple (Class I and Class IV represent ion channel blockers, Class II receptor blockers, Class III a change in a measured electrophysiologic variable).
2. Drugs may produce a Vaughn Williams class effect by multiple fundamental mechanisms.
3. Some drugs have multiple classes of action.
4. Classification only accounts for blockade of ion channels or currents. Antiarrhythmic action may be produced by activation of some of these processes.
5. Classification is incomplete. Adenosine, ATP, digitalis, cholinergic agonists, and α-adrenergic agents are not included.
6. Classification of electrophysiologic characteristics is based upon action in *in vitro* isolated normal cardiac tissue. Profound alterations may occur in diseased myocardium, often where antiarrhythmic agents are most needed.

This chapter, because of its review nature, will describe agents and relate them to their Vaughn Williams classification. It is hoped and anticipated that the next edition of this text will be based on more fundamental knowledge of antiarrhythmic drug action and more fundamental knowledge of how various basic processes change with advancing age. Thus, the classification scheme such as the Sicilian gambit may allow a broader overview of cardiac pharmacology and how the effects and toxicities of various agents might change (in a more general way) with advancing age.

A. LIDOCAINE

Lidocaine, administered only in intravenous form and utilized for short-term management of ventricular arrhythmias, is one of the most widely used antiarrhythmics.[3] It is considered a class IA drug, and its major effects are mediated by a blockade of the fast sodium channel. This results in shortening of both the action potential duration and effective refractory, particularly the former. Conduction velocity is not appreciably affected.[4]

			Electrophysiologic Effects			Electrocardiographic Effects		
Class	Drug	Action	Conduction Velocity	Effective Refractory Period	Action Potential Duration	PR	QRS	JT
I		Depress Phase 0 repolarization						
IA	Quinidine		D	I	I	NC/I	NC/I	I
	Procainamide		D	I	I	NC/I	NC/I	I
	Disopyramide		D	I	D	NC/I	NC/I	I
IB	Tocainide		D	NC/D	D	NC	NC	NC/D
	Mexiletine		D	NC/D	D	NC	NC	NC/D
IC	Flecainide		D	I	I	I	I	NC
	Encainide		D	NC	I	I	I	NC
III	Amiodarone	Prolong repolarization	D	NC/I	D	I	NC	I

I = Increase D = Decrease NC = No change

FIGURE 5.1. Adapted from the Vaughn Williams Antiarrhythmic Drug Classification.

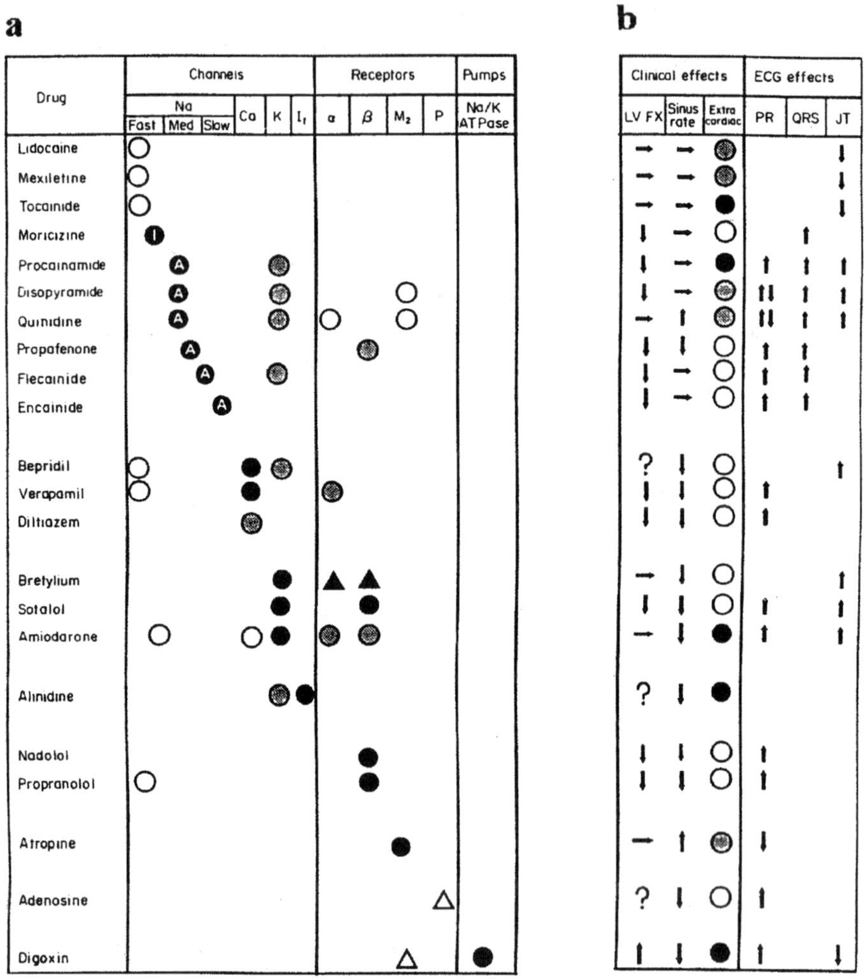

FIGURE 5.2. Adapted from The Sicilian Gambit: Evolution and Perspectives.

There are many questions that remain to be answered concerning the pharmacokinetics of lidocaine in the elderly. Perhaps the only clear difference is that protein binding of lidocaine in the elderly is increased, as is the elimination half-life.[5] Three studies have been published which compare lidocaine pharmacokinetics in young and elderly patients. The results of these studies are all different. The first study, published in 1977, administered a lidocaine bolus dose to four young males (22 to 26 years) and six elderly males (62 to 77 years).[5] A significant increase in Vd_{ss} in the elderly subjects was reported (1.127 L/kg vs. 0.652 L/kg). This accounted for the significant increase in the half-life of the parent compound, as clearance was not different between the two groups. The second study, published in 1983, evaluated the effects of both age and sex on lidocaine pharmacokinetics.[6] A single bolus dose was administered to 15 young males (x = 29), 9 young females (x = 28), 6 elderly males (x = 70) and 7 elderly females (x = 72). Contrary to the first study, no age-related differences in Vd were detected, although Vd was significantly greater in female patients compared to male patients in both age groups. Clearance, however, was significantly reduced in the elderly male population, but not in the elderly females. The reduced clearance did result in a significant prolongation of the half-life of lidocaine in the elderly males. The third study, published in 1985, enrolled four males and two females in each group.[7] The mean age of the young group was 27, while that for the elderly group was 80. Interestingly, this study found no significant differences in clearance or Vd. However, the elimination half-life was significantly prolonged in the elderly group.

The results of these studies leave several questions unanswered. What is the role of gender in the pharmacokinetics of lidocaine? Is the prolongation in half-life due to a change in volume or clearance or a combination of both? Further studies are needed to clearly evaluate these questions.

It should be noted that congestive heart failure is known to cause a decrease in clearance of lidocaine due to the decrease in liver blood flow. Lidocaine is a drug with a high intrinsic clearance, and therefore clearance is dependent on liver blood flow.[8] It is important to exclude these types of patients from pharmacokinetic studies in order to answer the above questions.

Age-related electrophysiologic effects of lidocaine have been studied in rat hearts by Goldberg et al.[9–11] Action potential duration at 95% repolarization was prolonged to a greater extent in 20-month-old Fischer 344 (F-344) rats than at younger ages. Utilizing a Langendorff preparation with surgical atrioventricular block, lidocaine reduction in atrial and ventricular pacemaker activity was measurable. The results in the two tissues were discordant, with depression of pacemaker activity being more profound in the atria with advancing age, while lidocaine was less potent in the ventricles.

Clinical studies have demonstrated an increased incidence of lidocaine side effects, primarily neurologic, in the elderly. These are likely secondary to changes in pharmacokinetic variables which in turn may be secondary to alterations in cardiac output and liver blood flow.[12,13] Whether or not the central nervous system per se is more sensitive to a given concentration of lidocaine with advancing age is incompletely defined.

B. TOCAINIDE AND MEXILETINE

Two lidocaine congeners, tocainide and mexiletine, are available for oral use. Although both agents block the fast sodium channel and have reasonable efficacy in short-term trials, they are not particularly effective to the majority of patients with chronic ventricular ectopy.[14] They have little significant effect on atrial tissue.

Tocainide is classified as a Vaughn Williams IB agent. Peak plasma concentrations of tocainide are reached in 30 to 90 min after oral administration; there is approximately a 50% protein binding of the drug; and the drug is cleared by both renal and hepatic mechanisms. In middle-aged adults, approximately 40% is excreted unchanged in the urine while 60% undergoes hepatic metabolism. Though these may be expected to be altered in the elderly, extensive data are not available.[15]

Mexiletine is available for experimental use in intravenous form and clinically in oral form. In middle-aged adults, peak blood levels occur 2 to 4 hr after oral dosing. Oral bioavailability is high at 80 to 88%. The drug is lipophilic with a volume of distribution of 500 to 600 L. Hepatic metabolism is the major route of elimination. There is a slight impairment in total body clearance of mexiletine in the setting of severe renal insufficiency. Decreased hepatic and renal blood flow by chronic congestive heart failure and/or acute myocardial infarction may dramatically prolong the half-life of this agent.[16,17] Limited data suggest that mexiletine is less effective in those over age 65 vs. younger patients (17 vs. 37%), as well as more likely to cause side effects (62 vs. 32%).[18] Irrespective of age, mexiletine has demonstrated limited success in the clinical treatment of patients with life-threatening sustained ventricular tachyarrhythmias.

C. QUINIDINE

Quinidine is an agent that blocks the sodium channel with an intermediate time course of recovery, as well as interacting with the potassium channel. It has effects on muscarinic and α-adrenergic receptors as well. It is classified as a Vaughn Williams IA agent and is one of the most widely used drugs in the clinical treatment of ventricular and supraventricular arrhythmias. Quinidine has high oral availability, with maximal effects 1 to 3 hr after administration.[19,20]

Also, 60 to 80% of quinidine is bound to total plasma proteins.[21] Quinidine is metabolized in the liver to 3-hydroxyquinidine, an active metabolite.[22] Less than 20% of the orally administered dose of quinidine is excreted unchanged in the urine. Metabolism of both quinidine and its metabolites is affected by changes in hepatic blood flow and function.[23–25] Limited data suggest a prolonged half-life of quinidine in the elderly and perhaps, therefore, diminished dosage requirements.[26,27] How much of this is due to aging effects per se vs. increased prevalence of factors that affect hepatic metabolism with advancing age is unclear.

D. PROCAINAMIDE

Procainamide is another widely prescribed Vaughn Williams IA agent that prolongs repolarization. It has prominent effects on the sodium channel, as well as on the potassium channel. It does not interact significantly with α-adrenergic or muscarinic receptors. It is utilized for the treatment of ventricular and supraventricular arrhythmias.[14] Procainamide is clinically available for intravenous or oral administration. It is well absorbed from the small intestine with peak plasma levels occurring approximately 60 min after oral intake. Plasma half-life of procainamide in normal middle-aged adults is 3 to 4 hr. Approximately half of the dose is excreted unchanged in the urine; the remainder is acetylated in the liver to *N*-acetyl-procainamide.[19,28,29]

With the age-related decline in renal function, it is not surprising that the renal clearance of procainamide is decreased in elderly individuals. However, two studies suggest that the decrease in renal clearance is greater than that which can be accounted for by age alone.[30,31] This is hypothesized to be due to a decrease in tubular secretion of procainamide. Further studies are needed to determine what role glomerular filtration and secretion play in the elimination of procainamide. Additionally, congestive heart failure, a common disorder in the elderly, results in decreased renal clearance of procainamide. However, the mechanisms have not been well described.

A late-occurring side effect of procainamide, the lupus-like syndrome, appears to occur more frequently with advancing age.[32] Thus, the therapeutic/toxic ratio is altered in the elderly.

E. DIISOPYRAMIDE

Diisopyramide is another IA agent which is available for the clinical treatment of ventricular or supraventricular arrhythmias.[14] It interacts with both the sodium channel as well as the potassium channel and muscarinic receptors. There is no discernible interaction with α-adrenergic receptors. It is metabolized predominantly in the liver, and there appears to be an age-associated decline in its hepatic metabolism with advancing age. It has been suggested that diisopyramide dosages be reduced by approximately one third in the elderly vs. middle-aged adults. Interestingly, smoking augments hepatic clearance of diisopyramide such that the age-associated effect was no longer present.[33] Studies of diisopyramide in isolated rabbit tissue suggest no age-associated change in the diastolic threshold for stimulation or the effective refractory period.[34] Unfortunately, anticholinergic side effects (e.g., difficulty with urination, visual changes, and dry mouth) impair the widespread use of this agent in the elderly.

F. MORICIZINE

Moricizine (also known as Ethmozine) has been available in the U.S. for a relatively brief period of time. It was originally developed in the U.S.S.R. and is chemically related to phenothiazines.[35] It blocks the sodium channel with a medium time course of recovery.[1] It is available for experimental use in intravenous form and commercially in oral form. There is essentially complete absorption of oral moricizine, but there is high first-pass hepatic metabolism via multiple mechanisms. Moricizine sulfoxide is approximately equally potent to the parent compound. Like other drugs metabolized primarily via the hepatic route, there does not appear to be significant alteration in dosage requirement with age.[36] Limited preliminary data suggested no alteration in adverse affects with advancing age.[18] Results from the prospective Cardiac Arrhythmia Suppression Trial, involving 2371 patients, many of whom received moricizine, showed that adverse events did in fact increase as a function of age. The moricizine results were similar to those found with flecainide and encainide. Similar efficacy as a function of advancing age in conjunction with altered toxicity suggests a definite change in the therapeutic/toxic ratio in the elderly.[37]

G. FLECAINIDE

Flecainide, encainide, and propafenone are Vaughn Williams class IC drugs that are effective in the treatment of ventricular and supraventricular arrhythmias.[14] All three agents interact with the sodium channel, though the time course of block varies. Flecainide also blocks the potassium channel, while propafenone has modest β-adrenergic antagonist effects. These drugs generally prolong the PR, as well as the QRS interval.[1,2]

Flecainide is well absorbed after oral administration. Approximately 27% of a single dose is excreted unchanged in the urine, secondary to both glomerular filtration and active tubular secretion. The drug is also biotransformed in the liver to meta-*O*-dealkylated flecainide and its lactam; both of these drugs are less active than the parent compound. These metabolites are subsequently renally excreted. Serum protein binding of flecainide appears unchanged with age.[38,39] Early clinical data suggested no difference in adverse cardiac effects of flecainide with advancing age, and perhaps a minimal increase in the incidence of nausea.[18] More recent data from the prospective randomized Cardiac Arrhythmia Suppression Trial suggest that adverse effects of flecainide (as well as encainide and moricizine; see below) are indeed more common in the elderly. This is true even if potential cofounders (such as prior infarction, ejection fraction, digitalis therapy, and density of ventricular arrhythmias) are controlled for. This large study suggested that older age is indeed associated with a significantly increased risk of adverse events, with a relative risk of 1.30 per decade. Importantly, this trial demonstrated similar efficacy of suppression of ventricular dysrhythmia and thus implied marked alteration in the therapeutic/toxic ratio with advancing age.[37]

H. ENCAINIDE

Encainide is another IC drug used for treatment of ventricular and supraventricular arrhythmias.[14] It undergoes more extensive hepatic metabolism than flecainide. It is chemically related to lysergic acid. It has high oral absorption and is extensively metabolized, principally to the two active metabolites *O*-desmethyl encainide and 3-methoxy-*O*-desmethyl encainide. There is genetic polymorphism in the hepatic enzymes, controlling this transformation, and thus considerable heterogeneity among individuals.[40,41] Importantly, after results of the Cardiac Arrhythmia Suppression Trial were disseminated, the manufacturer ceased production of this agent.[37]

I. PROPAFENONE

Propafenone is clinically utilized in the treatment of ventricular and supraventricular dysrhythmias.[14] It is hypothesized that the β-adrenergic effects of propafenone may be synergistic with its effects on the sodium channel such that it is particularly useful in supraventricular dysrhythmias (by blockade of the AV node) as well as potentially fewer episodes of ventricular proarrhythmia (by blunting the heart rate, there may be a minimization of use dependence). These theoretically attractive properties have not been proven to have a clinical advantage. Gastrointestinal absorption is nearly complete, though there appears to be saturable first-pass hepatic clearance. Thus, increasing doses of propafenone result in a disproportionate increase in serum drug levels. There is high (97%) protein binding and nearly total hepatic metabolism. The principal metabolite, 5-hydroxypropafenone, is even more potent than the parent compound. Similar to encainide, there appears to be genetic heterogeneity in propafenone metabolism.[42] Limited clinical data suggest no appreciable difference between efficacy or side effects in young and elderly patients.[18,43]

J. SOTALOL

Sotalol is a potent Vaughn Williams class III drug that has found wide clinical application in the treatment of ventricular and supraventricular arrhythmias. It blocks the potassium channel and the levorotatory isomer also has potent nonselective β-blocking effects.[1] While sotalol is clinically available in racemic form, recent investigation of the pure dextrorotatory isomer has shown that this agent has significant potential for clinical use, without the potentially troublesome β-blocking side effects of the racemate. Sotalol is completely absorbed after oral administration and excreted unchanged in the urine. The maximal concentration of sotalol occurs somewhere between 2 and 3 hr after oral administration with a half-life of 7 to 15 hr in middle-aged normal volunteers.[44] Clearly, the sotalol dose must be reduced in the elderly, secondary to the age-associated decline in glomerulofiltration rate. On a per milligram basis, racemic sotalol appears to have approximately one third the β-blocking potency of propranolol.[44] Adverse events appear to increase in frequency with increasing age, particularly heart failure, bradycardia, and proarrhythmia.[45] This may simply be due to the age-associated decline in renal clearance. Wide-scale clinical trials of this agent in ventricular and supraventricular arrhythmias are currently ongoing, and its use in the elderly, therefore, remains incompletely defined. Perhaps comparison of clinical and *in vitro* studies of the dextrorotatory isomer and the racemate will clarify how much of the age-associated alterations in drug effects are secondary to changes in the interaction with the potassium channel vs. interaction with the sympathetic nervous system (with there being a clearly documented generalized decline in β-adrenergic responsiveness of the myocardium with advancing age).

K. AMIODARONE

Amiodarone is a class III antiarrhythmic which has multiple fundamental mechanisms of action. It blocks the sodium, calcium, and potassium channels, as well as having modest α-adrenergic and β-adrenergic receptor blocking effects.[46] It is the most effective clinically available antiarrhythmic,[14] and its spectrum of activity includes supraventricular as well as ventricular dysrhythmias.[47] The drug will slow the sinus rate and prolong conduction through the AV node. It prolongs repolarization in both atrial and ventricular tissue. Clinical studies have revealed antiarrhythmic efficacy in two thirds or more of all patients treated, and it is not infrequently effective when essentially all other drugs have been ineffective.[14] It is poorly absorbed, has a large volume of distribution (approximately 5000 L at steady state), and has a terminal elimination half-life of approximately 1 month after a single oral dose. It is metabolized to desethylamiodarone, which has pharmacologic action similar to the parent compound. It has frequent side effects involving many major organ systems, principally thyroid (hyper- and hypothyroidism),[48] hepatic (hepatitis), pulmonary (interstitial fibrosis), skin (photosensitivity), as well as corneal pigmentation and neurologic and gastrointestinal toxicity. The thyroid side effects appear to be due to the large iodine content of the drug. Data indicate that amiodarone-associated hypothyroidism increases in prevalence with advancing age. The pharmacology of amiodarone is sufficiently complex and unusual that there are no reliable data regarding the alteration of pharmacokinetics in the elderly.[46,47]

There is an increased incidence of amiodarone-associated bradycardia with advancing age. This may be secondary to the interaction of amiodarone with the sympathetic nervous system (which changes with age) or secondary to actual degeneration of the conduction system with increasing age (independent of autonomic effects). This distinction has not been completely elucidated.

IV. DIGOXIN

Digoxin is one of the most commonly prescribed medications for the elderly population. In fact, in the National Nursing Home Survey of 1977, 32.3% of patients were taking digoxin.[49] A more recent survey of Kentucky Nursing Homes in 1985 found that 36.6% of patients were receiving digoxin.[50] As the elderly population is on the rise, digoxin is likely to remain a frequently prescribed medication for the elderly population.

Much remains to be learned about the use of digoxin in the elderly. Perhaps the best starting point is the pharmacokinetics of digoxin in the elderly patient. Digoxin is a drug with a narrow therapeutic window, and many of the physiologic changes of aging will affect the pharmacokinetics of digoxin.

Studies of digoxin bioavailability and pharmacokinetics in the elderly often produce seemingly conflicting results. While limitations peculiar to an individual study may explain part of the variance, the small sample sizes and clinical (and subclinical) heterogeneity of the elderly are likely cofounders.

A. ABSORPTION

When assessing the absorption of digoxin in the elderly, it is important to consider the dosage form, drug interactions, and the underlying health of the individual. The elderly are a heterogenous population, in various states of health, and on various medications. Therefore, clinical studies must be of sufficient size to overcome these variables.

In young healthy volunteers, digoxin capsules (Lanoxicaps®) are about 90 to 100% bioavailable. The tablets (Lanoxin®) are about 60 to 80% bioavailable.[53] Therefore, the manufacturer recommends that 125% of the capsule dosage be administered in the tablet form. In elderly individuals, however, two studies have suggested that this ratio may be inappropriate.[51,52] In the first study, nursing home patients were switched from capsules to tablets due to a change in the formulary of the supplier pharmacy. The recommended ratio listed above was used to determine the patients' new dosage. Steady-state serum digoxin concentrations obtained before and after the change in dosage form were compared. Despite using the suggested conversion ratio, paired comparisons of digoxin concentrations were significantly higher for the tablet form. The mean concentration during capsule therapy was 0.92+/–0.26 ng/mL and for the tablets 1.03+/–0.29 ng/mL. A second study utilized a crossover comparison to measure steady-state trough concentrations for each formulation. This study confirmed the results of the first study, finding lower serum concentrations for the capsule formulation (mean 0.9+/–0.4 nmol/L) compared to the tablets (1.3+/–0.5 nmol/L). Both of these studies found lower steady-state serum concentrations obtained with the capsules, despite using the recommended dosage adjustment ratio of 1.25:1. This suggests that in contrast to healthy adults, in elderly patients the bioavailability of the capsules and tablets is not different. It is possible that the decrease in gastric emptying and intestinal transit rates which occurs in the elderly may have resulted in increased absorption of the tablets. It has been shown that drugs which enhance gastric emptying result in a decreased absorption from tablets without affecting the absorption of digoxin from capsules.[54] One investigation suggests the bioavailability of digoxin in the patients >70 years old is closer to 60% while for patients <70 years old it is closer to 80%.[55] Another study which measured the absolute bioavailability of digoxin tablets in both the young and old found no significant differences in the absorption of the tablets. However, the plasma measurements were carried out for less than one half-life of the drug.[56] More studies are needed to determine the absolute bioavailability of tablets and capsules in the elderly population.

Many drugs which are administered in the elderly population can also decrease digoxin absorption.[53] Additionally, disease states may have an effect on digoxin absorption. Patients who are malnourished or undergoing chemotherapy may have decreased absorption of digoxin from the tablet forms.[57] It is important to remember that the elderly are a very diverse population. Therefore, studies should attempt to enroll large numbers of subjects or limit themselves to homogenous subgroups when assessing digoxin absorption.

B. DISTRIBUTION

About 20 to 30% of digoxin binds to plasma proteins in humans, and this does not appear to change with age. The major determinant of digoxin distribution is the location in the body of the enzyme Na-K-ATPase, the enzyme to which digoxin binds.[58] Similar to plasma protein binding of digoxin, the concentration of digitalis binding sites in skeletal muscle does not appear to depend on age.[59,60] However, the concentration of binding sites is increased in the presence of hyperthyroidism and decreased in patients with hypothyroidism.

In the elderly, there is a decrease in total body water and skeletal muscle mass. Taken together, these factors result in a decreased fraction of bound digoxin and a decrease in the apparent volume of distribution. One study comparing elderly and young subjects found no difference in the apparent volume of digoxin when the volume of digoxin was adjusted for weight. They found that the apparent volume of distribution correlated with age and was significantly reduced in older individuals when the data were not weight corrected. This suggests that the decrease in apparent volume of distribution is directly related to the decrease in the body mass, rather than changes in binding affinity. Elderly individuals are known to have a decrease in lean body mass which is where most digoxin is distributed. Therefore it is important to base the dosage of digoxin on body weight and to correct pharmacokinetic parameters for weight.

C. METABOLISM

Approximately 12% of digoxin is excreted in the urine as intact metabolites.[61] The primary site of metabolism is considered to be the liver. Although there are decreases in liver blood flow and liver function with increasing age, digoxin metabolism is not considered to change with age.[60–63]

One recent study[64] compared digoxin tablet and capsule excretion in elderly subjects who had known gastrointestinal disorders. The subjects were evaluated at steady state in a randomized-crossover fashion. Total urinary and fecal elimination of both parent drug and metabolites were measured. This study found no statistically significant differences with respect to total drug eliminated, urinary excretion, or fecal excretion when subjects were given digoxin 0.125-mg tablets or 0.1-mg capsules. This study did not simultaneously evaluate younger patients or disease-free patients. Further research is needed to clarify whether or not there is a decrease in metabolism and to identify whether or not the metabolite profile changes with age.

D. EXCRETION

Approximately 70% of digoxin is excreted by the kidneys. The majority of the excreted digoxin is cleared via glomerular filtration. However, tubular secretion does account for a portion of renally cleared digoxin, and this is a potential site for drug interactions. It is well known that creatinine clearance and tubular function decline with age, and therefore it is not unexpected to have a decline in renal elimination and overall clearance of digoxin in the elderly. It is important to note that serum creatinine alone is not a good measure of renal function in the elderly. Therefore, when undertaking clinical pharmacokinetic studies in the elderly, creatinine clearance should be measured.

Nonrenal clearance mechanisms include biliary excretion and possible intestinal secretion with subsequent fecal elimination. It appears that the decrease in plasma clearance is most likely a result of the decline in renal function with age. The alteration in body weight with age does not seem to be a factor, as both total clearance and weight-adjusted clearance were found to be significantly different between young and old patients.[56]

E. SUMMARY OF DIGOXIN PHARMACOKINETICS

In conclusion, absorption of digoxin in the elderly may be different from that of the younger patients and is probably dependent on the dosage form. Volume of distribution is decreased due to a decrease in body mass and clearance is decreased due to a decline in renal function. This decreased clearance results in a prolongation of the serum $t_{1/2}$ from 30 to 40 hr in younger patients to 70 hr in the 8th and 9th decades of life.[63]

F. PHARMACODYNAMICS

While differences in the pharmacokinetics of digoxin in the young and old have been well documented, there is little evidence to suggest that the pharmacodynamics differ between the young and old. In 1980, Cokkinos and co-workers[66] published the results of a study which evaluated the inotropic effects of digitalis using systolic time intervals. A dose of 1.2 mg of the cardiac glycoside deslanoside was administered to healthy "elderly" volunteers (mean age 65.3) and young volunteers (mean age 34.3). The changes seen in the systolic time intervals were very similar in the two groups. Unfortunately, deslanoside concentrations were not measured, so it can not be certain whether or not pharmacokinetic differences influenced the outcome of the study.

On the other hand, one animal study using isometric trabeculare carneae obtained from young and senescent rats found that at the same concentration of ouabain, the developed tension and maximal rate of tension development was four times greater in the young myocardium.[67] However, the mechanism for this difference is not clear. It was not due to the inability of the myocardium to respond nor was it due to differences in Na-K ATPase inhibition.

G. EFFICACY

Many questions remain regarding the clinical usage of digoxin in the elderly. Digoxin is currently recommended for use for congestive heart failure and for chronic atrial fibrillation. Digoxin concentrations to treat atrial fibrillation in young and elderly appear to be the same.[68] Of course, lower dosages will be required in the elderly due to the pharmacokinetic differences described above.

Use of digoxin for the treatment of congestive heart failure is somewhat controversial.[69] There are other modalities on the market such as angiotensin converting enzyme inhibitors which may be used to treat this condition. Currently, there are no definite data to state which medication class would be best suited for the elderly population.

Many studies have been published that suggest that digoxin use may be unnecessary in the elderly population.[69–74] Digoxin maintenance therapy was withheld from elderly patients who had been placed on digoxin therapy for treatment of congestive heart failure. Anywhere from 60 to 90% of patients could be removed from digoxin treatment without any deleterious effects on their cardiac function. This result is important, as digoxin has a narrow therapeutic index and elderly patients may be exposed to unnecessary toxicity.

However, this is not to say that digoxin has no role in the treatment of congestive heart failure. It does appear to have some benefit in the treatment of patients with chronic congestive heart failure secondary to systolic dysfunction. This was recently demonstrated in the PROVED trial.[75] This was a randomized, double-blind study which compared withdrawal of digoxin treatment with the continuation of digoxin treatment in patients with chronic congestive heart failure. Those patients who had their digoxin withdrawn had a significant worsening of their exercise performance and an increased incidence of treatment failure. There is currently a large NIH-sponsored trial to better elucidate the use of digoxin in a broad spectrum of patients with congestive heart failure.

H. TOXICITY

Although the general impression is that digoxin toxicity occurs more frequently in the elderly, there is little clinical evidence to support that this is due to digoxin alone.[76] There are several reasons why digoxin toxicity might be expected to occur more frequently in the elderly. These would include its more frequent use in the elderly population, alterations in pharmacokinetics, hypokalemia, polypharmacy, and medication errors. The incidence of both congestive heart failure and atrial fibrillation increases with age, leading to an increase in digoxin use among the elderly population. This population has a decreased clearance of digoxin and must have their dosage carefully titrated.

Digoxin toxicity can be divided into three major types: cardiac, gastrointestinal, and neurologic manifestations. A post-marketing study of patients being treated with digoxin immune FAB evaluated patients older than 55 with serum digoxin concentrations >2.5 nmol/L. These patients were further divided into four groups: 55 to 64, 65 to 75, 75 to 84, and >85 years old. No differences in AV block between the age groups were noted, suggesting that the aged heart is not more sensitive to cardiac toxicity.[77] Another study of 52 elderly patients and 54 young patients found that conduction disturbances occurred in 42.1% of elderly and 22.2% of the younger patients.[78] Arrhythmias were seen in 40.1% of the elderly and 31.5% of the younger patients. Unfortunately, statistical analysis of these results was not performed. Gastrointestinal complaints are common among the elderly, and it is difficult to determine whether or not digoxin itself contributes to an increased incidence of gastrointestinal complaints. In the post-marketing study described above, no statistically significant difference in nausea/vomiting was found. The neurotoxic side effects of digoxin such as hallucinations, visual disturbances, headache, and dizziness have not been well described in the elderly population. This is an area that requires further evaluation.

V. CONCLUSION

It is hoped that as a greater understanding of the ***fundamental*** basis of cardiovascular drug actions is elucidated and as basic pathophysiologic processes and their alteration with age are better delineated, the pharmacology of antiarrhythmic drugs as a function of age will be both predictable (via a schema such as a Sicilian Gambit) and ultimately verified.

REFERENCES

1. **Task Force of the Working Group on Arrhythmias of the European Society of Cardiology,** The Sicilian Gambit, a new approach to the classification of antiarrhythmic drugs based on their actions on arrhythmogenic mechanisms, *Circulation*, 84, 1831, 1991.
2. **Zaza, Z.,** The Sicilian Gambit: evolution and perspectives, *CVR & R*, 8, 1994.
3. **Frieden, J.,** Lidocaine as an antiarrhythmic agent, *Am. Heart J.*, 70, 713, 1965.
4. **Bigger, J. T., Jr. and Mandel, W. J.,** Effect of lidocaine on the electrophysiological properties of ventricular muscle and Purkinje fibers, *J. Clin. Invest.*, 49, 63, 1970.
5. **Davis, D., Grossman, S. H., Kitchell, B. B., Shand, D. G., and Routledge, P. A.,** Age related changes in the plasma protein binding of Lidocaine (L) and Diazepam, *Clin Res.*, 28, 234A, 1980.
6. **Nation, R. L., Triggs, E. J., and Selig, M.,** Lignocaine kinetics in cardiac patients and aged subjects, *Br. J. Clin. Pharmacol.*, 4, 439, 1977.
7. **Abernathy, D. R. and Greenblatt, D. J.,** Impairment of lidocaine clearance in elderly male subjects, *J. Cardiol. Pharm.*, 5, 1093, 1983.
8. **Hunt, C. M., Westerkam, W. R., and Stave, G. M.,** Effect of age and gender on the activity of human hepatic CYP3A, *Biochem. Pharm.*, 44(2), 275, 1992.
9. **Goldberg, P. B. and Roberts, J.,** Age effects on atrial and ventricular sensitivity to quinidine and lidocaine. II, *Gerontologist*, 15, 24, 1975.
10. **Goldberg, P. B., Stoner, S.A., and Roberts, J.,** Influence of age on activity of antiarrhythmic drugs in rat heart, *Adv. Exp. Med. Biol.*, 97, 309, 1978.
11. **Goldberg, P. B. and Roberts, J.,** Physiological and pharmacological changes of rat cardiac pacemakers with increasing age, *Adv. Exp. Med. Biol.*, 97, 315, 1978.
12. **Cusson, J., Nattel, S., Mattews, C., Talajic, M., and Lawand, S.,** Age-dependent lidocaine disposition in patients with acute myocardial infarction, *Clin. Pharm. Ther.*, 37(4), 381, 1985.
13. **Cusack, B., O'Malley, K., Lavan, J., Noel, J., and Kelly, J. G.,** Protein binding and disposition of lignocaine in the elderly, *Eur. J. Clin. Pharmacol.*, 29(3), 323, 1985.
14. **Salerno, D. M., Gillingham, K. J., Berry, D. A., and Hodges, M.,** A comparison of antiarrhythmic drugs for the suppression of ventricular ectopic depolarizations: a meta-analysis, *Am. Heart J.*, 120, 340, 1990.
15. **Kutalek, S. P., Morganroth, J., and Horowitz, L.,** Tocainide: a new oral antiarrhythmic agent, *Ann. Intern. Med.*, 103, 387, 1985.

16. **Podrid, P. J. and Lown, B.,** Mexilitine for ventricular arrhythmias, *Am. J. Cardiol.*, 47, 895, 1981.
17. **Fenster, P. E. and Comess, K. A.,** Pharmacology and clinical use of mexiletine, *Pharmacotherapy*, 6(1), 1, 1986.
18. **Podrid, P. J., Levine, P. A., and Klein, M. P.,** Effect of age on antiarrhythmic drug efficacy and toxicity, *Am. J. Cardiol.*, 63, 735, 1989.
19. **Mason, D. T., DeMaria, A. N., Amsterday, E. A., Vismara, L. A., Miller, R. R., Vera, Z., Lee, G., Zelis, R., and Massumi, R. A.,** Antiarrhythmic agents: mechanisms of action, clinical pharmacology and therapeutic considerations, *Cardiovascular Drugs*, Vol. 1, Avery, G. S., Ed., University Park Press, Baltimore, 1977, 75.
20. **Harrison, D. C., Meffin, R. J., and Winkle, R. A.,** Clinical pharmacokinetics of antiarrhythmic drugs, *Progr. Cardiovasc. Dis.*, 20, 217, 1977.
21. **Conn, H. J. and Luchi, R. J.,** Some quantitative aspects of binding by quinidine and related quinoline compounds by human serum albumin, *J. Clin. Invest.*, 40, 504, 1961.
22. **Drayer, D. E., Lowenthal, D. T., Restivo, K. M., Schwartz, A., Cooke, C. E., and Reidenberg, M. M.,** Steady state serum levels of quinidine and active metabolites in cardiac patients with varying degrees of renal function, *Clin. Pharmacol. Ther.*, 24, 31, 1978.
23. **Ueda, C. T. and Dzindzio, B. S.,** Quinidine kinetics in congestive heart failure, *Clin. Pharmacol. Ther.*, 23, 158, 1978.
24. **Ueda, C. T., Hirshfeld, D. S., Scheinman, M. M., Rowland, M., Williamson, B. J., and Dzindzio, B. S.,** Disposition kinetics of quinidine, *Clin. Pharmacol. Ther.*, 19, 30, 1976.
25. **Ochs, H. R., Greenblatt, D. J., and Woo, E.,** Clinical pharmacokinetics of quinidine (review), *Clin. Pharmacokinetics*, 5(2), 150, 1980.
26. **Drayer, D. E., Hughes, M., Lorezo, B., and Reidenberg, M. M.,** Prevalence of high (3S)-3-hydroxyquinidine/quinidine rations in serum, and clearance of quinidine in cardiac patients with age, *Clin. Pharm. Ther.*, 27(1), 72, 1980.
27. **Ochs, H. R., Greenblatt, D. J., Woo, E., and Smith, T. W.,** Reduced quinidine clearance in elderly persons, *Am. J. Cardiol.*, 42(3), 481, 1978.
28. **Lucchesi, B. R.,** Antiarrhythmic drugs, *Cardiovascular Pharmacology*, Antonaccio, M., Ed., Raven Press, New York, 1977, 269.
29. **Karlsson, E.,** Clinical pharmacokinetics of procainamide, *Clin. Pharmacokinetics*, 3, 97, 1978.
30. **Reidenberg, M. M. et al.,** Aging and renal clearance of procainamide and acetyl procainamide, *Clin. Pharmacol. Ther.*, 28, 732, 1980.
31. **Baver, L. A. et al.,** Influence of age, renal function and heart failure on procainamide clearance and n-acetylprocainamide serum concentrations, *Int. J. Clin. Pharmacol. Ther. Toxicol.*, 27, 213, 1989.
32. **Heningsen, N. C., Cederberg, A., and Hansom, A.,** Effects of long-term treatment with procaine amide, *Acta. Med. Scand.*, 198, 475, 1975.
33. **Bonde, J., Pedersen, L. E., Bodtker, S., Angelo, H. R., Svendsen, T. L., and Kampmann, J. P.,** The influence of age and smoking on the elimination of diisopyramide, *Br. J. Clin. Pharmacol.*, 20(5), 453, 1985.
34. **Mokler, C. M.,** Lack of an aging effect on responses to diisopyramide in rabbit ventricle, *Mech. Ageing Dev.*, 18(2), 111, 1982.
35. **Rosenshtraukh, L. V., Shugushev, K. K., and Smetnev, A. S.,** Ethacizin: a new efficacious Soviet antiarrhythmic drug of the phenothiazine group, *Electrophysiol. Heart, U.S.S.R.*, 112, 932, 1986.
36. **Woosley, R. L., Morganroth, J., Fogoros, R. N., McMahon, F. G., O'Neal Humphries, J., Mason, D. T., and Williams, R. L.,** Pharmacokinetics of moricizine HCl, *Am. J. Cardiol.*, 60, 35F, 1987.
37. **Akiyama, T., Pawitan, Y., Campbell, W. B., Papa, L., Barker, A. H., Rubbert, P., Friedman, L., Keller, M., Josephson, R. A., and the CAST Investigators,** Effects of advancing age on the efficacy and side effects of antiarrhythmic drugs in post-myocardial infarction patients with ventricular arrhythmias, *J. Am. Geriatr. Soc.*, 40, 666, 1992.
38. **Roden, D. M. and Woosley, R. L.,** Drug therapy flecainide, *N. Engl. J. Med.*, 315, 36, 1986.
39. **Zordan, R., Padrini, R., Bernini, V., Piovan, D., and Ferrari, M.,** Influence of age and gender on the in vitro serum protein binding of flecainide, *Pharmacol. Res.*, 28(3), 259, 1993.
40. **Somberg, J. C., Zanger, B. A., Levine, E., and Tepper, D.,** Encainide: a new and potent arrhythmic, *Am. Heart J.*, 114, 826, 1987.
41. **Oates, J. A., Wood, A., JJ., Woosley, R. L., and Roden, D. M.,** Drug therapy encainide, *N. Engl. J. Med.*, 318, 1107, 1988.
42. **Salerno, D. M. and Hodges, M.,** New therapy focus: propafenone, *Cardiovasc. R & R*, 6, 924, 1985.
43. **Zehender, M., Hohnloser, S., Geibel, A., Furtwangler, A., and Olschewski, M.,** Short-term and long-term treatment with propafenone: determinants of arrhythmia suppression, persistence of efficacy, arrhythmogenesis, and side effects in patients with symptoms, *Br. Heart J.*, 67(6), 491, 1992.
44. **Antonaccio, M. J. and Gomoll, A.,** Pharmacology, pharmacodynamics and pharmacokinetics of sotalol, *Am. J. Cardiol.*, 65, 12A, 1990.

45. **Antonaccio, M. J. and Gomoll, A.,** Pharmacology, pharmacodynamics and pharmacokinetics of sotalol, *Am. J. Cardiol.*, 65, 14A, 1990.
46. **Zipes, D. P., Prystowsky, E. N., and Heger, J. J.,** Amiodarone: electrophysiologic actions, pharmacokinetics and clinical effects, *JACC*, 3, 1059, 1984.
47. **Oates, J. A., Wood, A. J. J., and Mason, J. W.,** Drug therapy amiodarone, *N. Engl. J. Med.*, 316, 455, 1987.
48. **Borowski, G. D., Garofano, C. D., Rose, L. I., Spielman, S. R., Rotmensch, H. R., Greenspan, A. M., and Horowitz, L. N.,** Effect of long-term amiodarone therapy on thyroid hormone levels and thyroid function, *Am. J. Med.*, 78(3), 443, 1985.
49. United States Center for Health Statistics: The National Nursing Home Survey 1977. Summary for the United States Vital and Health Statistics Series 13, 51, 1977.
50. **Chen, L. H., Liu S., Cookwell, M. E., et al.,** Survey of drug use by the elderly and possible impact of drugs on nutritional status, *Drug-Nutr. Interact.*, 3, 73, 1985.
51. **Drinka, P. J., Nickel, D. Z., and Schomisch, G. W.,** Transition from Lanoxin capsules to Lanoxin tablets in the debilitated elderly, *DICP, Ann. Pharmacol. T her.*, 24, 381, 1990.
52. **Pouwels, M. J., Hooymans, P. M., van der Aa, G. C., and Gribnau, F. W.,** Comparison of steady-state serum concentrations of digoxin in tablets (Lanoxin) and capsules (Lanoxicaps) in the elderly, *DICP Ann. Pharmacother.*, 10, 1043, 1991.
53. **Reuning, R. H., Geraets, D. R., Rocci, M. L., and Vlasses, P. H.,** Digoxin, in *Applied Pharmacokinetics, Principles of Therapeutic Drug Monitoring*, Evans, W. E., Schentag, J. J., and Jusko, W. J., Eds., Applied Therapeutics, Vancouver, 1992, chap. 20.
54. **Johnson, B. F., Brusrack, J. A., Urbach, D. R., Hull, J. H., and Marwaha, R.,** Effect of metoclopramide on digoxin absorption from tablets and capsules, *Clin. Pharmacol. Ther.*, 36, 724, 1984.
55. **Grimm, R., Elliot, C., and Paulus, L.,** Estimated versus measured serum digoxin levels, *Am. J. Hosp. Pharm.*, 35, 1346, 1978.
56. **Cusack, B., Kelly, J., O'Malley, K., Noel, J., Lavan, J., and Horgan, J.,** Digoxin in the elderly: pharmacokinetic consequences of old age, *Clin. Pharmacol. Ther.*, 23, 772, 1979.
57. **Bjornsson, T. D., Huang, A. T., Roth, P., Jacob, D. S., and Christenson, R.,** Effects of high-dose chemotherapy on the absorption of digoxin in two different formulations, *Clin. Pharmacol. Ther.*, 39, 25, 1986.
58. **Aronson, J. K. and Gruhame-Smith, D. G.,** Monitoring digoxin therapy. II. Determinants of the apparent volume of distribution, *Br. J. Clin. Pharmacol.*, 4, 23, 1977.
59. **Kjeldsen, K.,** Regulation of the concentration of 3H-oubain binding sites in mammalian skeletal muscle — effects of age, potassium depletion, thyroid status and hypertension, *Dan. Med. Bull.*, 34, 15, 1987.
60. **Tsang, P. and Gerson, B.,** Understanding digoxin use in the elderly patient, *Clin. Lab. Med.*, 10, 479, 1990.
61. **Mooradain, A. D., Grieff, V. L., Bressler, R., Reed, R. L., and Marcus, F. I.,** Digitalis in the elderly, *JAGS*, 37, 873, 1989.
62. **Algeo, S., Fenster, P. D., and Marcus, F. I.,** Digitalis therapy in the elderly, *Geriatrics*, 38, 93, 1983.
63. **Stults, B. M.,** Digoxin use in the elderly, *JAGS*, 30, 158, 1982.
64. **Hui, J., Wang, Y. C., Chandrasekaran, A., Gereats, D. R., Caldwell, J. H., Robertson, L. W., and Reuning, R. H.,** Disposition of tablet and capsule formulations of digoxin in the elderly, *Pharmacotherapy*, 14, 607, 1994.
65. **Mayerson, M. B.,** Special pharmacokinetic considerations in the elderly, in *Applied Pharmacokinetics, Principles of Therapeutic Drug Monitoring*, Evans, W. E., Schentag, J. J., and Jusko, W. J., Eds., Applied Therapeutics, Vancouver, 1992, chap. 9.
66. **Cokkinos, D. V., Tsartsalis, G. D., Heimonas E. T., and Gardikas, C. D.,** Comparison of the inotropic action of digitalis and isoproterenol in younger and older individuals, *Am. Heart. J.*, 100, 802, 1980.
67. **Gerstenblith, G., Spurgeon, H. A., Froehlich, J. P., Weisfelt, M. L., and Lakutta, E. G.,** Diminished inotropic responsiveness to oubain in aged rat myocardium, *Circulation*, 44, 517, 1979.
68. **Chamberlain, D. A., et al.,** Plasma digoxin concentrations in patients with atrial fibrillation, *Br. Med. J.*, 3, 429, 1970.
69. **Murlow, C. D., Feussner, J. R., and Velez, R.,** Reevaluation of digitalis efficacy, *Ann. Intern. Med.*, 101, 113, 1984.
70. **Krakauer, R. and Peterson, B.,** The effects of discontinuing maintenance digoxin therapy: a study of elderly cardiac patients in sinus rhythm, *Dan. Med. Bull.*, 26, 10, 1979.
71. **Gheorghiade, M. and Beller, G. A.,** Effects of discontinuing maintenance digoxin therapy in patients with ischemic heart disease and congestive heart failure in sinus rhythm, *Am. J. Cardiol.*, 51, 1243, 1983.
72. **Boman, K., Allgulander, S., and Skoglund, M.,** Is maintenance digoxin necessary in geriatric patients, *Acta Med. Scand.*, 210, 493, 1981.
73. **Forman, D. E., Coletta, D., Kenny, D., Kosowsky, B. D., Stoukides, J., Rohrer, M., and Pastore, J. O.,** Clinical issues related to discontinuing digoxin therapy in nursing home patients, *Arch. Intern. Med.*, 151, 2194, 1991.

74. **Bowman, K.,** Digoxin and the geriatric in-patient, a randomized trial of digoxin and placebo, *Acta Med. Scand.*, 214, 353, 1983.
75. **Uretsky, B. F., Young, J. B., Shahidi, F. E., Yellen, L. G., Harrison, M. C., and Jolly, M. K.,** Randomized study assessing the effect of digoxin withdrawal in patients with mild to moderate chronic congestive heart failure: results of the PROVED trial, *J. Am. Coll. Cardiol.*, 22, 955, 1993.
76. **Wofforf, J. L. and Ettinger, W. H.,** Risk factors and manifestations of digoxin toxicity in the elderly, *Am. J. Emer. Med.*, 9 (Suppl. 1), 11, 1991.
77. **Wofford, J. L., Hickey, A. R., Ettinger, W. H., and Furberg, C. D.,** Lack of age-related differences in the clinical presentation of digoxin toxicity, *Arch. Intern. Med.*, 152, 2261, 1992.
78. **Durakovic, Z., Durakovic, A., and Durakovic, S.,** Does any correlation exist between a high plasma digoxin concentration and an electrocardiogram in younger and older patients, *Indian Heart J.*, 45, 37, 1993.

Chapter 6

USE OF DIURETIC AGENTS IN THE ELDERLY

Concetta Harakal

I. INTRODUCTION

Diuretics have been used for many clinical problems related to abnormal water or electrolyte metabolism. They find their greatest use in congestive heart failure, cirrhosis with ascites, and the nephrotic syndrome. They can be lifesaving in pulmonary edema. They can also be useful in acute, self-limited conditions such as toxemia of pregnancy and in periodic recurrent edema.

II. GENERAL ACTIONS OF DIURETICS

Diuretics promote primarily the excretion of sodium and either chloride or bicarbonate, those ions which are largely restricted to and which constitute the major electrolyte components

0-8493-8306-4/96/$0.00+$.50

of the extracellular fluid. Water is eliminated in an amount equivalent to the ions excreted, reducing the volume of extracellular fluid and resulting in loss of weight.

A. ACTION AT THE PROXIMAL TUBULE

Sodium bicarbonate, glucose, amino acids, and other organic solutes are reabsorbed in the proximal tubule on an isosmotic basis. The reabsorption of bicarbonate by the proximal tubule is dependent upon the activity of the enzyme carbonic anhydrase and upon a sodium/hydrogen exchanger located in the luminal membrane. As is true for all segments of the nephron, Na^+, K^+-ATPase in the basolateral membrane maintains the intracellular concentration of sodium low.

B. ACTION AT THE LOOP OF HENLE

The thick ascending limb of the loop of Henle is the site of Na^+ and Cl^- reabsorption. It is impermeable to water and is essentially a diluting segment. The medullary portions of the thick ascending limb are primarily responsible for urine concentration. The sodium chloride transport system in the luminal membrane of the thick ascending limb is a sodium/potassium/2-chloride cotransport mechanism.

C. ACTION AT THE DISTAL CONVOLUTED TUBULE

Potassium undergoes both tubular reabsorption and secretion. Reabsorption occurs in the proximal tubule and in the thick ascending limb; secretion occurs in the distal tubule. NaCl reabsorption in the distal convoluted tubule is effected by a neutral cotransporter.

D. ACTION AT THE COLLECTING TUBULE

In the presence of ADH, the collecting tubule becomes permeable to water. During dehydration, there is an increase in levels of ADH; a concentrated urine is excreted. During overhydration, there is a suppression of ADH secretion and an excretion of large volumes of dilute urine.

III. PHARMACOLOGY OF SPECIFIC DIURETIC AGENTS

Except for the osmotic diuretics, the drugs that are included in this discussion act directly on tubular epithelium.

A. OSMOTIC DIURETICS

The presence in the glomerular filtrate of poorly reabsorbed material tends to carry an osmotic equivalent of H_2O with it into the urine. Osmotic diuretics depend for their action on the limited capacity of the proximal tubule for reabsorbing Na and concentrating this ion against a high concentration gradient. Diuretic effect is primarily water; all must be given intravenously; large amounts must be administered; must be freely filterable. It is the increase in urine flow that constitutes the rationale for their use.

Prototype — Mannitol (Osmitrol).

Therapeutic uses — Prophylaxis of acute renal failure; for the reduction of cerebrospinal fluid pressure.

Toxicity — Headache, nausea, and vomiting are common.

B. CARBONIC ANHYDRASE INHIBITORS

Acetazolamide (Diamox) is the prototypical drug, a sulfonamide with significant carbonic anhydrase inhibitory action, resulting in an inhibition of H^+ secretion and a consequent decrease in the availability of H^+ for Na^+-H^+ exchange. Subsequent to the administration of acetazolamide, there is an increase in urinary volume, urinary pH, urinary concentration of

Na^+, K^+, and bicarbonate, and a decrease in the excretion of titratable acid and ammonia. With a decrease in the concentration of bicarbonate in the extracellular fluid, metabolic acidosis develops, which reduces the response of the kidney to acetazolamide.

The usefulness of acetazolamide as a diuretic is limited, but because of the high concentration of bicarbonate in aqueous humor, acetazolamide is used in glaucoma to reduce aqueous humor formation and consequently to reduce intraocular pressure.

Toxicity — Paresthesias and drowsiness have been reported with large doses. Otherwise, serious toxicity is rare.

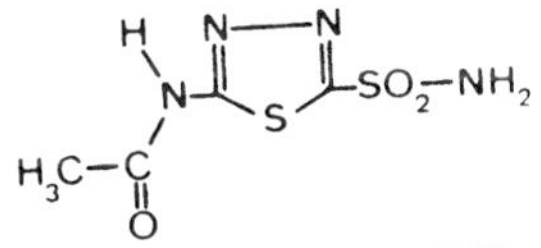

ACETAZOLAMIDE

C. BENZOTHIADIAZINE DERIVATIVES (THIAZIDES)

The synthesis of the thiazides yielded a class of drugs which retained an element of carbonic anhydrase inhibition, but which distinguished themselves primarily by significant increases in urinary chloride.[1]

Sulfonamide diuretics such as chlorthalidone, metolazone, quinethazone, and indapamide are structurally different, but have the same pharmacological effect as the thiazides. Thiazides act in the early distal renal tubule to increase urinary Na^+, Cl^-, H_2O, and K^+, due to blockade of electroneutral Na-Cl-cotransport.[2] Because of the wide range of carbonic anhydrase inhibition among the thiazides, bicarbonate excretion will vary accordingly. Thiazides decrease the renal excretion of calcium by direct action on the early distal tubule[3] and enhance the excretion of magnesium.

The toxic dose of the thiazides is significantly greater than the amount used for their pharmacological action. Hypersensitivity reactions are serious, but rare. However, diuretic-induced hypokalemia, hyperuricemia, and hyperglycemia may occur. Hypokalemia may be related to the hyperglycemia by inhibition of insulin secretion.[4]

By mechanisms as yet unexplained, thiazides cause an increase in the concentration of cholesterol and triglycerides in plasma. Thiazides have proved useful in congestive heart failure, hypertension, and in hypercalciuria. In hypertension due to renal abnormalities, fluid retention may occur. Here, a thiazide may be considered a first-line drug. Clinically, all thiazides are virtually equivalent except for the dose in milligrams.

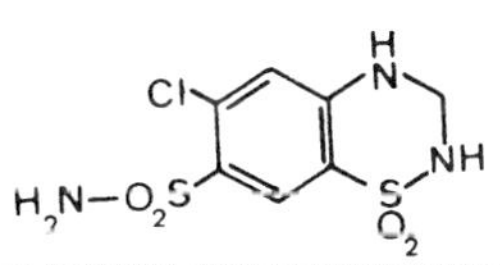

HYDROCHLOROTHIAZIDE

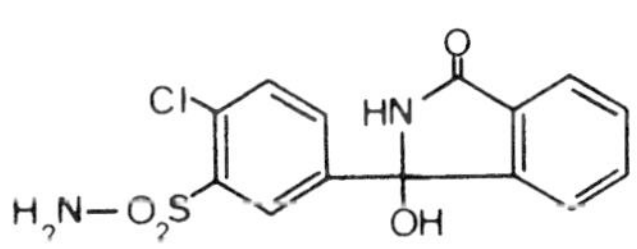

CHLORTHALIDONE

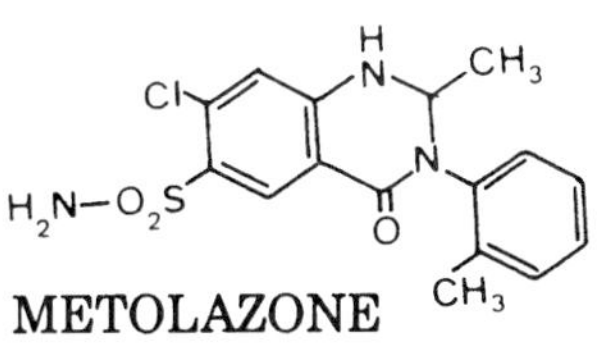

METOLAZONE

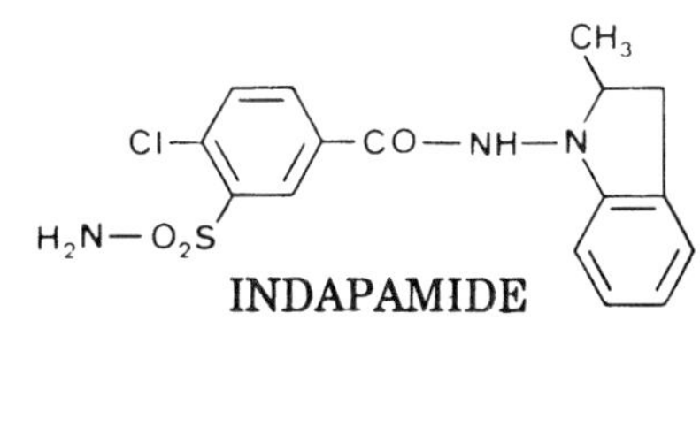

INDAPAMIDE

D. AGENTS ACTING AT THE LOOP OF HENLE (LOOP DIURETICS)

These agents result in a diuresis that is much greater than that noted with other agents; thus they are often referred to as "high-ceiling" diuretics. Because of their major site of action, the thick ascending limb of the loop of Henle, they are known as "loop diuretics" and include ethacrynic acid (Edecrin), furosemide (Lasix), and bumetanide (Bumex).

Pharmacologically they are similar and are thus grouped into one class; structurally they differ. Ethacrynic acid is an unsaturated derivative of phenoxyacetic acid; furosemide is an anthranilic acid derivative; bumetanide is an aminobenzoic acid derivative which is more potent than furosemide, but otherwise similar. Both furosemide and bumetanide are sulfonamides.

These compounds are characterized by a rapid onset, a short duration of action, and a profuse diuresis. They inhibit electrolyte reabsorption in the thick ascending limb of the loop of Henle by an action on the luminal surface of the epithelial cells to inhibit the Na^+-K^+-$2Cl^-$ cotransport mechanism.[5]

Furosemide and bumetanide, both sulfonamides, have weak carbonic anhydrase inhibitory action. The potassium loss and the hyperuricemia caused by these agents occur by the same mechanisms as with the thiazides. These loop diuretics cause an increased excretion of Ca^{2+}, Mg^{2+}, titratable acid, and ammonia, and the development of metabolic alkalosis.

High-ceiling diuretics are well absorbed from the gastrointestinal tract. They are strongly bound to plasma proteins. Excretion is by the kidneys and, to a lesser extent, by the liver.

Toxicity may include fluid and electrolyte imbalance, hyperuricemia, ototoxicity brought about by changes in the electrolyte composition of the endolymph,[6,7] as well as adverse interactions with other drugs. For example, furosemide, strongly bound to plasma albumin, may compete for sites on the protein with warfarin.

The high-ceiling diuretics are very useful for the treatment of serious edema states, and can be lifesaving in the treatment of acute pulmonary edema.

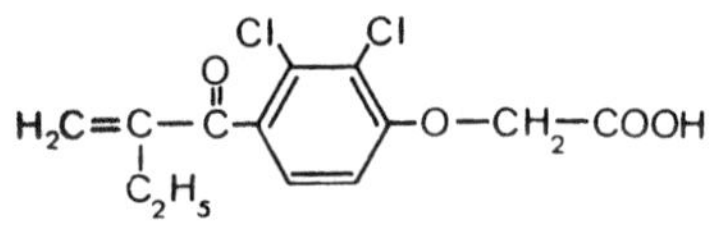

ETHACRYNIC ACID

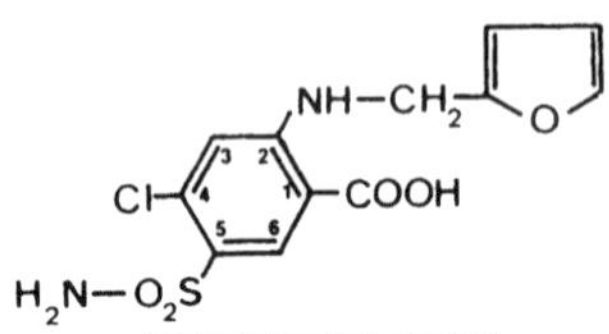

FUROSEMIDE

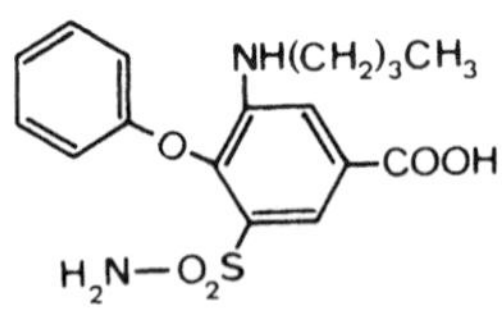

BUMETANIDE

E. POTASSIUM-SPARING DIURETICS: ALDOSTERONE ANTAGONISTS

The loss of potassium, characteristic of the action of the thiazides and the loop diuretics, stimulated interest in a group of 17-spirolactone steroids which manifested competitive inhibition of the sodium-reabsorptive and the potassium-secreting effects of mineralocorticoids such as aldosterone. Spironolactone appears to be most effective.

Mineralocorticoids act in the nucleus of responsive epithelial cells to cause the transcription of messenger RNA, which in turn codes for the production of proteins involved in Na^+ and K^+ transport. The hormones are carried to the nucleus while bound to a protein in the cytoplasm, and are also bound to a protein in the nucleus during their action. Spironolactone competitively inhibits binding of the mineralocorticoids to these proteins, and thus prevents the action of the hormones. The major sites of action are the distal tubule and the collecting duct. Spironolactone antagonism requires the presence of aldosterone, but may be overcome by high concentrations of aldosterone.

Spironolactone is well absorbed orally, is metabolized during its first passage through the liver, and binds readily to plasma proteins. A major metabolite of spironolactone is canrenone, which is also an active aldosterone antagonist.

Major toxic effects of spironolactone result from the hyperkalemia which it may produce. Other untoward effects include gynecomastia, impotence, and gastrointestinal disturbances, all of which are reversible when the drug is discontinued. An aldosterone antagonist has been used in combination with other diuretic agents to prevent loss of K^+. This is a valuable adjunct to therapy, but does raise the question of modification of actions of drugs which are administered simultaneously.

Preparations available include Spironolactone (Aldactone) and a fixed-dose combination of spironolactone and hydrochlorothiazide (Aldactazide).

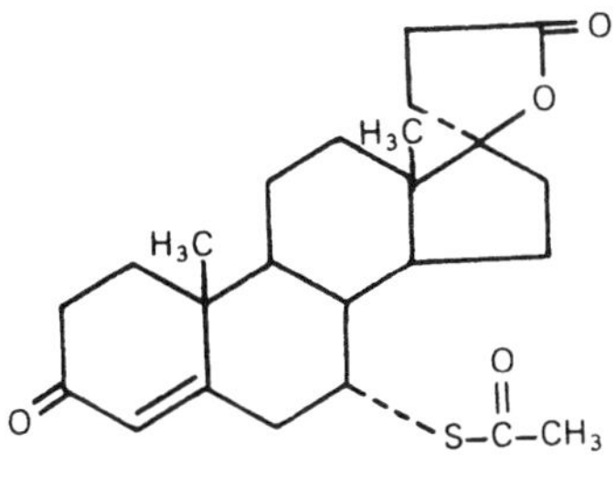

SPIRONOLACTONE

F. OTHER POTASSIUM-SPARING DIURETICS

The two drugs in this class are triamterene and amiloride, with the same "potassium-sparing" action as spironolactone, but completely independent of aldosterone antagonism. Triamterene and amiloride are organic bases. Triamterene is a pteridine; amiloride is a guanidine.

The drugs seem to have identical action. They act directly on tubular transport, independent of levels of aldosterone. They inhibit secretion of K^+ in the distal nephron; this is achieved by a primary reduction in Na^+ reabsorption, leading to a drop in transtubular electrical potential difference. The latter is normally the driving force for K^+ secretion. This reduction is the basis for the K^+-sparing effect.[8] The result is an increase in Na^+ excretion and a decrease in K^+ excretion in urine. Both amiloride and triamterene are given orally, resulting in a 50% absorption. Both undergo plasma protein binding. Amiloride is not metabolized; triamterene is completely metabolized. The chief toxic effect of both drugs is hyperkalemia, a result of their action. The preparations available (both for oral use) are Triamterene (Dyrenium) and Amiloride (Midamor).

Therapeutically, good results have been obtained using each of these preparations alone for edema. Their greatest use, however, is in combination with other diuretic agents so as to increase the natriuresis and reduce the K^+ loss. This reduction in K^+ loss is the more important end point.

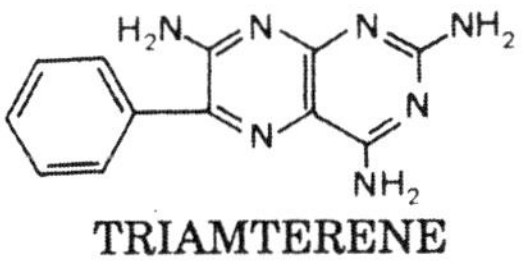

TRIAMTERENE

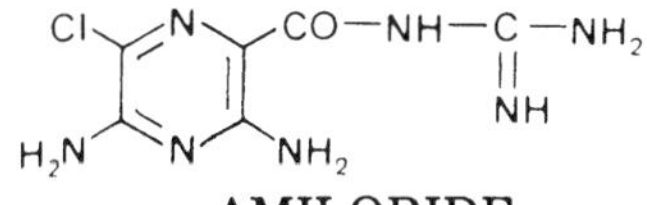

AMILORIDE

IV. DIURETICS IN THE ELDERLY: AN OVERVIEW

With increasing age, glomerular filtration rate, renal plasma flow, and tubular excretory capacity as well as creatinine and urea clearance are significantly reduced. The ability of the kidney to concentrate urine and to conserve sodium also declines with age.

Diuretics have an established record of usefulness in hypertension, congestive heart failure, and edema. As a result, they constitute one of the most frequently prescribed groups of drugs, especially in the elderly. A report from the Boston Collaborative Drug Surveillance Program revealed that, based on the pattern of diuretic use in the U.S., 64% of the furosemide which was prescribed was in patients over 60 years of age.[9] Furthermore, it has been reported that such agents as ethacrynic acid and furosemide, the "loop" diuretics, are more frequently prescribed than the thiazides.[10] With the paucity of information about diuretic pharmacokinetics in the elderly, a thorough knowledge of the indications for diuretic therapy and careful monitoring of the effects of therapy should be the key factors in avoiding complications.[11]

A. SIDE EFFECTS OF DIURETICS IN ELDERLY PATIENTS

Diuretics are among the most frequently prescribed medications for elderly patients. As a result, these agents constitute the most common group of drugs causing adverse reactions requiring hospital admission. Approximately 60% of all serious adverse reactions in elderly patients are due to diuretics.[12]

Hypokalemia — Among elderly patients taking diuretics, 1 in 20 develops hypokalemia[13] by virtue of the action of the diuretics, especially thiazides and loop diuretics. The problem is more critical for patients taking cardiac glycosides because hypokalemia accentuates the cardiotoxicity of these agents.[14] Furthermore, the diets of many elderly people are deficient in potassium; their body potassium stores may be low even before the initiation of diuretic therapy. It may prove useful to add a K-sparing agent provided that K levels are monitored. Hypokalemic patients have a higher risk of ventricular fibrillation after infarction,[15] and in the 24 hr after the infarction, patients receiving diuretics have an increased mortality. Hypokalemia was found to occur with hydrochlorothiazide alone or in combination with a K sparer, but it was much less common with a K sparer aboard.[16] However, K-retaining diuretics may be associated with an increased risk of hyponatremia.[17]

Hyponatremia — Diuretic-induced hyponatremia seems to be predisposed by age, sex, and body weight. Patients are usually old, female, and underweight.[18] Severe symptomatic hyponatremia was related to diuretic treatment, primarily the thiazides.

Hyperuricemia — The use of diuretics is the most important risk factor for hyperuricemia in the elderly.[19] The highest serum uric acid values are associated with the use of furosemide combined with spironolactone, or hydrochlorothiazide combined with amiloride. The lowest values are associated with the use of triamterene alone, or triamterene plus trichlormethiazide. Elderly women are particularly prone to diuretic-induced tophaceous gout, but less likely to have episodes of acute gout than men.[20]

Glucose intolerance — The diabetogenic effect of thiazide diuretics has also been described with loop diuretics. Glucose intolerance is worsened by potassium depletion and a low caloric intake. Both of these factors are critical in the elderly, whose potassium intake and caloric intake may be low.[11] In elderly patients with congestive heart failure, higher blood glucose levels developed in a furosemide-treated group (40 mg daily) than in a bumetanide-treated group (1 mg daily).[21]

Hypovolemia — The elderly are highly susceptible to this untoward effect of diuretic therapy. The glomerular filtration rate of the aged kidney decreases significantly; there is a marked reduction in the ability to reabsorb NaCl, resulting in volume depletion.[11]

Fatigue and weakness — This may occur in the elderly because of decreased perfusion of muscle, hypokalemia, and hyponatremia.

Postural hypotension — Elderly patients taking thiazide diuretics for mild cardiac failure are more likely to develop postural hypotension than those taking a loop diuretic such as furosemide. Although the mechanisms are not yet clear, the results indicate that loop diuretics may be a safer first treatment than thiazide diuretics for mild cardiac failure in the frail elderly.[22]

Effect on lipids — With the use of diuretics, plasma triglycerides, very low-density lipoproteins, and serum cholesterol may be elevated. This may increase coronary risk, especially in the elderly.

Effect on magnesium — Diuretics may induce magnesium depletion, particularly in the elderly with low magnesium intake. Digitalis, often prescribed in the elderly, induces arrhythmias more often in patients with hypomagnesemia.[23] Diuretic-associated hypomagnesemia is common in the elderly, with thiazide diuretics being most frequently implicated.[24,25] There is an impaired magnesium-conserving ability in hypomagnesemic patients on loop and thiazide diuretic therapy. However, the use of a K-sparing diuretic seems to protect the magnesium-conserving ability.[24] Magnesium is intimately involved in potassium transport. Magnesium depletion may exacerbate the effects of hypokalemia. Thus, the use of a potassium-magnesium-sparing diuretic in combination, which may reduce the risk of depletion, has been suggested.[25]

Ototoxicity — As was mentioned in Section II, the loop diuretics, in large doses, may bring about change in the electrolyte composition in the endolymph[6,7] which may result in temporary or permanent deafness.

Uremia — All diuretics can cause uremia and hyponatremia, but combinations of a diuretic and a potassium-sparing agent are likely to do so in the elderly.[26] Giving K-sparing agents or K supplements does not eliminate the need to check serum electrolyte concentrations. Some patients develop hyperkalemia, which is more likely to cause cardiac arrhythmia and sudden death than K depletion.

Stroke — Diuretic drugs may contribute to the development of cerebral ischemia or stroke when blood pressure is lowered too quickly. Drugs like the loop diuretic furosemide should be avoided in the treatment of hypertension because of their powerful hypovolemic action with the risk of a quick fall in blood pressure. In the aged, this relatively rapid reduction of blood pressure may induce stroke.[27]

Effect on renal clearance — In the elderly, there is a decrease in renal clearance due to a deterioration of renal function. In patients receiving amiloride and hydrochlorothiazide, the plasma concentration of each drug increased. The increased area under the curve after a single dose of amiloride and hydrochlorothiazide was the result of a reduction in the plasma clearance of these two drugs.[28] Similar findings were noted with the use of furosemide, spironolactone, and triamterene.[29]

Effect on elimination half-life — The elimination half-life of chlorthalidone was more than doubled in elderly patients.[30]

Effect on renin release — In the elderly, there was a reduction in plasma renin activity. With aging, the enzyme producing PGI_2 decreases in activity relative to that producing thromboxone A_2 (TXA_2). Therefore, a stimulus which releases arachidonic acid, such as furosemide, would lead to relatively more TXA_2 than PGI_2, resulting in a reduction of renin release.[31]

Rash — Since thiazide diuretics are sulfonamides, the elderly may develop rashes on initial treatment with thiazide diuretics.[23]

Other side effects — If severe constipation, fecal impaction, and large bowel obstruction are grouped together, they occur significantly more frequently in elderly patients on diuretic therapy.[32] Confusion, dehydration, and sexual dysfunction have been experienced by the elderly on diuretic therapy.[23] A less common side effect is an increased risk of acute pancreatitis or cholecystitis.[33,34]

B. SIDE EFFECTS AS THEY PERTAIN SPECIFICALLY TO THE USE OF DIURETICS AS ANTIHYPERTENSIVE AGENTS IN THE ELDERLY

Hypertension is very prevalent among individuals in the older age group. Diuretics have been found to be more effective in lowering blood pressure in older hypertensive individuals than in young patients. Administration of 25 mg of hydrochlorothiazide a day with or without 2.5 mg of amiloride proved effective. There was no further antihypertensive effect with the addition of amiloride. Adverse effects included hyperuricemia, hyponatremia, hypokalemia, and an increase in blood glucose and creatinine.[35] In those patients treated with chlorthalidone, 21% had serum potassium levels less than 3.5 mEq/L; 54% of them were on lower doses of chlorthalidone (25 mg/day). Thus, even low doses of diuretics may provoke hypokalemia in older hypertensive subjects. In another study, it was noted that 5% of the admissions to a large general hospital over a 2-month period were from iatrogenic causes. Diuretic therapy was the leading agent responsible for these admissions.[36] The mortality rate among elderly hypertensive patients treated with diuretics was found to be twice that of those treated with other antihypertensive agents.[37]

Diuretics appear to be more effective in lowering blood pressure in older hypertensives than in younger patients, but the risks of diuretic therapy cannot be ignored. Calcium channel blockers and serotonin antagonists have been suggested as useful and safe alternatives.[35]

C. MINIMIZING THE SIDE EFFECTS OF DIURETICS: THE VALUE OF "SLOW-RELEASE" PREPARATIONS

Loop diuretics such as furosemide are important in the treatment of acute pulmonary edema because of their rapid and potent action. Slow-release furosemide given to elderly patients with congestive heart failure was found to attenuate the diuresis in such a way as to avoid the peak effect without loss of the overall diuretic response, thus offering advantages in maintenance therapy.[38]

D. THE VALUE OF A SEROTONIN BLOCKER-DIURETIC COMBINATION

The combination of ketanserin, a 5-HT_2 blocker, plus hydrochlorothiazide at a dose of 20 + 25 mg, respectively, has proved to be an effective and well-tolerated antihypertensive treatment for patients in the >50-year-old age group. Few and mild side effects were encountered.[39]

E. THE VALUE OF A CENTRALLY ACTING ANTISYMPATHETIC AGENT-DIURETIC COMBINATION

A single daily dose of a combination of 500 mg of methyldopa, 25 mg of hydrochlorothiazide, and 2.5 mg of amiloride was used to test the efficacy and side effects in the aged. This regimen was found to be safe and effective for the elderly hypertensive patient. The lack of side effects was attributed to the small daily dose.[40]

F. THE RISK/BENEFIT OF COMBINATION DIURETICS IN THE ELDERLY

The introduction of a tablet containing a thiazide combined with a potassium-sparing diuretic improved the chances of drug compliance, but also prompted questions about the safety of such fixed combinations, especially in the elderly. The development of hypokalemia, azotemia, and hyponatremia in elderly patients during treatment with 50 mg hydrochlorothiazide combined with 5 mg amiloride daily suggested that a tablet of reduced strength would be more appropriate.[41]

V. CONCLUSION

Diuretics can be very useful in disorders of the elderly, but they cause side effects in this same age group. Prerequisites for using them are an accurate diagnosis, careful monitoring for efficacy and side effects, and regular review of the need for continued treatment.[42]

What is true for other classes of drugs pertains aptly to the diuretics: most drugs are studied in young, healthy, predominantly male volunteers in single-dose experiments. Most drugs are used by old, far from healthy, predominantly female patients on a chronic basis.[43]

REFERENCES

1. **Beyer, K. H.,** The mechanism of action of chlorothiazide, *Ann. N.Y. Acad. Sci.*, 71, 363, 1958.
2. **Velazquez, H.,** Thiazide diuretics, *Renal Physiol.*, 10, 184, 1987.
3. **Stier, C. T., Jr. and Itskovitz, H. D.,** Renal calcium metabolism, *Annu. Rev. Pharmacol. Toxicol.*, 26, 101, 1986.
4. **Tannen, R. L.,** Diuretic-induced hypokalemia, *Kidney Int.*, 28, 988, 1985.
5. **Greger, R. and Wangemann, P.,** Loop diuretics, *Renal Physiol.*, 10, 174, 1987.
6. **Rybak, L. P.,** Pathophysiology of furosemide ototoxicity, *J. Otolaryngol.*, 11, 127, 1982.
7. **Rybak, L. P.,** Ototoxicity of ethacrynic acid (a persistent clinical problem), *J. Laringol. Otol.*, 102, 518, 1988.
8. **Horisberger, J. D. and Giebisch, G.,** Potassium-sparing diuretics, *Renal Physiol.*, 10, 198, 1987.
9. **Greenblatt, D. J., Duhme, D. W., Allen, M. D., and Koch-Weser, J.,** Clinical toxicity of furosemide in hospitalized patients, *Am. Heart J.*, 94, 6, 1977.
10. **Portnoi, V. A. and Paulson, L. G.,** Abuse of diuretic therapy in nursing homes, *J. Chronic Dis.*, 34, 363, 1981.
11. **Smith, W. E. and Steele, T. H.,** Avoiding diuretic-related complications in older patients, *Geriatrics*, 38, 117, 1983.
12. **Lye, M.,** Diuretics and the elderly, *Nursing Elderly*, 2, 24, 1990.
13. **Sunderam, S. G. and Mankikar, G. D.,** Hyponatraemia in the elderly, *Age Ageing*, 12, 77, 1983.
14. **Steiners, E.,** Diuretics, digitalis and arrhythmias, *Acta Med. Scand. (Suppl.)*, 647, 75, 1981.
15. **Calcott, R., Dobson, A. J., and Gibberd, R. W.,** Antihypertensive treatment, body mass and survival after myocardial infarction, *Med. J. Aust.*, 141, 419, 1984.
16. **Myers, M. G.,** Hydrochlorothiazide with or without amiloride for hypertension in the elderly, *Arch. Intern. Med.*, 147, 1026, 1987.
17. **Byatt, C. M., Millard, P. H., and Levin, G. E.,** Diuretics and electrolyte disturbances in 1000 consecutive geriatric admissions, *J. R. Soc. Med.*, 83, 704, 1990.
18. **Ashouri, O. S.,** Severe diuretic-induced hyponatremia in the elderly, *Arch. Intern. Med.*, 146, 1355, 1986.
19. **Takala, J., Anttila, S., Gref, C. G., and Isomaki, H.,** Diuretics and hyperuricemia in the elderly, *Scand. J. Rheumatol.*, 17, 155, 1988.
20. **Macfarlane, D. G. and Dieppe, P. A.,** Diuretic-induced gout in elderly women, *Br. J. Rheumatol.*, 24, 155, 1985.
21. **Datta Chaudhuri, M. L. and Cantania, J.,** A comparison of the effects of bumetanide (Burinex) and frusemide on carbohydrate metabolism in the elderly, *Br. J. Clin. Pract.*, 42, 427, 1988.
22. **Heseltine, D. and Bramble, M. G.,** Loop diuretics cause less postural hypotension than thiazide diuretics in the frail elderly, *Curr. Med. Res. Opinion*, 11, 232, 1988.
23. **Lamy, P.,** Side effects of diuretics a danger for aged, *J. Gerontol. Nursing*, 11, 44, 1985.
24. **Martin, B. J. and Milligan, K.,** Diuretic-associated hypomagnesemia in the elderly, *Arch. Intern. Med.*, 147, 1768, 1987.
25. **Petri, M., Cumber, P., Grimes, L., Treby, D., Bryant, R., Rawlins, D., and Ising, H.,** The metabolic effects of thiazide therapy in the elderly: a population study, *Age Ageing*, 15, 151, 1986.
26. **Borland, C., Amadi, A., Murphy, P., and Shallcross, T.,** Biochemical and clinical correlates of diuretic therapy in the elderly, *Age Ageing*, 15, 257, 1986.
27. **Jansen, A. A., Schulte, B. P., Meyboom, R. H., and Gribnau, F. W.,** Antihypertensive treatment as a possible cause of stroke in the elderly, *Age Ageing*, 15, 129, 1986.

28. **Ismail, Z., Triggs, E. J., Smithurst, B. A., and Parke, W.,** The pharmacokinetics of amiloride-hydrochlorothiazide combination in the young and elderly, *Eur. J. Clin. Pharmacol.*, 37, 167, 1989.
29. **Muhlberg, W.,** Pharmacokinetics of diuretics in geriatric patients, *Arch. Gerontol. Geriatr.*, 9, 283, 1989.
30. **Colussi, D., Schoeller, J. P., Richard, A., and Sioufi, A.,** Pharmacokinetics of chlorthalidone in the elderly after single and multiple doses, *Br. J. Clin. Pharmacol.*, 16, 755, 1983.
31. **Wilson, T. W., McCaulay, F. A., and Walsen, T. A.,** Effects of aging on responses to furosemide, *Prostaglandins*, 38, 675, 1989.
32. **Borland, C., Amadi, A., Murphy, P., and Shallcross, T.,** Biochemical and clinical correlates of diuretic therapy in the elderly, *Age Ageing*, 15, 357, 1986.
33. **Eckhauser, M. L., Dokler, M. A., and Imbembo, A. L.,** Diuretic-associated pancreatitis: a collective review and illustrative cases, *Am. J. Gastroenterol.*, 82, 865, 1987.
34. **Van der Linden, W., Ritter, B., and Edlund, G.,** Acute cholecystitis and thiazide, *Br. Med. J.*, 289, 654, 1984.
35. **Weinberger, M. H.,** Diuretic responsiveness of blood pressure in the elderly, *J. Cardiovasc. Pharmacol.*, 12, S60, 1988.
36. **Lakshmanan, M. C., Hershey, C. O., and Breslan, D.,** Hospital admissions caused by iatrogenic disease, *Arch. Intern. Med.*, 146, 1931, 1986.
37. **Morgan, T., Adam W., and Carney, S.,** Treatment of mild hypertension in elderly males, *Clin. Sci. Mol. Med.*, 57, S355, 1979.
38. **Verneulen, A. and Chadha, D. R.,** Diuretic effect of slow-release furosemide in elderly patients, *Eur. J. Clin. Pharmacol.*, 24, 449, 1983.
39. **Ferrara, L. A., Fasano, M. L., Soro, S., Pasanisi, F., and Mancini, M.,** Antihypertensive efficacy of the combination of ketanserin + thiazide in hypertensives older than 50 years, *J. Cardiovasc. Pharmacol.*, 10, S124, 1987.
40. **Fidel, J. and Glickberg, F.,** The effect of a single daily low dose of methyldopa and K^+ sparing diuretic on blood pressure in the elderly, *Br. J. Clin. Pract.*, 42, 491, 1988.
41. **Donaldson, M.,** Combination diuretics in the elderly, *Med. J. Aust.*, 1, 106, 1983.
42. **MacLennan, W. J.,** Diuretics in the elderly: how safe?, *Br. Med. J.*, 296, 1551, 1988.
43. **Kerremans, A. L. and Gribnau, F. W.,** Changes in pharmacokinetics and in effect of furosemide in the elderly, *Clin. Exp. Hyper. Theory Pract.*, 5, 271, 1983.

Chapter 7

THE EFFECT OF AGE ON BRONCHODILATORS USED TO TREAT ASTHMA

Jay Roberts, David L. Snyder, and Mark D. Johnson

CONTENTS

I. INTRODUCTION

A. PATHOPHYSIOLOGY OF ASTHMA

Asthma is a constriction of the bronchial smooth muscles, resulting in a dramatic reduction in airway passage. The bronchospasm associated with asthma can be precipitated by exposure to one or more of a wide variety of stimuli, including allergens, exercise, infections, and emotional stress. Typical asthma symptoms are recurrent bouts of shortness of breath, episodic wheezing, and intermittent cough. A lessening of airflow obstruction in response to bronchodilator therapy is a definitive characteristic of this disease.[1] Asthma prevalence in the general population is 7 to 8%.[2]

A rational approach to the pharmacotherapy of asthma must take into account the fact that asthma involves IgE antibodies bound to mast cells in the airway mucosa. Additional exposure to the antigen triggers release of mediators stored in the granules of the cells of the muscles and the release of other mediators. The substances released include histamine, tryptase and other neutral proteases, leukotrienes C_4 and D_4, prostaglandin D_2, eosinophil chemotactic factor, neutrophil chemotactic factor, neutral proteases, and other compounds. These agents diffuse throughout the airway wall and cause contraction of muscle, edema, cellular infiltration, and a change in mucous secretion either by altering neurohumoral

0-8493-8306-4/96/$0.00+$.50

influences or by direct action. Asthmatic bronchospasm results from a combined release of mediators and an exaggeration of the response to these agents.[3]

Allergens are less important in provoking asthma in the elderly compared to younger subjects.[1] Viral respiratory infections, cigarette smoke, and β-adrenoceptor antagonists (β-blockers) are common agents which may precipitate an asthma attack in the elderly.[4]

B. PREVALENCE OF ASTHMA IN THE ELDERLY

Asthma in the elderly is usually chronic with persistent airflow obstruction and only partial reversibility with maximum therapy.[5] The prevalence of asthma in the elderly has been estimated to be between 6.5 and 17%.[5–7] General population studies by Dodge and Burrows[7] indicate that approximately 7% of people over 70 report asthma symptoms. After age 40, 40% of people with asthma develop the condition.[8] Burr et al.[6] examined 27 asthmatic patients over the age of 70. In this group 37% had developed asthma after 50 and 19% after 70. Braman et al.[5] reported that of 25 asthma patients over 70, 48% developed the condition after age 65, and these patients were 17% of all patients over 70 seen in their chest clinic. Evans et al.[2] reported on asthma prevalence in the U.S. from 1964 to 1984 based on data from the National Center for Health Statistics. The prevalence of active asthma in the 65- to 74-year-old group was 10.4% compared to 5.7% in younger teenagers, 6.9% in the 18- to 44-year-old group, and 9.6% in the 45- to 64-year-old group. These studies suggest that development of asthma in the elderly is not uncommon. Therefore, the effect of aging on therapeutic interventions is an important consideration when dealing with elderly asthmatic patients.

C. COMMON ASTHMA TREATMENTS FOR THE ELDERLY

In 1982, Ziment[9] reported that theophylline was the therapy of choice in managing asthma in the elderly. Today, β-agonists have become the drugs of choice as first-line therapy for asthma. The use of β-agonists in the elderly should be monitored closely because of diminished β-receptor function with age (see below). Inhaled ipratropium, an anticholinergic agent, may be considered in the elderly when β-agonist therapy is no longer effective.[10] β-Agonists and anticholinergic therapy have generally replaced the use of methylxanthines, such as aminophylline and theophylline, as first-line therapy because they are less toxic and more effective.[11] However, sustained-release formulations of theophylline are still useful in patients with uncontrolled asthma symptoms, but who are already using maximum bronchodilator and steroid inhalation therapy.

II. BRONCHODILATORS

A. THEOPHYLLINE

The capacity of the xanthines to relax airway smooth muscle has been of help in the treatment of asthmatic conditions. The three most important methylxanthines are theophylline, theobromine, and caffeine. The most commonly used asthma treatment among the xanthines is the theophylline-ethylene-diamine complex (aminophylline). As previously mentioned, the importance of theophylline as a therapeutic agent is waning, as inhaled sympathomimetic agents for acute asthma and inhaled anti-inflammatory agents for chronic asthma have replaced theophylline.

1. Mechanism of Action of Theophylline

The mechanism of action of theophylline has been attributed to its inhibition of the enzyme phosphodiesterase (PDE), which hydrolyzes cyclic nucleotides. This inhibition results in higher concentrations of intracellular cAMP, resulting in relaxation of bronchial and vascular smooth muscles. There is still some question as to whether or not therapeutic theophylline levels are sufficient to increase cAMP levels.

Changes in PDE activity with age have been variously reported. In extracts of the prostate and the heart, PDE activity has been reported to decrease.[12] A decline in the low K_m-PDE activity in the epididymis and prostate of aged rats was also observed by Razaboni and Terner.[13] Bylund et al.[14] reported that PDE activity in erythrocyte membranes was reduced in those taken from 13.5-month-old rats compared to 1.5-month-old animals. Hoskins and Ho[15] noted that PDE activity decreases in cerebellum of aged male rats. However, a significant rise in high KM-PDE activity was observed in the cerebral cortex, hypothalamus, and hippocampus in aged rats while the low KM form did not change.[16] PDE activity increases with age in adipocytes in rats fed *ad libitum* and to a greater extent than that found in dietary-restricted rats.[17] In adrenal cortical cells from Sprague-Dawley rats, hydrolysis of cAMP by low and high KM-PDE did not change significantly with advancing age.[18] Dax et al.[19] also showed that PDE activity in the presence or absence of isoproterenol did not change with age in the isolated rat adipocyte preparation. Since age-related changes in bronchial PDE activity have not been studied, the effect of age on the capacity of theophylline to inhibit PDE activity is uncertain.

While the cellular basis for the response to xanthine derivatives is much debated, adenosine receptor antagonism has been suggested as an important mode of action.[20] Adenosine receptor activation results in decreased adenylyl cyclase activity and cAMP production. Since increased intracellular cAMP levels cause airway smooth muscle relaxation, adenosine may be a contributing factor in bronchoconstriction. Adenosine does induce isolated airway muscle contraction and enhances histamine release in the lung.[3] Some of the adverse effects of theophylline in the CNS are attributed to adenosine receptor antagonism. Enprofylline, a much weaker adenosine receptor antagonist, is thought to be free of such effects and, unlike theophylline, does not produce seizures in experimental animals.[20] However, enprofylline and theophylline exhibit similar pulmonary effects, suggesting that the capacity of theophylline to relax airways involves other mechanisms in addition to adenosine antagonism.[21]

The interaction of theophylline with adenosine receptors as a function of age has not been examined. Studies in the rat heart indicate that adenosine levels are higher in older animals, rendering them less responsive to β-adrenergic stimulation.[22,23] If this were to occur at the bronchial level, then theophylline antagonism of adenosine receptors could have a greater effect in older bronchi. However, studies with bronchial tissue obtained from young and old rats are needed to determine the extent of the interaction between theophylline and adenosine receptors as a function of age.

Despite the wide variability within individuals, when compared to young subjects (22 to 33 years), elderly subjects (62 to 78 years) demonstrated a lower absolute change in bronchodilator response to equal concentrations of theophylline. Heart rate increased progressively with increasing theophylline concentrations, but significant heart rate differences were not noted between age groups. Whether the differences in theophylline-induced bronchodilator response in the young and elderly groups are due to age or the severity of airway obstruction is not known.[24]

Theophylline induced neurotoxicity is apparently not age dependent.[25] Age did not influence the onset of general seizures in male Fischer rats (4, 14, and 22 months old) following intravenous administration of theophylline as aminophylline. However, theophylline kinetics did vary between young and old rats. Larger doses of theophylline were necessary to produce seizures in young rats and the CSF to brain theophylline concentration ratio was higher in young rats at the onset of seizures. The differences in kinetics were not due to age-related alterations in serum protein binding of the drug, since the serum free fraction of theophylline did not differ among the age groups. In human subjects 1 to 68 years, age does not influence the theophylline concentration at which seizures develop.[26]

Besides the effects on bronchial smooth muscle, other actions of methylxanthines in the CNS cause mild cortical arousal, increased alertness, and deferral of fatigue.[3] The caffeine contained in coffee and other beverages may be responsible for these CNS effects and account for the large consumption of coffee. The methylxanthines also have a direct positive chronotropic and inotropic effect on the heart. This may be due to increased catecholamine release following inhibition of presynaptic adenosine receptors by high concentrations of methylxanthines. Also, theophylline impairs calcium sequestration by the sarcoplasmic reticulum, and calcium availability may increase, resulting in higher intracellular concentrations and increased muscle contractility.[3] These actions on the heart must be taken into account in considering the use of methylxanthines for the treatment of asthma.[3]

Methylxanthines also decrease blood viscosity and may improve blood flow under certain conditions. One of the more important agents for this effect is pentoxifylline. Methylxanthine increases gastric acid and digestive enzyme secretion, and this effect must be considered in the older person. Methylxanthines seem to affect striated muscle function, improving contractility. The methylxanthines are also weak diuretics.[3]

2. Theophylline Pharmacokinetics in the Elderly

Theophylline base is only slightly water soluble, so a number of different salts containing various amounts of theophylline base are used instead. Most preparations are well absorbed from the gastrointestinal tract. When a rapid action of theophylline is required, an I.V. or rapidly absorbed liquid is preferable to rectal administration.[27] In addition there are several sustained-release preparations such as So-Phyllin and Theo-Dur which can produce therapeutic levels of theophylline for up to 12 hr. These preparations offer less frequent administration, which may be particularly desirable in the elderly.

Therapeutic and toxic effects of theophylline increase with plasma concentrations of the drug greater than 20 mg/mL.[27] The initial or loading dose of a drug is determined by its distribution and the subsequent maintenance dose by the rate of plasma clearance. The apparent volume of distribution (V_d) for theophylline is proportional to the lean body weight, but otherwise varies only slightly among individuals.[3] Thus, with the reduction in lean body weight and relative increase in fat in the elderly, the volume distribution for theophylline would be expected to decrease. However, changes in theophylline V_d with age have been variously reported.[28] Cusack et al.[29] reported similar V_d in young and older groups, while Jusko et al.[30] and Neilsen-Kudsah et al.[31] reported a decreased V_d in the elderly. While no significant differences in V_d and overall plasma clearance were observed when calculations were based on total plasma theophylline, a 37% reduction in V_d and a 30% reduction in overall plasma clearance (*P*) in the elderly became apparent when plasma protein binding was taken into account.[32] A decrease in 3-methylxanthine was also detected in the urine specimens of geriatric subjects, indicating decreased theophylline metabolism. For these reasons, Antal et al.[32] recommended a reduction in theophylline dosages, despite the apparent normal total theophylline clearance in geriatric patients.

Theophylline kinetics in the elderly were examined by Fox et al.[28] Theophylline elixir, given as a single standard dose (5 mg/kg of lean body weight), was administered in all subjects. A sustained-release theophylline tablet was given to young and geriatric subjects 1 week later. Theophylline elimination ($t_{1/2}$ β) was shorter in the geriatric group (6.93 vs. 8.14 hr); total body theophylline clearance was greater in the geriatric group (44.39 vs. 32.97 mL/kg/hr); and the apparent volume of distribution was also greater in the geriatric group than in the young group (26.29 vs. 22.97). Gender and smoking did not influence any of the parameters studied. In 93% of the geriatric subjects, serum theophylline levels of 8 to 20 μg/mL were reached at steady state with the slow-release tablets. These concentrations are below toxic levels.[27] Since the clinical efficacy and toxicity of theophylline are directly related to serum concentrations,[33–35] Fox et al.[28] concluded that theophylline dose reduction based on an arbitrary age limit is not invariably indicated, although the current practice is to lower the dose in the elderly. Blouin et al.[36] came to the same conclusions after examining total body clearance, elimination half-life, volume of distribution, and protein binding of theophylline. They found that there were no statistically significant differences in these kinetic parameters between the elderly and young subjects. Bauer and Blouin[37] and Cusak et al.[29] also found no change in theophylline clearance.

Other investigations have found age-related differences in theophylline clearance. Au et al.[38] reported a decrease in theophylline clearance in old age. In this study, 39 adult patients with chronic obstructive pulmonary disease (COPD) received an intravenous dose of aminophylline. Theophylline clearance declined significantly between middle aged and older patients, the $t_{1/2}$ of older patients being somewhat longer (11 vs. 7.4 hr). Jusko et al.[39] demonstrated similar decreases in theophylline elimination in the elderly.

Further studies of the relationship between theophylline clearance and age were performed by Jackson et al.[40] using Theo-Dur, a slow-release form of theophylline. Mean theophylline clearance was 0.53 mL/min/kg in a group with a mean age of 70 years, 0.72 for the middle-age group (47 years), and 0.73 for the young group (26 years). There were no significant age-related changes in volume of distribution per kilogram corrected for body weight, but the $t_{1/2}$ did increase with age. This was observed in both patients with asthma and normal volunteers analyzed separately. Thus, although clearance may not fall with increasing age up to adult life, clearance does fall during late adult life, becoming apparent in the seventh, eighth, and ninth decades. These findings suggest that theophylline clearance only falls in the upper third of the age distribution, i.e., in the range of 58 to 87 years of age. Thus, the study by Jackson et al.[40] provides additional evidence to support the clinical impression that patients older than 70 years need a lower weight-related dose of theophylline than young and middle-aged adults.

Shin et al.[41] showed that both the renal and metabolic elimination processes for theophylline are less active in the normal elderly. The unbound faction of theophylline was significantly raised in the elderly and was correlated with serum albumin levels. Theophylline nonrenal clearance does not change, but the total unbound clearance is significantly reduced in elderly subjects (31%) as compared with younger subjects. Creatinine clearance was reduced in the elderly, and this was significantly correlated with unbound renal clearance of theophylline. There was no age-related difference in urinary excretion of theophylline, 1-methyluric acid, 3-methylxanthine, or 1,3-dimethyluric acid. As in the case of unbound renal theophylline clearance, the unbound metabolic clearance of 1,3-dimethyluric acid, 3-methylxanthine, and 1-methyluric acid was reduced in the elderly subjects. These observations indicate that both renal and metabolic elimination processes for theophylline are less active in the normal elderly. In contrast to Shin et al.,[41] Vestal et al.[42] showed that total clearance (bound plus unbound theophylline) in the elderly was 33% less than in younger groups. As Shin et al.[41] pointed out, the smaller sample size (6 vs. 10) in their study compared with Vestal et al.[42] was the most likely explanation for this discrepancy.

While total theophylline clearance is often used as an index of hepatic drug metabolizing enzyme activity, only unbound drug enters the hepatocytes or becomes filtered by the glomerulus. Because the total (hepatic and renal) unbound clearance values take into account changes in distribution volume and protein binding, total unbound clearance is a more direct assessment of the eliminating capacity of the excretory organs of the body. The total unbound clearance, not the total systemic clearance, has more pharmacological and clinical importance.[41]

Studies in humans have shown theophylline metabolism to be decreased,[38,43] increased,[28] or unchanged.[29,32,44] These conflicting reports may have been confounded by other variables such as liver disease, heart disease, smoking, obesity, viral infections, and concomitant use of other drugs known to influence theophylline disposition.[41] Except for Vestal et al.,[42] Antal et al.,[32] and Shin et al.,[41] the effect of age on protein binding and urinary metabolism has not been determined. Although intravenous administration would have provided more definitive quantitative data, theophylline was given orally in most studies. Differences in plasma clearance, renal clearance, and the amount of unchanged drug recovered in the urine have been reported between oral and intravenous theophylline given to the same subjects. The autoinduction phenomenon, whereby theophylline induces enzymes for its own metabolism, complicates interpretation of these studies.[45] Some studies were performed in institutionalized subjects, which limits the applicability of these results to the general elderly population. The studies by Shin et al.[41] were performed in noninstitutionalized people and were designed to include elements lacking in some of the previously mentioned studies: strict control of methylxanthine intake, intravenous drug administration, assessment of protein binding under physiologic conditions, and measurement of theophylline metabolites in urine.

Shin et al.[41] observed that both the N-demethylation and C-oxidation pathways for theophylline become less active in the elderly. These observations are consistent with the age-related impairment of phase I metabolic pathways responsible for the elimination of many drugs.[46] Figure 7.1, taken from Shin et al.,[41] provides a summary of the effects of age-related physiological changes on theophylline pharmacokinetics.

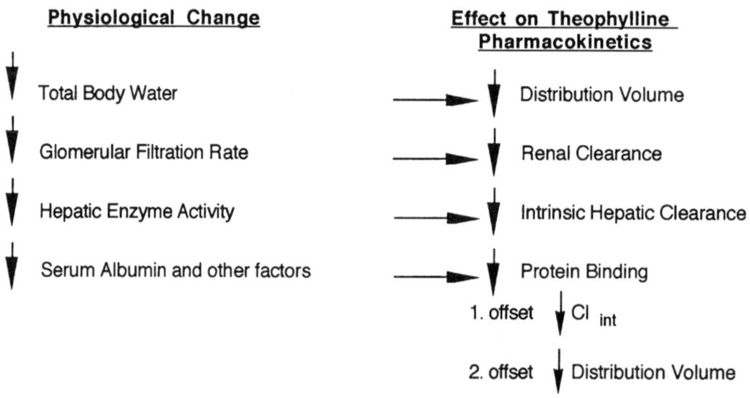

FIGURE 7.1. Summary of effects of physiologic changes on theophylline pharmacokinetics associated with aging. Cl_{int} = unbound theophylline hepatic clearance. (From Shin, S. G., Juan, D., and Rammohan, M., *Clin. Pharmacol. Ther.*, 44, 522, 1988. With permission.)

The effects of dietary protein restriction and age on theophylline pharmacokinetics in rats have been investigated by Jung and Nanavaty.[47] Dietary protein restriction in 2- and 14-month-old rats led to a significant reduction in total clearance from 73 to 45 mL/hr/kg. Interestingly, although there appeared to be a diet-related impairment of theophylline metabolism in younger rats, theophylline clearance was approximately 45 mL/hr/kg in 20-month-old rats irrespective of dietary protein. Thus, in older rats, dietary protein restriction did not appear to affect theophylline clearance.

3. Theophylline and Cimetidine Drug Interaction in the Elderly

Cimetidine is an H_2 histamine receptor blocker which may be prescribed in the elderly for the treatment of gastric and duodenal ulcers. Cimetidine inhibits the P450 enzymes responsible for theophylline metabolism, and therefore the combination of these two drugs may result in an increased theophylline action. The effect of age and cimetidine dose on this interaction was studied by Cohen et al.[48] These authors noted that cimetidine-induced alterations in theophylline pharmacokinetics appear to be dose related and of similar magnitude in the elderly and young healthy adults. Vestal et al.[49] have shown that there is no age difference in the inhibition of theophylline metabolism by cimetidine and ciprofloxin administered in combination to healthy male and female nonsmokers. Vestal et al.[49] also found an age-associated reduction in the basal capacity to oxidize theophylline in the liver, presumably due to changes in at least two isozymes of cytochrome P450 (CYP_1A_2, $CYP2E_1$, and possibly CYP_3A) in healthy male nonsmokers. Despite this both the induction of theophylline metabolism by smoking and the inhibition of theophylline metabolism by cimetidine are preserved in the elderly. The effects of age, smoking, and cimetidine on theophylline pharmacokinetics are presented in Table 7.1 (Vestal et al.).[49] Theophylline metabolism was induced by phenytoin

TABLE 7.1.
Effects of Age, Smoking, and Cimetidine on Pharmacokinetics of Theophylline

Group	N	Age (years)	$T_{1/2}$ (hr)		Vd_{ss} (L/kg)		CL_{iv} (mL/hr/kg)		Mean plasma cimetidine (μg/mL
			Control	Cimetidine	Control	Cimetidine	Control	Cimetidine	
Young subjects									
Nonsmokers	10	27 ± 1	7.7 ± 0.7	10.6 ± 1.1**	0.45 ± 0.03	0.45 ± 0.02	45.6 ± 4.0	32.3 ± 2.7**	0.94 ± 0.08
Smokers	10	28 ± 1	5.4 ± 0.4	7.0 ± 0.4**	0.48 ± 0.02	0.46 ± 0.01	67.8 ± 6.3	48.1 ± 3.4**	0.80 ± 0.05
p^a			<0.05	<0.01	NS	NS	<0.05	<0.01	NS
Old subjects									
Nonsmokers	10	76 ± 2	10.2 ± 0.5	13.5 ± 0.5**	0.42 ± 0.02	0.41 ± 0.02	30.9 ± 2.9	22.0 ± 1.5**	1.46 ± 0.11
Smokers	10	70 ± 1	6.1 ± 0.4	8.6 ± 0.5*	0.44 ± 0.02	0.46 ± 0.03	54.7 ± 4.7	38.0 ± 2.2**	1.06 ± 0.11
p^a			<0.001	<0.001	NS	NS	<0.001	<0.001	<0.05

Note: Data are mean ± SE. Vd_{ss} = Volume of distribution at steady state. CL_{iv} = clearance of drug given intravenously. Statistical comparisons between control and cimetidine within each age group (paired analysis) are as follows: $*p < 0.01$; $**p < 0.001$.

[a] Statistical comparisons between nonsmokers and smokers (unpaired analysis). Two-factor analysis of variance with interaction showed main effects of age and smoking to be significant (p at least <0.01) for $T_{1/2}$ and CL_{iv}, but not Vd_{ss}.

From Vestal, R. E., Cusack, B. J., Crowley, J. J., and Loi, C.-M., *Exp. Ger.*, 28, 42[illegible], 1993. With permission.

to an equal extent in both young and old age groups and in smokers. These studies also showed a reduction in basal capacity to oxidize theophylline in elderly nonsmoking males. In addition, the study demonstrated that the ability of smoking or phenytoin to induce theophylline metabolism and the ability of theophylline to induce cortisol metabolism are maintained in old age.

B. β-AGONISTS

1. β_2-Adrenoceptor Function and Aging

β_2-adrenoceptors are located in the smooth muscle of the bronchi as well as vascular smooth muscle. When stimulated by epinephrine, norepinephrine, or a β_2-adrenoceptor agonist the receptor couples to a G protein in the membrane. The agonist-receptor-G protein complex is then capable of exchanging the GDP connected to the G protein for GTP. The complex then becomes destabilized and releases the G protein-GTP part of the complex. The G protein-GTP activates the catalytic unit of adenylyl cyclase, which then converts ATP to cyclic AMP (cAMP). Increases in intracellular cAMP reduce bronchial smooth muscle contraction and open the airways.[3]

Vasodilation in response to β_2-adrenergic stimulation has been reported to be reduced in the elderly[50] or not to change.[51] The reduction in responsiveness may be related to a reduction in β-adrenoceptor affinity or a reduced number of receptors in the high-affinity state. Abnormal postreceptor events may also be responsible for an age-related reduction in cAMP production. Reduced β-adrenergic agonist affinity and reduced adenylyl cyclase activity have been reported in the senescent rat lung.[52] β-adrenoceptor responsiveness in other organ systems also tends to decline with age.[53,54]

β_2-adrenoceptor function in women may also be influenced by the menstrual cycle. A report by Wheeldon et al.[55] suggests that lymphocyte β_2-adrenoceptor density and maximal cAMP production in response to isoprenaline increases when sex steroid hormones are high and declines when these hormones are low. The authors believe that the connection between phases in the menstrual cycle and β_2-adrenoceptor function may explain premenstrual deterioration in asthmatic women.

2. β_2-Adrenoceptor Function in Asthma

β-Adrenoceptor dysfunction has been linked to increased nonspecific bronchial responsiveness and to asthma.[56] This observation has led to several studies looking for a connection between asthma and β-adrenoceptor function in the lung and other tissues, especially peripheral blood mononuclear lymphocytes. β-adrenergic responses, measured using lymphocyte membranes, are reduced with age[57] and in asthmatics.[58,59] Lymphocyte β-adrenergic receptors are classified as the β_2 subtype, and their densities and responses are similar to those in the human lung.[60,61] Further evidence for the connection between β-adrenoceptor function and asthma was seen in PET scans using β-antagonist radioligands. These studies have shown that pulmonary β-adrenoceptor density is reduced in asthmatics compared to control subjects.[62]

There are similarities between the β-adrenergic abnormalities associated with aging and those seen in asthma. Abnormalities in the β-adrenoceptor adenylyl cyclase signal transduction pathway of asthmatics, and their similarity to alterations in these pathways in the elderly have been reviewed by Connolly.[63] Hyper-responsiveness to methacholine inhalation challenge has been correlated with significantly lower β_2-adrenoceptor affinity on peripheral mononuclear cells.[64] This study suggests that there is a relationship between the extent of the β-adrenoceptor abnormality in juvenile-onset asthma and the severity of the asthma. Connolly et al.[65] postulated that a reduction in β-adrenoceptor function with age could be associated with an increasing prevalence of nonspecific bronchial responsiveness. They tested this hypothesis by examining nonspecific bronchial responsiveness to methacholine and mononuclear leukocyte β_2-adrenoceptor affinity and density in elderly late-onset asthmatics and elderly nonasthmatics and in young asthmatics and nonasthmatics. Receptor density did not change with age, but receptor affinity was highest in young nonasthmatics and lowest in elderly asthmatics. Elderly nonasthmatics had intermediate values. Receptor affinity and bronchial responsiveness had a significant inverse relationship. The authors concluded that late-onset asthma may be due to age-associated β-adrenoceptor dysfunction.

3. Effect of Age on β_2-Adrenoceptor Agonists Used as Bronchodilators

There are now considerable data to suggest that the bronchodilator response to β_2-adrenoceptor agonists declines with age. Ullah et al.[66] reported that the response to inhaled salbutamol, a selective β_2-adrenoceptor agonist, in older asthmatics declined significantly compared to younger asthmatics (mean age 54 vs. 35). The age of onset of asthma in the old-age group was 47 compared to 12 in the younger group of asthmatics. An age-associated decline in bronchodilator response to salbutamol was also reported by Barros and Rees,[67] Van Schayck et al.,[68] and Connolly et al.[69] *In vivo* and *in vitro* β_2-adrenergic receptor responsiveness to terbutaline has been assessed in young and elderly asthmatics by Hamelin et al.[70] A single subcutaneous dose of terbutaline was less effective in the elderly asthmatics in producing bronchodilation, but the difference was not statistically significant. Lymphocyte cAMP production was also lower in the elderly asthmatics.

Not all studies confirm the age-associated decline in β_2-adrenergic receptor responsiveness in the lung. Bambuterol, a long-acting prodrug of terbutaline, was found to have similar efficacy in young and old asthmatics, but the apparent plasma clearance of terbutaline was lower in the elderly asthmatics (mean age 72 vs. 29).[71] Bambuterol tablets taken once daily were effective in improving pulmonary function in elderly asthmatics (mean age 70) and produced few cardiovascular side effects. In another study the bronchodilator response to inhaled albuterol did not decline in a group of asthmatics older than 65.[72] When compared to young asthmatics, age 18 to 25, there were no differences in either the magnitude of response or in the time and dose needed to reach peak response.

The conflicting evidence for an age-associated loss of bronchodilator response to β_2-adrenoceptor agonists parallels the conflicting evidence for age-associated losses of β_2-adrenoceptor agonist response in other tissues.

C. OTHER BRONCHODILATOR AGENTS

1. Antimuscarinic Agents

Antimuscarinic cholinergic blocking drugs such as ipratropium have bronchodilator effects and are used in the treatment of reversible obstructive lung disease. The bronchodilator effects of ipratropium may be less pronounced than those of β_2-adrenergic antagonists, particularly on the small-diameter airways. Thus β_2-adrenergic antagonists are often the drug of first choice for treatment of asthma.[73–75] Anticholinergic agents may preferentially dilate larger airways, making them more suited to the treatment of COPD complicated by emphysema or bronchitis.[10,77] In contrast to the age-related decline in the bronchodilator response to β_2-adrenergic agonists, the bronchodilator effects of ipratropium do not appear to decrease with age, leading to the suggestion that it may be a more suitable choice in geriatric patients.[66–68] However, other investigators report that both β-adrenergic agonists and antimuscarinic drugs remain effective as bronchodilators in elderly patients, with little or no effect of age on the response to either class of drug.[73,78]

2. Corticosteroids

Corticosteroids have anti-inflammatory actions which make them useful for the treatment of asthma and COPD. While a lower percentage of patients respond to corticosteroids compared to β_2-agonists or muscarinic cholinergic antagonists, corticosteroids may be effective in some patients who are refractory to β_2-agonists or muscarinic antagonists. Furthermore, corticosteroids may produce additional therapeutic effects in patients who do respond to these other agents.[79,80] There have been no systematic studies examining these effects of corticosteroids in young and old patients. There is some evidence to suggest that the age-related decline in pulmonary function may be related to the levels of endogenous cortisol in the plasma.[81]

3. Histamine Receptor Antagonists

Antagonists to the H_1 histamine receptor have bronchodilator effects which are due in large part to inhibition of muscarinic cholinergic receptors by some of these agents.[82] The older H_1 receptor antagonists, such as diphenhydramine, are the most likely to produce these effects. Newer agents, such as terfenadine and astemizole, have no effect on muscarinic cholinergic receptors. H_1 receptor antagonists are metabolized by hepatic microsomal oxidation, and a decrease in elimination by this route has been reported with age for many different drugs.[46,83] Decreased elimination of several H_1 receptor antagonists including doxylamine, diphenhydramine, and hydroxyzine has been reported in the elderly, and is thought to be responsible for the increased duration of antihistaminergic effects in these individuals.[84–86] There is some evidence that these effects may be gender specific, occurring in elderly men, but not in women.[84]

III. SUMMARY

Table 7.2 provides a summary of the age-associated changes in the pharmacokinetic and pharmacodynamic properties of the therapeutic agents commonly used to treat asthma in the elderly. Except for the antimuscarinic agent ipratropium there appears to be conflicting information on the occurrence of age-associated changes in the response to bronchodilators. Differences in the age and physical condition of the individuals examined in each study may account for these discrepancies. In general, there appears to be sufficient information indicating that bronchodilator responses may change with age, but there is a limited understanding of the basis for these age-associated changes.

TABLE 7.2.
Summary of the Age-Associated Changes in the Pharmacokinetic and Pharmacodynamic Properties of Therapeutic Agents Commonly Used to Treat Asthma in the Elderly

Therapeutic agent	Pharmacokinetic change	Ref.	Pharmacodynamic change	Ref.
Theophylline				
Aminophylline	Decreased volume of distribution	30–32	Reduced bronchodilator response	24
	Decreased plasma clearance	32, 38–42		
	No change in volume of distribution	28, 29, 36, 40		
	No change in plasma clearance	28, 29, 36, 37		
β_2-Adrenoceptor agonists				
Salbutamol			Reduced bronchodilator response	66–69
Terbutaline			Reduced bronchodilator response	70
Bambuterol	Decreased plasma clearance	71	No change in bronchodilator response	71
Albuterol			No change in bronchodilator response	72
Antimuscarinic agents				
Ipratropium			No change in bronchodilator response	66–68, 72

REFERENCES

1. **Braman, S. S.,** Asthma in the elderly patient, *Clin. Chest Med.,* 14, 413, 1993.
2. **Evans, R., Mullally D. I., and Wilson, R. W.,** National trends in the morbidity and mortality of asthma in the US, *Chest*, 91, 65S, 1987.
3. **Katzung, B. G.,** *Basic & Clinical Pharmacology*, 6th ed., Appleton & Lange, Norwalk, 19, 311, 1995.
4. **Tattersfield, A. E. and Harrison, R. N.,** Effect of β-blocker therapy on airway function, *Drugs*, 25, 227, 1983.
5. **Braman, S. S., Kaemmerlen, J. T., and Davis, S. M.,** Asthma in the elderly. A comparison between patients with recently acquired and long-standing disease, *Am. Rev. Respir. Dis.,* 143, 336, 1991.
6. **Burr, M. L., Charles, T. J., Roy, K., and Seaton, A.,** Asthma in the elderly: an epidemiological survey, *Br. Med. J.*, 1, 1041, 1979.
7. **Dodge, R. R. and Burrows, B.,** The prevalence and incidence of asthma and asthma-like symptoms in a general population sample, *Am. Rev. Respir. Dis.*, 122, 567, 1980.
8. **Dodge, R. R., Cline, M. G., and Burrows, B.,** Comparisons of asthma, emphysema and chronic bronchitis diagnosis in a general population sample, *Am. Rev. Respir. Dis.*, 133, 981, 1986.
9. **Ziment, I.,** Management of respiratory problems in the aged, *J. Am. Geriatr. Soc.*, 30, 536, 1982.
10. **Gross, N. J. and Skorodin, M. S.,** Anticholinergic, antimuscarinic bronchodilators, *Am. Rev. Respir. Dis.*, 129, 856, 1984.
11. **Lam, A. and Newhouse, M. T.,** Management of asthma and chronic airflow limitation: are methylxanthines obsolete?, *Chest*, 98, 44, 1990.
12. **Moses, M. A., Szabo, E. I., and Terner, C.,** Control of low K_m cyclic adenosine 3′,5′-monophosphate-phosphodiesterase in prostate and heart of adult and aged rats, *Mech. Age Dev.,* 39, 103, 1987.
13. **Razzaboni, B. and Terner, C.,** Cyclic adenosine 3′,5′monophosphate-phosphodiesterases in epididymis and prostate of castrate and of aged rats, *Mech. Age Dev.,* 61, 1988.
14. **Bylund, D. B., Tellez-Inon, M. T., and Hollenberg, M. D.,** Age-related parallel decline in β-adrenergic receptors, adenylate cyclase and phosphodiesterase activity in rat erythrocyte membranes, *Life Sci.*, 21, 403, 1977.
15. **Hoskins, B. and Ho, I. K.,** Effects of maturation and aging on calmodulin and calmodulin-regulated enzymes in various regions of mouse brain, *Mech. Age Dev.,* 36, 173, 1986.
16. **Stancheva, S. L. and Alova, L. G.,** Age-related changes of cyclic AMP phosphodiesterase activity in rat brain regions and a new phosphodiesterase inhibitor-nootropic agent adafenoxate, *Gen. Pharmacol.*, 22, 955, 1991.
17. **Voss, K. H., Masoro, E. J., and Anderson, W.,** Modulation of age-related loss of glucagon-promoted lipolysis by food restriction, *Mech. Age Dev.*, 18, 135, 1982.
18. **Popplewell, P. Y., Tsubokawa, M., Ramachandran, J., and Azhar, S.,** Differential effects of aging on adrenocorticotropin receptors, adenosine 3′5′-monophosphate response, and corticosterone secretion in adrenocortical cells from Sprague-Dawley rats, *Endocrinology*, 119, 2206, 1986.
19. **Dax, E. M., Partilla, J. S., and Gregerman, R. I.,** Mechanism of the age-related decrease of epinephrine-stimulated lipolysis in isolated rat adipocytes: β-adrenergic receptor binding, adenylate cyclase activity, and cyclic AMP accumulation, *J. Lipid Res.*, 22, 934, 1981.
20. **Arnold, J. D., Courtenay-Evans, R. J., Whitfield, R., O'Reilly, J. F., Petries, G. R., Higgins, A. J., and Swift, C. G.,** Comparative assessment of enprofylline and theophylline for chronic obstructive airway disease in the elderly, *Respir. Med.,* 84, 211, 1990.
21. **Howell, R. E.,** Multiple mechanisms of xanthine actions on airway reactivity, *J. Pharm. Exp. Ther.*, 225, 1008, 1990.
22. **Dobson, J. G., Jr., Fenton, R. A., and Romano, F. D.,** Increased myocardial adenosine production and reduction of β-adrenergic contractile response in aged hearts, *Circ. Res.*, 66, 1381, 1990.
23. **Dobson, J. G., Jr. and Fenton, R. A.,** Adenosine inhibition of β-adrenergic induced responses in aged hearts, *Am. J. Physiol.*, 265, H494, 1993.
24. **Chandler, M. H. H., Clifton, G. D., Burki, N. K., Hunt, B. A., and Blouin, R. A.,** Pulmonary function in the elderly: response to theophylline bronchodilation, *J. Clin. Pharmacol.,* 30, 330, 1990.
25. **Yashuhara, M. and Levy, G.,** Effect of age on neurotoxicity of theophylline, *J. Pharm. Sci.,* 77, 645, 1988.
26. **Gaudreault, P. and Guay, J.,** Theophylline poisoning: pharmacological considerations and clinical management, *J. Med. Toxicol.*, 1, 169, 1986.
27. Facts and Comparisons, *Drug Facts and Comparisons*, 1991 ed., J. B. Lippincott, St. Louis, 1991, 622.
28. **Fox, R. W., Samaan, S., Bukantz, S. C., and Lockey, R. F.,** Theophylline kinetics in a geriatric group, *Clin. Pharmacol. Ther.*, 34, 60, 1983.
29. **Cusack, B., Kelly, J. G., Lavan, J., Noel, J., and O'Malley, K.,** Theophylline kinetics in relation to age: the importance of smoking, *Br. J. Clin. Pharmacol.*, 10, 109, 1980.
30. **Jusko, W. J., Gardner, M. J., Mangione, A., Schentag, J. J., Koup, J. R., and Vance, J. W.,** Factors affecting theophylline clearances: age, tobacco, marijuana, cirrhosis, congestive heart failure, obesity, oral contraceptives, benzodiazepines, barbiturates and ethanol, *J. Pharm. Sci.*, 68, 1358, 1979.

30. **Jusko, W. J., Gardner, M. J., Mangione, A., Schentag, J. J., Koup, J. R., and Vance, J. W.,** Factors affecting theophylline clearances: age, tobacco, marijuana, cirrhosis, congestive heart failure, obesity, oral contraceptives, benzodiazepines, barbiturates and ethanol, *J. Pharm. Sci.*, 68, 1358, 1979.
31. **Neilsen-Kudak, F., Magnussen, I., and Jakobsen, P.,** Pharmacokinetics of theophylline in ten elderly patients, *Acta Pharmacol. Toxicol.*, 42, 226, 1978.
32. **Antal, E. J., Kramer, P. A., Mercik, S. A., Chapron, D. J., and Lawson, I. R.,** Theophylline pharmacokinetics in advanced age, *Br. J. Clin. Pharmacol.*, 12, 637, 1981.
33. **Ellis, E. F.,** Theophylline and derivatives, Middleton, B., Reed, E. E., and Ellis, E. F., Eds., *Allergy, Principles and Practice*, C.V. Mosby, St. Louis, 1978, 434.
34. **Hendeles, L., Weinberger, M., and Johnson, G.,** Monitoring serum theophylline levels, *Clin. Pharmacokinet.*, 3, 294, 1978.
35. **Ogilvie, R. I.,** Clinical pharmacokinetics of theophylline, *Clin. Pharmacokinet.*, 3, 267, 1978.
36. **Blouin, R. A., Erwin, W. G., Foster, T. S., and Scott, S.,** Pharmacokinetics of theophylline in young and elderly subjects, *Gerontology*, 28, 323, 1981.
37. **Bauer, L. A. and Blouin, R. A.,** Influence of age on theophylline clearance in patients with chronic obstructive pulmonary disease, *Clin. Pharmacokinet.*, 6, 469, 1981.
38. **Au, W. Y. W., Dutt, A. K., and DeSoyza, N.,** Theophylline kinetics in chronic obstructive airway disease in the elderly, *Clin. Pharmacol. Ther.*, 37, 472, 1985.
39. **Jusko, W. J., Koup, J. R., Vance, J. W., Schentag, J. J., and Kuritzky, P.,** Intravenous theophylline therapy: nomogram guidelines, *Ann. Intern. Med.*, 86, 400, 1977.
40. **Jackson, S. H. D., Johnston, A., Woollard, R., and Turner, P.,** The relationship between theophylline clearance and age in adult life, *Eur. J. Clin. Pharmacol.*, 36, 29, 1989.
41. **Shin, S. G., Juan, D., and Rammohan, M.,** Theophylline pharmacokinetics in normal elderly subjects, *Clin. Pharmacol. Ther.*, 44, 522, 1988.
42. **Vestal, R. E., Cusack, B. J., Mercer, G. D., Dawson, G. W., and Park, B. K.,** Aging and drug interactions. 1. Effect of cimetidine and smoking on the oxidation of theophylline and cortisol in healthy men, *J. Pharm. Exp. Ther.*, 24, 488, 1987.
43. **Talseth, T., Kornstad, S., Boye, N. P., and Bredesen, J. E.,** Individualization of oral theophylline dosage in elderly patients, *Acta Med. Scand.*, 210, 489, 1981.
44. **Riegelman, S. L.,** Theophylline disposition in acutely ill hospitalized patients: the effect of smoking, heart failure, severe airway obstruction and pneumonia, *Am. Rev. Respir. Dis.*, 118, 229, 1978.
45. **Denlinger, C. L., Stryker, K. K., Slusher, L. B., and Vesell, E. S.,** Studies on theophylline metabolism: autoinduction and inhibition by antipyrine, *Clin. Pharmacol. Ther.*, 41, 522, 1987.
46. **Schmucker, D. L.,** Aging and drug disposition: an update, *Pharmacol. Rev.*, 37, 133, 1985.
47. **Jung, D. and Nanavaty, M.,** The effects of age and dietary protein restriction on the pharmacokinetics of theophylline in the rat, *Pharm. Toxicol.*, 66, 361, 1990.
48. **Cohen, I. A., Johnson, C. E., Berardi, R. R., Hyneck, M. L., and Achem, S. R.,** Cimetidine-theophylline interaction: effects of age and cimetidine dose, *Ther. Drug Monitoring*, 7, 426, 1985.
49. **Vestal, R. E., Cusack, B. J., Crowley, J. J., and Loi, C.-M.,** Aging and the response to inhibition and induction of theophylline metabolism, *Exp. Ger.*, 28, 421, 1993.
50. **Ford, G. A., Dachman, W. E. D., Blaschke, T. F., Tewari, A., Flokas, K. L., Starnes, H. F., and Hoffman, B. B.,** Effect of aging on B_2 mediated uptake of potassium, free fatty acids and glycerol into human forearms, *Age Ageing*, 21 (Suppl. 2), P12, 1992.
51. **Klein, C., Hiatt, W. R., Gerber, J. G., and Nies, A. S.,** Age does not alter human vascular and nonvascular β_2-adrenergic responses to isoproterenol, *Clin. Pharmacol. Ther.*, 44, 573, 1988.
52. **Scarpace, P. J. and Abrass, I. B.,** Decreased β-adrenergic agonist affinity and adenylate cyclase activity in senescent rat lung, *J. Gerontol.*, 38, 143, 1983.
53. **Vestal, R. E., Wood, A. J., and Shand, D. G.,** Reduced β adrenoceptor sensitivity in the elderly, *Clin. Pharmacol. Ther.*, 26, 181, 1979.
54. **Gurdal, H., Friedman, E., and Johnson, M. D.,** Beta adrenoceptor-G_s coupling decreases with age in the rat aorta, *Mol. Pharmacol.*, in press.
55. **Wheeldon, N. M., Newnham, D. M., Coutie, W. J., Peters, J. A., McDevitt, D. G., and Lipworth, B. J.,** Influence of sex-steroid hormones on the regulation of lymphocyte β_2-adrenoceptors during the menstrual cycle, *Br. J. Clin. Pharm.*, 37, 583, 1994.
56. **Szentivanyi, A.,** The β-adrenergic theory of the atopic abnormality in bronchial asthma, *J. Allergy*, 40, 203, 1968.
57. **Rutledge, D. R. and Steinberg, J. D.,** Effect of age on lymphocyte β-2 adrenergic responsiveness, *Drug Intell. Clin. Pharm.*, 25, 532, 1991.
58. **Connolly, M. E. and Greenacre, J. K.,** The lymphocyte β-adrenergic receptor in normal subjects and patients with bronchial asthma, *J. Clin. Invest.*, 58, 1307, 1976.

61. **Liggett, S. B., Marker, J. C., Shah, S. D., Roper, C. L., and Cryer, P. E.,** Direct relationship between mononuclear leukocyte and lung β-adrenergic receptors and apparent reciprocal regulation of extravascular, but not intravascular, α- and β-adrenergic receptors by the sympathochromaffin system in humans, *J. Clin. Invest.*, 82, 48, 1988.
62. **Qing, F., Sriskandan, S., Rhodes, C. G., Ueki, J., Ind, P. W., Brown, D. J., Waters, S., Jones, T., and Hughes, J. M. B.,** Alveolar β adrenergic receptor density in asthmatic subjects before and during corticosteroid and β agonist therapy: preliminary studies using positron emission tomography (PET) and ^{11}C-S-CGP 12177, *Thorax,* 47, 871, 1992.
63. **Connolly, M. J.,** Ageing, late-onset asthma and the β-adrenoceptor, *Pharmac. Ther.*, 60, 389, 1994.
64. **Connolly, M. J., Crowley, J. J., Nielson, C. P., Charan, N. B., and Vestal, R. E.,** Relationship between nonspecific bronchial responsiveness to methacholine and peripheral mononuclear leukocyte β-adrenergic receptor function in young drug-naive subjects, *Am. Rev. Respir. Dis.*, 146, 592, 1992.
65. **Connolly, M. J., Crowley, J. J., Nielson, C. P., Charan, N. B., and Vestal, R. E.,** Peripheral mononuclear leucocyte B adrenoceptors and nonspecific bronchial responsiveness to methacholine in young and elderly normal subjects and asthmatic patients, *Thorax*, 49, 26, 1994.
66. **Ullah, M., Newman, G. B., and Saunders, K. B.,** Influence of age on response to ipratropium and salbutamol in asthma, *Thorax*, 36, 523, 1981.
67. **Barros, M. J. and Rees, P. J.,** Bronchodilator responses to salbutamol followed by ipratropium bromide in partially reversible airflow obstruction, *Respir. Med.,* 84, 371, 1990.
68. **Van Schayck, C. P. L., Folgering, H., Harbers, H., Maras, K. L., and van Weel, C.,** Effects of age and allergy on responses to salbutamol and ipratropium bromide in moderate asthma and chronic bronchitis, *Thorax*, 46, 355, 1991.
69. **Connolly, M. J., Crowley, J. J., Nielson, C. P., Charan, N. B., and Vestal, R. E.,** Airway β-receptor dysfunction in normal elderly subjects, *Age Ageing,* 21 (Suppl. 1), P29, 1991.
70. **Hamelin, B. A., Blouin, R. A., Wolf, K. M., Clifton, G. D., and Chandler, M. H.,** In vivo and in vitro β_2-adrenergic receptor responsiveness in young and elderly asthmatics, *Pharmacotherapy*, 12, 376, 1992.
71. **Sitar, D. S., Warren, C. P., and Aoki, F. Y.,** Pharmacokinetics and pharmacodynamics of bambuterol, a long-acting bronchodilator pro-drug of terbutaline, in young and elderly patients with asthma, *Clin. Pharmacol. Ther.*, 52, 297, 1992.
72. **Kradjan, W. A., Driesner, N. K., Abuan, T. H., Emmick, G., and Schoene, R. B.,** Effect of age on bronchodilator response, *Chest*, 101, 1545, 1992.
73. **Barnes, P. J., Basbaum, C. B., and Nael, J. A.,** Autoradiographic localization of autonomic receptors in airway smooth muscle: marked differences between large and small airways, *Am. Rev. Respir. Dis.*, 127, 758, 1983
74. **Ruffin, R. E., Fitzgerald, J. D., and Rebuck, A. S.,** A comparison of the bronchodilator activity of SCH 1000 and salbutamol, *J. Allergy Clin. Immunol.*, 59, 139, 1977.
75. **Easton, P., Jadue, C., Dhingra, S., and Anthonisen, N. R.,** A comparison of the bronchodilating effects of a β-2 adrenergic agent (albuterol) and an anticholinergic agent (ipratropium bromide) given by aerosol alone or in sequence, *N. Engl. J. Med.*, 315, 735, 1986.
76. **Gross, N. J. and Skorodin, M. S.,** Role of the parasympathetic system in airway obstruction due to emphysema, *N. Engl. J. Med.*, 311, 421, 1984.
77. **Storms, W., Bodman, S., Nathan, R., Busse, W., Bush, R., and Falliers, C.,** Use of ipratropium bromide in asthma, *Am. J. Med.*, 81 (Suppl. 5A), 61, 1986.
78. **Nissar, M., Earis, J. E., Pearson, M. G., and Calverley, P. M. A.,** Acute bronchodilator trials in chronic obstructive pulmonary disease, *Am. Rev. Respir. Dis.*, 146, 555, 1992.
79. **Mendella, L. A., Manfreda, J., Warren, C. P. N., and Anthonisen, N. R.,** Steroid response in stable chronic obstructive pulmonary disease, *Ann. Intern. Med.*, 96, 17, 1982.
80. **Sahn, S. A.,** Corticosteroids in chronic bronchitis and pulmonary emphysema, *Chest*, 73, 389, 1978.
81. **Sparrow, D., O'Connor, G. T., Rosner, B., Demolles, D., and Weiss, S. T.,** A longitudinal study of plasma cortisol concentration and pulmonary function decline in men. The normative aging study, *Am. Rev. Respir. Dis.*, 147, 1345, 1993.
82. **Garrison, J. C.,** Histamine, bradykinin, 5-hydroxytryptamine, and their antagonists, in *Goodman and Gilman's The Pharmacological Basis of Therapeutics,* 8th ed., Gilman, A. G., Ral, T. W., Nies, A. S., and Taylor, P., Eds., Pergamon Press, New York, 1990, chap. 23.
83. **Montamat, S. C., Cusack, B. J., and Vestal, R. E.,** Management of drug therapy in the elderly, *N. Engl. J. Med.*, 321, 303, 1989.
84. **Friedman, H., Greenblatt, D. J., Scavone, J. M., Burstein, E. S., Ochs, H. R., Harmatz, J. S., and Shader, R. I.,** Clearance of the antihistamine doxylamine reduced in elderly men but not in elderly women, *Clin. Pharmacokinet.*, 16, 312, 1989.
85. **Simons, K. J., Watson, W. T. A., Chen, X. Y., and Simons, F. E. R.,** Pharmacokinetic and pharmacodynamic studies of the H_1-receptor antagonist hydroxyzine in the elderly, *Clin. Pharmacol. Ther.*, 45, 9, 1989.
86. **Simons, K. J., Watson, W. T. A., Martin, T. J., Chen, X. Y., and Simons, F. E. R.,** Diphenhydramine: pharmacokinetics and pharmacodynamics in elderly adults, young adults and children, *J. Clin. Pharmacol.*, 30, 665, 1990.

85. **Simons, K. J., Watson, W. T. A., Chen, X. Y., and Simons, F. E. R.,** Pharmacokinetic and pharmacodynamic studies of the H_1-receptor antagonist hydroxyzine in the elderly, *Clin. Pharmacol. Ther.*, 45, 9, 1989.
86. **Simons, K. J., Watson, W. T. A., Martin, T. J., Chen, X. Y., and Simons, F. E. R.,** Diphenhydramine: pharmacokinetics and pharmacodynamics in elderly adults, young adults and children, *J. Clin. Pharmacol.*, 30, 665, 1990.

Chapter 8

SEDATIVES, HYPNOTICS, ALCOHOL, AND ANTICONVULSANTS

Philip I. Markowitz

CONTENTS

I. INTRODUCTION

This chapter deals with classes of pharmacologic agents which share one important property — the ability to cause sedation. The implications in the elderly are obvious: impairment of psychomotor performance, cognitive impairment, and increased risk of untoward adverse effects directly related to sedation, in particular, falls and long bone fractures. Elderly individuals taking psychotropic medication appear to be a high-risk population; compared to those not in need of these drugs they are older, more likely to be widowed and therefore socially isolated, and more likely to be taking various other medications. By both subjective and objective measures they appear more impaired physically and mentally.[1] Numerous studies have associated use of psychotropic medications in the aged and femoral fractures. The possibility of an increased risk of motor vehicle accidents exists as well. Even if catastrophic events are avoided, impaired quality of life due to attenuated mental acuity can result. Finally, the interaction of the neuropharmacologic effects of these drugs with the neurobiologic sequelae of aging such as dementia and cerebrovascular disease demand attention, as the interaction of the two may be additive and avoidably increase the morbidity of the primary central nervous system (CNS) disorder. For these reasons special attention needs to be paid to the use of sedating medications in the aged, and an understanding of age related differences in pharmacokinetic and pharmacodynamic effects is essential if these agents are to be employed properly.

II. PHYSIOLOGIC CHANGES UNIQUE TO THE ELDERLY

Independent of disease processes, normal aging induces physiological changes which will effect drug disposition and actions. For most medications non-neurologic factors affecting drug absorption, distribution, metabolism, protein binding, and elimination are most pertinent. Aging produces a variety of general changes which hypothetically could alter pharmacologic effects. Basal metabolic rate decreases at age 90 to 80% of the value in young adulthood.

0-8493-8306-4/96/$0.00+$.50

This could potentially influence psychodynamic activity. Cardiac index decreases by 30%, altering systemic and organ-specific perfusion with consequences for drug distribution and elimination. Pulmonary vital capacity decreases by 50%. Respiratory drive decreases and results in decreased responses to hypoxia and hypercapnia. The implications for a fatal overdose of a respiratory depressant medication in the elderly are obvious. Glomerular filtration rate is also markedly decreased, resulting in decreased clearance and an increased half-life for most medications.

Age-induced neurologic changes may also alter pharmacodynamic response. Brain weight and absolute numbers of neurons are decreased. Cerebral blood flow and oxygen consumption decrease. Total brain mass decreases by 10 to 15%. Nerve conduction velocity decreases. Cortical-evoked responses show decreased amplitude and increased latency of response.[2] The EEG shows generalized slowing of electrical activity and a decrease in the mean alpha rhythm. Focal changes are noted as well, particularly in the anterior temporal regions.[3] All of these changes are consistent with a shift toward greater end-organ sensitivity.

Focal age-related neurologic changes may also be relevant to the function of the classes of drugs discussed in this chapter. A 19 to 43% decrease in hippocampal neurons has been demonstrated.[4] This would render the elderly more susceptible to memory impairment produced by hypnotic and anxiolytic drugs. Neuronal loss on the order of 28 to 40% in the frontal cortex[5,6] may predispose older individuals to benzodiazepine-induced disinhibition. Decreased cerebellar Purkinje cells[7] may underlie the increased sensitivity to benzodiazepines which can lead to the alterations in balance and gait often noted in the elderly.[7] Cell loss and decreased norepinephrine receptors[8,9] may decrease cortical arousal levels and thus alter sensitivity to sedative/hypnotic agents. Age-related changes in the serotonergic system,[10] which plays a prominent role in the activity of both anxiolytic and antidepressant agents, may also contribute to altered drug effect. For example, the 70% decline in 5-HT_1 receptor density seen with age[10] may affect response to anxiolytic agents, such as buspirone, which interact with this site. The loss of GABAergic and acetylcholine receptors in Alzheimer's-type dementia and normal aging[11–14] would be expected to alter the response to drugs like the benzodiazepines that interact with this receptor complex. Although the above data base is extremely preliminary and inferences highly speculative, a neuroanatomical and neurochemical foundation for understanding differential age-related drug effects is clearly emerging.

III. ANXIOLYTICS AND HYPNOTICS

Anxiety disorders occur in the elderly and are a significant cause of morbidity. What is not clear is the actual prevalence of these disorders in this population and to what extent, if any, it differs from younger cohorts. The literature is contradictory in this regard. Older studies suggested that prevalence peaked in early adulthood and declined with age.[15] Recent studies suggest that 10 to 22% of the elderly, irrespective of gender, demonstrate anxiety of sufficient degree to warrant treatment,[16,17] although large-scale epidemiologic studies indicate a progressive decrease in anxiety disorders such as phobias and panic disorder from the age of 65 on.[18,19] There is also a significant difference between the 45 to 64 age bracket and the 65 and above. Comparing these two groups, the prevalence of panic disorder decreases from 1.10 to 0.04%, obsessive-compulsive disorder from 2.01 to 1.54%, and generalized anxiety disorder from 3.10 to 1.90%. Whether this represents a real decrease in risk for an anxiety disorder or differential attrition due to mortality or other confounding factors is not clear. Additionally, the data from the Epidemiologic Catchment Area (ECA) study have been criticized on various methodologic grounds and thus may not reflect the true prevalence of psychopathology.

The diagnosis of an anxiety disorder in the elderly may be more difficult than in younger patients. Little is known about phenomenology in the geriatric group, as it has not been systematically studied. The elderly with anxiety states are more likely to present with somatic complaints or with a mixed picture of anxiety and depression. Data like those obtained by the ECA study do not assess the institutionalized segment of this population, which increases from 1.5% of the population aged 65 to 74 to 21.6% of those over 85.[20] Excessive use of psychotropic medications in the institutionalized aged has been well documented. Contrariwise, there does not appear to be an epidemic of tranquilizer use in the elderly residing in community settings. Of the 25 most commonly prescribed drugs to those over 75, only phenobarbital is included, at a rate of 1.7/100 medical visits.[21] Nor does there appear to be an increase in self-medication, as alcohol use actually decreases in the aged. What clearly does increase with age is the prevalence of cognitive impairment, with a rate of 3.0% in the 65 to 74-year-old bracket and 9.3% in those over 75.[22] Associated symptoms of agitation and restlessness are common and often require psychopharmacologic management. Thus, anxiolytic therapy is often resorted to in the geriatric population. Such treatment is complicated by the aging process itself, concomitant diseases, polypharmacy, and patient confusion regarding appropriate compliance with medical regimens. Therefore, special attention is required when prescribing for this more vulnerable and less resilient group of individuals.

Insomnia is a common complaint in the elderly; 5 million older people suffer a disorder of sleep.[23] With aging, sleep changes quantitatively, qualitatively, and neurophysiologically. The average duration of sleep decreases to 5.75 hr/d at the age of 90. Paradoxically, the actual amount of time spent in bed increases by almost an hour, which may partially contribute to the perception of decreased sleep quality. As a result, sleep efficiency, or the time spent asleep divided by the time spent in bed, decreases from 0.95 in early adulthood to 0.77 after the age of 70. Those over 70 are much more likely to report difficulty getting to sleep; 26% compared to 6.2% at age 19. Sleep in the aged is experienced as shorter, lighter, and more broken. Dissatisfaction is increased. Sleep EEG changes occur as well. Interestingly, sleep onset latency changes little with age, although individual variability increases greatly. The frequency and total duration of wakefulness increase steadily with advancing age. The number of stage shifts increase as well, and a greater proportion of time is spent in stage 1 sleep (drowsiness). Both of these correlate well with sleep satisfaction. Total sleep time decreases proportionally between REM and NREM sleep, although stages 3 and 4 sleep decline disproportionately, producing a reduction in depth of sleep.[24]

Not only are the elderly more prone to experience insomnia, but they may also be more likely to experience the adverse effects of the medications used to treat the problem. These include daytime drowsiness, or the "hangover" effect, rebound effects, such as rebound insomnia, rebound anxiety, REM rebound, and daytime withdrawal effects, particularly with very short half-life preparations. Drug dependence is also a greater concern, as elderly individuals tend to be more habitual users of hypnotics. This prolonged use coupled with drug tolerance and dose escalation may initiate a drug dependency due to the disordered sleep that frequently follows attempts at abrupt discontinuation of hypnotics. This can obviously be mitigated by proper medical supervision, but this, for a variety of sociodemographic and economic reasons, is often absent.

Until recently, the only class of anxiolytic/hypnotic medication available was the benzodiazepines. Sedative hypnotics such as barbiturates and chloral hydrate are rarely used today. Therefore, this will be the focus of discussion. Although the elderly comprise only 12% of the U.S. population, they account for 35 to 40% of the prescriptions written for hypnotic agents.[23] Thus, the geriatric population appears to be overly represented amongst benzodiazepine users. For the elderly living at home, prevalence rates for use of an hypnotic agent range from 5.9 to 33%.[24] The rate is considerably higher in the institutionalized geriatric population, between 22.6 and 54%.[25] One consistent finding in the literature is the overrepresentation of women among those using benzodiazepines. Adverse effects, particularly hip fractures, can be a serious consequence in the elderly, although this appears to be a greater risk with long vs. short half-lived benzodiazepines. It should also be noted that this increased risk is present with multiple psychotropic drugs, not only the benzodiazepines.

What, then, should guide prescribing of benzodiazepines in the elderly? Both pharmacokinetic and pharmacodynamic factors need to be considered. The major pharmacokinetic variable is drug clearance, which is affected by distribution, metabolism, elimination, and plasma protein binding capacity. Some general principles apply. Benzodiazepines are primarily, if not exclusively, cleared by biotransformation in the liver. Age-related changes in biotransformation are most evident for drugs with high hepatic clearance such as triazolam and midazolam. Most benzodiazepines are low-clearance drugs, such that hepatic clearance is considerably lower than hepatic blood flow. Because of this, aging effects on the liver will less prominently affect drug elimination. Although age-related decreases in hepatic microsomal enzyme oxidation may occur, direct evidence for this is sparse. With age, plasma clearance of free diazepam decreases,[25–28] leading to the inference that hepatic drug metabolizing capacity is impaired.[29,30] Animal studies are conflicting.[31,32] This will, to a large extent, be mitigated by the degree of hepatic clearance of a drug. Low hepatic clearance will manifest itself differently pharmacokinetically, producing a lower area under the curve for plasma concentration. This translates into prolongation of elimination half-life with elevated steady-state concentrations as opposed to the elevation in peak plasma concentrations that one might expect with a high hepatic clearance drug. Age-related decrements in hepatic clearance are irrelevant for benzodiazepines such as oxazepam, lorazepam, and temazepam, which are metabolized by glucuronidation, a process not affected by aging.

Volume of distribution of a drug also affects clearance. Lipid-soluble drugs like the benzodiazepines preferentially distribute in adipose tissue. With aging there is an increase in percent body weight attributible to fat, going from 15% at age 20 to 36% at age 55 in males and 33% at age 20 to 48% at age 55 in females.[33] Thus, increased lipid deposits with age decrease the percentage of drug in the water compartment and thus accessible for elimination. This will result in longer elimination half-lives in the elderly and potential drug accumulation with long half-life medications such as diazepam and chlordiazepoxide. Drugs exist in blood in equilibrium between the protein-bound and free form. A drug can only exert its pharmacologic effect or be biologically cleared in its unbound state. Thus, drugs which are highly protein bound will be significantly affected by changes in plasma protein binding capacity, particularly albumin. Aging independent of disease leads to a reduction in plasma albumin concentration. Pathology, such as malnutrition or liver disease, will compound this. Benzodiazepines are significantly, although not highly, protein bound. Increases in the free fraction with age may result in both increased end-organ availability as well as increased hepatic clearance.

In general, the data for the benzodiazepines are consistent with what would be predicted pharmacokinetically. Age-related changes in drug disposition were first demonstrated with diazepam and are very dramatic. Between the ages of 15 and 82 the elimination half-life of the parent compound increases from 20 to 90 hr.[34] Its major metabolite, desmethyldiazepam, demonstrates a threefold increase in half-life. Additionally, with advancing age initial appearance of this metabolite is delayed.[35] Thus, accumulation of both the parent compound and its major active metabolite increases the potential for drug toxicity, and may not be readily apparent until weeks into therapy. Chlordiazepoxide manifests an even greater increase in half-life with age, increasing from 6 hr at age 20 to 36 hr at age 80.[36] To a great extent a two- to threefold increase in volume of distribution is responsible for this increase in elimination time, although decreased systemic clearance is a contributory factor as well.

Recently the trend has been to prescribe shorter half-life and less sedating benzodiazepines like alprazolam. Studies evaluating age effects have been conflicting. Greenblatt et al.[37] demonstrated a 50% decrease in systemic clearance in the elderly, but only in male subjects. Kroboth et al.[38] also found an increase in the elimination half-life, but this was not gender related. The discrepancy may be due to the single-dose paradigm used in the former study as opposed to a multiple-dose regimen employed in the latter. As expected, studies of drugs primarily glucuronidated have not demonstrated significant age-related differences.

Age-related pharmacodynamic effects also exist with the benzodiazepines. Increased target organ sensitivity is demonstrable independent of pharmacokinetic factors. For instance, epidemiologic studies have demonstrated an increased incidence of drowsiness in hospitalized geriatric medical patients,[39] although the effect of illness, per se, may be a contributory factor. Elderly patients require a significantly lower dose of intravenous diazepam or midazolam to produce the same degree of sedation. Numerous studies have demonstrated that acceptable bedtime sedation can be obtained at lower hypnotic doses, often half that required in younger individuals.[40] Experimental studies have used various measures of "sensitivity", including self-rating instruments, psychomotor testing such as reaction time or tracking, and physiologic measures such as changes in EEG rhythm or postural sway. Performance on all of these tasks has been shown to be negatively influenced by acute doses of benzodiazepines, but surprisingly not nearly as consistently and to the extent that one might hypothesize. Results have often been confounded by differential plasma concentrations so that pharmacokinetic factors may have been operative. Additionally, free drug concentrations are usually not measured. Recent studies have indicated increased unbound fractions for both oxazepam[41] and diazepam[42] in elderly subjects, suggesting the possibility of increased drug end-organ availability. To date no comparative differences in either benzodiazepine receptor density or affinity have been demonstrable using rodents of different ages.[40] Some data are available to suggest a decrease in GABA receptors with age,[43–46] which could partially underlie increased pharmacodynamic sensitivity.

Given the above, it would seem prudent to observe the following guidelines when prescribing benzodiazepines in the elderly:

1. Begin with lower doses and titrate upward gradually.
2. Observe particular caution in individuals with hepatic disease or a medical condition that could lead to lowered plasma protein binding. Direct measurement of plasma albumin levels may be useful.
3. Renal function will be a factor for benzodiazepines with active metabolites, such as diazepam, since renal elimination of these compounds will be delayed.
4. Dosing should be influenced by patient body habitus. One should anticipate a greater likelihood of drug accumulation in the obese. Conversely, physically frail individuals may also be at greater risk.
5. Short half-life drugs are preferable to long half-life medications. The risk of serious falls and hip fractures appears to be less with their use. This should be tempered by the understanding that short half-life benzodiazepines such as alprazolam need to be dosed more often, an inconvenience at any age, but particularly inconvenient for the elderly who are often on complicated medication schedules which can easily be confused. Additionally, terminating therapy with short half-life drugs is often more difficult because of more prominent withdrawal symptoms.
6. Consideration should be given to the preferential use of benzodiazepines that undergo glucuronidation, since these are less likely to be affected by age-related changes in hepatic microsomal enzyme capacity.

Nonbenzodiazepine hypnotics and anxiolytics are now just becoming available for clinical use. They fall into two major drug classes: the imidazopyridines such as zolpidem and alpidem, and the cyclopyrrolones, such as zopiclone and suriclone. Like benzodiazepines, they affect the benzodiazepine-GABA-chloride channel complex and have a high affinity for benzodiazepine receptors. It is still unclear whether they modulate GABA receptor function by directly interacting with any or all of the three identified benzodiazepine receptor subtypes, or if they act at a site separate from, but pharmacologically related to, the benzodiazepine receptor.

The efficacy of these medications as anxiolytics and hypnotics has been well established; good hypnotic activity has been demonstrated in more than 80% of patients.[47,48] They are more selective in their pharmacologic activity than are the benzodiazepines, possessing no myorelaxant properties. Unlike different benzodiazepines, which are nonspecific both as anxiolytics and hypnotics, different agents in these new classes may act selectively as either a hypnotic or anxiolytic.[49,50] In comparison to benzodiazepines, they would appear to offer certain advantages. They do not disturb sleep architecture, in particular exerting no effect on stages 3 and 4 and REM sleep.[51,52] This is especially pertinent in the elderly given the aforementioned effects of aging on sleep architecture. Thus, use of the newer hypnotic agents may be less perturbing of an already perturbed process. Additionally, rebound insomnia is less likely to occur,[53] making discontinuation easier and less traumatic. They appear to have less behavioral toxicity, evincing little effect on psychomotor performance across age groups, including the elderly.[54] Both animal models[55] and large-scale clinical trials[56] suggest less likelihood of producing physical dependence.

Mention should also be made of the azapirone class of anti-anxiety medications, exemplified by buspirone. This drug has demonstrated anxiolytic efficacy both in general[57,58] and geriatric populations.[59] Its pharmacokinetic profile does not differ across age groups.[60] Unlike the benzodiazepines, buspirone is nonsedating. It has no effect on cognitive or psychomotor performance in the elderly.[61] It may also be useful in the treatment of agitation and aggression in the elderly, particularly in those with organic brain syndromes and dementia.[62] Its main disadvantage is its delayed onset of action as opposed to benzodiazepine anxiolytics. This may be particularly problematic in an elderly population less able to tolerate a delay in therapeutic effect. Another drawback is the frequent occurrence of dizziness, an obvious concern in the aged who are already predisposed to orthostasis due to cardiac, psychotropic, and other medications. Low initial doses with very gradual upward titration of dose will decrease this particular risk and premature treatment termination due to unacceptable side effects.

In summary, anxiolytic/hypnotic drugs are commonly, although not excessively, used by the elderly. Judicious prescribing can increase their safety and decrease unwanted side effects. Additionally, thoughtful dispensing can decrease unnecessary and prolonged use. Attention to and education of patients regarding normal sleep patterns with age and reassurance as to the normalcy of the situation is clearly preferable to the reflexive prescription of an hypnotic in response to the complaint of insomnia. Nonpharmacological approaches to improved sleep hygiene can also decrease the indiscriminate use of these medications. Finally, time-limited use will allow the above to occur as well as decrease the risk of tolerance and addiction.

IV. ANTICONVULSANTS

Geriatric epilepsy and its pharmacologic management is to date a much understudied area considering its considerable prevalence in the elderly. It has an annual incidence of 1.34% in persons over the age of 65,[63] with an estimated 41,700 new cases annually.[64] In the aged, epilepsy is always secondary to an underlying CNS pathological process, although the actual cause is often not identifiable. Cerebrovascular disease is thought to account for 17 to 52% of cases, while tumor is responsible in 11 to 65%. Head trauma and metabolic encephalopathy are other frequent contributors. Alcoholism and dementia can also cause seizure disorders, although these are far less common etiologies. Given the increased frequency of underlying neuropathology, it is not unexpected that partial seizures predominate. Recurrence after a first seizure is the rule rather than the exception.

Few studies of antiepileptic drug elimination in the elderly have been performed, so that little empirical evidence is available to guide therapy. Phenytoin is probably the most commonly prescribed anticonvulsant in the elderly.[65] Some reports suggest a weakly positive correlation between age and phenytoin plasma concentration,[66] although one study found this to be the case only in women.[67] A single oral dose study found phenytoin clearance to be increased in the elderly.[68] This was attributed to decreased plasma albumin levels. One study in the literature suggests that oral loading doses in the elderly may need to be higher to achieve plasma concentrations equivalent to that in younger subjects.[69] Less is known about carbamazepine. One oral single-dose study of 11 healthy volunteers suggests no age-related differences in pharmacokinetics.[70] Multiple-dosing studies have not been performed. For phenobarbital, higher plasma levels may be attainable at lower doses in the elderly, again only in women.[71] Conflicting results have been obtained in two studies of sodium valproate pharmacokinetics after a single oral dose; both an increase[72] and no difference[73] in volume of distribution and half-life have been found in the elderly. However, free valproate concentration and clearance were increased and decreased, respectively, in the latter study, and this has been confirmed in one other study.[74]

There are no data to suggest differential efficacy of various anticonvulsants in the elderly. Data are also extremely limited regarding adverse effects. One might expect increased neurocognitive side effects in the aged, but objective data are lacking. Phenobarbital has been found to be an independent risk factor for falls and hip fractures in the elderly.[75] There are reports of increased risk of cardiac arrhythmias with the use of carbamazepine in older individuals.[76,77] Drug-drug interactions are an important consideration because of their high prevalence with antiepileptic drugs and the increased number of medications the average geriatric patient takes. Documented interactions can be found in Table 8.1.

Given the profound neurobiologic changes that occur in the brain with aging, one would expect alterations in the geriatric response to anticonvulsant medications. Although it is frequent practice to use lower doses of antiepileptic drugs in the elderly, especially at the initiation of treatment, there is no empirical evidence in humans to support this practice. The aged do appear to be more sensitive to the sedating effects of these medications, but the question of whether or not the dose-response curve is shifted has not been addressed. The earlier mentioned electrophysiologic changes that occur in the aged would suggest an intrinsic decrease in paroxysmal epileptic potential. Although the liability for the development of epilepsy may increase due to structural changes in the brain, the ability to mount and sustain an epileptiform discharge might be decreased due to decreased neuronal excitability. Studies in rodents suggest that the threshold for both electroshock[78] and pentylenetrazole[79]-induced seizures is decreased with age. Clinical experience with human patients with depression treated with electroconvulsive therapy suggests this as well. Studies in rodents have also indicated that the minimal effective anticonvulsant plasma concentration needed to abolish electroshock-induced seizures is lower with aging for a variety of antiepileptic drugs including phenobarbital,[80,81] phenytoin,[82] valproate,[83] oxazepam,[84] and zonisamide.[85] Increased sensitivity to the ataxic effects of these medications has also been demonstrated.[81,84,86] Increased sensitivity to the benzodiazepine midazolam as assessed by EEG parameters has also been found.[87]

V. ALCOHOL

Controversy continues to rage regarding the salutory vs. deleterious effects of alcohol consumption in the elderly. Most arguments tend to be polemical and nondata based. Long-term pathological effects are clouded by the confounding effects of duration and magnitude of exposure. Unlike the emerging body of literature pertaining to middle-aged males, few data regarding the cardiovascular implications of modest alcohol use in the elderly are available. Regular but moderate alcohol consumption, defined as up to two drinks per day, appears to decrease the risk of coronary artery disease in males.[88] Alcohol increases the level of high-density lipoprotein (HDL) cholesterol, including HDL_3, a subfraction with antiatherogenic properties. It can also decrease blood platelet aggregation. Whereas this is clearly beneficial during the developmental stages of atherogenesis, it is not clear that protection would continue to be afforded once atherosclerosis has proceeded to an advanced stage. It is also unclear whether or not attendant risks would outweigh any potential benefits.

TABLE 8.1.
Some Reported Interactions between Antiepileptic Drugs and Other Medications

Drug class drug	Antiepileptic drug[a]	Interaction or effect[b]
Analgesics/antipyretics	PHT, VPA	Transient ↑ free AED concentration, may result in PHT concentration high and ASA treatment prolonged
Aspirin		
Ibuprofen	PHT	Possible ↑ PHT Concentration
Propoxyphene	CBZ	↑↑ CBZ concentration, rapid
Antimicrobials		
Erythromycin	CBZ	↑↑ CBZ concentration, rapid
Isoniazid	CB, PB, PHT	Possible AED accumulation
Rifampin	PHT	↓ PHT concentration
Sulfa drugs	PHT	↑ PHT concentration
Gastrointestinal drugs		
Antacids	PHT, VPA, ? others	Variable; ↓ PHT absorption; ? ↑ VPA absorption↑
Cimetidine	CBZ, PHT	↑ ↑ PHT concentration; transient ↑ CBZ concentration
Ranitidine	PHT	↑ PHT concentration (only one case)
Sucralfate	PHT	↓ PHT absorption (? effect on other AEDs)
Antiasthmatic drugs		
Theophylline	CBZ, PB, PHT	Theophylline may lower seizure threshold in susceptible persons; AEDs cause ↓ theophylline concentration
Cardiovascular drugs		
Digoxin	PHT	↓ Digoxin concentration
Dilitazem	CBZ	↑ to x CBZ concentration
Disopyramide	PHT	↓ Disopyramide concentration
Lidocaine	PB, PHT	↓ Lidocaine concentration
Nifedepine	PHT	↑ PHT concentration
Quinidine	PB, PHT	↓ Quinidine concentration
Verapamil	CBZ	↑ to ↑ ↑ CBZ concentration
Warfarin	CBZ, PB, PHT	↓ Warfarin effect with CBZ and PB, possibly ↑ effect with PHT
Immunosuppressants		
Steroids	CBZ, PB	↑ Steroid elimination
Cyclosporin A	PHT, CBZ	↑ Cyclosporin concentration
Psychotropic drugs		
Chlorpromazine	PH, VPA	↑ PHT and ↑ VPA concentration
Desipramine	PHT	↓ Desipramine concentration
Haloperidol	CBZ, PB, PHT, VPA	↓ Haloperidol concentration with CBZ, PB, or PHT; no effect with VPA
Imipramine	PHT	↑ PHT concentration
Thioridazine	PB, PHT	↓ Concentration thioridazine active metabolite
Lithium	CBZ	Encephalopathy and tremor at acceptable drug concentrations

[a] AED = antiepileptic drug; ASA = acetylsalicylic acid; CBZ = carbamazepine; PB = phenobarbital; PHT = phenytoin; VPA = valproic acid.

[b] ↑ = increased; ↑ ↑ = marked increase; ↓ = decreased; ↓ ↓ marked decrease.

From Scheurer, M. L. and Cohen, J., *Neurol. Clin.*, 11, 800, 1993. With permission.

Although the number of individuals consuming alcohol decreases with age, heavy and problematic use occur in 6 to 14% and 1 to 17% of the elderly population, respectively. This depends to a large extent on the population surveyed, ranging from 4% in a general outpatient medical setting to 11% in nursing home admissions and 23% in geriatric psychiatry residential treatment units.[89] When defined by widely accepted diagnostic criteria, the ECA study indicated that 1.8% of men over the age of 65 suffered from alcohol abuse disorder compared to 0.3% of women.[90] Although drinking habits tend to become well established by the early adult years, it has recently become evident that alcohol abuse can begin late in life. This can be a *de novo* problem or the reactivation of a problem long in remission. Late-onset alcoholism tends to be more benign in its presentation and course[91] and more amenable to treatment.[92]

A discussion of alcohol and aging needs to address two primary issues: changes with age in the biological response of the organism to acute or short-term exposure to alcohol, e.g., pharmacokinetics, sensitivity, and tolerance, and the relationship, if any, between chronic alcohol exposure and the aging process. The former will be of greater interest to the clinician, the latter to the basic scientist, but together they illustrate the interface between neuroscience and the practice of medicine.

In general, the elderly are less tolerant of any given dose of alcohol. Both pharmacokinetic and pharmacodynamic factors play a role. For any given dose of alcohol, blood alcohol levels will be higher in the elderly, primarily due to changes in distribution. Alcohol, being hydrophilic in nature, will distribute in the body water compartment. As previously noted, this compartment shrinks with age due to the increased percentage of body fat present. Absorption from the stomach remains unchanged with age so that time to reach peak plasma concentration is similar. But actual peak plasma level will be higher in the elderly because the ethanol is distributing in a relatively smaller compartment. Similarly, peak levels will be higher in females than males due to gender-related differences in body habitus. Because the elderly possess less tissue water per body mass, organ ethanol concentrations, including the brain, will be higher as well.[93,94] In essence, the elderly are more likely to become intoxicated with similar levels of alcohol consumption. Relatively few age-related differences in metabolism appear to exist. Alcohol dehydrogenase, the enzyme responsible for converting ethanol to acetaldehyde, shows no change in activity with age. Elimination time is therefore no different.[95]

Over the past 10 years, gastric first-pass metabolism of alcohol has been recognized as a potentially important metabolic pathway. Alcohol dehydrogenase is abundant in the epithelial cells of the gastric mucosa. The magnitude of this first-pass effect is controversial, although under social drinking conditions it may account for as much as 28% of the metabolism of a given dose.[96] It is affected by many factors including age, sex, ethnicity, and stomach content. It is less in alcoholics and the elderly.[97] Thus, older individuals may experience higher blood alcohol levels not only because of differences in volume of distribution, but also because of diminished first-pass metabolism capacity, particularly if drinking occurs on an empty stomach. This may be potentiated by the administration of H_2-antagonists such as cimetidine and ranitidine, which inhibit gastric ADH activity,[96] although the clinical significance of this well-established pharmacologic phenomenon is controversial. Age-related decrements in hepatic microsomal function in the cytochrome P450 ethanol oxidizing system, as well as aniline hydroxylation and mitochondrial low K_m-acetaldehyde dehydrogenase activity, have been demonstrated,[98–101] although the significance of these findings may relate more to potential differences in tissue toxicity than the issue of intoxication, per se. It has become increasingly clear that end-organ toxicity in heart, liver, and brain is not solely related to dietary deficiencies. Redox changes produced by the NADH generated by the alcohol dehydrogenase pathway are directly hepatotoxic. Ethanol-inducible cytochrome P450 2E1 is partially involved in ethanol metabolism and responsible for the activation of xenobiotics to toxic radicals.[102] Acetaldehyde, an intermediary metabolite, may be cytotoxic via adduct formation with various tissue constituents resulting in damage to microtubule-associated proteins.[103] Thus, the elderly may be more vulnerable than their younger counterparts to the cytotoxic effects of alcohol.

Pharmacodynamic differences are purported to exist in the elderly as well, yet the literature is sparse and in humans less than rigorous. Studies have found decrements in memory[104] and psychomotor performance[105–107] in aged adults as compared to younger individuals, but pharmacokinetic factors may be partially responsible. Animal studies are more convincing, but few in number. The righting response is more impaired at similar brain ethanol concentrations in aged mice and is eventually regained at lower levels.[108–110] Chronic ethanol administration produces more behavioral evidence of intoxication and withdrawal in aged male mice,[111] and passive avoidance learning and regional brain choline acetyltransferase activity are affected to a greater degree.[112] Neurobiologic evidence is sparse. Neuroanatomic evidence of increased vulnerability in aged mice is suggested by the presence of increased cell loss and mitochondrial and nerve-ending damage in aged, ethanol-treated mice.[113] Human brain tissue of aged individuals obtained at autopsy shows greater inhibition by ethanol of synaptosomal (Na+)-(K+)-ATPase activity.[114]

Some evidence points to increased biochemical sensitivity as well. Allyl alcohol hepatotoxicity is increased in aged male rats.[115,116] Female rats acutely exposed to ethyl alcohol demonstrate delayed restitution of hepatic glutathione levels with increased age.[117] Chronic ethanol intake in humans exacerbates normal physiologic age-related decrements in cerebral blood flow and metabolism. This has been elegantly demonstrated using positron emission tomography (PET), a neuroradiologic imaging procedure that evaluates functional CNS parameters. This has been demonstrated both with acute ethanol challenges as well as in chronic alcoholics. Administration of 1 g/kg of ethyl alcohol to normal and alcoholic subjects produced inhibition of cortical and cerebellar metabolism in both groups, but was more pronounced in alcoholics.[118] Chronic alcoholics who had been abstinent for anywhere from 6 to 32 d show significantly decreased whole-brain metabolism on PET scanning using [18F]-fluorodeoxyglucose.[119,120] During acute alcohol withdrawal, brain metabolism increases and then gradually decreases and reaches a baseline lower than that of nonalcoholic controls. This return to basal function occurred over a 16 to 30-d period,[121] suggesting that elderly binge drinkers may spend much of their time in a state of CNS disequilibrium, even if they are refraining from alcohol at the moment. In summary, the evidence to date suggests the presence of alcohol-induced CNS impairment in the elderly that persists beyond the stage of acute intoxication.

Excessive alcohol intake potentiates other age-related functional impairments. With age, blood pressure increases, glucose tolerance decreases, gastrointestinal atrophic changes appear, water and solute homeostasis becomes impaired, bone mass decreases, and, in males, androgenic steroid production decreases. Alcohol produces a multitude of physiologic alterations that are intrinsically detrimental and may interact with the aging process. Mention has already been made of the protective effect of moderate alcohol intake on the atherogenic process. This is due to increases in HDL_2/HDL_3 cholesterol and apolipoprotein A-I/B and decreases in low-density lipoprotein (LDL) cholesterol. But the same amount of alcohol consumed in binge cycles has the opposite effect[122] and may predispose to acute vascular thrombosis and stroke. Alcohol has been demonstrated to produce changes in the Na(+)-K(+)ATPase, Na(+)-Li+ countertransport, and Na(+)-K(+)-Cl(–) cotransport systems conducive to a hypertensive response that dissipates with cessation of drinking.[123] These changes may mediate the observed pressor response of alcohol and additionally contribute to the acute cardiovascular and CNS morbidity of binge drinking. Additionally, chronic alcoholics demonstrate reduced lymphocyte β-adrenoreceptor levels with abrupt increase in the number and function of these receptors during acute alcohol withdrawal, resulting in a state of acute adrenergic hypersensitivity.[124] This is particularly salient given the increased circulating levels of catecholeamines present in the elderly, as well as compromised vasodilation with exercise in response to β-adrenergic stimulation and decreased β-adrenergic modulation of myocardial contractility.[125]

Age-related gastrointestinal changes include decreased motility, secretion, and absorption. Functional reserve usually compensates for this with no resultant measurable loss in overall function. Alcohol produces similar alterations in intestinal function, including decreased brush border enzyme activity and decreased activity of Na(+)-K(+)-ATPase. Bacterial flora is increased, leading to increased metabolism of alcohol to acetaldehyde.[126] This, coupled with the common use of broad-spectrum antibiotics, which also alter bacterial flora, may produce changes which are additive and potentially toxic. Although not a universal finding, many studies have demonstrated insulin resistance in the elderly. Chronic alcoholism is also associated with insulin resistance. This may be due to direct decreases in cell-surface insulin receptors as well as postreceptor changes in enzymes modulated by insulin.[127,128] Finally, alcohol-induced hypoglycemia may be compounded by the frequent treatment of the elderly with oral hypoglycemic agents.

Fluid and electrolyte imbalance is exceedingly common in the elderly, particularly those living alone or with cognitive impairment. Alcohol profoundly inhibits antidiuretic hormone release, allowing a diuresis that can lead to fluid depletion and hypernatremia. This is compounded by the renal tubular changes that occur with aging that impair the ability to handle water and solute loads and renal concentrating and diluting capacity. Bone density decreases with aging, particularly in postmenopausal women, markedly increasing the risk of serious fractures. Chronic alcohol consumption also produces decreased bone mineral density as measured by decreased serum osteocalcin and bone gla protein levels, suggesting decreased osteoblast activity as well as an uncoupling of osteoblastic and osteoclastic activity,[129–131] which appear partially reversible with abstinence. Acute alcohol intoxication causes transitory hypoparathyroidism with hypocalcemia and hypercalciuria. Prolonged drinking, even if only moderate in nature, increases serum parathyroid hormone levels. This secondary hyperparathyroidism can also contribute to bone demineralization. Severe chronic alcohol consumption results in vitamin D deficiency, hypocalcemia, and hypocalciuria.[132] Lastly, aging in men is associated with a progressive decline in serum testosterone levels, which has been dubbed the "andropause". Chronic alcohol consumption may exacerbate this both at the level of the testes and hypothalamus by inhibiting luteinizing hormone (LH) binding to Leydig cells, inhibition of steroidogenesis, and inhibition of LH release by the pituitary.[133–135]

Special attention has to be paid to drug-alcohol interactions in the elderly due to the increased number of medications they are taking and the decreased therapeutic index present. Short-term consumption of alcohol will result in competition for P450 hepatic microsomal enzymes, thereby elevating the concentration of many drugs metabolized through this pathway. This may be particularly important with benzodiazepines and barbiturates, especially if dosing errors occur. Long-term alcohol consumption will have the opposite effect, producing microsomal enzyme induction, resulting in a decrease in the plasma concentrations of such commonly used medications as warfarin, phenytoin, tolbutamide, and propranolol. Alcohol will enhance the potential hepatotoxicity of acetaminophen, a drug often consumed in excessive quantities by the elderly due to the presence of arthritis and other musculoskeletal ailments.

In conclusion, alcohol, particularly in the elderly, should be viewed as a drug, with a risk-benefit profile that deserves careful consideration in the clinical care of the geriatric population.

VI. ALCOHOL AND THE AGING PROCESS

Alcohol in sufficient quantity is a potent toxin capable of producing multi-organ damage. The effect is cumulative and at times resembles that produced by normal aging itself. This has lead to attempts to relate alcohol-induced changes to the aging process and to explain that process by phenomena that occur with chronic alcohol exposure. Neuropsychological findings in alcoholism are variable and have led to two main theses regarding the effect of alcohol on neurocognition: the premature aging hypothesis, i.e., that alcohol induces performance decrements throughout the life span that are similar to those found in individuals of an older age, and the increased vulnerability with age hypothesis, i.e., that older individuals are more susceptible to neurocognitive deficits than are younger ones. Of interest, age rather than duration of alcohol exposure appears to better predict degree of cognitive deficit.[136] This is consistent with earlier cited evidence suggesting increased psychodynamic sensitivity to alcohol in the elderly. Although neuropsychological deficits often improve with sobriety, age is again an important predictor of the extent of improvement.[137] Neuroradiologic abnormalities such as cortical atrophy and reduced regional blood flow do not appear to correlate well with neuropsychologic outcome.

Alcohol produces a number of effects that may simulate or interact with the aging process. One is its effect on biological membranes. Acutely, alcohol fluidizes or disorders cell and organelle membranes. With continued exposure the membrane becomes resistant to this disordering effect. This correlates with behavioral tolerance in animals, but adult animals, which are more sensitive to the behavioral effects of alcohol, demonstrate less membrane disordering effect. On the other hand, membranes of animals chronically exposed to alcohol are more rigid and have higher cholesterol/phospholipid ratios.[138] Similar membrane changes are found with aging. Membranes become stiffer, cholesterol content increases, and saturated fatty acid content increases. The latter may be related to increased lipid peroxidation.[139]

Lipofuscin accumulation in neurons is a reliable correlate of aging, increasing from 7% of neurons in the first decade of life to 35% in the fifth.[140] Chronic alcohol exposure in rats has been found to produce premature lipofuscin deposition in the cerebellum[141] and hippocampus[142] which can be ameliorated by treatment with piracetam[143] and 2-ethyl-6-methyl-3-hydroxypyridine.[144] Additionally, the latter agent was also able to counteract the deleterious effects of alcohol exposure on behavior, memory, and learning. Increased myocardial lipofuscin formation has also been found in chronic alcoholics.[145] Human alcoholic brains at autopsy show an acceleration of the normal loss of myelin associated with the aging process.[146] Lipofuscin has also been hypothetically related to lipid peroxidation.

Comparisons between alcohol toxicity and normal aging have also been attempted on the neurochemical level. This has been examined at the level of the neurotransmitter, neuroreceptor, and intracellular second messenger pathways. Results are both very preliminary and contradictory, although similarities may exist. Normal aging is associated with reductions in the levels of all major neurotransmitters, although to variable degrees across individuals and the specific neurotransmitter in question. Striatal dopamine levels decrease by 1% per year in humans. Alcoholism has been found to markedly accelerate that process, with depression of striatal and hypothalamic dopamine levels by 50 and 100% compared to controls 20 years older.[147] Animal studies have yielded mixed results, with reports of increased,[148] decreased,[149] and unchanged[150] dopamine brain content. The same investigators[147] also reported marked decreases in norepinephrine and serotonin levels in their alcoholic subjects. The findings in animals have been totally contradictory[148,150–158] for these two neurotransmitters. Whereas human aging is associated with decreased CNS acetylcholine levels secondary to decreased choline acetyltransferase activity, studies in alcoholics have not been performed and the animal literature is once again inconsistent.[159–164]

Due to the central role played by cholinergic mechanisms in memory and neurocognitive aging, the differential effects of aging and chronic alcohol exposure on muscarinic binding sites have also been examined. Muscarinic receptor density measured by [3H]quinuclidinyl benzilate was found to be decreased in the putamen and hippocampus of alcoholics compared to controls.[165,166] Contrariwise, rats chronically treated with alcohol were found to demonstrate an age-related decline in receptors, but an increase in receptors with chronic exposure to alcohol.[167]

The hallmark of the aged brain is a decreased capacity to learn. The cause of this is undoubtedly multifactorial and can not be attributed to dysfunction in any particular neurotransmitter pathway. Excitatory neurotransmitters are thought to play a role in kindling, long-term potentiation, and possibly learning and memory.[168] [3H]MK-801 binding sites have been shown to progressively decline in human frontal cortex[169] and to be decreased in density in senescent rat hippocampus.[170] Antagonism of *N*-methyl-D-aspartate (NMDA) receptors in young animals has been shown to produce effects on learning similar to those found in older animals. Alcohol potently antagonizes the NDA receptor,[171] an effect not influenced by animal age.[172] Chronic administration results in receptor up-regulation,[173,174] perhaps making the organism more vulnerable to neuroexcitotoxicity and neuronal death.[175] Inhibitory GABA receptors have been reported to decrease or remain the same in aged rat brains (previously referenced). Chronic alcohol treatment has been reported to increase,[176] decrease,[177,178] or not change [3H]GABA binding sites.[159,179]

Interest has also recently been focused on the role of the phosphoinositol pathway in learning, memory, and neuronal plasticity. Involvement in cellular aging or the sequelae of aging is possible as well. Although not universal, there is mounting evidence to suggest alteration in brain protein kinase C activity and translocation in aging animals.[180] Abnormalities have also been identified in the intracellular calcium mobilizing agent inositol 1,4,5-triphosphate (increased),[181] phospholipase C and diacylglycerol activity (increased),[182] and phosphoinositol turnover (decreased).[183] Chronic alcohol exposure has been found to inhibit norepinephrine-stimulated phosphoinositol hydrolysis in rat liver slices[184] and brain[185]

The interaction between age and ethanol exposure has yet to be addressed. Theories of aging can be divided into two major categories: the stochastic and the developmental-genetic. Biological effects of chronic alcohol exposure share characteristics with many of the theoretical mechanisms postulated to date. Stochastic theories argue that aging is the result of random damage to organs and the molecules, membranes, organelles, and cells they comprise. The somatic mutation theory holds that environmentally produced genetic damage results in loss of physiological integrity. These insults can arise from both the internal and external milieu. The error catastrophe theory suggests that alterations in "template" molecules involved in protein or DNA synthesis can occur and produce a multiplier effect due to abnormal protein synthesis. Post-translational errors may also be involved in the aging process, particularly the cross linking of collagen and DNA molecules. Finally, free radical formation secondary to aerobic metabolism has also been proposed as a mechanism of molecular damage leading to cell senescence.

The other major theoretical orientation, the developmental-genetic model of aging, holds that aging is part of a genetically programmed process of deterioration. The neuroendocrine hypothesis argues that the hypothalamic-pituitary-adrenal (HPA) axis is a "master regulator" of cell function and that hormonal changes over time induce cellular changes resulting in aging. The intrinsic mutagenesis theory maintains that progressive compromise in the fidelity of genetic transcription and replication leads to deleterious or lethal gene mutations. The immunologic theory of aging considers impaired immune surveillance as responsible for external or autoimmune damage.

Chronic alcohol exposure can produce a variety of biological insults similar to those associated with the aging process. As already stated, chronic exposure also appears to result in premature aging both psychologically and physiologically. The question then arises as to whether or not alcohol is an aetatic agent. Myriad biological observations suggest that in sufficient quantity it may very well be. Chronic exposure can produce lipofuscin formation, a hallmark biological marker of aging. Cell-mediated immune function is compromised in alcoholics, although it would be premature to suggest that the mechanism or actual changes overlap with those seen in aging.[186–188] The risk of carcinoma, particularly of the esophagus, stomach, liver, and breast, is increased tenfold, and after cardiovascular disease is the most common cause of death in chronic alcoholics.[189] Carcinomatous change in cells appears to be an inevitable occurrence with time. Glucocorticoids are neurotoxic and may play a role in natural senescense.[190,191] Hyperactivity of the HPA axis with increased levels of circulating corticosteroids has been well documented in chronic alcoholics and during acute alcohol withdrawal.[192–196] Aging is associated with a decrease in blood levels of growth hormone (GH) and insulin-like growth factors.[197,198] The plasma GH response to stimulation by sodium valproate has been reported to be blunted in normal aging.[199] Ethanol ingestion in healthy humans has been found to blunt the nightly peak of GH secretion.[200] Additionally, alcoholics demonstrate a blunted GH response to biological challenge with clonidine[201] and apomorphine.[202] Acute ethanol exposure has been shown to quickly decrease GH synthesis as assessed by a decrease in GH mRNA.[203] Melatonin, a hormone produced by the pineal gland, demonstrates a number of characteristics that may relate to aging. The circadian rhythm of secretion deteriorates with age and can be restored in animals by caloric deprivation, a process which has been well established to increase longevity. Exogenous administration has been reported to increase longevity and have immunoenhancing and oncostatic properties.[204] Alcohol reduces nocturnal melatonin production both with acute ingestion by healthy human subjects[205,206] and in chronic alcoholics.[207] Thus, although very preliminary in nature, there is accumulating evidence to link alcohol and aging-related neuroendocrine changes.

Chronic alcohol exposure produces multiple biological insults consistent with stochastic theories of aging. Metabolism of ethanol by alcohol dehydrogenase generates NADH, which favors free radical formation and alters the metabolism of lipids, proteins, and purines. It induces cytochrome P450 2E1, a microsomal enzyme important in the metabolism of xenobiotics such as drugs, solvents, and carcinogens. Activation of this enzyme may result in an increase in the production of potentially carcinogenic substances and toxic radicals.[208] It depresses levels of the antioxidants vitamin A[209] and vitamin E.[210,211] Rats fed a chronic ethanol low-vitamin E diet demonstrate more hepatic lipid peroxidation than controls.[212] Chronic ethanol intake may increase microsomal production of superoxide and hydrogen peroxide, both of which are potent oxidants capable of initiating lipid peroxidation, particularly in the presence of iron.[213] Alcohol abuse is associated with disturbances in iron homeostasis. Hepatocytes of alcohol-fed rats demonstrate increased ferritin uptake.[214] Acetaldehyde, its immediate metabolite, is capable of protein adduct formation by covalently binding to microsomal proteins, collagen, and blood proteins such as albumin, hemoglobin, and lipoproteins.[215–222] By complexing with various proteins it can create antigens that induce an autoimmune response.[223–226] It also induces glutathione depletion,[227–230] a substance important in the detoxification of carcinogens and free radicals. Finally, deletions in mitochondrial DNA increase markedly with advanced age, possibly due to the action of free radicals.[231,232] Thus, alcohol may also be responsible for the progressive accumulation of deleterious genetic mutations. Aging is also associated with a decline in mitochondrial oxidative phosphorylation.[233] Chronic alcohol exposure does the same,[234] although this effect may be specific to liver and not occur in brain.[235]

REFERENCES

1. **Jones, D.,** Characteristics of elderly people taking psychotropic medication, *Drugs Aging*, 2, 389, 1992.
2. **Kok, A. and Zeef, E. J.,** *Event-Related Brain Research*, EEG Suppl. 42, Elsevier Science Publishers, Amsterdam, 1991, 324.
3. **Visser, S. L.,** *Event-Related Brain Research*, EEG Suppl. 42, Elsevier Science Publishers, Amsterdam, 1991, 289.
4. **Dam, A. M.,** The density of neurons in the human hippocampus, *Neuropathol. Appl. Neurobiol.*, 5, 249, 1979.
5. **Terry, R. D., Hansen, L. A., and DeTeresa, R.,** Senile dementia of the Alzheimer type without neocortical neurofibrillary tangles, *Neuropathol. Exp. Neurol.*, 5, 249, 1979.
6. **Coleman, P. D. and Flood, D. G.,** Neuron numbers and dendritic extent in normal aging and Alzheimer's disease, *Neurobiol. Aging*, 8, 521, 1987.
7. **Hall, T. C., Miller, A. K. H., and Corsellis, J. A. N.,** Variations in human Purkinje cell population according to age and sex, *Neuropathol. Appl. Neurobiol.*, 1, 267, 1975.

8. **Mann, D. M. A., Yates, P. O., and Hawkes, J.**, The pathology of the human locus ceruleus, *Clin. Neuropathol.*, 2, 1, 1983.
9. **Tejani-Butt, S. M. and Ordway, G. A.**, Effect of age on [3H]nisoxetine binding to uptake sites for norepinephrine in the locus coeruleus of humans, *Brain Res.*, 583, 312, 1992.
10. **Coffey, C. E. and Cummings, J. L.**, *Textbook of Geriatric Neuropsychiatry*, American Psychiatric Press, London, 1994, 55.
11. **DeBlasi, A., Cotecchia, S., and Mennini, T.**, Selective changes of receptor binding in brain regions of aged rats, *Life Sci.*, 31, 335, 1982.
12. **Govoni, S., Memo, M., Saiani, L., Spano, P. F., and Trabucchi, M.**, Impairment of brain neurotransmitter receptors in aged rats, *Mech. Ageing Dev.*, 12, 39, 1980.
13. **Maggi, A., Schmidt, M. J., Ghetti, B., and Enna, S. J.**, Effect of aging on neurotransmitter receptor binding in rat and human brain, *Life Sci.*, 24, 367, 1979.
14. **Kendall, D. A., Strong, R., and Enna, S. J.**, *The Aging Brain: Cellular and Molecular Mechanisms of Aging in the Nervous System*, Raven Press, New York, 1982, 211.
15. **Shepherd, M. and Gruenberg, E. M.**, The age for neuroses, *Milbank Mem. Fund.*, 35, 258, 1957.
16. **Turnbull, J. M. and Turnbull, S. K.**, Management of specific anxiety disorders in the elderly, *Geriatrics*, 8, 75, 1985.
17. **Himmelfarb, S. and Murrell, S. A.**, The prevalence and correlates of anxiety symptoms in older adults, *J. Psychol.*, 116, 159, 1984.
18. **Myers, J. K., Weissman, M. M., and Tischler, G. L.**, *Arch. Gen. Psychiatry*, 41, U.S. Government Printing Office, Washington, D.C., 1984, 959.
19. **Robins, N., Helzer, J.E., and Weissman, M. M.**, *Arch. Gen. Psychiatry*, U.S. Government Printing Office, Washington, D.C., 1984, 949.
20. **Brody, J. A. and Foley, D. J.**, *The Teaching Nursing Home*, Raven Press, New York, 1983.
21. **White, L. R. and Cartwright, W. S.**, Geriatric epidemiology, *Annu. Rev. Gerontol. Geriatr.*, 6, 215, 1986.
22. **Kramer, M., German, P. S., and Anthony, J. C.**, Patterns of mental disorders among the elderly residents of eastern Baltimore, *J. Am. Geriatr. Soc.*, 33, 236, 1985.
23. **Gottlieb, G. L.**, Sleep disorders and their management, *Am. J. Med.*, 88, 3A-29S, 1990.
24. **Morgan, K.**, *Sleep and Aging*, John Hopkins University Press, Baltimore, 1987, 23.
25. **Greenblatt, D. J., Allen, M. D., Harmatz, J. S., and Shader, R. I.**, Diazepam disposition determinants, *Clin. Pharmacol. Ther.*, 27, 301, 1980.
26. **Divoll, M., Greenblatt, D. J., and Ochs, H. R.**, Absolute bioavailability of oral and intramuscular diazepam: effect of age and sex, *Anesth. Analg.*, 62, 1, 1983.
27. **Macklon, A. F., Barton, M., James, O., and Rawlins, M. D.**, The effect of age on the pharmacokinetics of diazepam, *Clin. Sci.*, 59, 479, 1980.
28. **Kanto, J., Maenpaa, M., Mantyla, R., Sellman, R., and Valovirta, E.**, Effect of age on the pharmacokinetics of diazepam given in conjunction with spinal anesthesia, *Anesthesiology*, 51, 154, 1979.
29. **Greenblatt, D. J., Sellers, E. M., and Shader, R. I.**, Drug disposition in old age, *N. Engl. J. Med.*, 306, 1081, 1982.
30. **Greenblatt, D. J., Divoll, M., Abernathy, D. R., Harmatz, J. S., and Shader, R. I.**, Antipyrine kinetics in the elderly: prediction of age related changes in benzodiazepine oxidizing capacity, *J. Pharmacol. Exp. Ther.*, 220, 120, 1982.
31. **Tsang, C. F. C. and Wilkinson, G. R.**, Diazepam disposition in mature and aged rabbits and rats, *Drug. Metab. Dispos.*, 10, 413.
32. **Fujita, S., Tatsuno, J., Kitani, K., and Suzuki, T.**, Age-associated alterations in diazepam metabolizing enzyme activities in male and female rats, *Drug Metab. Dispos.*, 18, 812, 1990.
33. **Forbes, G. B. and Reian, J. C.**, Adult lean body mass declines with age: some longitudinal observations, *Metabolism*, 19, 653, 1970.
34. **Klotz, U., Avant, G. R., Hoyumpa, A., Schenker, S., and Wilkinson, G. R.**, The effects of age and liver disease on the disposition and elimination of diazepam in man, *J. Clin. Invest.*, 55, 347, 1975.
35. **Klotz, U. and Muller-Seydlitz, P.**, Altered elimination of desmethyldiazepam in the elderly, *Br. J. Clin. Pharmacol.*, 7, 119, 1979.
36. **Shader, R. I., Greenblatt, D. J., Harmatz, J. S., Franke, K., and Koch-Weser, J.**, Absorption and disposition of chlordiazepoxide in young and elderly male volunteers, *J. Clin. Pharmacol.*, 17, 709, 1977.
37. **Greenblatt, D. J., Divoll, M., Abernathy, D. R., Moschitto, I. J., and Smith, R. B.**, Alprazolam kinetics in the elderly: relation to antipyrine disposition, *Arch. Gen. Psychiatry*, 40, 287, 1983.
38. **Kroboth, P. D., McAuley, J. W., and Smith, R. B.**, Alprazolam in the elderly: pharmacokinetics and pharmacodynamics during multiple dosing, *Psychopharmacology*, 100, 477, 1990.
39. **Greenblatt, D. J. and Divoll, A. M.**, Toxicity of nitrazepam in the elderly: a report from the Boston Collaborative Drug Surveillance Program, *Br. J. Clin. Pharmacol.*, 5, 407, 1978.
40. **Greenblatt, D. J., Harmatz, J. S., and Shader, R. I.**, Clinical pharmacokinetics of anxiolytics and hypnotics in the elderly, *Clin. Pharmacokinet.*, 21, 262, 1991.

41. **Sonne, J., Loft, S., Dossing, M., Boesgaard, S., and Andreasen, F.,** Single dose pharmacokinetics and pharmacodynamics of oral oxazepam in very elderly institutionalized subjects, *Br. J. Clin. Pharmacol.*, 1, 719, 1991.
42. **Viani, A., Rizzo, G., Carrai, M., and Pacifica, G. M.,** The effect of ageing on plasma albumin and plasma protein binding of diazepam, salicylic acid and digitoxin in healthy subjects and patients with renal impairment, *Br. J. Clin. Pharmacol.*, 33, 299, 1992.
43. **Kendall, D. A., Strong, R., and Enna, S. J.,** *The Aging Brain: Cellular and Molecular Mechanisms of Aging in the Nervous System*, Raven Press, New York, 1982, 211.
44. **DeBlasi, A., Cotecchia, S., and Mennini, T.,** Selective changes of receptor binding in brain regions of aged rats, *Life Sci.*, 31, 335, 1982.
45. **Govoni, S., Memo, M., Saiani, L., Spano, P. F., and Trabucchi, M.,** Impairment of brain neurotransmitter receptors in aged rats, *Mech. Ageing Dev.*, 12, 39, 1980.
46. **Maggi, A., Schmidt, M. J., Ghetti, B., and Enna, S. J.,** Effect of aging on neurotransmitter receptor binding in rat and human brain, *Life Sci.*, 24, 367, 1979.
47. **Delahaye, C., Gerrand, B., Pieddeloup, C., and Musch, B.,** Post marketing surveillance of zopiclone: interim analysis on the first 10,000 cases in a clinical study in general practice, *Int. Clin. Psychopharmacol.*, 5, 131, 1990.
48. **Roger, M., Attali, P., and Coquelin, J. P.,** Multicenter, double-blind, controlled comparison of zolpidem and triazolam in elderly patients with insomnia, submitted.
49. **Stutzmann, J. M., Piot, O., Reibaud, M., Doble, A., and Blanchard, J. C.,** Pharmacological properties and mechanism of action of the cyclopyrrolones, *L'Encephale*, XVIII, 393, 1992.
50. **Langer, S. Z., Arbilla, S., Benavides, J., and Scatton, B.,** Zolpidem and alpidem: two imidazopyridines with selectivity for omega 1- and omega 3- receptor subtypes, *Adv. Biochem. Psychopharmacol.*, 46, 61, 1990.
51. **Lavoisky, J., Zivkovic, B., Benavides, J., Perrault, G. H., and Robert, P.,** Contribution of zolpidem in the management of sleep disorders, *Encephale*, 18, 379, 1992.
52. **Stutzmann, J. M., Delahaye, C., and Allain, H.,** Zopiclone. Data of experimental pharmacology and clinical use, *Therapie*, 48, 33, 1993.
53. **Shapiro, C. M., Macfarlane, J. G., and MacLean, A. W.,** Alleviating sleep-related discontinuance symptoms associated with benzodiazepine withdrawal: a new approach, *J. Psychosomatic Res.*, 37, 55, 1993.
54. **Jackson, H. C., Ramsay, E., and Nutt, D. J.,** Effect of the cyclopyrrolones suriclone and RP on 59037 on body temperature in mice, *Eur. J. Pharmacol.*, 216, 23, 1992.
55. **Piot, O., Betschart, J., Stutzmann, J. M., and Blanchard, J. C.,** Cyclopyrrolones, unlike some benzodiazepines, do not induce physical dependence in mice, *Neurosci. Lett.*, 117, 140, 1990.
56. **Wadworth, A. N. and McTavish, D.,** Zopiclone. A review of its pharmacological properties and therapeutic efficacy as an hypnotic, *Drugs Aging*, 3, 441, 1993.
57. **Enkelmann, R.,** Alprazolam versus buspirone in the treatment of outpatients with generalized anxiety disorder, *Psychopharmacology*, 105, 428, 1991.
58. **Strand, M., Hetta, J., Rosen, A., Sorensen, S., Malmstrom, R., Fabian, C., Marits, K., Vetterskog, K., Liljestrand, A. G., and Hegen, C.,** A double-blind, controlled trial in primary care patients with generalized anxiety: a comparison between buspirone and oxazepam, *J. Clin. Psychiatry*, 51, 40, 1990.
59. **Bohm, C., Robinson, D. S., Gammans, R. E., Shortriya, R. C., Alms, D. R., Leroy, A., and Placchi, M.,** Buspirone therapy in anxious elderly patients: a controlled clinical trial, *J. Clin. Psychopharmacol.*, 10, 47S, 1990.
60. **Gammans, R. E., Westrick, M. L., Shea, J. P., et al.,** Pharmacokinetics of buspirone in elderly subjects, *J. Clin. Pharmacol.*, 29, 72, 1989.
61. **Hart, R. P., Colenda, C. C., and Hamer, R. M.,** Effects of buspirone and alprazolam on the cognitive performance of normal elderly subjects, *Am. J. Psychiatry*, 148, 73, 1991.
62. **Yudofsky, S. C., Silver, J. M., and Hales, R. E.,** Pharmacologic management of aggression in the elderly, *J. Clin. Psychiatry*, 51, 29, 1990.
63. **Hauser, W. A., Annegers, J. F., and Kurland, L. T.,** Incidence of epilepsy and unprovoked seizures in Rochester, Minnesota, *Epilepsia*, 34, 453, 1993.
64. **Scheuer, M. L. and Cohen, J.,** Seizures and epilepsy in the elderly, *Neurol. Clin.*, 2, 787, 1993.
65. **Cohen, J. and Scheuer, M. L.,** Antiepileptic drug use in elderly patients with epilepsy, *Epilepsia*, 32, 53, 1991.
66. **Houghton, G. W., Richens, A., and Leighton, M.,** Effect of age, height, weight and sex on serum phenytoin concentration in epileptic patients, *Br. J. Clin. Pharmacol.*, 2, 251, 1975.
67. **Sherwin, A. L., Loynd, J. S., and Bock, G. W.,** Effects of age, sex, obesity, and pregnancy on plasma diphenylhydantoin levels, *Epilepsia*, 15, 507, 1974.
68. **Hayes, M. J., Landman, M. J. S., and Short, A. H.,** Changes in drug metabolism with increased age, *Br. J. Clin. Pharmacol.*, 2, 73, 1975.
69. **LoGerfo, F. W., Quist, W. C., Cantelmo, N. L., and Haudenschild, C. C.,** Integrity of vein grafts as a function of initial intimal and medial preservation, 68, 117, 1983.

70. **Hockings, N., Pall, A., Moody, J., Davidson, A. V., and Davidson, D. L.,** The effects of age on carbamazepine pharmacokinetics and adverse effects, *Br. J. Clin. Pharmacol.*, 22, 725, 1986.
71. **Furlanut, M., Benetello, P, and Testa, G.,** The effects of dose, age and sex on the serum levels of phenobarbital and diphenylhydantoin in epileptic patients, *Pharmacol. Res. Commun.*, 10, 85, 1978.
72. **Bryson, S. M., Verma, N., and Scott, P. J. W.,** Pharmacokinetics of valproic acid in young and elderly subjects, *Br. J. Clin. Pharmacol.*, 16, 104, 1983.
73. **Perucca, E., Grimaldi, R., and Gatti, G.,** Pharmacokinetics of valproic acid in the elderly, *Br. J. Clin. Pharmacol.*, 17, 665, 1984.
74. **Bauer, L. A., Davis, R., and Wilensky, A.,** Valproic acid clearance: unbound fraction and diurnal variation in young and elderly adults, *Clin. Pharmacol. Ther.*, 37, 697, 1985.
75. **Grisso, J. A., Kelsey, J. L., and Strom, B. L.,** Risk factors for falls as a cause of hip fracture in women, *N. Engl. J. Med.*, 324, 1326, 1991.
76. **Kenneback, G., Bergfeldt, L., and Vallin, H.,** Electrophysiologic effects and clinical hazards of carbamazepine treatment for neurologic disorders in patients with abnormalities of the cardiac conduction system, *Am. Heart J.*, 121, 1421, 1991.
77. **Takayanagi, K., Yamaguchi, H., and Hayashi, T.,** Carbamazepine-induced bradycardiatachycardia syndrome with pharmacological analysis and concurrent ECG monitoring, *J. Electrocardiol.*, 23, 85, 1990.
78. **Kitani, K., Sato, Y., Kanai, S., Nokubo, M., and Masuda, Y.,** Age related increased threshold for electroshock seizure in BDF1 mice, *Life Sci.*, 36, 657, 1985.
79. **Nokubo, M., Kitani, K., Ohta, M., Kanai, S., Sato, Y., and Masuda, Y.,** Age-dependent increase in the threshold for pentylenetetrazol induced maximal seizure in mice, *Life Sci.*, 38, 1999, 1986.
80. **Kitani, K., Sato, Y., Kanai, S., Nokubo, M., Ohta, M., and Masuda, Y.,** The effect of age on the adaptation of the brain to the anticonvulsant effect of phenobarbital in mice, *Life Sci.*, 39, 483, 1986.
81. **Stijnen, A. M., Danhof, M., and Van Bezooijen, C. F.,** Increased sensitivity to the anesthetic effect of phenobarbital in aging BM/BiRij rats, *J. Pharmacol. Exp. Ther.*, 261, 81, 1992.
82. **Kitani, K., Masuda, Y., Kanai, S., Ohta, M., and Nokubo, M.,** Increased anticonvulsant effect of phenytoin in aging BDF1 mice, *J. Pharmacol. Exp. Ther.*, 229, 231, 1984.
83. **Stijnen, A. M., Hovinga, S., Langemeijer, M. W., Hoogerkamp, A., van Bezooijen, C. F., and Danhof, M.,** Increased sensitivity to the anticonvulsant effect of valproate in aging BN/BiRij rats, *Pharmaceutical Res.*, 10, 1046, 1993.
84. **Kitani, K., Klotz, U., Kanai, S., Sato, Y., Ohta, M., and Nokubo, M.,** Age-related differences in the coordination disturbance and anticonvulsant effect of oxazepam in mice, *Arch. Gerontol. Geriatr.*, 31, 1989.
85. **Kitani, K., Sato, Y., Kanai, S., Nokubo, M., Ohta, M., and Masuda, Y.,** Increasing anticonvulsant effect of AD-810 (zonisamide) in aging BDFI mice, *Life Sci.*, 41, 1339, 1987.
86. **Kitani, K., Sato, Y., Kanai, S., Ohta, M., Nokubo, M., and Masuda, Y.,** The neurotoxicity of phenobarbital and its effect in preventing pentylenetetrazol-induced maximal seizure in aging mice, *Arch. Gerontol. Geriatr.*, 7, 261, 1988.
87. **Hovinga, S., Stijnen, A. M., Langemeijer, M. W. E., Mandema, J. W., van Bezooijen, C. F. A., and Danhof, M.,** Pharmacokinetic-EEG effect relationship of midazolam in aging BN/BiRij rats, *J. Pharmacol.*, 107, 171, 1992.
88. **Gaziano, J. M., Buring, J. E., Breslow, J. L., Goldhaber, S. Z., Rosner, B., VanDenbrugh, M., Willett, W., and Hennekens, C. H.,** Moderate alcohol intake increased levels of high-density lipoprotein and its subfractions, and decreased risk of myocardial infarction, *N. Engl. J. Med.*, 329, 1829, 1993.
89. **Coffey, C. E. and Cummings, J. L.,** *Textbook of Geriatric Neuropsychiatry*, American Psychiatric Press, Washington, D.C., 1994, 301.
90. **Eaton, W. W., Kramer, M., and Anthony, J. C.,** The incidence of specific DIS/DSM-III mental disorders: data from the NIMH epidemiologic catchment area program, *Acta Psychiatric Scand.*, 79, 163, 1989.
91. **Moos, R. H., Brennan, P. L., and Moos, B. S.,** Short-term processes of remission and nonremission among late life problem drinkers, *Alcoholism*, 15, 948, 1991.
92. **Atkinson, R. M., Tolson, R. L., and Turner, J. A.,** Factors affecting outpatient treatment compliance of older male problem drinkers, *J. Stud. Alcohol*, 54, 102, 1993.
93. **Ernst, A. J., Dempster, J. P., Yee, R., St. Dennis, C., and Nahans, L.,** Alcohol toxicity, blood alcohol concentration and body water in young and adult rats, *J. Stud. Alcohol*, 37, 347, 1976.
94. **Wood, W. G. and Armbrecht, H. J.,** Behavioral effects of ethanol in animals: age differences and age changes, *Alcoholism*, 6, 3, 1982.
95. **Vestal, R. E., McGuire, E. A., Tobin, J. D., Adres, R., Norris, A. H., and Mezey, E.,** Aging and ethanol metabolism, *Clin. Pharmacol. Ther.*, 21, 343, 1977.
96. **Gentry, R. T., Baraona, E., and Lieber, C. S.,** Agonist: gastric first pass metabolism of alcohol, *J. Lab. Clin. Med.*, 123, 21, 1994.
97. **Gugler, R.,** H2-Antagonist and alcohol. Do they interact?, *Drug Safety*, 10, 271, 1994.
98. **Seitz, H. K., Xu, Y., Simanowski, U. A., and Osswald, B.,** Effect of age and gender on in vivo ethanol elimination, hepatic alcohol dehydrogenase activity, and NAD+ availability in F344 rats, *Res. Exp. Med.*, 192, 205, 1992.

99. **Fernandez, V., Kriz, A., and Videla, L. A.,** Age-dependent changes in *in vivo* ethanol metabolism and in the activity of hepatic enzymes involved in ethanol oxidation and microsomal functions, *Cell Biochem. Function*, 6, 7, 1988.
100. **Seitz, H. K., Meydani, M., Ferschke, I., Simanowski, U. A., Boesche, J., Bogusz, M., Hoepker, W. W., Blumberg, J. B., and Russell, R. M.,** Effect of aging on *in vivo* and *in vitro* ethanol metabolism and its toxicity in F344 rats, *Gastroenterology*, 97, 446, 1989.
101. **Rikans, L. E., Snowden, C. D., and Moore, D. R.,** Influence of aging on ethanol and acetaldehyde oxidation in female rat liver, *Gerontology*, 36, 185, 1990.
102. **Lieber, C. S.,** Alcohol and the liver, *Gastroenterology*, 106, 1085, 1994.
103. **Lieber, C. S.,** Alcohol, liver, and nutrition, *J. Am. Coll. Nutr.*, 10, 602, 1991.
104. **Jones, M. K. and Jones, B. M.,** The relationship of age and drinking habits to the effects of alcohol on memory in women, *J. Stud. Alcohol*, 41, 179, 1980.
105. **Vogel-Sprott, M. and Barrett, P.,** Age, drinking habits and the effects of alcohol, *J. Stud. Alcohol*, 45, 517, 1984.
106. **Parker, E. S. and Noble, E. P.,** Alcohol consumption and cognitive functioning in social drinkers, *J. Stud. Alcohol*, 38, 1224, 1977.
107. **Linnoila, M., Erwin, C. W., Ramm, D., and Cleveland, W. P.,** Effects of age and alcohol on psychomotor performance of men, *J. Stud. Alcohol*, 41, 488, 1980.
108. **Ritzmann, R. F. and Springer, A.,** Age differences in brain sensitivity and tolerance to ethanol in mice, *Age*, 3, 15, 1980.
109. **Wood, W. G. and Armbrecht, H. J.,** Age differences in ethanol-induced hypothermia and impairment in mice, *Neurobiol. Aging*, 3, 243, 1982.
110. **Abel, E. L.,** Effects of ethanol and pentobarbital in mice of different ages, *Physiol. Psychol.*, 6, 366, 1978.
111. **Wood, W. G., Armbrecht, H. J., and Wise, R. W.,** Ethanol intoxication and withdrawal among three age groups of C57BL/6NNIA mice, *Pharmacol. Biochem. Behav.*, 17, 1037, 1982.
112. **Samorajski, T., Strong, R., Volpendesta, D., Miller-Soule, D., and Hsu, L.,** *Alcoholism and Aging: Advances in Research*, CRC Press, Boca Raton, FL, 1982, 115.
113. **Samorajski, T., Persson, K., Bissell, C., Brizzee, L., Lancaster, F., and Brizzee, K. R.,** *Alcoholism in the Elderly*, Raven Press, New York, 1984, 43.
114. **Sun, A. Y. and Samorajski, T.,** The effects of age and alcohol on (Na^+ + K^+)-ATPase activity of whole homogenate and synaptosomes prepared from mouse and human brain, *J. Neurochem.*, 24, 161, 1975.
115. **Rikans, L. E. and Hornbrook, K. R.,** Isolated hepatocytes as a model for aging effects on hepatotoxicity: studies with allyl alcohol, *Toxicol. Appl. Pharmacol.*, 84, 634, 1986.
116. **Rikans, L. E. and Moore, D. R.,** Effect of age and sex on allyl alcohol hepatotoxicity in rats: role of liver alcohol and aldehyde dehydrogenase activities, *J. Pharmacol. Exp. Ther.*, 243, 20, 1987.
117. **Rikans, L. E. and Snowden, C. D.,** Effects of acute ethanol administration on female rat liver as a function of aging, *Life. Sci.*, 45, 1373, 1989.
118. **Volkow, N. D., et al.,** Acute effects of ethanol on regional brain glucose metabolism and transport, *Psychiatry Res.*, 35, 39, 1990.
119. **Volkow, N. D., Hitzemann, R., Wang, G. J., Fowler, J. S., Burr, G., Pascani, K., Dewey, S. L., and Wolf, A. P.,** Decreased brain metabolism in neurologically intact healthy alcoholics, *Am. J. Psychiatry*, 149, 1016, 1992.
120. **Wang, G. J., Volkow, N. D., Roque, C. T., Cestaro, V. L., Hitzemann, R. J., Cantos, E. L., Levy, A. V., and Dhawan, A. P.,** Functional importance of ventricular enlargement and cortical atrophy in healthy subjects and alcoholics as assessed with PET, MR imaging, and neuropsychologic testing, *Radiology*, 186, 59, 1993.
121. **Volkow, N. D., Wang, G. J., Hitzemann, R., Fowler, J. S., Overall, J. E., Burr, G., and Wolf, A. P.,** Recovery of brain glucose metabolism in detoxified alcoholics, *Am. J. Psychiatry*, 151, 178, 1994.
122. **Hojnacki, J. L., Deschenes, R. N., Cluette-Brown, J. E., Mulligan, J. J., Osmolski, T. V., and Rencricca, N. J.,** Effect of drinking pattern on plasma lipoproteins and body weight, *Atherosclerosis*, 88, 49, 1991.
123. **Coca, A., Aguilera, M. T., de la Sierra, A., Sanchez, M., Picado, M. J., Lluch, M. M., and Urbano-Marquez, A.,** Chronic alcohol intake induces reversible disturbances on cellular Na + metabolism in humans: its relationship with changes in blood pressure, *Alcoholism*, 16, 714, 1992.
124. **Maki, T., Kontula, K., and Harkonen, M.,** The beta-adrenergic system in man: physiological and pathophysiological response. Regulation of receptor density and functioning, *Scand. J. Clin. Lab. Invest.*, 201, 25, 1990.
125. **Geokas, M.C.,** The aging process, *Ann. Intern. Med.*, 113, 455, 1990.
126. **Persson, J.,** Alcohol and the small intestine, *Scand. J. Gastroenterol.*, 26, 3, 1991.
127. **Patel, B. C., D'Arville, C., Iwahashi, M., and Simon, F. R.,** Impairment of hepatic insulin receptors during chronic ethanol administration, *Am. J. Physiol.*, 261, G199, 1991.
128. **Broughton, D. and Taylor, R.,** Review: deterioration of glucose tolerance with age: the role of insulin resistance, *Age Aging*, 20, 221, 1991.

129. **Laitinen, K., Tahtela, R., Luomanmaki, K., and Valimaki, M. J.,** Mechanisms of hypocalcemia and markers of bone turnover in alcohol-intoxicated drinkers, *Bone Min.*, 24, 171, 1994.
130. **Pepersack, T., Fuss, M., Otero, J., Bergmann, P., Valsamis J., and Corvilain, J.,** Longitudinal study of bone metabolism after ethanol withdrawal in alcoholic patients, *J. Bone Miner. Res.*, 7, 383, 1992.
131. **Laitinen, K., Lamberg-Allardt, C., Tunninen, R., Harkonen, M., and Valimak, M.,** Bone mineral density and abstention-induced changes in bone and mineral metabolism in noncirrhotic male alcoholics, *Am. J. Med.*, 93, 642, 1992
132. **Laitinen, K. and Valimaki, M.,** Alcohol and bone, *Calcified Tissue Int.*, 49, S70, 1991.
133. **Van Steenbergen, W.,** Alcohol, liver cirrhosis and disorders in sex hormone metabolism, *Acta Clin. Belg.*, 48, 269, 1993.
134. **Orpana, A. K., Harkonen, M., and Erikkson, C. J.,** Ethanol-induced inhibition of testosterone biosynthesis in rat Leydig cells: role of mitochondrial substrate shuttles and citrate, *Alcohol Alcoholism*, 25, 499, 1990.
135. **Orpana, A. K., Orava, M. M., Vihko, R. K., Harkonen, M., and Eriksson, C. J.,** Role of ethanol metabolism in the inhibition of testosterone biosynthesis in rats in vivo: importance of gonadotropin stimulation, *J. Steroid Biochem. Mol. Biol.*, 37, 273, 1990.
136. **Ryan, C. and Butters, N.,** *The Neuropsychology Handbook*, Wedding, D., Horton, A., Webster, J., Eds., New York, 1986, 376.
137. **Schafer, K., Butters, N., and Smith, T.,** Cognitive performance of alcoholics: a longitudinal evaluation of the role of drinking history, depression, liver function, nutrition, and family history, *Alcoholism*, 15, 653, 1991.
138. **Goldstein, D. B.,** Effect of alcohol on cellular membranes, *Ann. Emerg. Med.*, 15, 43, 1986.
139. **Wood, W. G.,** *Homeostatic Function and Aging*, Raven Press, New York, 1985, 125.
140. **Beregi, E.,** *Aging*, 18, Raven Press, New York, 1982, 15.
141. **Tavares, M. A., Paula-Barbosa, M. M., Barroca, H., and Volk, B.,** Lipofuscin granules in cerebellar interneurons after long-term alcohol consumption in the adult rat, *Anat. Embryol.*, 171, 61, 1985.
142. **Borges, M. M., Paula-Barbosa, M. M., and Volk, B.,** Chronic alcohol consumption induces lipofuscin deposition in the rat hippocampus, *Neurobiol. Aging*, 7, 347, 1986.
143. **Paula-Barbosa, M. M., Brandao, F., Pinho, M. C., Andrade, J. P., Madeira, M. D., and Cadete-Leite, A.,** The effects of piracetam on lipofuscin of the rat cerebellar and hippocampal neurons after long-term alcohol treatment and withdrawal: a quantitative study, *Alcoholism*, 15, 834, 1991.
144. **Voronina, T. A., Nerobkova, L. N., Kutepova, O. A., and Gugutcidse, D. A.,** Pharmacological correction of CNS functional disorders and parkinsonian syndrome in old animals, *Ann. Ist. Super. Sanita*, 26, 55, 1990.
145. **Jaatinen, P., Saukko, P., and Hervonen, A.,** Chronic ethanol exposure increases lipopigment accumulation in human heart, *Alcohol Alcoholism*, 28, 559, 1993.
146. **Wiggins, R. C., Gorman, A., Rolsten, C., Samorajski, T., Ballinger, W. E., Jr., and Freund, G.,** Effects of aging and alcohol on the biochemical composition of histologically normal human brain, *Metab. Brain Dis.*, 3, 67, 1988.
147. **Carlsson, A., Adolfusson, R., Aquilonius, S. M., Gottfries, C. G., Oreland, L., Svennerholm, L., Winblad, B.,** *Ergot Compounds and Brain Function. A Neuroendocrine and Neuropsychiatric Aspects*, Raven Press, New York, 1980, 295.
148. **Mena, M. A. and Herrera, E.,** Monoamine metabolism in rat brain regions following long term alcohol treatment, *J. Neural Transm.*, 47, 227, 1980.
149. **Fadda, F., Argiolas, A., Melis, M. R., Serra, G., and Gessa, G. L.,** Differential effect of acute and chronic ethanol on dopamine metabolism in frontal cortex, caudate nucleus and substantia nigra, *Life Sci.*, 27, 979, 1980.
150. **Liljequist, S., Ahlenius, S., and Engel, J.,** The effects of chronic ethanol treatment on behavior and central monoamines in the rat, *Naunyn-Schmiedeberg's Arch. Pharmacol.*, 300, 205, 1977.
151. **Rawat, A. K.,** Brain levels and turnover rates of presumptive neurotransmitters as influenced by administration and withdrawal of ethanol in mice, *J. Neurochem.*, 22, 915, 1974.
152. **Pohorecky, L. A.,** Effect of ethanol on central and peripheral noradrenergic neurons, *J. Pharmacol. Exp. Ther.*, 189, 380, 1974.
153. **Pohorecky, L. A., Jaffe, L. S., and Berkeley, H.,** Effects of ethanol on serotonergic neurons in the rat brain, *Res. Commun. Chem. Pathol. Pharmacol.*, 8, 1, 1974.
154. **Tabakoff, B. and Boggan, W. O.,** Effect of ethanol on serotonin metabolism in brain, *J. Neurochem.*, 22, 759, 1974.
155. **Moscatelli, E. A., Fujimoto, K., and Gilfoil, T. C.,** Effects of chronic consumption of ethanol and sucrose on rat whole brain 5-hydroxytryptamine, *J. Neurochem.*, 25, 273, 1975.
156. **Gothoni, P. and Ahtee, L.,** Chronic administration of ethanol decreases 5-HT and increases 5-HIAA concentration in rat brain, *Acta Pharmacol. Toxicol.*, 48, 113, 1980.
157. **Kuriyama, K., Rauscher, G. E., and Sze, P. Y.,** Effect of acute and chronic administration of ethanol on the 5-hydroxytryptamine turnover and tryptophan hydroxylase activity of the mouse brain, *Brain Res.*, 26. 450, 1971.
158. **Ahtee, L. and Svartstrom-Fraser, M.,** Effect of ethanol dependence and withdrawal on the catecholamines in rat brain and heart, *Acta Pharmacol. Toxicol.*, 36, 289, 1975.

159. **Hunt, W. A. and Dalton, T. K.,** Neurotransmitter-receptor binding in various brain regions in ethanol or rendered ethanol-dependent rats, *Pharmacol. Biochem. Behav.*, 14, 733, 1981.
160. **Muller, P., Britton, R. S., and Seeman, P.,** The effects of long-term ethanol on brain receptors for dopamine, acetylcholine, serotonin and noradrenaline, *Eur. J. Pharmacol.*, 65, 31, 1980.
161. **Pelham, R. W., Marquis, J. K., Kugelmann, K., and Munsat, T. L.,** Prolonged ethanol consumption produces persistent alterations of cholinergic function in rat brain, *Cancer Chemother. Pharmacol.*, 4, 282, 1980.
162. **Pietrzak, E. R., Wilce, P. A., and Shanley, B. C.,** Plasticity of brain muscarinic receptors in aging rats: the adaptive response to scopolamine and ethanol treatment, *Neurosci. Lett.*, 104, 331, 1989.
163. **Rabin, R. A., Wolfe, B. B., Dibner, M. D., Zahniser, N. R., Melchior, C. L., and Molinoff, P. B.,** Effect of ethanol administration and withdrawal on neurotransmitter receptor systems in C57 mice, *J. Pharmacol. Exp. Ther.*, 213, 491, 1980.
164. **Tabakoff, B., Munoz-Marcus, M., and Fields, J. Z.,** Chronic ethanol feeding produces an increase in muscarinic cholinergic receptors in mouse brain, *Life Sci.*, 25 2173, 1979.
165. **Freund, G. and Ballinger, W. E., Jr.,** Neuroreceptor changes in the putamen of alcohol abusers, *Alcoholism*, 13, 213, 1989.
166. **Freund, G. and Ballinger, W. E., Jr.,** Loss of muscarinic and benzodiazepine neuroreceptors from hippocampus of alcohol abusers, *Alcohol*, 6, 23, 1989.
167. **Pietrzak, E. R., Wilce, P. A., and Shanley, B. C.,** Interaction of chronic ethanol consumption and aging on brain muscarinic cholinergic receptors, *J. Pharmacol. Exp. Ther.*, 252, 869, 1990.
168. **Davies, S. N., Lester, R. A. J., Reymann, K. G., and Collingridge, G. L.,** Temporally distinct pre and post synaptic mechanisms maintain long-term potentiation, *Nature*, 338, 500, 1989.
169. **Piggott, M. A., Perry, E. K., Perry, R. H., and Court, J. A.,** [3H]MK-801 binding to the NMDA receptor complex, and its modulation in human frontal cortex during development and aging, *Brain Res.*, 588, 277, 1992.
170. **Bonhaus, D. W., Perry, W. B., and McNamara, J. O.,** Decreased density, but not number, of N-methyl-D-aspartate, glycine and phencyclidine binding sites in hippocampus of senescent rats, *Brain Res.*, 532, 82, 1990.
171. **Lovinger, D. M., White, G., and Weight, F. F.,** Ethanol inhibits NMDA activated ion currents in hippocampal neurones, *Science*, 243, 1721, 1989.
172. **Brown, L. M., Trent, R. D., Jones, T. W., Gonzales, R. A., and Leslie, S. W.,** Alcohol inhibition of NMDA-stimulated catecholamine efflux in aging brain, *Alcohol*, 9, 555, 1992.
173. **Grant, K. A., Valverius, P., Hudspith, M., and Tabakoff, B.,** Ethanol withdrawal seizures and the NMDA receptor complex, *Eur. J. Pharmacol.*, 176, 289, 1990.
174. **Michaelis, E. K., Michaelis, M. L., Freed, W. J., and Foye, J.,** *Advances in Biomedical Alcoholism Research*, Pergamon Press, Oxford, in press.
175. **Lovinger, D. M.,** Excitotoxicity and alcohol-related brain damage, *Alcoholism*, 17, 19, 1993.
176. **Reggiani, A., Barbaccia, M. L., Spano, P. F., and Trabucchi, M.,** Acute and chronic ethanol administration on specific ^{3}H-GABA binding in different rat brain areas, *Psychopharmacology*, 67, 261, 1980.
177. **Ticku, M. K. and Burch, T.,** Alteration in γ-aminobutyric acid receptor sensitivity following acute and chronic ethanol treatments, *J. Neurochem.*, 34, 417, 1980.
178. **Volicer, L. and Biagioni, T. M.,** Effect of ethanol administration and withdrawal on benzodiazepine receptor binding in rat brain, *Neuropharmacology*, 21, 283, 1982.
179. **Ticku, M. K.,** The effects of acute and chronic ethanol administration and its withdrawal on γ-aminobutyric acid receptor binding in rat brain, *Br. J. Pharmacol.*, 70, 403, 1980.
180. **Battaini, F., Lucchi, L., Bergamaschi, S., Ladisa, V., Trabucchi, M., and Govoni, S.,** Intracellular signalling in the aging brain, the role of protein kinase C and its calcium-dependent isoforms, *Ann. N.Y. Acad. Sci.*, 719, 271, 1994.
181. **Igwe, O. J. and Ning, L.,** Inositol 1,4,5-trisphosphate arm of the phosphatidylinositide signal transduction pathway in the rat cerebellum during aging, *Neurosci. Lett.*, 164, 167, 1993.
182. **Strosznajder, J., Samochocki, M., Wikiel, H., and Malecki, A.,** Aging modulates calcium-dependent phosphatidylinositol degradation by cerebral cortex synaptic plasma membrane phospholipases, *Mol. Chem. Neuropathol.*, 21, 95, 1994.
183. **Ohnuki, T. and Nomura, Y.,** M1 acetylcholine receptor-mediated phosphatidylinositol turnover in adult and senescent rat brain slices, *J. J. Pharmacol.*, 57, 483, 1991.
184. **Gonzales, R. A. and Crews, F. T.,** Chronic ethanol inhibits receptor-stimulated phosphoinositide hydrolysis in rat liver slices, *Alcohol*, 8, 131, 1991.
185. **Kuriyama, K. and Ohkuma, S.,** Alteration in the function of cerebral neurotransmitter receptors during the establishment of alcohol dependence: neurochemical aspects, *Alcohol Alcoholism*, 25, 239, 1990.
186. **Kronfol, Z., Nair, M., Hill, E., Kroll, P., Brower, K., and Greden, J.,** Immune function in alcoholism: a controlled study, *Alcoholism*, 17, 279, 1993.
187. **Irwin, M., Caldwell, C., Smith, T. L., Brown, S., Schuckit, M. A., and Gillin, J. C.,** Major depressive disorder, alcoholism, and reduced natural killer cell cytotoxicity. Role of severity of depressive symptoms and alcohol consumption, *Arch. Gen. Psychiatry*, 47, 713, 1990.

188. **Grossman, C. J., Nienaber, M., Mendenhall, C. L., Hurtubise, P., Roselle, G. A., Rouster, S., Weber, N., Schmitt, G., and Gartside, P. S.**, Sex differences and the effects of alcohol on immune response in male and female rats, *Alcoholism*, 17, 832, 1993.
189. **Wilson, J. D., et al.**, *Principles of Internal Medicine*, McGraw-Hill, New York, 1991, 2148.
190. **McEwen, B. S., Spencer, R. L., Chapman, S., Ganem, J., and O'Steen, W. K.**, Neuroendocrine aspects of cerebral aging, *Int. J. Clin. Pharmacol. Res.*, 10, 7, 1990.
191. **Stein-Behrens, B. A. and Sapolsky, R. M.**, Stress, glucocorticoids, and aging, *Aging (Milano)*, 4, 197, 1992.
192. **Stewart, P. M., Burra, P., Shackleton, C. H., Sheppard, M. C., and Elias, E.**, 11 beta-Hydroxysteroid dehydrogenase deficiency and glucocorticoid status in patients with alcoholic and non-alcoholic chronic liver disease, *J. Clin. Endocrinol. Metabol.*, 76, 748, 1993.
193. **Fonzi, S., Murialdo, G., Bo, P., Filippi, U., Costelli, P., Parodi, C., Maurelli, M., Polleri, A., and Savoldi, F.**, [The neuroendocrine aspects of chronic alcoholism: the effect of alcohol intake and its withdrawal]. *Ann. Ital. Med. Intern.*, 7, 87, 1992.
194. **Wilkins, J. N., Gorelick, D. A., Nademanee, K., Taylor, A., and Herzberg, D. S.**, Hypothalamic-pituitary function during alcohol exposure and withdrawal and cocaine exposure, *Recent Dev. Alcoholism*, 10, 57, 1992.
195. **Valimake, M., Tuominen, J. A., Huhtaniemi, I., and Ylikahri, R.**, The pulsatile secretion of gonadotropins and growth hormone, and the biological activity of luteinizing hormone in men acutely intoxicated with ethanol, *Alcoholism*, 14, 928, 1990.
196. **Adinoff, B., Risher-Flowers, D., De Jong, J., Ravitz, B., Bone, G. H., Nutt, D. J., Roehrich, L., Martin, P. R., and Linnoila, M.**, Disturbances of hypothalamic-pituitary-adrenal axis functioning during ethanol withdrawal in six men, *Am. J. Psychiatry*, 148, 1023, 1991.
197. **Cohen, P., Ocrant, I., Fielder, P. J., Neely, E. K., Gargosky, S. E., Deal, C. I., Ceda, G. P., Youngman, O., Pham, H., and Lamson, G.**, Insulin-like growth factors (IGFs); implications for aging, *Psychoneuroendocrinology*, 17, 335, 1992.
198. **O'Neill, P. A.**, Neuroendocrinology and ageing, *Med. Lab. Sci.*, 49, 283, 1992.
199. **Monteleone, P., Iovino, M., Orio, F., and Steardo, L.**, Impaired growth hormone response to sodium valproate in normal aging,
200. **Nielsen, H. K., Lindby, L., Rasmussen, K., Charles, P., and Hansen, C.**, Alcohol decreases serum osteocalcin in a dose-dependent way in normal subjects, *Calcified Tissue Int.*, 46, 173, 1990.
201. **De Marinis, L., Mancini, A., Fiumara, C., Conte, G., Iacona, T., Ianiri, L., Zeppetelli, E., Gobbi, G., and Tempesta, E.**, Growth hormone response to growth hormone-releasing hormone in early abstinent alcoholic patients, *Psychoneuroendocrinology*, 18, 475, 1993.
202. **Balldin, J., Berggren, U., Lindstedt, G., and Sundkler, A.**, Further neuroendocrine evidence for reduced D2 dopamine receptor function in alcoholism, *Drug Alcohol Dependence*, 32, 159, 1993.
203. **Emanuele, M. A., Tentler, J. J., Kirsteins, L., Emanuele, N. V., Lawrence, A., and Kelley, M. R.**, The effect of "binge" ethanol exposure on growth hormone and prolactin gene expression and secretion, *Endocrinology*, 131, 2077, 1992.
204. **Reiter, R. J.**, The ageing pineal gland and its physiological consequences, *Bioessays*, 14, 169, 1992.
205. **Ekman, A. C., Leppaluoto, J., Huttunen, P., Aranko, K., and Vakkuri, O.**, Ethanol inhibits melatonin secretion in healthy volunteers in a dose-dependent randomized double blind cross-over study, *J. Clin. Endocrinol. Metab.*, 77, 780, 1993.
206. **Rojdmark, S., Wikner, J., Adner, N., Anderson, D. E., and Wetterberg, L.**, Inhibition of melatonin secretion by ethanol in man, *Metab. Clin. Exp.*, 42, 1047, 1993.
207. **Muriadlo, G., Filippi, U., Costelli, P., Fonzi, S., Bo, P., Polleri, A., and Savoldi, F.**, Urine melatonin in alcoholic patients: a marker of alcohol abuse?, *J. Endocrinol. Invest.*, 14, 503, 1991.
208. **Lieber, C. S.**, Biochemical factors in alcoholic liver disease, *Semin. Liver Dis.*, 13, 136, 1993.
209. **Leo, M. A. and Lieber, C. S.**, Hepatic vitamin A depletion in alcoholic liver injury, *N. Engl. J. Med.*, 307, 597, 1982.
210. **Bjorneboe, G. E. A., Bjorneboe, A., Hagen, B. F., Morland, J., and Drevon, C. A.**, Reduced hepatic α-tocopherol content after long-term administration of ethanol to rats, *Biochem. Biophys. Acta*, 918, 236, 1987.
211. **Bjorneboe, G. E. A., Johnsen, J., Bjorneboe, A., Marklund, S. L., Skylv, N., Hoiseth, A., Bache-Wiig, J. E., Morland, J., and Drevon, C. A.**, Some aspects of antioxidant status in blood from alcoholics, *Alcoholism Clin. Exp. Res.*, 12, 806, 1988.
212. **Kawase, T., Kato, S., and Lieber, C. S.**, Lipid peroxidation and antioxidant defense systems in rat liver after chronic ethanol feeding, *Hepatology*, 10, 815, 1989.
213. **Cederbaum, A. I.**, Microsomal generation of reactive oxygen species and their possible role in alcohol hepatoxicity, *Alcohol Alcoholism*, 1, 291, 1991.
214. **Zhang, H., Loney, L. A., and Potter, B. J.**, Effect of chronic alcohol feeding on hepatic iron status and ferritin uptake by rat hepatocytes, *Alcoholism*, 17, 394, 1993.

215. **Nomura, F. and Lieber, C. S.,** Binding of acetaldehyde to rat liver microsomes: enhancement after chronic alcohol consumption, *Biochem. Biophys. Res. Commun.*, 100, 131, 1981.
216. **Behrens, U. J., Hoerner, M., Lasker, J. M., and Lieber, C. S.,** Formation of acetaldehyde adducts with ethanol-inducible P4501lEl in vivo, *Biochem. Biophys. Res. Commun.*, 154, 584, 1988.
217. **Lin, R. C., Smith, R. S., and Lumeng, L.,** Detection of a protein-acetaldehyde adduct in the liver of rats fed alcohol chronically, *J. Clin. Invest.*, 81, 615, 1988.
218. **Baraona, E., Liu, W., Ma, X. L., Svegliati-Baroni, G., and Lieber, C. S.,** Acetaldehyde-collagen adducts in N-nitrosodimethylamine-induced liver cirrhosis in rats, *Life Sci.*, 52, 1249, 1993.
219. **Svegliati-Baroni, G., Baraona, E., Rosman, A. S., and Lieber, C. S.,** Collagen-acetaldehyde adducts in alcoholic and non-alcoholic liver disease, *Hepatology*, in press.
220. **Donahue, T. M., Jr., Tuma, D. J., and Sorrell, M. F.,** Acetaldehyde adducts with protein: binding of [^{14}C]acetaldehyde to serum albumin, *Arch. Biochem. Biophys.*, 220, 239, 1983.
221. **Stevens, V. J., Fantl, W. J., Newman, C. B., Sims, R. V., and Peterson, C. M.,** Acetaldehyde adducts with hemoglobin, *J. Clin. Invest.*, 67, 361, 1981.
222. **Wehr, H., Rodo, M., Lieber, C. S., and Baraona, E.,** Acetaldehyde adducts and autoantibodies against VLDL and LDL in alcoholics, *J. Lipid Res.*, 34, 1237, 1993.
223. **Israel, Y., Hurwitz, E., Niemela, O., and Arnon, R.,** Monoclonal and polyclonal antibodies against acetaldehyde-containing epitopes in acetaldehyde-protein adducts, *Proc. Natl. Acad. Sci. U.S.A.*, 83, 7923, 1986.
224. **Hoerner, M., Behrens, U. J., Worner, T., and Lieber, C. S.,** Humoral immune response to acetaldehyde adducts in alcoholic patients, *Res. Commun. Chem. Pathol. Pharmacol.*, 54, 3, 1986.
225. **Hoerner, M., Behrens, U. J., Worner, T. M., Blacksberg, I., Braly, L. F., Schaffner, F., and Lieber, C. S.,** The role of alcoholism and liver disease in the appearance of serum antibodies against acetaldehyde adducts, *Hepatology*, 8, 569, 1988.
226. **Niemela, O., Klajner, F., Orrego, H., Vidins, E., Blendis, L., and Israel, Y.,** Antibodies against acetaldehyde-modified protein epitopes in human alcoholics, *Hepatology*, 7, 1210, 1987.
227. **Shaw, S., Rubin, K. P., and Lieber, C. S.,** Depressed hepatic glutathione and increased diene conjugates in alcoholic liver disease: evidence of lipid peroxidation, *Dig. Dis. Sci.*, 28, 585, 1983.
228. **Morton, S. and Mitchell, M. C.,** Effects of chronic ethanol feeding on glutathione turnover in the rat, *Biochem. Pharmacol.*, 34, 1559, 1985.
229. **Speisky, H., MacDonald, A., Giles, G., Orrego, H., and Israel, Y.,** Increased loss and decreased synthesis of hepatic glutathione after acute ethanol administration, *Biochem. J.*, 225, 565, 1985.
230. **Hirano, T., Kaplowitz, N., Tsukamoto, H., Kamimura, S., and Fernandez-Checa, J. C.,** Hepatic mitochondrial glutathione depletion and progression of experimental alcoholic liver disease in rats, *Hepatology*, 6, 1423, 1992.
231. **Martin, G. R., Danner, D. B., and Holbrook, N. J.,** Aging — causes and defenses, *Ann. Rev. Med.*, 44, 419, 1993.
232. **Richter, C.,** Reactive oxygen and DNA damage in mitochondria, *Mutat. Res.*, 275, 249, 1992.
233. **Schapira, A. H. and Cooper, J. M.,** Mitochondrial function in neurodegeneration and ageing, *Mutat. Res.*, 275, 133, 1992.
234. Comparative effects of chronic ethanol consumption on the properties of mitochondria from rat brain and liver, *Alcoholism*, 16, 1, 1992.
235. **Seitz, H. K., Simanowski, U. A., Egerer, G., Waldherr, R., and Oertl, U.,** Human gastric alcohol dehydrogenase: in vitro characteristics and effect of cimetidine, *Digestion*, 51, 80, 1992.

Chapter 9

PARKINSON'S DISEASE AND AGING: PHARMACOLOGICAL APPROACHES TO UNDERSTANDING THE DISEASE

David R. Lynch and Howard Hurtig

CONTENTS

I. INTRODUCTION

Idiopathic Parkinson's disease (PD) is a progressive, degenerative disorder of unknown cause characterized by resting tremor, rigidity, bradykinesia, and postural instability. PD is mainly a disease of the elderly population. It affects 1% of people older than 55, and the incidence increases with advancing age.[1,2] Secondary parkinsonism, resulting from dopaminergic blocking medications (such as neuroleptics and metaclopramide) and structural lesions such as stroke, is also more common in the elderly. Moreover, PD is frequently associated with other central nervous system (CNS) conditions of older people, including depression and dementia of the Alzheimer type. These facts make successful pharmacotherapy of PD in the elderly extraordinarily difficult.

However, the age dependence of PD and its uneven response to therapy also provide insight on the pathogenesis of PD and potential methods for its prevention. By examining

0-8493-8306-4/96/$0.00+$.50

the scientific observations on PD, it may be possible to better understand the aging process. To accomplish this goal, this review will discuss factors in aging which may contribute to PD and also how aging influences the responsiveness of patients with PD to treatment.

II. NEURODEGENERATIVE DISORDERS AND AGE RELATED CHANGES IN THE BRAIN

The age dependence of PD is shared by at least two other neurodegenerative disorders: Alzheimer's disease (AD) and amyotrophic lateral sclerosis (ALS). However, each has a distinct clinical picture. The primary difference between these diseases is the selective vulnerability of particular neuronal populations for each disorder. AD causes loss of many neurons, particularly the cholinergic neurons originating in the nucleus basalis of Meynert in the basal forebrain, while ALS affects motor neurons of the spinal cord and motor cortex.[3,4] However, it is likely that current and future research may uncover mechanisms of neuronal death common to all of these disorders. Although age-related cell death is a likely contributor to all of these diseases, none appears to be caused by aging alone.

Many chemical changes take place in the aging brain involving many different types of molecules. For example, lipid composition of the brain changes with age as the content of cerebral cortical phospholipids and cholesterol decreases linearly from ages 20 to 100.[5] In contrast, gangliosides, which may have protective roles in neurodegenerative disorders, change in quality, but not quantity with aging.[5] Selective changes most likely occur for all types of molecules in the brain, including proteins and nucleic acids. Monoamine oxidase (MAO), an enzyme involved in degrading catecholamines and in oxidative stress, ***increases*** with age.[6] DNA in the brain can accumulate age-dependent mutations which could conceivably induce neurodegeneration. In one degenerative disorder, the sporadic, rapidly progressive dementia of Creutzfeldt-Jakob disease, spontaneous somatic mutation has been proposed as the mechanism which begins its rapid clinical course.[7]

One clear difference between the aging process in the brain compared with other tissues is the inability of neurons to divide.[8] This difference may be reflected in the different types of disorders in neurons compared with other cells. The degenerative properties of the CNS may be an alternative to tumorigenesis seen in aging nonneuronal cells. In nonneuronal cells, DNA mutations are passed from one generation of cells to the next. Some of these mutations may induce abnormal cell growth, leading to neoplasia. In contrast, as neurons age, they do not replicate nor are new stem cells created. Mutations which might induce neoplasia are not passed to subsequent generations of cells. However, mutations which cause cell death or loss of a key enzyme would be more noticeable as no new cells are generated from precursor cells to replace them. This hypothesis is supported by the low frequency of neuron-derived tumors, but the high incidence of neurodegenerative disorders.[9] Loss of a critical number of neurons (80%) in one specific region of the brain may be sufficient to cause or induce pathophysiological changes which produce a specific disorder.[8]

The analogy between central nervous degeneration and peripheral tissue neoplasia is substantiated by a variety of genetic syndromes. Chromosomal abnormalities such as Down's syndrome and velocardiofacial syndrome and the genetic disease neurofibromatosis are associated with neoplasia or maldevelopment peripherally.[10–12] Though disorders like neurofibromatosis cause glial neoplasia, in neurons they are associated with degenerative disorders or neuronal atrophy, not tumorigenesis. Degenerative disorders and tumors share one feature which makes their study difficult: the time of the inciting event may precede the development of the illness by many years. This analogy suggests that the mechanisms of neurodegeneration and the age dependence of PD may be the consequence of one or more events occurring over a lifetime, and not events which immediately precede the clinical presentation, as acute onset of PD from stroke or encephalitis is rare.

III. SCIENTIFIC BASIS OF PARKINSON'S DISEASE

A. NEUROANATOMY AND NEUROCHEMISTRY OF THE BASAL GANGLIA

PD and parkinsonism from other causes result from dysfunction of the basal ganglia of the brain. Knowledge of the chemical neuroanatomy of the basal ganglia and how it is disturbed in parkinsonism has increased dramatically in recent years. Unfortunately, it is still not completely clear what function the basal ganglia performs in normal people. While its primary function may involve initiation and modification of motor acts (motor planning and motor programming), it also plays a role in executive cognitive function.

Much of what is understood about the basal ganglia results from studies of patients with PD and of animal models. The traditional view of parkinsonism emphasizes the loss of the dopaminergic pathway originating in the zona compacta of the substantia nigra and projecting to the corpus striatum (caudate and putamen). The dopaminergic input inhibits GABAergic pathways from the striatum which project back to the cortex through the thalamus. The loss of the nigrostriatal pathway causes an inability to initiate movements, and traditional therapy emphasized restoring the dopamine to this pathway by administering exogenous L-dopa.[13]

However, the anatomy of the basal ganglia is now better elucidated and offers more avenues for successful therapy.[13] There are two parallel neuroanatomic pathways through the basal ganglia (Figure 9.1); one of these is direct and the other is indirect from the striatum through the globus pallidus to the thalamus. Dopamine from the substantia nigra inhibits the indirect pathway and excites the direct pathway. Thus, dopaminergic loss increases the inhibitory output through the indirect pathway from the globus pallidus to the thalamus. Inhibition of the motor nuclei of the thalamus with consequent diminished output to the primary and supplementary motor cortex is the best explanation for the bradykinesia and rigidity of PD. Although the cause of PD is unknown, the primary site of pathology is the pigmented neurons of the substantia nigra. However, the increased understanding of basal ganglia circuitry allows for other possible ways in which the syndrome of parkinsonism may be produced and for novel ways to treat parkinsonism. For example, agents which interfere with glutamatergic neurotransmission should be excellent antiparkinsonian agents based on the new model of basal ganglia circuitry (see below). Understanding such novel therapies is particularly important in treating elderly patients, who may be particularly sensitive to any specific pharmacological intervention because of coexistent age-related pathology. Having multiple possible targets for intervention allows a treating physician to adjust medications to best fit the patient's complex medical problems.

B. PATHOLOGY AND PATHOPHYSIOLOGY OF PARKINSON'S DISEASE

Both chemical and morphological changes in the basal ganglia contribute to the pathobiology of PD. Parkinsonian symptoms develop when levels of the neurotransmitter dopamine drop to less than 20% of normal as a result of death of the melanin containing substantia nigra neurons. As the disease progresses, neuronal numbers decline further so that few if any pigmented neurons remain at the time of death in advanced disease. This basic pathology has been validated in animal models using a variety of chemical lesions.[1,2,14–16]

Loss of neurons in the substantia nigra also occurs as a result of normal aging. Thus, in some ways, the pathology of PD may be viewed as a variant of normal aging. About 35% of substantia nigra neurons have been estimated to die in normal aging; this value is much higher than suggested for other areas of the CNS.[8] In normal elderly individuals and in parkinsonian patients, substantia nigra size correlates with motor performance.[17] Even Lewy bodies, the intracytoplasmic inclusions which are the pathologic hallmark of PD, may occur in up to 10% of normal individuals over age 50.[18] What brings patients to clinical attention is the magnitude of the nigral cell loss. Conceivably, this could result from a variety of reasons, all possibly under genetic control (Figure 9.2):

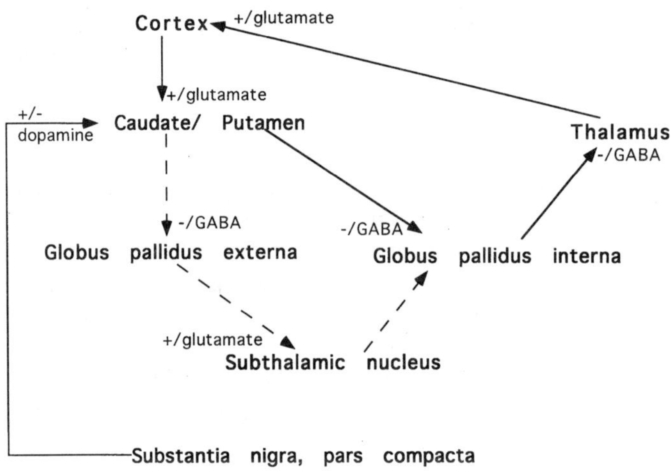

FIGURE 9.1. Chemical neuroanatomy of the basal ganglia. The dopaminergic cells of the substantia nigra are excitatory (+) on the cells of direct basal ganglia pathway, and inhibitory (–) on the cells of the indirect pathway (through the subthalamic nucleus, shown by dotted lines). (Adapted from Delong, M. R., *Trends Neurosci.*, 13, 281, 1990. With permission.)

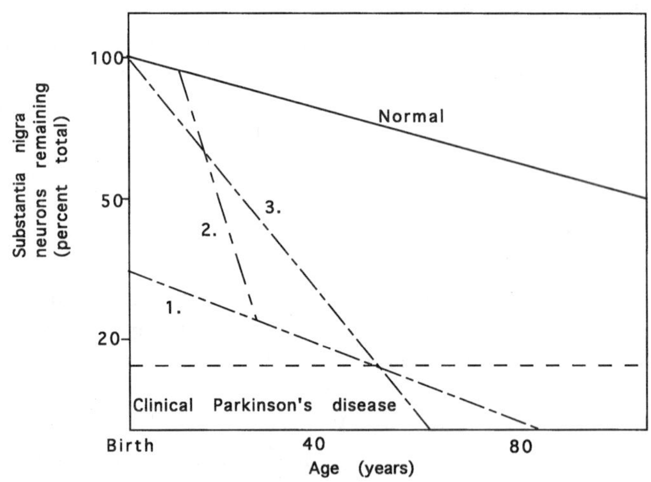

FIGURE 9.2. Comparison of neuronal loss in PD and aging. Theoretically, loss of nigral neurons in PD could result from aging in conjunction with a failure of nigral neurons to develop (1), a fixed injury early in life (2), or an accelerated rate of loss of nigral neurons (3). PD develops clinically when less than 20% of nigral neurons remain, compared with the age-dependent loss of about 30% of nigral neurons.

1. A large, one-time loss of neurons early in life with subsequent insidious, age-dependent loss.
2. A congenitally low number of substantia nigra neurons and subsequent age-dependent loss.
3. Accelerated loss of substantia nigra neurons throughout life.
4. Some combination of all of these.

The hypothesis that PD is merely a variant of normal aging is overly simplistic. A number of factors might also be important.

1. Akiyama and McGeer[14] have shown microglia phagocytosing neurons in the substantia nigra of patients with PD, suggesting an ongoing active component to the disorder.[14]

2. The microanatomical distribution of substantia nigra neurons lost in PD differs from those lost with aging.[19] In PD, cells of the lateral, ventral portion of the substantia nigra are most affected, while in aging this subdivision of the substantia nigra is least affected.
3. Analysis of the natural history of PD suggests that the rate of cell loss is not fixed in PD, but is highest early in the disease process.[20] Mathematical models suggest that some event, remote in time from the onset of PD, either damages substantia nigra neurons such that their life expectancy is reduced beyond normal aging or starts a process which kills neurons at a rate above the age-expected rate. Both of these scenarios would rationalize the observation that later onset PD may progress faster.[20,21]

Thus, while aging contributes to the loss of substantia nigra neurons, aging alone does not explain the evolution of PD. The most likely scenario is an interaction between aging and other causes.

A few other CNS nuclei besides the substantia nigra are affected in PD and in animal models of PD. The dorsal motor nucleus of the vagus and the locus coeruleus, two noradrenergic nuclei of the brain stem, suffer modest cell loss in PD.[22] However, no age-related changes in these nuclei have been noted in humans, suggesting more than a simple age-related process in their loss in PD.[22–24] Adrenergic nuclei of the brain stem which do not contain melanin do not degenerate in PD. Other areas of modest cell loss when compared with controls include the serotonergic raphe, the cholinergic nucleus basalis of Meynert, and a few other subcortical nuclei.[22]

Although the pathological findings of PD are limited to the substantia nigra and a few other nuclei, clues to the age dependence and etiology may be found in the association of PD with other disorders, including AD and also depression.[25] When these disorders coexist with PD, patients tend to have more cell loss outside the substantia nigra.[22] Depression likely has many causes biochemically, but much research has focused on biogenic amines such as norepinephrine and serotonin, which share common synthetic and metabolic pathways with dopamine. Dopamine is the precursor of norepinephrine and epinephrine, so abnormalities of dopamine synthesis may also create abnormal synthesis of these amines. Amino acid decarboxylase functions as a synthetic enzyme both for dopamine and for serotonin, thus linking their synthetic pathways. Thus, common pathophysiological mechanisms could be reflected in the association between depression and PD. Once this is better understood, more rational therapies may be directed toward these two disorders when they coexist.

IV. AGE-RELATED PATHOLOGY WHICH COULD CONTRIBUTE TO PARKINSON'S DISEASE

A. GENETIC FACTORS

Whether or not PD has a genetic basis is a much debated subject. Although a positive family history of PD is obtained in 15 to 20% of patients, this may simply reflect the high frequency of the disease and nongenetic familial aggregation. However, there are a few reported kindreds with autopsy confirmation where PD follows an autosomal dominant pattern.[26,27] In some, but not all families, the age of onset is lower than in sporadic cases, but the patients respond to typical therapies. As yet, full pathology is available on only a few individuals, but classic Lewy bodies have been noted in the substantia nigra in some kindreds. Genetic PD may represent the same underlying, age-dependent pathophysiology seen in idiopathic PD, but the evidence is only suggestive.

B. OXIDATIVE DAMAGE

The age dependence of PD in conjunction with other factors has led to speculation that PD may represent the end product of oxidative damage to the nervous system. It has been proposed that the aging process creates circumstances leading to oxidative stress with consequent damage to susceptible tissues. In patients with mitochondrial myopathy, a peripheral nervous system degeneration, pathologic changes in the complex I cytochrome oxidase enzymes of oxidative phosphorylation may lead to cell death.[28] At least one toxin known to cause parkinsonism in humans and experimental animals (1-methyl-4-phenylpyridinium ion[MPP^+]) inhibits mitochondrial complex I oxidative function, suggesting that abnormal mitochondrial function could underlie the phenotype of PD.[29] This observation that MPP^+ causes mitochondrial damage and oxidative stress has prompted a variety of investigations to document abnormal oxidative function in PD. Glutathione SH, an index of cellular reducing agents, is reduced in the substantia nigra early in the course of PD.[30] Mitochondria isolated from platelets, muscle, or on occasion substantia nigra of patients with PD have abnormal electron transport properties, particularly in complex I.[28,31,32] This occurs against age-matched controls in some cases, but the results have not been consistent.[33–36] In some studies, such changes have been suggested in presymptomatic patients, ruling out an effect of therapy as a cause of mitochondrial dysfunction. Although results have been inconsistent, such studies have directed much attention to mitochondria as the source of the pathophysiology of PD.

Abnormal oxidative phosphorylation could reflect abnormalities of proteins coded by the mitochondrial genome, which codes for several (though not all) of the enzymes of oxidative phosphorylation;[37] for example, mitochondrial DNA codes for 3 of the 13 subunits in cytochrome oxidase, with the nuclear genome coding for the other polypeptide chains.[38] If an enzyme of oxidative phosphorylation were abnormal, it most likely would not lead to abnormal cell growth, as seen in cancer, but instead to premature cell death. Mitochondrial DNA has a much higher somatic mutation rate than nuclear DNA so that mutations could accumulate with time. A critical number of mutations could lead to clinical disease and to cell death. This could explain the age dependence of PD, although direct evidence substantiating this hypothesis is lacking at present. It is true that mutations accumulate in mitochondrial DNA of the substantia nigra.[33] However, it is not clear that they affect mitochondrial function, nor do they clearly represent variations from normal.[36] One study which demonstrated abnormalities in oxidative phosphorylation in patients with PD did not find reproducible abnormalities in mitochondrial DNA.[33] Still, if evidence for involvement of mitochondria could be found, it would be a clue to the age dependence of PD.

C. TOXINS

It has also been proposed that the clinical expression of PD represents the end result of long-term poisoning of the substantia nigra by environmental toxins. Evidence for this model of PD is still circumstantial.[39] A large number of possible toxins have been created since the industrial revolution. Epidemiologic studies have identified specific environmental factors associated with PD (e.g., use of pesticides, consumption of well water, head injury), but none has been shown to play a causal role.[2,39]

MPTP, a by-product of the home synthesis of the reverse ester of meperidine, produces parkinsonism in humans and animals by destroying pigmented neurons in the substantia nigra.[2,29,39] It is taken up into the brain and metabolized by MAO type B to MPP^+. MPP^+ is taken up selectively into dopaminergic neurons, where it causes cell death by poisoning complex I of the mitochondria.[40] MAO B is a necessary component of the mechanism, and MAO levels clearly increase with age.[6] If a toxin like MPTP were responsible for most PD, then variations in the levels of MAO with aging could contribute to the age dependence of PD. Inhibitors of MAO B prevent the toxicity associated with MPTP and are capable of increasing life span in animals independent of toxin exposure.[6] This represents circumstantial evidence that toxins like MPTP may exist and perhaps play a role in the aging process of the brain by enhancing oxidative stress. However, no epidemiological studies to date have incriminated any specific agents. In experimental animals, the toxicity of MPTP and aging in the substantia nigra can interact to cause more cell damage than with either alone.[41] This finding would fit with the observed slow, age-dependent onset of PD in humans. Though

MPTP has caused few cases of parkinsonism in humans and produces a different pathology than idiopathic PD with no Lewy bodies, it is possible that more subtle, indolent toxins kill substantia nigra cells slowly over the course of years or that they begin a self-sustaining process. This would link the slow course of PD to an environmental event encountered early in life.

Oxygen-derived free radicals have been implicated in the pathogenesis of PD, but the evidence is not firm. Though there are many sources of free radicals, they can form as by-products of L-dopa synthesis.[42] They kill cells by causing lipid peroxidation of the cell membrane or by other oxidative damage to cellular respiration. Thus, their role as potential toxins links closely with the oxidative hypothesis and with the selective vulnerability of nigral neurons to oxidative damage. Free radicals are normally inactivated by the enzyme superoxide dismutase (SOD), and animals which overproduce this enzyme in their brains are resistant to MPTP and other oxidative toxins.[43] Furthermore, mutations in SOD cause familial ALS, another neurodegenerative disorder characterized by death of a selected population of neurons.[44] However, the exact relation between altered SOD activity and the disease process is unclear.

Another interesting aspect of the proposed toxic hypothesis is the interaction of putative toxins with the pigment melanin. Melanin is the product of long-term oxidation of catecholamines, and it accumulates in specific brain stem neurons over the course of a lifetime. The substantia nigra pars compacta (mesencephalon) is the major nucleus in the brain with melanin deposition; however, the locus coeruleus (pons) and dorsal motor nucleus of the vagus (medulla) also contain melanin. Cell loss is also present in each of the latter two nuclei in idiopathic PD and in the MPTP model of PD, though not to the same degree as in the substantia nigra. Noradrenergic nuclei without melanin production are spared in PD. It is not known which symptoms if any in PD are produced by the modest cell loss of these other nuclei. That these nuclei degenerate suggests that melanin or the metabolic processes which synthesize it are critical to the pathogenesis of PD. Though the age-related increase of melanin correlates with the age dependence of PD, melanin itself is not toxic. However, melanin binds specific drugs, and in particular it binds MPP^+, the toxic metabolite of MPTP.[29,45] Melanin could serve as a reservoir for a toxin which kills substantia nigra neurons in the pathogenesis of PD.

Melanin also binds metals experimentally, and this binding varies with the age of the experimental animal.[46] Metals are closely associated with the oxidative hypothesis of PD because they are capable of creating oxidative stress by depleting glutathione SH from tissues. Iron is a metal with a heterogeneous distribution in the brain, and is normally abundant in the basal ganglia, especially the globus pallidus. This distribution correlates with the distribution of transferrin receptors.[47] Iron is particularly well bound by melanin, and intrastriatal injection of iron can produce an animal model of PD.[48] Pretreatment of animals with iron chelators can lessen the damage in other oxidative stress models of PD.[48] Iron accumulates in the globus pallidus with normal aging and is present at higher levels in the substantia nigra of patients with PD, suggesting a pathogenic role of basal ganglia iron handling in the disease.[49] If some of the pathology of PD were related to metals, such as production of free radicals by their interaction with oxygen or by their interaction with melanin, then melanized nuclei like the substantia nigra would be most at risk. Metal toxicity clearly is capable of producing neurodegeneration, as is seen in mercury and arsenic ingestion and in the copper-mediated destruction of neurons in the putamen found in Wilson's disease. Still, there is no definitive evidence that melanin-metal interactions are important in the pathogenesis of PD.

D. EXCITOTOXICITY

Initially described in tissue culture studies, excitotoxicity has been proposed as a contributing mechanism for a variety of neurological disorders.[50] Glutamate is the major excitatory neurotransmitter in the brain, and almost every neuron has glutamate receptors. At high levels, glutamate can kill neurons by overstimulation. This occurs in experimental conditions where an induced injury (e.g., stroke or status epilepticus) causes cells to release glutamate at toxic levels, leading to cell death. This further increases extracellular glutamate levels, leading to further cell death and an expanding cascade. Such secondary damage can be blocked by antagonists of glutamate receptors, particularly the *N*-methyl-D-aspartate (NMDA) receptor. This receptor, a ligand-gated cation channel, allows calcium to enter the cell when the channel is open and leads to cell death when calcium entry is excessive.

Though it is easy conceptually to understand how excitotoxicity can contribute to acute neuronal destruction, its link to chronic illness ("slow excitotoxicity") is less clear.[50] It is crucial to understand the ways in which calcium entering through the NMDA receptor kills cells. In some systems, NMDA receptor activation can cause synthesis of nitric oxide, an intercellular messenger, but also a possible source of free radicals.[51] NMDA receptor activation also activates a variety of cell proteases (called calpains) and the prostaglandin synthesis pathways.[52] These changes all lead to physiological modification of cell function under normal conditions, and these events may contribute to the cellular basis of memory. However, the same enzymes produce toxic molecules under excitotoxic conditions. The cumulative buildup of toxic molecules such as glutamate over the course of a lifetime could lead to a slowly progressive disorder rather than the acute changes seen in stroke or neuronal trauma, especially in genetically or otherwise susceptible individuals at increased risk under conditions of high stimulation.[50]

Morphological evidence from various sources shows that neuronal pathology identical to acute excitotoxic lesions occurs in chronic neurological disorders. The pathology of Huntington's disease in the caudate and putamen is an example, with a preservation of small NADPH diaphorase containing neurons and loss of larger projection neurons.[50] Metabolic disorders such as glutaric acidemia, hyperammonemia, and nonketotic hyperglycinemia produce pathologies matching excitotoxic lesions.[53,54] ALS is characterized both by abnormalities of glutamate metabolism and by abnormalities of calcium handling, suggesting that it too has an excitotoxic component.[50,52] In animals, various metabolic toxins produce lesions which are slowly progressive in nature, but can be selectively blocked by glutamate receptor antagonists, suggesting that such lesions also represent slow excitotoxicity. One of these toxins is MPTP, the agent which produces severe parkinsonism in animals and humans.[50]

Does excitotoxicity play any role in PD? The classic loss of substantia nigra neurons is difficult to link with excitotoxicity. Glutamate receptors are found in the substantia nigra, but they are not present in exceptionally high levels. However, if the pathophysiology of PD involves excessive glutamatergic activation in conjunction with other abnormalities limited to the substantia nigra, then PD could evolve as a slow excitotoxic process. Direct evidence for such a model is lacking at present, but the excitotoxic hypothesis continues to hold the attention of researchers.

V. PHARMACOLOGICAL THERAPY FOR PARKINSON'S DISEASE

A. INTRODUCTION

Until the late 1980s, relief of symptoms was the principal purpose of antiparkinsonian therapy. Symptomatic therapies have been available since Charcot used anticholinergic agents in the 1800s. However, with the introduction of L-dopa in the late 1960s, the principle of pharmacological replacement therapy was successfully established. The advent of drugs like deprenyl (Eldepryl) gave credence to the concept of "protective therapy" which might slow the progression of PD or other chronic neurodegenerative illness.[50] Early notions that L-DOPA therapy cured PD have withered in the face of incontrovertible evidence that PD continues to progress despite an initial beneficial response. However, despite the success of L-dopa and several other symptomatic therapies, it has been suggested that L-dopa increases the speed of progression of PD by enhancing oxidative stress, and that preventative and symptomatic therapies may need to be used concurrently.

B. PREVENTATIVE THERAPIES

At present, no drug has clearly been shown to slow the progression of PD, nor to prevent the onset of symptoms. However, promising leads have developed as a result of the proposed pathophysiologies of PD discussed in association with aging. Much attention has been paid to the possibility that exogenous toxins in the pattern of MPTP kill neurons of the substantia nigra as a result of enzymatic oxidation and the subsequent formation of free radicals. MPTP is converted by MAO B to the toxic compound MPP^+.[55] If PD is caused by oxidation of a similar compound, preventing its formation would slow or prevent PD. Animal data show that MAO B inhibitors like deprenyl prevent destruction of substantia nigra neurons by MPTP and may facilitate recovery in injured neurons.[6] These observations and the uncontrolled clinical observation that patients taking deprenyl tended to live longer led to the DATATOP (**D**eprenyl **A**nd **T**ocopherol **A**ntioxidant **T**herapy **O**f **P**D) study in the late 1980s — a double blind, randomized clinical trial, which initially suggested that deprenyl might slow the progression of PD.[56,57] Patients with early untreated PD were randomized to deprenyl or placebo and examined serially to the endpoint of requiring levodopa therapy for symptomatic relief. Patients treated with deprenyl were found to reach the endpoint significantly later (approximately 9 months) than those receiving placebo. However, with longer followup a definite protective effect appears less distinct.[58] This may result from a small, but significant symptomatic effect of deprenyl and its dopamine-enhancing metabolites or from a smaller magnitude of protection than initially thought. These data suggest that oxidation does not have a large role in the ongoing pathogenesis of PD, although more clinical and basic research is needed before a major conclusion can be drawn.

With the proposed role of oxidative stress in PD, attempts to slow the progression of PD through antioxidants such as vitamin E have also been attempted. A second arm of the DATATOP study examined the effect of vitamin E on PD progression.[59] By preventing membrane lipid peroxidation, vitamin E could theoretically slow progression by blocking free radical damage. This correlates indirectly with the knowledge that vitamin E deficiency causes neurodegenerative disease of the dorsal columns of the spinal cord. However, vitamin E had no effect on the rate of progression in patients with early PD.[60]

Although neither of the protective agents in DATATOP clearly slowed disease progression, the study itself successfully demonstrated how animal models of human disease can generate therapeutically relevant hypotheses, which can in turn be tested in a randomized clinical trial. This offers the possibility of not only aiding the patient, but also increasing the basic understanding of disease mechanisms. Such linked studies represent the future of investigations in PD.

C. SYMPTOMATIC THERAPY

Just as the critical neurochemical abnormality of PD is a depletion of dopamine from the nigrostriatal pathway, the critical therapeutic intervention is restoration of dopamine levels in the brain. Carbidopa/levodopa (Sinemet) is the principal drug used to replenish brain stores of dopamine. It is now available in controlled release and regular preparations and remains one of the most impressive success stories in clinical neuropharmacology. Other attempts to replace deficient neurotransmitters in neurodegenerative disorders (restoration of GABA in HD, and acetylcholine in AD) have generally been unsuccessful. This suggests that the dopaminergic system of the nigrostriatal pathway may be a more tonically active system. However, not all symptoms of advancing PD respond well to simple restoration of dopamine levels, postural instability and cognitive dysfunction in the late stages of the illness being notable examples. Thus, the key to understanding the complex pathophysiology of PD is to know that the underlying problem is not simply dopamine loss, which can be reversed by exogenous replacement therapy, but the more mystifying effects of dopamine loss on cortical and basal ganglia neuronal systems downstream from the nigra.

Progressive clinical disability in PD is associated with a change in the response to individual doses of levodopa. Initially, the response to Sinemet given two to three times per day is smooth and sustained. After several years, the long duration response gives way to short, fluctuating, and variable periods of benefit. Ordinarily, the short 90-min half-life of L-dopa is offset by the capacity of the brain to store L-dopa in the remaining neurons of the substantia nigra.[61] The L-dopa is then converted to dopamine enzymatically by DOPA decarboxylase for tonic release in the striatum. As PD progresses, more nigral neurons die, leading to diminished capacity to synthesize and store dopamine at the synapse. This leads to a diminished duration of action of each dose, producing the typical end-of-dose wearing-off effects. Whereas early in PD, the "on" response is sustained without fluctuations, as the disease progresses, the "on" response is shorter and contaminated by unmodulated overactivity in the form of adventitious movements (dyskinesias) of the head, limbs, and body. As each dose wears off, the patient feels slow, stiff, and tremulous. Controlled-release L-dopa (Sinemet CR) and direct dopaminergic agonists decrease the intensity of motor fluctuations to some extent, but motor fluctuations frequently continue to be a significant problem in advanced PD.[61] Such fluctuations imply changes in the neuronal or receptor responsiveness with time. Agonist-induced changes in receptor characteristics have been characterized in many *in vitro* systems, and it seems likely that loss of agonist sensitivity at dopaminergic receptors is a characteristic of prolonged L-dopa therapy *in vivo* as well.[62,63]

Do these fluctuations result from L-dopa therapy or do they represent the evolution of PD? Though such fluctuations were not seen before the introduction of L-dopa therapy, the general success of dopaminergic therapy may simply allow individuals to survive to a point where new aspects of the underlying disease process are noted. The hypothesis of decreased storage of dopamine in later PD leading to motor fluctuations has been validated in both patients and animal experiments, so that the advancing pathology of PD is at least partially responsible for the motor fluctuations. In addition, the group of patients with another disorder — hereditary dystonia with diurnal fluctuation — illustrates that long-term L-dopa alone does not cause the motor fluctuations commonly seen in PD.[64] These patients present at an early age with parkinsonism and dystonia, which are responsive to small amounts of L-dopa. The genetic and biochemical defect is the absence of an enzyme which synthesizes biopterin, the cofactor for tyrosine hydroxylase, which in turn synthesizes L-dopa from tyrosine.[65,66] No cell loss is seen pathologically in such patients,[67] who require many years of L-dopa therapy, but do not experience motor fluctuations, possibly because of intact storage and release mechanisms. This suggests that the development of motor fluctuations requires more than simple exposure to prolonged L-dopa.

It is possible that L-dopa could accelerate the development of motor fluctuations in the presence of an underlying pathology. L-dopa is oxidized to create oxygen and hydroxyl free radicals. If the underlying pathophysiology of PD involves a susceptibility to free radical damage in conjunction with aging, then L-dopa may paradoxically accelerate nigral cell death, even though it reverses clinical disability early in the disease. Although L-dopa is the most effective drug in relieving parkinsonian symptoms, an alternative strategy is the use of direct dopaminergic agonists such as pergolide and bromocriptine. These agents work therapeutically by stimulating dopaminergic receptors directly, thus bypassing the oxidative steps in the dopaminergic metabolic pathway. Although they stimulate different subtypes of dopamine receptors, both have similar clinical profiles. Their use decreases endogenous dopamine turnover and the exposure of nigral neurons to potentially toxic levels of L-dopa or dopamine. In addition, they do not produce free radicals on oxidation that could theoretically promote the pathogenesis of PD.

While the oxidative stress hypothesis lacks definitive proof in humans, animal models substantiate these predictions.[68] In animals, the dopamine agonist pergolide prevents damage from oxidative by-products of L-dopa synthesis and leads to a stability of substantia nigra neurons. This finding suggests that pergolide, designed as a symptomatic treatment in humans, is potentially capable of a protective role. Clinical trials are needed to explore this possibility.

Other treatment strategies may also be effective in reducing the amount of exogenous L-dopa needed by the brain in therapy of PD, including the use of dopamine uptake blockers or catabolic enzyme inhibitors. These could potentiate the effects of released dopamine, reduce the need for its synthesis, and decrease the need for exogenous L-dopa and the production of potentially toxic free radicals. At present, the therapeutic potency of dopamine agonists or uptake blockers is exceeded by L-dopa, which remains the drug of choice despite the theoretical disadvantages of its use.

D. OTHER SYMPTOMATIC AGENTS

Based on the biochemical anatomy of the basal ganglia, a variety of other agents have been used in PD with some success. Cholinergic neurons are thought to counteract the actions of dopaminergic neurons in the basal ganglia. Therefore, anticholinergic drugs have long been in use. However, the low potency and frequent occurrence of side effects, especially in elderly patients, limit their practical utility in a majority of patients.

The new frontier in both symptomatic and protective therapy for PD is represented by NMDA receptor blocking agents, which theoretically protect neurons from glutamate-derived cell damage. The effects of glutamate could promote any of the possible mechanisms of PD. NMDA receptor antagonists could also be effective symptomatic therapies in PD, since lesioning of the glutamatergic pathway from the subthalamic nucleus to the globus pallidus interna reverses the parkinsonism caused by MPTP treatment in monkeys. Amantadine, a relatively weak antiparkinsonian agent, has NMDA receptor-blocking properties, although it also releases dopamine and blocks acetylcholine receptors in the striatum. Thus, NMDA receptor blockers may eventually have roles both as symptomatic and neuroprotective agents in PD.[69] While some NMDA receptor blocking agents (such as amantadine and dextromethorphan) are well tolerated clinically, others, such as the street drug phencyclidine, cause profound psychosis.[70] This correlates with *in vitro* studies demonstrating multiple types of NMDA receptor.[70] Clearly, further research of drugs in this class is needed before their widespread clinical use in PD is possible.

E. SIDE EFFECTS OF ANTIPARKINSONIAN MEDICATIONS

Antiparkinsonian medications may be associated with side effects, particularly in the aged. These include orthostatic hypotension, hallucinations, delirium/confusion, depression, and slowed gastrointestinal motility (i.e., constipation, delayed gastric emptying). Increased basic science knowledge allows us to separate the various side effects into two groups: those which result from overstimulation of dopaminergic receptors on cells which remain normal in PD, and those resulting from aggravation of the underlying disease process. The first category includes L-dopa-induced hallucinations, which presumably represent stimulation of dopaminergic receptors in the mesolimbic dopamine pathway in the brain, and L-dopa-induced nausea, which results from stimulation of dopamine receptors in the area postrema in the medulla of the brain stem. These effects can be managed pharmacologically: nausea can be abolished through the use of inhibitors of DOPA decarboxylase to prevent peripheral conversion of L-dopa to dopamine or by use of the peripheral dopaminergic receptor blocker domperidone, which does not enter the CNS but acts at receptors outside the blood-brain barrier in the area postrema.[71] Hallucinations from L-dopa can be treated with clozapine, an atypical neuroleptic that blocks subtypes of the serotonin receptor and dopamine receptors in the mesolimbic pathway.[72]

In contrast, other "side effects " of antiparkinsonian medications may represent not only medication effects, but manifestations of the disease itself. A modest amount of neuronal loss in PD is seen in nuclei outside the substantia nigra including the locus coeruleus and dorsal motor nucleus of the vagus, nucleus basalis of Meynert, and the serotonergic nuclei of the central brain stem. In a few patients with PD, memory loss, depression, and autonomic dysfunction can be apparent as intrinsic components of the disease, not as an effect of medication. Depression can be treated with tricyclic antidepressants or the more modern serotonin reuptake inhibitors, while flucortisone can be used for orthostatic hypotension.

Cognitive dysfunction may be associated with PD or as a medication side effect.[73–75] Up to 40% of patients with PD develop a dementia which is distinguished clinically from AD because of the rarity of language dysfunction in the dementia associated with PD.[71] For this reason, the dementia of PD is designated as "subcortical" compared with the "cortical dementia" of AD. AD pathology is found in the brains of demented PD patients in up to 50% of patients, although the role of neurofibrillary tangles and plaques in the pathogenesis of PD is debated. Some patients with PD and dementia will have Lewy body inclusions in cortical neurons (diffuse Lewy body disease) as an explanation of the association of parkinsonism and dementia.[75] However, many brains of demented PD patients lack a definitive histopathology.

If cognitive dysfunction is a component of the disease or its treatment in a patient with PD, there is no good pharmacologic therapy. Despite the use of clozapine in controlling the more serious psychiatric symptoms, most confused or demented parkinsonian patients will need to have their drug burden reduced. Inevitably, lower doses of levodopa and other potentially helpful medications result in unsatisfactory motor control in the context of advancing disease.

VI. CONCLUSIONS

A wide variety of hypotheses linking aging and PD have been proposed and have many therapeutic implications. Therapies initially thought to be preventative have symptomatic effects (e.g., deprenyl), and those designed as symptomatic treatments may have preventative capabilities (e.g., pergolide). At some point, a full understanding of the disease process may offer the possibility of pharmacologically stopping and reversing the underlying disease process. However, the pathophysiology of PD may not be a single mechanism, but a variety of mechanisms with a single phenotype. Future research should help elucidate the role of these various mechanisms and therapies in PD as they relate to aging.

ACKNOWLEDGMENTS

This work was written while Dr. Lynch was a Pfizer postdoctoral fellow and is supported by NIDA grant RO1-07130.

REFERENCES

1. **Stern, M. B.,** The clinical characteristics of Parkinson's disease and Parkinsonian syndromes: diagnosis and assessment, in *The Comprehensive Management of Parkinson's Disease*, Stern, M. B. and Hurtig, H., Eds., PMA Publishing, New York, 1988, chap 1.
2. **Golbe, L. I. and Duvoisin, R. C.,** The epidemiology and natural history of Parkinson's disease, in *The Comprehensive Management of Parkinson's Disease*, Stern, M. B. and Hurtig, H., Eds., PMA Publishing, New York, 1988, chap 2.
3. **Whitehouse, P. J., Price, D. L., Struble, R. J., Clark, A. W., Coyle, J. T., and Delong, M. R.,** Alzheimer's disease and senile dementia: loss of neurons in the basal forebrain, *Science*, 215, 1237, 1982.
4. **Kuncl, R. W., Crawford, T. O., Rothstein, J. D., and Drachman, D. B.,** Motor neuron diseases, in *Disease of the Nervous System*, 2nd ed., Asbury, A. K., McKhann, G. M., and McDonald, W. I., Eds., W. B. Saunders, Philadelphia, 1992, chap 89.

5. **Svennerholm, L., Bostrom, K., Jungber, B., and Olsson, L.,** Membrane lipids of adult human brain: lipid composition of frontal and temporal lobe in subjects of age 20 to 100 years, *J. Neurochem.*, 63, 1802, 1994.
6. **Knoll, J.,** Deprenyl: a strategy to modulate the age related decline of the striatal dopaminergic system, *J. Am. Geriatr. Soc.*, 40, 839, 1992.
7. **Hsiao, K. and Prusiner, S. B.,** Human prion diseases, *Neurology*, 40, 1820, 1990.
8. **Calne, D. B.,** Is idiopathic parkinsonism the consequence of an event or a process?, *Neurology*, 44, 5, 1994.
9. **Shapiro, W. R. and Shapiro, J. R.,** Primary brain tumors, in *Disease of the Nervous System*, 2nd ed., Asbury, A. K., McKhann, G. M., and McDonald, W. I., Eds., W. B. Saunders, Philadelphia, 1992, chap 81.
10. **Baraitser, M,.** Neurocutaneous disorders, in *Disease of the Nervous System*, 2nd ed., Asbury, A. K., McKhann, G. M., and McDonald, W. I., Eds., W. B. Saunders, Philadelphia, 1992, chap 89.
11. **Burger, P. C. and Vogel, F. S.,** The development of pathologic changes of Alzheimer's disease and senile dementia in patients with Downs syndrome, *Am. J. Pathol.*, 73, 457, 1973.
12. **Lynch, D. R., McDonald-McGinn, D. M., Zackai, E. H., Emanuel, B. S., Driscoll, D. A., Whitaker, L. A., and Fischbeck, K. H.,** Cerebellar atrophy in a patient with velocardiofacial syndrome, *J. Med. Genet.*, in press.
13. **Delong, M. R.,** Primate models of movement disorders of basal ganglia origin, *Trends Neurosci.*, 13, 281, 1990.
14. **Akiyama, H. and McGeer, P. L.,** Microglial response to 6-hydroxydopamine-induced substantia nigra lesions, *Brain Research*, 489, 247, 1989.
15. **McGeer, P. L., Itagaki, S., Akiyama, H., and McGeer, E. G.,** Rate of cell death in parkinsonism indicates active neuropathological process, *Ann. Neurol.*, 24, 574, 1988.
16. **McGeer, P. L., Itagaki, S., Boyes, B. E., and McGeer, E. G.,** Reactive microglia are positive for HLA-DR in the substantia nigra of Parkinson's and Alzheimer's disease brains, *Neurology*, 38, 1285, 1988
17. **Pujol, J., Junque, C., Vendrell, P., Grau, J. M., and Capdevila, A.,** Reduction of the substantia nigra width and motor decline in aging and Parkinson's disease, *Arch. Neurol.*, 49, 1119, 1992.
18. **Koller, W. C.,** When does Parkinson's disease begin?, *Neurology*, 42, 27, 1992.
19. **Fearnley, J. M. and Lees, A. J.,** Aging and Parkinson's disease: substantia nigra regional selectivity, *Brain*, 114, 2283, 1991.
20. **Schulzer, M., Lee, C. S., Mak, E. K., Bingerhoets, F. J., and Calne, D. B.,** A mathematical model of pathogenesis in idiopathic parkinsonism, *Brain*, 117, 509, 1994.
21. **Ruberg, Y., Scherman, D., Javoy-Agid, F., and Agid, Y.,** Dopamine denervation, age of onset and Parkinson's disease, *Neurology*, 45, 392, 1995.
22. **Jellinger, K. A.,** Pathology of Parkinson's disease: changes other than the nigrostriatal pathway, *Mol. Chem. Neuropathol.*, 14, 153, 1991.
23. **Gai, W. P., Blumbergs, P. C., Geffen, L. B., and Blessing, W. W.,** Age related loss of dorsal vagal neurons in Parkinson's disease, *Neurology*, 42, 2106, 1992.
24. **Malessa, S., Hirsch, E. C., Cervera, P., Duyckaerts, C., and Agid, Y.,** Catecholaminergic systems in the medulla oblongata in parkinsonian syndromes: a quantitative immunohistochemical study in Parkinson's disease, progressive supranuclear palsy and striatonigral degeneration, *Neurology*, 40, 1739, 1990.
25. **Brown, A. S. and Gershon, S.,** Dopamine and depression, *J. Neural Trans.*, 91, 75, 1993.
26. **Wszolek, Z. K., Pfeiffer, B., Filgham, J. R., Parisi, J. E., Thompson, B. M., Uitti, R. J., Calne, D. B., and Pfeiffer, R. F.,** Western Nebraska family (family D) with autosomal dominant parkinsonism, *Neurology*, 45, 502, 1995.
27. **Lazzarini, A. M., Myers, R. H., Zimmerman, T. R., Jr., Mark, M. H., Golbe, L. I., Sage, J. I., Johnson, W. G., and Duvoisin, R. C.,** A clinical genetic study of Parkinson's disease: evidence for dominant transmission, *Neurology*, 44, 499, 1994.
28. **Cooper, J. M., Mann, V. M., Krige, D., and Schapira, A. H.,** Human mitochondrial complex I dysfunction, *Biochim. Biophys. Acta*, 1101, 198, 1992.
29. **Tipton, K. F. and Singer, T. P.,** Mechanisms of MPTP neurotoxicity, *J. Neurochem.*, 61, 1195, 1993.
30. **Jenner, P., Schapira, A. H., and Marsden, C. D.,** New insights into the cause of PD, *Neurology*, 42, 2241, 1992.
31. **Cardellach, F., Marti, M. J., Fernandez-Sola, J., Marin, C., Hoek, J., Tolosa, E., and Urbano-Marquez, J.,** Mitochondrial respiratory chain activity in skeletal muscle from patients with PD, *Neurology*, 43, 2258, 1993.
32. **Shoffner, J. M., Watts, R. L., Juncos, J. L., Torroni, A., and Wallace, D. C.,** Mitochondrial oxidative phosphorylation defects in Parkinson's disease, *Ann. Neurol.*, 30, 332, 1991.
33. **Didonato, S., Zeviani, M., Giovanni, P., Savarese, N., Eimoldi, M., Mariotti, C., Girotti, and Caraceni, T.,** Respiratory chain and mitochondrial DNA in muscle and brain in patients with PD, *Neurology*, 43, 2262, 1993.
34. **Yoshino, H., Nakagawa-Hattori, Y., Kondo, T., and Mizuno, Y.,** Mitochondrial complex I and II activities of lymphocytes and platelets in PD, *J. Neural Transm.*, 4, 27, 1992.

35. **Schapira, A. H. and Cooper, J. M.,** Mitochondrial function in neurodegeneration and aging, *Mutat. Res.*, 275, 133, 1992.
36. **Dimauro, S.,** Mitochondrial involvement in PD: the controversy continues, *Neurology*, 43, 2170, 1993.
37. **Wallace, D.,** Mitochondrial genetics: a paradigm for aging and degenerative diseases?, *Science*, 256, 628, 1992.
38. **Lombes, A., Nakase, H., Tritschler, H.-J., Kadenbach, B., Bonilla, E., Devivo, D. C., Schon, E. A., and Dimauro, S.,** Biochemical and molecular analysis of cytochrome c oxidase deficiency in Leigh's syndrome, *Neurology*, 41, 491, 1991.
39. **Rajput, A. H.,** Environmental causation of PD, *Arch. Neurol.*, 50, 651, 1993.
40. **Javitch, J. A., D'Amato, R. J., Strittmatter, S. M., and Snyder, S. H.,** Parkinsonism-inducing neurotoxin, N-methyl-4-phenyl-1,2,3,6 tetrahydropyridine: uptake of the metabolite N-methyl-4-phenylpyridine by dopamine neurons explains selective toxicity, *Proc. Natl. Acad. Sci. U.S.A.*, 82, 2173, 1985.
41. **Tatton, W. G., Greenwood, C. E., Seniuk, N. A., and Sato, P. T.,** Interactions between MPTP induced parkinsonism and age related neuronal death in a murine model of parkinsons disease, *Can. J. Neurol. Sci.*, 19, 124, 1992.
42. **Olanow, C. W.,** Oxidation reactions in Parkinson's disease, *Neurology*, 40S1, 32, 1990
43. **Przedborski, S., Kostic, V., Jackson-Lewis, V., Naini, A. B., Simonetti, S., Fahn, S., Carlson, E., Epstein, C. J., and Cadet, J. L.,** Transgenic mice with increased Cu/Zn-superoxide dismutase activity are resistant to N-methyl-4-phenyl-1,2,3,6-tetrahydropyridine-induced neurotoxicity, *J. Neurosci.*, 12, 1658, 1992.
44. **Borchelt, D. R., Lee, M. K., Slunt, H. S., Guarnieri, M., Xu, Z. S., Wong, P. C., Brown, R. H., Jr., Price, D. L., Sisodia, S. S., and Cleveland, D. W.,** Superoxide dismutase 1 with mutations linked to familial amyotrophic lateral sclerosis possesses significant activity, *Proc. Natl. Acad. Sci. U.S.A.*, 91, 8292, 1994.
45. **D'Amato, R. J., Alexander, G. M., Schwartzman, R. J., Kitt, C. A., Price, D. L., and Snyder, S. H.,** Evidence for neuromelanin involvement in MPTP-induced neurotoxicity, *Nature*, 327, 324, 1987
46. **Beard, J. L., Connor, J. R., and Jones, B. C.,** Iron in the brain, *Nutr. Rev.*, 51, 157, 1993.
47. **Youdim, M. B. and Riederer, P.,** The role of iron in senescence of dopaminergic neurons in PD, *J. Neural Transm.*, 40, 57, 1993.
48. **Antonini, A., Leenders, K. L., Meier, D., Oertel, W. H., Boesiger, P., and Anliker, M.,** T2 relaxation time in patients with PD, *Neurology*, 43, 697, 1993
49. **Hirsch, E. C., Brandel, J. P., Galle, P., Javoy-Agid, F., and Agid, Y.,** Iron and aluminum increase in the substantia nigra of patients with Parkinson's disease: an X-ray microanalysis, *J. Neurochem.*, 56, 446, 1991.
50. **Beal, M. F.,** Does impairment of energy metabolism result in excitotoxic neuronal death in neurodegenerative illnesses, *Ann. Neurol.*, 31, 119, 1992.
51. **Dawson, V. L., Dawson, T. M., Bartley, D. A., Uhl, G. R., and Snyder, S. H.,** Mechanisms of nitric oxide-mediated neurotoxicity in primary brain cultures, *J. Neurosci.*, 13, 2651, 1993.
52. **Lynch, D. R. and Dawson, T. M.,** Secondary mechanisms in neuronal trauma, *Curr. Opin. Neurol.*, 7, 510, 1994.
53. **Heyes, M. P.,** Hypothesis: a role for quinolinic acid in the neuropathology of glutaric aciduria, type I, *Can. J. Neurol. Sci.*, 14, 441, 1987.
54. **Batshaw, M. L., Robinson, M. B., Hyland, K., Djali, S., and Heyes, M. P.,** Quinolinic acid in children with congenital hyperammonemia, *Ann. Neurol.*, 34, 676, 1993.
55. **Bradbury, A. J., Costall, B., Domeney, A. M., Jenner, P., Kelly, M. E., Marsden, C. D., and Naylor, R. J.,** *Nature*, 319, 56, 1986.
56. **Kieburtz, K., McDermott, M., Como, P., Growdon, J., Brady, J., Carter, J., and Huber,** The effect of deprenyl and tocopherol on cognitive performance in early untreated Parkinson's disease. Parkinson Study Group, *Neurology*, 44, 1756, 1994.
57. **Birkmayer, W. and Birkmayer, G. D.,** Effect of (–) deprenyl in long-term treatment of Parkinson's disease. A 10 years experience, *J. Neural Transm.*, 22, 219, 1986.
58. **The Parkinson Study Group,** Effect of deprenyl on the progression of disability in early Parkinson's disease, *N. Engl. J. Med.*, 321, 1364, 1989.
59. **Ward, C. D.,** Does selegiline delay progression of Parkinson's disease? A critical re-evaluation of the DATATOP study, *J. Neurol. Neurosurg. Psychiatry*, 57, 217, 1994
60. **LeWitt, P. A.,** Clinical trials of neuroprotection in Parkinson's disease: long-term selegiline and alpha-tocopherol treatment, *J. Neural Transm.*, 43, 171, 1994.
61. **Chase, T. N., Fabbrini, G., Juncos, J. L., and Mouradian, M. M.,** Motor response complications with chronic levodopa therapy, *Adv. Neurol.*, 53, 377, 1990.
62. **Mouradian, M. M., Heuser, I. J., Baronti, F., and Chase, T. N.,** Modification of central dopaminergic mechanisms by continuous levodopa therapy for advanced Parkinson's disease, *Ann. Neurol.*, 27, 18, 1990.
63. **Mouradian, M. M., Heuser, I. J., Baronti, F., Fabbrini, G., Juncos, J. L., and Chase, T. N.,** Pathogenesis of dyskinesias in Parkinson's disease, *Ann. Neurol.*, 25, 523, 1989.

64. **Nygaard, T. G., Wilhelmsen, K. C., Risch, N. J., Brown, D. L., Trugman, J. M., Gilliam, T. C., Fahn, S., and Weeks, D. E.,** Linkage mapping of dopa-responsive dystonia (DRD) to chromosome 14q, *Nature Genet.*, 5, 386, 1993.
65. **Ludecke, B., Dworniczak, B., and Bartholome, K.,** A point mutation in the tyrosine hydroxylase gene associated with Segawa's syndrome, *Hum. Genet.*, 95, 123, 1995.
66. **Ichinose, H., Ohye, T., Takahashi, E., Seki, N., Hori, T., Segawa, M., Nomura, Y., Endo, K., Tanaka, H., and Tsuji, S.,** Hereditary progressive dystonia with marked diurnal fluctuation caused by mutations in the GTP cyclohydrolase I gene, *Nature Genet.*, 8, 236, 1994.
67. **Rajput, A. H., Gibb, W. R., Zhong, X. H., Shannak, K. S., Kish, S., Chang, L. G., and Hornykiewicz, O.,** Dopa-responsive dystonia: pathological and biochemical observations in a case, *Ann. Neurol.*, 35, 396, 1994.
68. **Felten, D. L., Felten, S. Y., Steece-Collier, K., Date, I., and Clemens, J. A.,** Age related decline in the dopaminergic nigrostriatal system: the oxidative hypothesis and protective strategies, *Ann. Neurol.*, 32, S133, 1992.
69. **Greenamyre, J. T. and O'Brien, C. F.,** N Methyl-D-aspartate antagonists in the treatment of Parkinson's disease, *Arch. Neurol.*, 48, 977, 1991.
70. **Porter, R. H. and Greenamyre, J. T.,** Regional variations in the pharmacology of NMDA receptor channel blockers: implications for therapeutic potential, *J. Neurochem.*, 64, 614, 1995.
71. **Stoessl, A. J.,** Prevention and management of late stage complications in Parkinson's disease, *Can. J. Neurol. Sci.*, 19, 113, 1992.
72. **Factor, S. A., Brown, D., Molho, E. S., and Podskalny, G. D.,** Clozapine: a 2-year open trial in Parkinson's disease patients with psychosis, *Neurology*, 44, 544, 1994.
73. **Grossman, M.,** Alzheimer's disease and parkinsonism, in *Parkinsonian Syndromes*, Stern, M. B. and Koller, W. C., Eds., Marcel Dekker, New York, 1993, chap. 16.
74. **Levin, B. E. and Katzen, H. L.,** Early cognitive changes and nondementing behavioral abnormalities in Parkinson's disease, in *Behavioral Neurology of Movement Disorders*, Weiner, W. J. and Lang, A. E., Eds., Advances in Neurology, vol. 65, Raven Press, New York, 1995.
75. **Mohr, E., Mendis, T., and Grimes, J. D.,** Late cognitive changes in Parkinson's disease with an emphasis on dementia, in *Behavioral Neurology of Movement Disorders*, Weiner, W. J. and Lang, A. E., Eds., Advances in Neurology, vol. 65, Raven Press, New York, 1995.

Chapter 10

ANTIPSYCHOTIC DRUGS

Ashiwel S. Undie and Eitan Friedman

CONTENTS

I. INTRODUCTION

Disturbances in thought, perception, affect, and cognition are common and general characteristics of psychotic illness. Depending on the specific clinical features, the psychosis may be further categorized into syndromes of depression, schizophrenia, or bipolar disorder. The drugs discussed in this chapter are those used predominantly in the treatment of schizophrenia — a psychotic disorder that is associated with delusions, hallucinations, disordered thought, affective flattening, paucity of speech, and bizarre and incomprehensible associations. It is generally believed that clinical manifestations of schizophrenic dysfunction result from an interplay of genetic vulnerability and environmental or psychosocial factors, but the exact etiology of this disorder remains unknown. Nevertheless, intensive research efforts have focused on understanding the pathophysiology and neurochemistry of the disorder with the aim of developing drugs that would control the symptoms of disease and permit affected individuals to function in society.

The neuropathology of schizophrenia encompasses a number of brain structural and functional changes, some of which may underlie the clinical symptoms of the disorder. Studies using computed tomography, magnetic resonance imaging, and direct examination of post-mortem brain suggest the presence of increased ventricular size, dilatation of cortical sulci, abnormalities of the temporal lobe, and overall reduction in brain size and weight.[1–5] Regionally selective reductions in neuron number and aberrations in neuronal cytoarchitecture were also observed by some workers.[6] It is important to note, however, that these changes may not necessarily be specific for schizophrenia, although the consistent presence of brain structural abnormalities could strongly support the notion of an organic basis for the disease.

0-8493-8306-4/96/$0.00+$.50

A number of studies have focused on neurochemical assessments of neuroactive substances in target brain tissues and in body fluids. Schizophrenia-related changes in the content, release, or metabolism of the neurotransmitters dopamine, serotonin, norepinephrine, GABA, excitatory amino acids, and several neuroactive peptides have been documented or postulated.[7] The content of important phospholipids such as the phosphoinositides and of phospholipid-metabolizing enzymes, such as phospholipase A_2, may be severely altered.[8–11] These alterations may in turn lead to abnormalities in membrane integrity or function or in signal transduction processes.[12–14] Various neurotransmitter receptors have been examined in post-mortem schizophrenia brains or by positron emission tomographic methods in schizophrenic patients, but the findings are generally inconsistent. In view of the reported bilateral asymmetries in the severity of the cytoarchitectonic abnormalities in schizophrenia, it may be necessary for future studies to match samples not only for age and sex, but also for laterality when performing assays such as receptor measurements. Inasmuch as the processes of thought, affect, cognition, and motivation are poorly understood, it remains uncertain if and how any of these structural and neurochemical alterations would contribute to the etiology or pathology of schizophrenia. Nevertheless, because of the demonstrated effectiveness of antipsychotic agents in this disorder, it is expected that any efforts at developing better drugs for schizophrenia will concomitantly contribute to a better understanding of the disease in particular and of brain function in general.

II. MECHANISM OF ANTIPSYCHOTIC DRUG ACTION

Antipsychotic drugs are commonly classified on the basis of their chemical structure as phenothiazines (e.g., chlorpromazine, fluphenazine, and thioridazine), thioxanthines (e.g., chlorprothixene, flupenthixol, and thiothixene), butyrophenones (e.g., haloperidol and spiperone), dihydroindolones (e.g., molindone), diphenylbutylpiperidines (e.g., pimozide), benzamides (e.g., sulpiride), dibenzoxazepines (e.g., loxapine), and dibenzodiazepines (e.g., clozapine, fluperlapine, and tilozepine). While this chemical classification may be useful in predicting drug pharmacokinetics and certain adverse reactions, the most clinically useful classification divides the drugs into classical and atypical neuroleptics. Atypical neuroleptics include sulpiride, remoxipride, clozapine, and the clozapine congeners fluperlapine and tilozepine. Most of the remaining agents fall into the classical category. The utility of this scheme will become more apparent when we discuss the actions and side effects of the drugs.

A. THE DOPAMINE HYPOTHESIS OF SCHIZOPHRENIA

The most widely accepted hypothesis for the etiology of schizophrenia — the Dopamine Hypothesis — suggests that schizophrenic psychosis results from an overactivity of dopamine in the mesolimbic and mesocortical dopaminoceptive areas of the brain.[15] While several variants of the dopamine hypothesis are in circulation, the primary thesis implicating aberrations in dopamine neurotransmission in schizophrenia is supported by both basic and clinical data.[16] Drugs such as amphetamine that increase dopamine activity in the brain induce psychotic behaviors that are qualitatively indistinguishable from clinical psychosis.[17,18] Pharmacological agents that are effective in schizophrenia are compounds with high antagonistic activity at dopamine receptors,[19–22] or compounds that act through some other mechanism to reduce dopaminergic neurotransmission.[23] Moreover, the potency of antipsychotic drugs in blocking dopamine receptors, particularly the D_2 dopamine receptor, correlates with the clinical effectiveness of the drugs.[24,25] Measurements of brain regional transmitter content and of cerebrospinal fluid levels of the dopamine metabolite homovanillic acid (HVA) have produced rather inconsistent results. On the other hand, plasma HVA concentrations appear to consistently reflect brain dopamine activity as studied in animals and humans. Thus, in schizophrenia, the plasma concentration of HVA is correlated with psychopathology,[26,27] increases with acute antipsychotic drug treatment,[27,28] decreases during chronic drug treatment,[29,30] and rises again following discontinuation of neuroleptic administration.[31,32] Hence, measurement of plasma HVA has provided another line of support for the antidopaminergic mechanism of antipsychotic drug action. The procedure is also becoming a very useful tool for studying the pathophysiology of schizophrenia and for evaluating the clinical pharmacology of antipsychotic drugs.

At clinically effective doses, virtually all available antipsychotic drugs are capable of interacting with multiple receptors besides the D_2 dopamine receptor. These interactions may include blockade of dopamine D_1, D_3, or D_4 receptors, as well as serotonergic, muscarinic, histaminergic, and α-adrenergic receptors. While antagonism of muscarinic and α-adrenergic receptors may contribute to the adverse effects of antipsychotic drugs, recent studies suggest that inhibition of the serotonin 5-HT_2 receptor may play a role in the antipsychotic effectiveness of the drugs.[33,34] Observations such as this would seriously argue against the sufficiency of the dopamine hypothesis as the model of schizophrenic pathophysiology and pharmacotherapy. Nevertheless, it remains to be clarified whether these nondopaminergic systems are central in the mechanism of antipsychotic drug action, or if they are influential only because of their ability to interact with dopaminergic systems.

B. ACTIONS IN DOPAMINERGIC SYSTEMS

Brain dopaminergic systems are differentiated with regard to neuroanatomical or biochemical characteristics. Based on their source, course, and terminal areas, fibers containing dopamine as the primary neurotransmitter may be divided into four major pathways:

1. The *nigrostriatal dopamine system* is composed of neurons with cell bodies located in area A9 of the substantia nigra pars compacta and projecting rostrally to give a wide and dense innervation of the caudate nucleus and putamen.
2. In the *mesolimbic system*, the dopaminergic fibers arise from region A10 of the ventral tegmental area and project to the nucleus accumbens, amygdala, pyriform cortex, and lateral septum.
3. Neurons of the *mesocortical system* also arise from region A10 of the ventral tegmental area, and innervate primarily the frontal cortex and the hippocampus.
4. The *tuberoinfundibular system* consists of neurons which originate in the arcuate nucleus of the hypothalamus and project to the median eminence and pituitary gland. This dopamine system is primarily involved in the regulation of neuroendocrine function.

The physiological effects of dopamine are mediated through activation of specific dopamine receptors, of which at least five subtypes, D_1 to D_5, have been identified. On the basis of similarities in their molecular structures, these receptors can be grouped into the D_1 receptor family (comprising D_1 and D_5 subtypes) and the D_2 receptor family (comprising D_2, D_3, and D_4 subtypes). The D_1 dopamine receptors are classically defined as those which are coupled to activation of adenylyl cyclase with consequent increased formation of cyclic AMP, while the D_2 receptors inhibit cyclic AMP formation. This early classification of dopamine receptors based on adenylyl cyclase stimulation, however, is becoming less useful because more recent evidence indicates that some dopamine receptors may couple to other second messenger systems besides adenylyl cyclase. For example, dopamine activates phospholipase C-mediated phosphoinositide hydrolysis with formation of the second messengers diacylglycerol and inositol phosphates in brain slices,[35–38] and membranes.[39] Dopamine may also stimulate phospholiapse A_2 as well as modulate ion channel gating in brain tissue.[40–43] As new studies continue to generate information on the coupling of specific dopamine receptor subtypes to these signal transduction mechanisms, a new understanding of dopamine receptor physiology should emerge.

One of the most intriguing observations in the study of dopamine neurotransmission and function is the interaction between the D_1 and D_2 receptor subtypes. This interaction occurs both at the biochemical and functional levels. While a discussion of the possible mechanisms of the interactions is outside the scope of this review, it is important to note that such receptor cross-talk makes it difficult to precisely delineate the roles of each receptor subtype in whole organisms.

Dopamine agonists stimulate grooming, hyperactivity, and stereotyped behavior in rodents, and these actions are blocked by antipsychotic drugs. In man, dopamine agonists induce stereotyped behavior, hallucinations, and disordered thought.[17,18] Antidopaminergic antipsychotic drugs, in turn, produce catalepsy in rodents and parkinsonian reactions following acute administration in man. The doses of neuroleptic drugs required to control psychotic symptoms in man correlate with the potency of the drugs in blocking dopamine D_2 receptors.[24,44] Hence, the conventional notion is that neuroleptics produce their antipsychotic effect by blocking D_2 dopamine receptors in areas innervated by the mesocortical and mesolimbic dopamine pathways. However, post-mortem assessments as well as recent imaging studies in man have not consistently demonstrated dopamine receptor proliferation in schizophrenic patients. As a result of these inconsistencies, much current research activity is being focused on the more recently identified dopamine receptors, particularly the D_4 subtype, as well as on neurotransmitter systems other than dopamine.

The classical neuroleptics have an antiemetic effect, and some have been used for this purpose in humans. This action is mediated by dopamine receptor antagonism in the chemoreceptor trigger zone. The tuberoinfundibular dopamine system regulates prolactin secretion by exerting a tonic inhibitory effect on pituitary function. Thus, these dopamine antagonists elicit significant, but reversible hyperprolactinemia when antipsychotic therapy is initiated. Neuroleptics may also interfere with gonadotropin release and growth hormone secretion.

C. ACTIONS IN NONDOPAMINERGIC SYSTEMS

In addition to effects on dopamine receptors, most neuroleptics interact with multiple neurotransmitter receptors in the central nervous system. These compounds variously block serotonin ($5\text{-}HT_2$), muscarinic acetylcholine, α-noradrenergic, and histamine receptors. The drugs may also interfere with opioid and excitatory amino acid receptor function in the brain. Some of these actions, such as the blockade of serotonin $5\text{-}HT_2$ and sigma opioid receptors, may contribute to the therapeutic activity of the drugs.[33,45–47] Other actions, such as blockade of α-, histamine, and muscarinic receptors, are thought to be instrumental in mediating some of the serious side effects of the drugs.[48]

D. CELLULAR AND MOLECULAR EFFECTS

Chronic neuroleptic treatment in animals is associated with modest and selective reductions in cell density within the striatum.[6,49,50] The neurons most affected are large, probably cholinergic, cells in the ventrolateral quadrant of the striatum. In one study this cell loss persisted for at least 16 weeks after the cessation of drug administration,[6] suggesting that the cytopathological effects may be irreversible.

There is evidence indicating that chronic neuroleptic treatment induces collateral sprouting of axon terminals in the substantia nigra,[51] induces both the formation of new synapses and structural modification of existing synapses in the striatum,[52–54] and causes a selective loss of excitatory asymmetric synapses in the prefrontal cortex.[54,55] These changes in neuronal architecture following haloperidol treatment are reminiscent of similar findings of abnormalities in large aspiny neurons in neuroleptic-treated schizophrenics compared to untreated schizophrenics or control subjects.[56,57] On the other hand, clozapine, an atypical neuroleptic, did not induce significant modifications of neuronal architecture in the studied brain areas.[53,55] This suggests that the observed neuronal changes following haloperidol or raclopride treatments may be more a reflection of toxicity than of the therapeutic action of the antipsychotic drugs.

Recent molecular studies suggest that neuroleptics may alter neuronal and synaptic organization by altering the expression of diverse genes in the brain. Indeed, neuroleptics have been shown to alter the expression of genes encoding cellular proto-oncogenes or immediate early genes,[58-60] diverse neuropeptides,[61–64] neurotransmitter-synthesizing or -metabolizing enzymes,[65–68] neuroreceptors,[61,69–72] cytoskeletal proteins, and various other cellular components.[73–75] The immediate early genes code for transcription factors that regulate the expression of specific genes involved in the synthesis and disposition of neurotransmitters, neuroreceptors, and various other cell components that are involved in signal transduction and neuronal function.[76] It is conceivable, therefore, that the long-term neurochemical and structural effects of neuroleptic administration are the cumulative results of multiple, incremental, or chronic drug-induced modulation of gene expression. Of even greater import to the pharmacology of antipsychotic drugs in aging is the observation that the ability of a neuroleptic to induce the expression of specific genes may be influenced by aging.[77,78] To the extent that any specific action of a neuroleptic is dependent on drug-induced modulation of gene expression, therefore, age may be a determining factor in the therapeutic response as well as the enduring untoward effects of antipsychotic drugs.

III. MODULATION OF ANTIPSYCHOTIC DRUG ACTION IN AGING

A. BRAIN STRUCTURE AND FUNCTION

Normal aging of the human central nervous system involves significant structural and functional changes that may progressively compromise the ability of the brain to regulate body functions.[79–81] All loci or levels of brain structure may be affected, although the rate and extent of the age-related changes may differ significantly between brain regions or between specific neural functions. While studies that measure specific indices of brain structure, composition, or function in aging have not always produced concordant results, it is nevertheless fairly well documented that aging is usually associated with moderate losses of nerve cells in especially the subcortical regions of the brain.[82–85] The remaining neurons may undergo significant perikaryal shrinkage.[86–88] There may be generalized reductions in dendritic arborizations and spines, as well as decreased numbers of synapses in discrete areas of the brain.[87,89] By measuring glial markers such as glial fibrillary acidic protein (GFAP) and glutamate synthetase, some workers have demonstrated net increases in the number or size of astrocytes in rodents or humans,[87,90,91] and there may be increased permissiveness of the tight junctions that constitute the blood-brain barrier.[87,92,93] Numerous studies have shown that aging may be associated with alterations in the synthesis, release, and metabolism of various neurotransmitters or their receptors.[81,84,94–99] These alterations frequently correlate with aging-related changes in the organismic functions or behaviors that are subserved by the respective transmitter systems.

More recently, much attention has focused on age-related alterations in signal transduction processes and associated intracellular trafficking and regulatory events. We and others have demonstrated marked deficits in receptor-coupled G protein activation, and in phosphoinositide hydrolysis in the hippocampus, striatum, and frontal cortex of the rodent brain.[100–102] The deficits in second messenger metabolism were associated with decrements in phospholipase C immunoreactivity and phosphoinositide content in the brain tissues.[101] However, there was no apparent change in the responsivity of the dopaminergic or muscarinic receptors that are coupled to phospholipase C activation.[101,103] These rodent data probably have relevance to human brain function because in human brain the levels of both phosphoinositides and free myo-inositol decrease progressively with age, the levels at age 90 being only 50% of levels found at age 20.[104] Similar to the phosphoinositide system, there have been observations of decreased dopaminergic stimulation of adenylyl cyclase in aging rodent brain.[105] Other aging-induced changes have been demonstrated beyond the level of second messenger formation as in decreased sensitivity of protein kinase C to direct or receptor-coupled activation,[101,106,107] impaired mobilization of intracellular calcium in response to inositol-1,4,5-trisphosphate,[108-110] possible alterations in the fidelity or efficiency of genomic expression, and selective alterations in RNA content and protein synthesis.[90,111,112] Further research will need to be accomplished in these areas in order to more fully understand the relationship between specific functional changes and their underlying structural or biochemical defects.

B. PHARMACOKINETICS

The bioavailability of many drugs is altered in senescence, and some of these aging-related pharmacokinetic changes are particularly relevant to the pharmacology of antipsychotic drugs in the geriatric population. Antipsychotic drugs are most commonly prescribed for administration by mouth, and gastrointestinal absorption of the drugs is usually very good. Some compounds, notably clozapine, undergo extensive first-pass metabolism, which severely limits drug bioavailability. The antipsychotic drugs are highly bound to serum proteins and are distributed widely with brain concentrations reaching severalfold over serum levels during chronic administration. Antipsychotic drugs are generally extensively metabolized by the liver to produce, as in the case of chlorpromazine, scores of metabolites, some of which may retain pharmacological activity. The primary route of elimination of chlorpromazine and related compounds is through renal excretion. Aging is associated with increased brain concentrations of antipsychotic drugs,[113] hence drug doses calculated by weight or age must be reduced to obtain comparable therapeutic effect in the elderly, at least during the early stages of therapy. Changes in plasma composition or in liver and kidney functions, as frequently found in old age, produce wide variations in therapeutic efficacy, complicate therapeutic monitoring, and predispose to diverse adverse drug effects.

C. PHARMACODYNAMICS

From the foregoing discussion, it should be apparent that several of the effects of antipsychotic drugs on brain structure and function are qualitatively similar to the changes which occur during normal aging of the brain. Thus, antipsychotic drug treatment could effectively accelerate the impact of aging on these target brain structures and functions. Key factors in the pharmacodynamic actions of antipsychotic drugs include receptor concentration and affinity, the presence of competing ligands, signal transduction efficiency, and the integrity of the physiological output systems. Numbers of specific receptors for the aminergic neurotransmitters norepinephrine, dopamine, acetylcholine, and serotonin either remain unchanged or decrease during aging. Receptor loss may result from decreased receptor gene expression, abnormal post-translational modification, increased receptor degradation, and decreased membrane fluidity. With time, the levels of receptor molecules could fall below the threshold necessary to respond adequately to physiological activation and thus maintain normal function. For receptor systems that contribute to a basal functional tone in subserved tissues, progressive receptor loss can be expected to produce corresponding losses in basal tone. Moreover, the sensitivity to receptor antagonists could increase as a consequence of the loss in receptor number. Thus, increased responsiveness to the pharmacological effects of antipsychotic drugs in geriatric populations probably results from both pharmacodynamic and pharmacokinetic factors.

An important parameter in understanding altered drug responsiveness is the fidelity of transmembrane signal transduction processes. Receptors for most aminergic neurotransmitters couple through a G protein to regulate the activity of enzymes that form specific intracellular second messengers. For example, the dopamine D_1 receptor couples through the G protein, Gs, to stimulation of adenylyl cyclase and formation of cyclic AMP, which subsequently activates protein kinase A. Similarly, phosphoinositide-specific phospholipase C can be activated through a Gq protein to stimulate phosphoinositide hydrolysis with formation of inositol phosphates and diacylglycerol. Inositol phosphates, specifically inositol-1,4,5-trisphosphate, regulate the mobilization of intracellular calcium, while diacylglycerol is the endogenous activator of protein kinase C. It is well known that these second messengers and protein phosphorylation systems play diverse roles in fundamental cell processes such as secretion, motility, neurotransmitter release, long-term potentiation, growth, and differentiation. Recent studies have documented significant changes in several indices of transmembrane signaling in the brain as a result of aging, and some of these changes may be relevant to the therapeutic or adverse actions of antipsychotic drugs. For example, we and others have demonstrated marked losses in receptor-G protein coupling efficiencies of catecholaminergic and cholinergic receptors in the cerebral cortex and basal ganglia of aged F-344 rats.[101,103,114,115] There were severe aging-related losses in the content and activity of phospholipase C,[101] in the levels of *myo*-inositol and phosphoinositides,[101,104] and in the formation of inositol phosphate and diacylglycerol second messengers.[101,103,116,117] Other studies have demonstrated that receptor-coupled activation of adenylyl cyclase also is decreased in aging.[105,115] Moreover, the effectiveness of inositol-1,4,5-trisphosphate in mobilizing intracellular calcium and of diacylglycerol in activating protein kinase C are curtailed in brains of aged animals.[101,106–110] To the extent that the pharmacological action of antipsychotic drugs is dependent on these receptor systems and signal transduction processes, significant alterations in drug effects would be expected to accompany these aging-related changes.

Increasing evidence suggests that the processes of protein phosphorylation, intracellular trafficking, and regulation of gene expression that intervene between second messenger mobilization and the ultimate physiological response are also subject to modifications by both aging and antipsychotic drugs. For example, aging has been associated with decreased basal and agonist-induced translocation and activation of protein kinase C in rodent brain.[101,106,107] The expression of genes encoding neurotransmitter-synthesizing enzymes, receptors, and G proteins may be decreased with age or following chronic antipsychotic drug administration.[6,81,90,100] Moreover, aging and antipsychotic drug treatment are associated with specific cellular and neuroarchitectonic abnormalities in the brain. Together, these qualitatively similar effects of aging and antipsychotic drugs on brain structure and function support the notion not only that aging may alter the response to antipsychotic drugs, but also that chronic administration of antipsychotic drugs may accelerate the effects of aging on brain organization and function.

D. ADVERSE REACTIVITY

Antipsychotic drugs are notorious for the variety and severity of adverse reactions the drugs engender following their use in humans. Among these reactions are the extrapyramidal syndromes of dystonia, akathisia, parkinsonism, and tardive dyskinesia.[22,48,118,119] In addition, the drugs are associated with induction of sedation, hypotension, seizures, neuroleptic malignant syndrome, hormonal and sexual dysfunctions, hemolytic and hepatic disturbances, and weight gain.[120] These reactions result either from the antidopaminergic actions of the compounds, or from the anticholinergic, antiadrenergic, and antihistaminergic effects that are frequently associated with these agents. Dopaminergic blockade in the hypothalamic-pituitary axis causes hyperprolactinemia, which leads to several hormonal disturbances including galactorrhea, dysmenorrhea, and sexual dysfunctions. Increased circulating levels of prolactin may also increase the risk of prolactin sustained breast cancers in susceptible females. The atypical antipsychotic drugs have low liability for inducing extrapyramidal reactions, and the drugs are efficacious in relieving negative schizophrenic symptoms even in patients that are resistant to classical antipsychotic drugs.

Acute movement disorders, namely dystonic reactions, akathisia, and parkinsonism, are thought to result directly or indirectly from the initial blockade of nigrostriatal dopamine receptors by neuroleptic drugs.[118] In acute dystonia, for example, blockade of dopamine receptors in the basal ganglia might cause a compensatory increase in the activity of the nigrostriatal dopamine system, leading to increased striatal dopamine release and overactivation of the remaining unoccupied striatal dopamine receptors. Akathisia, a syndrome of compulsive perambulation, fidgeting, and restlessness, appears to result directly from blockade of mesocortical dopamine receptors by antipsychotic drugs. Acute dystonias often respond to antiparkinsonian anticholinergic drugs, or may spontaneously resolve in the course of antipsychotic therapy. On the other hand, akathisia by itself waxes and wanes with continued drug use and responds variably to decreased neuroleptic drug dosage, to a switch to the low-potency compounds, or to the use of antiparkinsonian anticholinergic agents.

Parkinsonian reactions, which are characterized by bilateral tremor, rigidity, and bradykinesia, appear within several weeks to months following initiation of antipsychotic drug therapy. The occurrence of parkinsonian reactions in neuroleptic-treated psychotics has traditionally been attributed to excessive neuroleptic blockade of dopamine receptors in the basal ganglia. The reductions in dopamine receptor number seen during aging may in part predispose schizophrenic patients to the parkinsonian side effects that frequently emerge during treatment with neuroleptic drugs. Once uncovered, the parkinsonian symptoms could be effectively managed with antimuscarinic anticholinergic agents. In fact, those antipsychotic drugs which have appreciable anticholinergic activity appear to have reduced liability to induce parkinsonism. These observations led to the classical hypothesis of a reciprocal dopamine-acetylcholine balance in the control of movement at the level of the basal ganglia. This hypothesis postulates that parkinsonian symptoms result from either a decrease in dopamine transmission or an increase in cholinergic neurotransmission in the basal ganglia. Consequently, a drug could have antiparkinsonian action either by increasing dopamine activity (as do antiparkinsonian dopamine agonists such as amantadine and levodopa), or by decreasing cholinergic activity (as does trihexiphenidyl and the other antimuscarinic agents) in the caudate-putamen. This scheme, which has served well in the symptomatic management of drug-induced parkinsonian reactions, is supported by animal studies in which acute neuroleptic-induced catalepsy could be attenuated by either an anticholinergic drug or a dopamine agonist.[121,122]

Psychotic patients exposed to neuroleptics for extended periods of time may develop abnormal involuntary movements called tardive dyskinesia. These dyskinetic movements affect principally the orofacial musculature, are usually reduced during voluntary movements of the affected parts, are absent during sleep, and may be exacerbated by emotional arousal or by voluntary movement of the unaffected body parts.[48] Tardive dyskinesia occurs in up to 20% of patients treated with classical antipsychotic drugs, and the disorder may be reversible in some patients following discontinuation of antipsychotic drug administration. While the dose and duration of exposure to antipsychotic drugs is correlated with the incidence of the disorder in treated patients, the most important risk factor for tardive dyskinesia is age: the elderly have a markedly greater likelihood of developing dyskinesia than younger persons treated for the same duration with equivalent doses of antipsychotic drugs. Aging is also associated with more severe and persistent forms of tardive dyskinesia. Similarly, the risk of developing more severe forms of the disorder is greater in women than in men. Withdrawal of antipsychotic medication after the emergence of dyskinesia is generally associated with exacerbations of the dyskinetic movements followed by gradual remission of symptoms in many of the subjects.

The pathophysiology of tardive dyskinesia has been associated with dopamine receptor supersensitivity, which results from long-term blockade of, especially, the D_2 subtype of dopamine receptors in the caudate-putamen. This view developed from several clinical and experimental observations. Dyskinetic symptoms appear only after prolonged administration of neuroleptics. Upon emergence, the symptoms could be relieved at least temporarily by increasing the dose of neuroleptic medication. Administration of levodopa, a dopamine agonist, exacerbates the dyskinesia in patients treated long term with antipsychotic drugs. In primates, up to 50% of monkeys given haloperidol or fluphenazine for up to 6 years developed abnormal involuntary limb and trunk movements that resembled the abnormal movements in humans with tardive dyskinesia.[123] Furthermore, chronic treatment of rats with neuroleptic drugs produces an increase in the numbers of dopamine receptors in the striatum; administration of dopamine receptor agonists in the chronic neuroleptic-treated animals elicits stereotyped behaviors that may be analogous to the movement disorders in humans.[124,125]

Not all the features of this dopamine supersensitivity hypothesis, however, are consistent with the clinical condition.[118,126,127] For example, spontaneous stereotyped movements have not been demonstrated even after prolonged neuroleptic treatment in rodents. Receptor proliferation and behavioral supersensitivity are consistently observed in neuroleptic-treated animals, but only a fraction of patients treated with antipsychotic drugs ever develop tardive dyskinesia. Indeed, receptor supersensitivity has not been unequivocally demonstrated in humans. Further, both dopaminergic neurotransmission and the capacity of dopamine receptors to develop supersensitivity decline with age, whereas clinical tardive dyskinesia is more prevalent, more severe, and more persistent in the elderly. These apparent anomalies in the dopamine supersensitivity hypothesis of tardive dyskinesia and in the rat model of the disorder have instigated the search for alternate hypotheses and models of tardive dyskinesia. Notable among these emerging propositions is the possible involvement of abnormalities in central γ-aminobutyric acid neurotransmission.[127] On the other hand, Gerlach[128] has recently advanced a refinement of the dopamine supersensitivity hypothesis by proposing that neuroleptics produce parkinsonian reactions by blocking the postsynaptic D_2 receptor, while their simultaneous blocking of presynaptic D_2 autoreceptors increases the release of dopamine which then stimulates unoccupied postsynaptic D_1 receptors, thereby producing tardive dyskinesia. We suggest a further extension of this hypothesis to incorporate the known involvement of the cholinergic system in both tardive dyskinesia and parkinsonism. Now, blockade of postsynaptic D_2 receptors by neuroleptic drugs induces increased release of acetylcholine in the striatum.[129–132] Similarly, inhibition of presynaptic D_2 receptors by neuroleptics increases the release of dopamine and consequent stimulation of postsynaptic dopamine D_1 receptors, an action that is associated with increased release of acetylcholine.[133–135] At the early stages of antipsychotic therapy, the cumulative enhancement of acetylcholine release creates a hypercholinergic state in the caudate-putamen, thus producing parkinsonian symptoms. Prolonged antipsychotic drug administration, however, would be associated with loss of cholinergic interneurons, desensitization of cholinergic receptors, and overall hypofunctionality of the cholinergic system.[135–137] The resulting cholinergic hypofunction then constitutes the primal link to the emergence of late dyskinetic reactions. This view would explain the observation that tardive dyskinesia can be ameliorated by administration of agents that facilitate cholinergic neurotransmission. Further, envisioning a primary role for cholinergic hypofunction in persistent tardive dyskinesia is consistent with the age-associated risk for dyskinesia, and with the decreased levels of acetylcholine synthesis, release, and receptors that occur during aging in particularly the caudate nucleus. Our current view considers alterations in cholinergic function to be central to the emergence of both the early parkinsonian and the late dyskinetic reactions to antipsychotic drug treatment. Whether or not this is the ultimate model of these disorders would depend on how the model consistently accounts for factors underlying the emergence, severity, and potential irreversibility of tardive dyskinesia, as well as the possible interplay between the impacts of aging, disease, and neuroleptic-induced structural and functional changes in the brain.

IV. CONCLUSION

Aging, psychosis, and neuroleptics are each associated with the induction of significant structural and functional changes in the central nervous system. Inasmuch as the mechanism of antipsychotic drug action depends on dopamine receptor blockade, it is easily apparent how the clinical effectiveness of antipsychotic drugs may be altered by aging-related losses in dopamine receptors, deficiencies in dopamine neurotransmission and signal transduction, and departures from optimal drug biotransformation and elimination kinetics. An important issue in the clinical use of antipsychotic drugs is the variety and severity of adverse reactions induced by these drugs. Among these reactions, tardive dyskinesia appears to be most obnoxious: it places serious functional limitations on the patient, there is no medication available to relieve the symptoms, and the dyskinesia frequently persists even following withdrawal of the antipsychotic medication. With hope that new approaches in addressing this disorder will emerge, we have proposed a revision of the dopaminergic-cholinergic hypothesis of neuroleptic-induced tardive dyskinesia and parkinsonism to emphasize the centrality of alterations in cholinergic neurotransmission in these syndromes. The observations that age is an important predisposing factor to tardive dyskinesia and that the elderly are pharmacodynamically more sensitive to the antipsychotic effects of neuroleptics are indications that aging may be associated with qualitative changes in brain function in addition to currently held notions of aging-related decline in the degree of normal functioning. Also of fundamental relevance is the question of whether or not neuroleptics can accelerate the normal course of aging in any brain structure or function. As these issues are addressed through continued research, we can expect to see new models of schizophrenia and neuroleptic-induced syndromes as well as new therapeutic compounds or approaches that will more effectively treat the patient while incurring fewer or milder side effects.

REFERENCES

1. **Lewis, S. W.**, Computerised tomography in schizophrenia 15 years on, *Br. J. Psychiat. Suppl.*, 157, 16, 1990.
2. **Daniel, D. G., Goldberg, T. E., Gibbons, R. D., and Weinberger, D. R.**, Lack of bimodal distribution of ventricular size in schizophrenia, *Biol. Psychiat.*, 30, 887, 1991.
3. **Harvey, I., Ron, M. A., Du Boulay, G., Wicks, D., Lewis, S. W., and Murray, R. M,.** Reduction of cortical volume in schizophrenia on magnetic resonance imaging, *Psychol. Med.*, 23, 591, 1993.
4. **Waddington, J. L., O'Callaghan, E., Larkin, C., Redmond, O., Stack, J., and Ennis, J. T.**, Magnetic resonance imaging and spectroscopy in schizophrenia, *Br. J. Psychiat. Suppl.*, 157, 56, 1990.
5. **Waddington, J. L.**, Neurodynamics of abnormalities in cerebral metabolism and structure in schizophrenia, *Schizophr. Bull.*, 19, 55, 1993.
6. **Harrison, P. J.**, Effects of neuroleptics on neuronal and synaptic structure, in *Antipsychotic Drugs and their Side-Effects,* Barnes, T. R. E. Ed., Academic Press, London, 1993, 99.
7. **Lieberman, J. A. and Koreen, A. R.**, Neurochemistry and neuroendocrinology of schizophrenia: a selective review, *Schizophr. Bull.*, 19, 371, 1993.
8. **Yasaei, P., Yao, J. K., van Kammen, D. P., and Neylan, T. C,.** Abnormal turnover of platelet PI in schizophrenia, *Trans. Am. Soc. Neurochem.*, 21, 130, 1990.
9. **Rotrosen, J. and Wolkin, A.**, Phospholipid and prostaglandin hypotheses of schizophrenia, in *Psychopharmacology: The Third Generation of Progress,* Meltzer, H. Y., Ed., Raven Press, New York, 1987, 759.
10. **Gattaz, W. F., Kollisch, M., Thuren, T., Virtanen, T., and Kinnunen, P.**, Increased plasma phospholipase-A2 activity in schizophrenic patients: reduction after neuroleptic therapy, *Biol. Psychiat.*, 22, 421, 1987.
11. **Pettegrew, J., Keshavan, M., Panchalingram, K., Strychor, S., Kadlan, D., Tretta, M., and Allen, M.**, Alterations in brain high energy phosphate and membrane phospholipid metabolism in first-episode, drug-naive schizophrenics, *Arch. Gen. Psychiat.*, 48, 563, 1991.
12. **Hudson, C. J., Young, L. T., Li, P. P., and Warsh, J. J.**, CNS signal transduction in the pathophysiology and pharmacotherapy of affective disorders and schizophrenia, *Synapse*, 13, 278, 1993.
13. **Kaiya, H., Nishida, A., Imai, A., Nakashima, S., and Nozawa, Y.**, Accumulation of diacylgylcerol in platelet phosphoinositide turnover in schizophrenia: a biological marker of good prognosis?, *Biol. Psychiatry,* 26, 669, 1989.
14. **Essali, M. A. and Hirsch, S. R.**, Extending neurotransmitter hypotheses of neuroleptic action and schizophrenia beyond cell-surface receptors. The phosphoinositide signalling system provides a link between receptors and intracellular calcium, *J. Psychopharmacol.*, 6, 453, 1992.
15. **Matthysse, S.**, Antipsychotic drug actions: a clue to a neuropathology of schizophrenia?, *Fed. Proc., Fed. Am. Soc. Exp. Biol.*, 32, 200, 1973.
16. **Goldstein, M. and Deutch, A. Y.**, Dopaminergic mechanisms in the pathogenesis of schizophrenia, *FASEB J.*, 6, 2413, 1992.
17. **Randrup, A. and Munkvad, I.**, Special antagonism of amphetamine-induced abnormal behavior, *Psychopharmacology,* 7, 416, 1965.

18. **Snyder, S. H., Banergee, S., and Yamamura, H.**, Drugs, neurotransmitters and schizophrenia, *Science*, 184, 1243, 1974.
19. **Seeman, P., Wong, M., and Lee, T.**, Dopamine receptor-block and nigral impulse blockade by major tranquilizers, *Fed. Proc., Fed. Am. Soc. Exp. Biol.*, 33, 246, 1974.
20. **Carlsson, A.**, Antipsychotic drugs, neurotransmitters, and schizophrenia, *Am. J. Psychiatr.*, 135, 164, 1978.
21. **Ellenbroek, B. A.**, Treatment of schizophrenia: a clinical and preclinical evaluation of neuroleptic drugs, *Pharmacol. Ther.*, 57, 1, 1993.
22. **Meltzer, H. Y.**, New drugs for the treatment of schizophrenia, *Psychiatr. Clin. North Am.*, 16, 365, 1993.
23. **Wetzel, H. and Benkert, O.**, Dopamine autoreceptor agonists in the treatment of schizophrenic disorders, *Prog. Neuropsychopharmacol. Biol. Psychiatry*, 17, 525, 1993.
24. **Creese, I., Burt, D. R., and Snyder, S. H.**, Dopamine receptor binding predicts clinical and pharmacologic potencies of antischizophrenic drugs, *Science*, 192, 481, 1975.
25. **Seeman, P.**, Brain dopamine receptors, *Pharmacol. Rev.*, 32, 229, 1980.
26. **Davis, K. L., Davidson, M., Mohs, R. C., Kendler, K. S., Davis, B. M., Johns, C. A., DeNigris, Y., and Horvath, T. B.**, Plasma homovanillic acid concentration and the severity of schizophrenic illness, *Science*, 29, 1601, 1985.
27. **Pickar, D., Labarca, R., Doran, A. R., Wolkowitz, O. M., Roy, A., Breier, A., Linnoila, M., and Paul, S.**, Longitudinal measurement of plasma homovanillic acid levels in schizophrenic patients, *Arch. Gen. Psychiatry*, 43, 669, 1986.
28. **Harris, P. Q., Brown, S. J., Friedman, J., and Bacopoulus, N. G.**, Plasma drug and homovanillic acid levels in patients receiving neuroleptics, *Biol. Psychiatry*, 19, 849, 1984.
29. **Bowers, M. B., Swigar, M. E., Jatlow, P. I., and Goicoechen, N.**, Plasma catecholamine metabolites and early response to haloperidol, *J. Clin. Psychiatry*, 45, 248, 1984.
30. **Pickar, D., Labarca, R., Linnoila, M., Roy, A., Hommer, D., Everett, D., and Paul, S.**, Neuroleptic-induced decrease in plasma homovanillic acid and antipsychotic activity in schizophrenic patients, *Science*, 25, 954, 1984.
31. **Davidson, M., Kahn, R. S., Powchik, P., Warne, P., Losonczy, M. F., Kaminsky, R., Aptu, S., Jaff, S., and Davis, K. L.**, Changes in plasma homovanillic acid levels in schizophrenic patients following neuroleptic discontinuation, *Arch. Gen. Psychiatry*, 48, 73, 1991.
32. **Glazer, W. M., Bowers, M. B., J. ., Charney, D. S., and Heninger, G. R.**, The effect of neuroleptic discontinuation on psychopathology, involuntary movements, and biochemical measures in patients with persistent tardive dyskinesia, *Biol. Psychiatry*, 26, 224, 1989.
33. **Bleich, A., Brown, S. L., Kahn, R., and van-Praag, H. M.**, The role of serotonin in schizophrenia, *Schizophr. Bull.*, 14, 297, 1988.
34. **Wilmot, C. A. and Szczepanik, A. M.**, Effects of acute and chronic treatments with clozapine and haloperidol on serotonin (5-HT2) and dopamine (D2) receptors in the rat brain, *Brain Res.*, 487, 288, 1989.
35. **Undie, A. S. and Friedman, E.**, Dopamine stimulates phosphoinositide metabolism in rat brain, *Neurosci. Res. Commun.*, 6, 69, 1990.
36. **Undie, A. S. and Friedman, E.**, Stimulation of a dopamine D1 receptor enhances inositol phosphate formation in rat brain, *J. Pharmacol. Exp. Ther.*, 253, 987, 1990.
37. **Undie, A. S. and Friedman, E.**, Selective dopaminergic mechanism of dopamine and SKF38393 stimulation of inositol phosphate formation in rat brain, *Eur. J. Pharmacol.*, 226, 297, 1992.
38. **Martin, L. P. and Waszczak, B. L.**, D1 receptor stimulation enhances phosphoinositol (PI) hydrolysis in slices from rat substantia nigra (SN), *Soc. Neurosci. Abstr.*, 19, 82, 1993.
39. **Wallace, M. A. and Claro, E.**, Transmembrane signaling through phospholipase C in human cortical membranes, *Neurochem. Res.*, 18, 139, 1993.
40. **Piomelli, D., Pilon, C., Giros, B., Sokoloff, P., Martres, M.-P., and Schwartz, J.-C.**, Dopamine activation of the arachidonic acid cascade as a basis for D_1/D_2 receptor synergism, *Nature*, 353, 164, 1991.
41. **Benishin, C. G., Krueger, B. K., and Blaustein, M. P.**, Phenothiazines and haloperidol block Ca-activated K channels in rat forebrain synaptosomes, *Mol. Pharmacol.*, 33, 195, 1988.
42. **Memo, M.**, Pharmacological and molecular basis for dopamine D-2 receptor diversity, *Mol. Neurobiol.*, 4, 181, 1990.
43. **Surmeier, D. J. and Kitai, S. T.**, D_1 and D_2 dopamine receptor modulation of sodium and potassium currents in rat neostriatal neurons, *Prog. Brain Res.*, 99, 309, 1993.
44. **Seeman, P.**, Anti-schizophrenic drugs: membrane receptor sites of action, *Biochem. Pharmacol.*, 26, 1741, 1977.
45. **Gerlach, J.**, Future treatment of schizophrenia, *Psychopharmacol. Ser.*, 5, 94, 1988.
46. **Lindstrom, L. H., Besev, G., Gunne, L. M., and Terenius, L.**, CSF levels of receptor-active endorphins in schizophrenic patients: correlations with symptomatology and monoamine metabolites, *Psychiatry Res.*, 19, 93, 1986.
47. **Nemeroff, C. B. and Bissette, G.**, Neuropeptides, dopamine, and schizophrenia, *Ann. N.Y. Acad. Sci.*, 537, 273, 1988.

48. **Kane, J. M. and Lieberman, J.,** Tardive dyskinesia, in *Adverse Effects of Psychotropic Drugs,* Kane, J. M. and Lieberman, J. A., Eds., The Guilford Press, New York, 1994, 235.
49. **Najlerahim, A., Barton, A. J., Harrison, P. J., Heffernan, J., and Pearson, R. C.,** Messenger RNA encoding the D2 dopaminergic receptor detected by in situ hybridization histochemistry in rat brain, *FEBS Lett.*, 255, 335, 1989.
50. **Jeste, D. V., Lohr, J. B., and Manley, M.,** Study of neuropathologic changes in the striatum following 4, 8 and 12 months of treatment with fluphenazine in rats, *Psychopharmacology* (*Berlin*), 106, 154, 1992.
51. **Benes, F. M., Paskevich, P. A., and Domesick, V. B.,** Haloperidol-induced plasticity of axon terminals in rat substantia nigra, *Science*, 221, 969, 1983.
52. **Meshul, C. K. and Casey, D. E.,** Regional, reversible ultrastructural changes in rat brain with chronic neuroleptic treatment, *Brain Res.*, 489, 338, 1989.
53. **Meshul, C. K., Janowsky, A., Casey, D. E., Stallbaumer, R. K., and Taylor, B.,** Effect of haloperidol and clozapine on the density of "perforated" synapses in caudate, nucleus accumbens, and medial prefrontal cortex, *Psychopharmacology* (*Berlin*), 106, 45, 1992.
54. **Benes, F. M., Paskevich, P. A., Davidson, J., and Domesick, V. B.,** Synaptic rearrangements in medial prefrontal cortex of haloperidol-treated rats, *Brain Res.*, 348, 15, 1985.
55. **Vincent, S. L., McSparren, J., Wang, R. Y., and Benes, F. M.,** Evidence for ultrastructural changes in cortical axodendritic synapses following long-term treatment with haloperidol or clozapine, *Neuropsychopharmacology*, 5, 147, 1991.
56. **Jellinger, K.,** Neuropathologic findings after neuroleptic long-term therapy, in *Neurotoxicology,* Roizin, L., Shiraki, H., and Grcevic, N., Eds., Raven Press, New York, 1977, 25.
57. **Jellinger, K.,** Quantitative changes in some subcortical nuclei in aging, Alzheimer's disease and Parkinson's disease, *Neurobiol. Aging*, 8, 556, 1987.
58. **Merchant, K. M. and Miller, M. A.,** Coexpression of neurotensin and c-fos mRNAs in rat neostriatal neurons following acute haloperidol, *Brain Res. Mol. Brain Res.*, 23, 271, 1994.
59. **MacGibbon, G. A., Lawlor, P. A., Bravo, R., and Dragunow, M.,** Clozapine and haloperidol produce a differential pattern of immediate early gene expression in rat caudate-putamen, nucleus accumbens, lateral septum and islands of Calleja, *Brain Res. Mol. Brain Res.*, 23, 21, 1994.
60. **Rogue, P. and Malviya, A. N.,** Neuroleptics differentially induce jun family genes in the rat striatum, *Neuroreport*, 5, 501, 1994.
61. **Jaber, M., Tison, F., Fournier, M. C., and Bloch, B.,** Differential influence of haloperidol and sulpiride on dopamine receptors and peptide mRNA levels in the rat striatum and pituitary, *Brain Res. Mol. Brain Res.*, 23, 14, 1994.
62. **Mercugliano, M. and Chesselet, M. F.,** Clozapine decreases enkephalin mRNA in rat striatum, *Neurosci. Lett.*, 136, 10, 1992.
63. **Williams, F. G., Murtaugh, M. P., and Beitz, A. J.,** The effect of acute haloperidol treatment on brain proneurotensin mRNA: in situ hybridization analyses using a novel fluorescence detection procedure, *Brain Res. Mol. Brain Res.*, 7, 347, 1990.
64. **Augood, S. J., Kiyama, H., Faull, R. L., and Emson, P. C.,** Dopaminergic D1 and D2 receptor antagonists decrease prosomatostatin mRNA expression in rat striatum, *Neuroscience*, 44, 35, 1991.
65. **Stork, O., Hashimoto, T., and Obata, K.,** Haloperidol activates tyrosine hydroxylase gene-expression in the rat substantia nigra, pars reticulata, *Brain Res.*, 633, 213, 1994.
66. **Mercugliano, M., Saller, C. F., Salama, A. I., U'Prichard, D. C., and Chesselet, M. F.,** Clozapine and haloperidol have differential effects on glutamic acid decarboxylase mRNA in the pallidal nuclei of the rat, *Neuropsychopharmacology*, 6, 179, 1992.
67. **Palacios, M., Padron, J., Glaria, L., Rojas, A., Delgado, R., Knowles, R., and Moncada, S.,** Chlorpromazine inhibits both the constitutive nitric oxide synthase and the induction of nitric oxide synthase after LPS challenge, *Biochem. Biophys. Res. Commun.*, 196, 280, 1993.
68. **Murray, M.,** Inhibition and induction of cytochrome P450 2B1 in rat liver by promazine and chlorpromazine, *Biochem. Pharmacol.*, 44, 1219, 1992.
69. **Srivastava, L. K., Morency, M. A., Bajwa, S. B., and Mishra, R. K.,** Effect of haloperidol on expression of dopamine D2 receptor mRNAs in rat brain, *J. Mol. Neurosci.*, 2, 155, 1990.
70. **Buckland, P. R., O'Donovan, M. C., and McGuffin, P.,** Both splicing variants of the dopamine D2 receptor mRNA are up-regulated by antipsychotic drugs, *Neurosci. Lett.*, 150, 25, 1993.
71. **Buckland, P. R., O'Donovan, M. C., and McGuffin, P.,** Clozapine and sulpiride up-regulate dopamine D3 receptor mRNA levels, *Neuropharmacology*, 32, 901, 1993.
72. **Delfs, J. M., Yu, L., Ellison, G. D., Reisine, T., and Chesselet, M. F.,** Regulation of mu-opioid receptor mRNA in rat globus pallidus: effects of enkephalin increases induced by short- and long-term haloperidol administration, *J. Neurochem.*, 63, 777, 1994.
73. **Rogue, P. and Vincendon, G.,** Induction by neuroleptics of certain genes in the central nervous system, *Ann. Med. Psychol.* (*Paris*), 150, 124, 1992.

74. **Eastwood, S. L., Burnet, P. W., and Harrison, P. J.,** Striatal synaptophysin expression and haloperidol-induced synaptic plasticity, *Neuroreport*, 5, 677, 1994.
75. **Caboche, J., Vernier, P., Rogard, M., and Besson, M. J.,** Haloperidol increases PPE mRNA levels in the caudal part of the nucleus accumbens in the rat, *Neuroreport*, 4, 551, 1993.
76. **Hanley, M. R.,** Proto-oncogenes in the nervous system, *Neuron*, 1, 175, 1988.
77. **Dobie, D. J., Merchant, K. M., Hamblin, M. W., Vatassery, G. T., Dysken, M. W., and Dorsa, D. M.,** Blunting of the neurotensin mRNA response to haloperidol in the striatum of aging rats: possible relationship to decline in dopamine D2 receptor expression, *Brain Res.*, 616, 105, 1993.
78. **Dobie, D. J., Merchant, K. M., Raskind, M. A., and Dorsa, D. M.,** Neurotensin mRNA expression in response to haloperidol is decreased in the dorsolateral striatum of aged rats, *Ann. N.Y. Acad. Sci.*, 668, 339, 1992.
79. **Timiras, P. S.,** Aging of the nervous system: structural and biochemical changes, in *Physiological Basis of Geriatrics*, Timiras, P. S., Ed., Macmillan, New York, 1988, 123.
80. **Timiras, P. S.,** Aging of the nervous system: functional changes, in *Physiological Basis of Geriatrics*, Timiras, P. S., Ed., Macmillan, New York, 1988, 144.
81. **Powers, R. E.,** Neurobiology of aging, in *Textbook of Geriatric Neuropsychiatry*, Coffey, C. E. and Cummings, J. L., Eds., American Psychiatric Press, Washington, D.C., 1994, 35.
82. **Dam, A. M.,** The density of neurons in the human hippocampus, *Neuropathol. Appl. Neurobiol.*, 5, 249, 1979.
83. **Terry, R. D., DeTeresa, R., and Hansen, L. A.,** Neocortical cell counts in normal human adult aging, *Ann. Neurol.*, 21, 530, 1987.
84. **Coleman, P. D. and Flood, D. G.,** Neuron numbers and dendritic extent in normal aging and Alzheimer's disease, *Neurobiol. Aging*, 8, 521, 1987.
85. **Katzman, R., Terry, R., DeTeresa, R., Brown, T., Davies, P., and Fuld, P.,** Clinical, pathological, and neurochemical changes in dementia: a subgroup with preserved mental status and numerous neocortical plaques, *Ann. Neurol.*, 23, 138, 1988.
86. **Haug, H., Kuhl, S., Mecke, E., Sass, N. L., and Wasner, K.,** The significance of morphometric procedures in the investigation of age changes in cytoarchitectonic structures of human brain, *J. Hirnforsch.*, 25, 353, 1984.
87. **Haug, H. and Eggers, R.,** Morphometry of the human cortex cerebri and corpus striatum during aging, *Neurobiol. Aging*, 12, 336, 1991.
88. **Haug, H.,** Brain sizes, surfaces, and neuronal sizes of the cortex cerebri: a stereological investigation of man and his variability and a comparison with some mammals (primates, whales, marsupials, insectivores, and one elephant), *Am. J. Anat.*, 180, 126, 1987.
89. **Scheibel, M. E., Lindsay, R. D., Tomiyasu, U., and Scheibel, A. B.,** Progressive dendritic changes in aging human cortex, *Exp. Neurol.*, 47, 392, 1975.
90. **Finch, C. E. and Morgan, D. G.,** RNA and protein metabolism in the aging brain, *Annu. Rev. Neurosci.*, 13, 75, 1990.
91. **Frederickson, R. C.,** Astroglia in Alzheimer's disease, *Neurobiol. Aging*, 13, 239, 1992.
92. **Mooradian, A. D.,** Effect of aging on the blood-brain barrier, *Neurobiol. Aging*, 9, 31, 1988.
93. **Mooradian, A. D.,** Blood-brain barrier transport of choline is reduced in the aged rat, *Brain Res.*, 440, 328, 1988.
94. **Sherman, K. A. and Friedman, E.,** Pre- and post-synaptic cholinergic dysfunction in aged rodent brain regions: new findings and an interpretative review, *Int. J. Dev. Neurosci.*, 8, 689, 1990.
95. **Gottfries, C. G.,** Neurochemical aspects on aging and diseases with cognitive impairment, *J. Neurosci. Res.*, 27, 541, 1990.
96. **Mendelsohn, F. A. O. and Paxinos, G.,** *Receptors in the Human Nervous System*, Academic Press, San Diego, 1991.
97. **Muller, W. E., Stoll, L., Schubert, T., and Gelbmann, C. M.,** Central cholinergic functioning and aging, *Acta Psychiatr. Scand. Suppl.*, 366, 34, 1991.
98. **Giaquinto, S.,** *Aging and the Nervous System*, John Wiley & Sons, New York, 1988.
99. **Giacobini, E.,** Cholinergic receptors in human brain: effects of aging and Alzheimer disease, *J. Neurosci. Res.*, 27, 548, 1990.
100. **Wang, H.-Y., Pisano, M. R., and Friedman, E.,** Age-related alteration in G protein function in rat cortex, *Ann. N.Y. Acad. Sci.*, 663, 426, 1992.
101. **Undie, A. S., Wang, H.-Y., and Friedman, E.,** Decreased phospholipase C-β immunoreactivity, phosphoinositide metabolism, and protein kinase C activation in senescent F-344 rat brain, *Neurobiol. Aging*, 16, 19, 1995.
102. **Roth, G. S.,** Age changes in adrenergic and dopaminergic signal transduction mechanisms: parallels and contrasts, *Neurobiol. Aging*, 9, 63, 1988.
103. **Undie, A. S. and Friedman, E.,** Aging-induced decrease in dopaminergic-stimulated phosphoinositide metabolism in rat brain, *Neurobiol. Aging*, 13, 505, 1992.

104. **Stokes, C. E., Gillon, K. R., and Hawthorne, J. N.,** Free and total lipid myo-inositol concentrations decrease with age in human brain, *Biochim. Biophys. Acta*, 753, 136, 1983.
105. **May, T. and Sugawa, M.,** Altered dopamine receptor mediated signal transmission in the striatum of aged rats, *Brain Res.*, 604, 106, 1993.
106. **Battaini, F., Del Vesco, R., Govoni, S., and Trabucchi, M.,** Regulation of phorbol ester binding and protein kinase C activity in aged rat brain, *Neurobiol. Aging*, 11, 563, 1990.
107. **Friedman, E. and Wang, H. Y.,** Effect of age on brain cortical protein kinase C and its mediation of 5-hydroxytryptamine release, *J. Neurochem.*, 52, 187, 1989.
108. **Burnett, D. M., Daniell, L. C., and Zahniser, N. R.,** Decreased efficacy of inositol 1,4,5-trisphosphate to elicit calcium mobilization from cerebrocortical microsomes of aged rats, *Mol. Pharmacol.*, 37, 566, 1990.
109. **Gibson, G. E. and Peterson, C.,** Calcium and the aging nervous system, *Neurobiol. Aging*, 8, 329, 1987.
110. **Roth, G. S.,** Mechanisms of altered hormone-neurotransmitter action during aging: from receptors to calcium mobilization, in *Annual Review of Gerontology and Geriatrics*, vol. 10, Special Focus on the Biology of Aging, Cristofalo, V. J., Ed., Springer-Verlag, New York, 1990, 132.
111. **Rance, N. E. and Young, W. S., III,** Hypertrophy and increased gene expression of neurons containing neurokinin-B and substance-P messenger ribonucleic acids in the hypothalami of postmenopausal women, *Endocrinology*, 128, 2239, 1991.
112. **Ingvar, M. C., Maeder, P., Sokoloff, L., and Smith, C. B.,** Effects of ageing on local rates of cerebral protein synthesis in Sprague-Dawley rats, *Brain*, 108, 155, 1985.
113. **Tran-Johnson, T. K., Krull, A. J., and Jeste, D. V.,** Late life schizophrenia and its treatment: pharmacologic issues in older schizophrenic patients, *Clin. Geriatr. Med.*, 8, 401, 1992.
114. **Scarpace, P. J. and Armbrecht, H. J.,** Adenylate cyclase in senescence: catecholamine and parathyroid hormone pathways, *Rev. Clin. Basic Pharm.*, 6, 105, 1987.
115. **Scarpace, P. J. and Abrass, I. B.,** Alpha- and beta-adrenergic receptor function in the brain during senescence, *Neurobiol. Aging*, 9, 53, 1988.
116. **Joseph, J. A., Kowatch, M. A., Maki, T., and Roth, G. S.,** Selective cross-activation/inhibition of second messenger systems and the reduction of age-related deficits in the muscarinic control of dopamine release from perfused rat striata, *Brain Res.*, 537, 40, 1990.
117. **Kurian, P., Narang, N., and Crews, F. T.,** Decreased carbachol-stimulated inositol 1,3,4,5-tetrakisphosphate formation in senescent rat cerebral cortical slices, *Neurobiol. Aging*, 13, 521, 1992.
118. **Waddington, J. L.,** Mechanisms of neuroleptic-induced extrapyramidal side effects, in *Adverse Effects of Psychotropic Drugs,* Kane, J. M. and Lieberman, J. A., Eds., The Guilford Press, New York, 1994, 246.
119. **Barnes, T. R. E. and Edwards, J. G.,** The side effects of antipsychotic drugs. I. CNS and neuromuscular effects, in *Antipsychotic Drugs and their Side-Effects,* Barnes, T. R. E., Ed., Academic Press, London, 1993, 213.
120. **Edwards, J. G. and Barnes, T. R. E.,** The side effects of antipsychotic drugs. II. Effects on other physiological systems, in *Antipsychotic Drugs and their Side-Effects,* Barnes, T. R. E., Ed., Academic Press, London, 1993, 249.
121. **Undie, A. S. and Friedman, E.,** Differences in the cataleptogenic actions of SCH23390 and selected classical neuroleptics, *Psychopharmacology*, 96, 311, 1988.
122. **Butkerait, P. and Friedemann, E.,** Scopolamine modulates apomorphine-induced behavior in rats treated with haloperidol or SCH 23390, *Eur. J. Pharmacol.*, 148, 269, 1988.
123. **Gunne, L. M., Haggstrom, J.-E., and Sjoquist, B.,** Association with persistent neuroleptic-induced dyskinesia of regional changes in brain GABA synthesis, *Nature*, 309, 347, 1984.
124. **Klawans, H. L. and Rubovits, R.,** An experimental model of tardive dyskinesia, *J. Neural Transm.*, 33, 235, 1972.
125. **Jenner, P. and Marsden, C. D.,** Chronic pharmacological manipulation of dopamine receptors in brain, *Neuropharmacology*, 26, 931, 1987.
126. **Waddington, J. L.,** Schizophrenia, affective psychoses and other disorders treated with neuroleptic drugs: the enigma of tardive dyskinesia, its neurobiological determinants, and the conflict of paradigms, *Int. Rev. Neurobiol.*, 31, 297, 1989.
127. **Fibiger, H. C. and Lloyd, K. G.,** Neurobiological substrates of tardive dyskinesia: the GABA hypothesis, *Trends Neurosci.*, 7, 462, 1984.
128. **Gerlach, J.,** Current views of tardive dyskinesia, *Pharmacopsychiatry*, 24, 47, 1991.
129. **Stoof, J. C., Thieme, R. E., Vrijmoed-de Vries, M. C., and Mulder, A. H.,** In vitro acetylcholine release from the rat caudate nucleus as a new model for testing drugs with dopamine receptor activity, *Naunyn-Schmiedeberg's Arch. Pharmacol.*, 309, 119, 1979.
130. **Marien, M. R. and Richard, J. W.,** Drug effects on the release of endogenous acetylcholine in vivo: measurement by intracerebral dialysis and gas chromatography-mass spectrometry, *J. Neurochem.*, 54, 2016, 1990.
131. **Bertorelli, R. and Consolo, S.,** D_1 and D_2 dopaminergic regulation of acetylcholine release from striata of freely-moving rats, *J. Neurochem.*, 54, 2145, 1990.

132. **Damsma, G., de Boer, P., Westerink, B. H. C., and Fibiger, H. C.,** Dopaminergic regulation of striatal cholinergic interneurons: an in vivo microdialysis study, *Naunyn Schmiedeberg's Arch. Pharmacol.*, 342, 523, 1990.
133. **Damsma, G., Tham, C., Robertson, G. S., and Fibiger, H. C.,** Dopamine D1 receptor stimulation increases striatal acetylcholine release in the rat, *Eur. J. Pharmacol.*, 186, 335, 1990.
134. **Imperato, A., Obinu, M. C., Casu, M. A., Mascia, M. S., Dazzi, L., and Gessa, G. L.,** Evidence that neuroleptics increase striatal acetylcholine release through stimulation of dopamine D1 receptors, *J. Pharmacol. Exp. Ther.*, 266, 557, 1993.
135. **Friedman, E., Wang, H. Y., and Butkerait, P.,** Decreased striatal release of acetylcholine following withdrawal from long-term treatment with haloperidol: modulation by cholinergic, dopamine-D1 and -D2 mechanisms, *Neuropharmacology*, 29, 537, 1990.
136. **Friedman, E., Gianutsos, G., and Kuster, J.,** Chronic fluphenazine and clozapine elicit opposite changes in brain muscarinic receptor binding: implications for understanding tardive dyskinesia, *J. Pharmacol. Exp. Ther.*, 226, 7, 1983.
137. **Dunstan, R. and Jackson, D. M.,** The demonstration of a change in responsiveness of mice to physostigmine and atropine after withdrawal from long-term haloperidol treatment, *J. Neural Transm.*, 40, 181, 1977.

Chapter 11

PHARMACOLOGY OF ANTIDEPRESSANTS IN THE ELDERLY

Mitsuhiko Yamada and Elliot Richelson

CONTENTS

0-8493-8306-4/96/$0.00+$.50

I. INTRODUCTION

In this chapter, we review the pharmacology of antidepressants in the elderly and discuss changes in pharmacokinetics and pharmacodynamics that can occur in this population.

Depression is an abnormal mental condition associated with high medical morbidity and substantial (excess) mortality. Because of the high rate of suicide, depression must be treated. The primary form of treatment of depression is pharmacotherapy, usually in combination with some form of limited, supportive psychotherapy.

The population of elderly people, those 65 years and older, is growing rapidly in the U.S. Depression has been estimated to affect 13% of this group, two to three times that of a younger population. In the U.S., more than 3.5 million elderly people may be suffering from depression.

For several reasons, the diagnosis and treatment of depression in the elderly is a challenge for clinicians. First, elderly oftentimes present with atypical symptoms of depression, making the diagnosis difficult. Second, normal physiologic changes that occur with aging in the gastrointestinal, hepatic, renal, cardiovascular, and central nervous systems can affect the pharmacokinetics and pharmacodynamics of antidepressants. Third, the incidence of chronic physical illness and associated use of medication increases with age, making drug interactions a likely possibility. Finally, drug compliance is difficult for the elderly patient because of memory difficulties and possibly other symptoms of depression as well.

Until recently, the so-called tricyclic antidepressants had been the drugs of choice in treating depression. However, this has changed with the availability of newer, second-generation antidepressants that have more favorable side effect profiles and low toxicity in an overdose. These new drugs are important for treating depression in the elderly, because older patients are generally more susceptible than younger ones to adverse drug reactions.

There are at least two different hypotheses to explain this increase in drug sensitivity in the elderly patient. The first hypothesis states that the "thermostat" for the pharmacologic activity of a drug is shifted to a more sensitive "setting". The second hypothesis states that a reduced rate of elimination of drugs (as may be reflected in a prolonged elimination half-life) leads to higher blood levels in the elderly. Higher blood levels, in turn, lead to increased incidence of adverse effects.

Although the receptor site hypothesis is very attractive and may, in fact, be correct, to date there is very little evidence to support this hypothesis. On the other hand, there are data to support a role for pharmacokinetic changes in the elderly to explain their increased sensitivity to the adverse effects of drugs.

All available antidepressants can be classified as either blockers of the uptake of biogenic amine neurotransmitters or inhibitors of monoamine oxidase. Currently, over 20 drugs are available in the U.S. for treating depression. However, little is known about the efficacy and the side effects of the newer antidepressants used in the elderly. Therefore, it is important to understand the basics of the pharmacologic mechanisms of antidepressants to predict their effects in elderly patients. Ultimately, this information may help us understand some of the biochemical changes that occur with aging.

II. DEPRESSION IN THE ELDERLY

A. DIAGNOSIS

The criteria for the diagnosis of major depression have been established.[1] The core symptoms of depression include depressed mood, diminished pleasure or interest in activities, significant change in appetite or weight, alterations in sleep (insomnia or hypersomnia), psychomotor agitation or retardation, fatigue or loss of energy, inability to concentrate, indecisiveness, and thoughts of death, dying, or suicide. In the elderly, the classic neurovegetative symptoms of depression generally are rare. Important symptoms of depression especially found in the elderly patients are listed in Table 11.1. These patients typically present with apathy, dysphoria, agitation, anxiety, somatic complaints, and sleep disturbances.

Elderly patients often have symptoms atypical of depression, including cognitive deficits and disturbing behavioral changes that may be mistaken for dementia. Also, some of the symptoms for major depression, e.g., impaired ability to think or to concentrate, may mislead physicians about the diagnosis. If an elderly patient has a chief complaint of fatigue, pain, sleep disturbances, anxiety, irritability, or gastrointestinal problems, the physician should be alert to the possibility of depression. If no physical reason is found for these complaints, the patient should be evaluated for depression.

TABLE 11.1.
Important Signs and Symptoms of Depression in Elderly Patients

A. Typically observed:
- Apathy
- Dysphoria
- Agitation
- Anxiety
- Somatic complaints
- Sleep disturbances

B. Symptoms easily mistaken for dementia:
- Cognitive deficits
- Disturbing behavioral changes
- Impaired ability to think or to concentrate

C. Other symptoms of possible depression:
- Fatigue
- Pain
- Sleep disturbances
- Anxiety
- Irritability
- Gastrointestinal problems

In addition, some of the features of depression are found in other conditions in the elderly (Table 11.2). Psychiatric disorders (e.g., schizophrenia, schizoaffective disorder, and anxiety disorders) may also have symptoms of depression. Furthermore, depression may coexist with another disorder. Moreover, many nonpsychiatric disorders can present with complaints of fatigue, insomnia, and difficulty concentrating. Illnesses that suggest the diagnosis of depression include endocrinopathies (hyper- or hypothyroidism, hyperparathyroidism, and Cushing's disease), collagen diseases (systemic lupus erythematosus), cardiovascular disease (congestive heart failure, myocardial infarction), neurologic diseases (Huntington's disease, Parkinson's disease, Alzheimer's disease, frontal lobe disease, right hemisphere stroke, brain tumors, multiple sclerosis, and infections of the brain), and vitamin deficiencies (vitamin B_1, nicotinic acid).[2] Also, anemia, hypoglycemia, and hyperglycemia may appear clinically like depression.

The incidence of depression increases with age. Loss, grief, and sadness are inevitable experiences of late life and do not necessarily imply clinical depression. Elderly patients are exposed to increased stress stemming from life events. These include death of spouse, retirement, children leaving home, and financial difficulties. It has been suggested that an abnormal response to stress may occur in the elderly in the absence of a depression syndrome.[3] These factors complicate making an accurate diagnosis.

TABLE 11.2.
Other Conditions That May Masquerade as, Co-exist with, or Precipitate Depression in the Elderly

A. Psychiatric disorders
   Schizophrenia
   Schizoaffective disorder
   Anxiety disorders

B. Nonpsychiatric disorders
   Endocrinopathies
      (hyper- or hypothyroidism, hyperparathyroidism, and Cushing's disease)
   Collagen diseases
      (systemic lupus erythematosus)
   Cardiovascular disease
      (congestive heart failure, myocardial infarction)
   Neurologic diseases
      (Huntington's disease, Parkinson's disease, Alzheimer's disease, frontal lobe disease, right hemisphere stroke, brain tumors, multiple sclerosis, and infections of the brain)
   Vitamin deficiencies
      (vitamin B_1, nicotinic acid)
   Anemia
   Hypoglycemia
   Hyperglycemia

C. Life events
   Death of spouse
   Retirement
   Children leaving home
   Financial difficulties

B. MEDICAL COMPLICATIONS

Depression in the elderly may appear to be a response to a physical illness; for example, cancer, endocrine malfunction, heart disease, stroke, Parkinson's disease, or another neurologic disorder. Chronic medical disorders — even a bone fracture — can often lead to depression in elderly patients. Also, primary depression in the elderly may be complicated with physical illness.

Three or more prescription drugs are taken by 85% of elderly patients.[4] Many drugs, including antihypertensive agents, sedatives, narcotics, and anxiolytics, cause secondary depression in the elderly. The use of medications known to cause depression should be discontinued when possible. This may make treatment with an antidepressant unnecessary.

C. DRUG COMPLIANCE

Elderly patients generally are more noncompliant than younger ones. They forget to take their medication, or they take a drug at the wrong time, take a larger or smaller dose than prescribed, or they take a drug for the wrong reason. For elderly patients with depression, compliance issues can be a life or death matter, especially because of the risk of suicide in late life. The slow onset of the therapeutic action of antidepressants may be misunderstood by elderly patients as treatment failure. Consequently, they may stop taking the medication before its therapeutic effect is established. Thus, it is important to educate elderly patients about this slow onset and to explain that antidepressants cannot be taken on an "as-needed" basis. Physicians should remember that the symptoms of depression — loss of motivation, shortened attention span, loss of concentration, apathy, fatigue, and feelings of helplessness and hopelessness — interfere with drug compliance and "limit" the effectiveness of patient education.

D. USE OF ANTIDEPRESSANTS IN OTHER DISORDERS IN THE ELDERLY

Tricyclic antidepressants are used to treat some nonpsychiatric disorders, including allergic and dermatologic problems, urinary incontinence, peptic ulcer disease, chronic pain syndrome, irritable colon syndrome, emotional incontinence, sleep apnea, and narcolepsy.[5] Also, recent clinical data suggest that potent uptake blockade of serotonin is necessary to treat certain anxiety disorders[6] and obsessive-compulsive disorder.[7]

In many cases, treatments with tricyclic antidepressants are successful and may be ideal for elderly patients who have concurrent depression. However, the changes in pharmacokinetics of antidepressants and their side effects profile with age should be considered.

III. PHARMACODYNAMICS OF ANTIDEPRESSANTS IN THE ELDERLY

A. PHARMACOLOGICAL EFFECTS OF ANTIDEPRESSANTS

The main pharmacological effects of antidepressants occur at the level of the synapse. This is the likely site for their therapeutic effects, drug interactions, and certain side effects.

After norepinephrine, serotonin and dopamine are released from their respective axon terminals at their synapses; they are then taken back into that axon terminal. This process, called "uptake" or "re-uptake", is a mechanism that prevents overstimulation of receptors in the synapse. Neurotransmission can be enhanced acutely by blocking this uptake with a drug. However, blocking uptake can also diminish the effect of the neurotransmitter by desensitizing its receptors. Antidepressants of many types, probably acting by different mechanisms, can desensitize receptors for catecholamines and serotonin. This is the basis for one hypothesis about the mechanism of action of antidepressants.[8,9]

Desensitization of the receptors that inhibit the firing of action potentials (somatodendritic autoreceptors) or the synthesis and release of a neurotransmitter (presynaptic autoreceptors or presynaptic heteroreceptors) removes these inhibitory influences. As a result, neurotransmission can be markedly enhanced, especially in the continued presence of the antidepressant drug.

Antidepressants can block the uptake of biogenic amine neurotransmitters and antagonize certain receptors (Table 11.3). Also, some antidepressants inhibit the activity of monoamine oxidase, an ubiquitous enzyme important in the degradation of catecholamines, serotonin, and other biogenic amines. In axon terminals, the inhibition of monoamine oxidase causes an increase in the concentration of neurotransmitter available for release.

The classic tricyclic antidepressants desipramine and protriptyline are the most potent agents for blocking the uptake of norepinephrine (Table 11.3).[10] Paroxetine, a new antidepressant, is most potent at blocking the uptake of serotonin (Table 11.3).[10] Most antidepressants are more potent at blocking uptake of norepinephrine than of serotonin. However, the newer antidepressants (serotonin selective uptake inhibitors, SSRIs) are generally more potent and more selective than the older ones at blocking uptake of serotonin over norepinephrine. Some antidepressants (e.g., bupropion and trimipramine) weakly block the uptake of norepinephrine, serotonin, and dopamine. Sertraline, a new antidepressant, is the most potent of the antidepressants at blocking uptake of dopamine, although it is much weaker than amphetamine (Table 11.3).[10]

Selectivity does not equate with potency, because selectivity is derived from a ratio of potencies. For example, sertraline is more selective than paroxetine at blocking serotonin uptake, but it is only about one-fourth as potent as paroxetine at this blockade.[10] Of the newer second-generation compounds, only bupropion is not potent or selective for blocking serotonin uptake.

Evidence suggests that the efficacy of antidepressants is not related to their selectivity or potency for blocking the uptake of norepinephrine, serotonin, or dopamine, but this is a point of controversy. This evidence is from clinical and basic science studies that show that

TABLE 11.3.
Antidepressant Blockade of Re-Uptake and of Neurotransmitter Receptors[10,29,45]

	Potency of uptake blockade[a]			Affinity for receptor blockade[b]			
Drug	**Norepinephrine**	**Serotonin**	**Dopamine**	**Histamine H_1**	**Muscarinic**	**α_1-Adrenoceptor**	**Dopamine D_2**
Amitriptyline	4.2	1.5	0.043	91	5.6	3.7	0.1
Amoxapine	23	0.21	0.053	4	0.1	2	0.62
Bupropion	0.043	0.0064	0.16	0.015	0.0021	0.0217	0.00048
Clomipramine[c]	3.6	18	0.057	3.2	2.7	2.63	0.53
Desipramine	110	0.29	0.019	0.91	0.5	0.77	0.03
Doxepin	5.3	0.36	0.018	420	1.2	4.17	0.042
Fluoxetine	0.36	8.3	0.063	0.016	0.05	0.0169	0.015
Fluvoxamine[c]	0.2	14	0.02	0.00092	0.0042	0.013	0.13
Imipramine	7.7	2.4	0.020	9.1	1.1	1.11	0.05
Maprotiline	14	0.030	0.034	50	0.18	1.11	0.29
Nefazodone	0.18	0.73	0.042	0.0044	0.0091	2.1	0.11
Nortriptyline	25	0.38	0.059	10	0.67	1.67	0.083
Paroxetine	3.0	136	0.059	0.0045	0.93	0.029	0.0031
Protriptyline	100	0.36	0.054	4	4	0.77	0.043
Sertraline	0.46	29	0.38	0.0041	0.16	0.26	0.0093
Trazodone	0.020	0.53	0.0070	0.29	0.00031	2.78	0.026
Trimipramine	0.20	0.040	0.029	370	1.7	4.17	0.56
Venlafaxine	0.48	2.6	0.019	0	0	0	0
Reference compounds[d]							
Amphetamine			1.2				
Diphenhydramine				7.1			
Atropine					42		
Phentolamine						6.7	
Haloperidol							26

[a] $10^{-7} \times 1/K_i$, where K_i = inhibitor constant in molarity.

[b] $10^{-7} \times 1/K_d$, where K_d = equilibrium dissociation constant in molarity. Data can be compared both vertically, horizontally, and across the table to find the most potent drug for a specific property and to find the most potent property for a specific drug.

[c] Not marketed in the U.S. as antidepressants.

[d] These are not antidepressants, but are shown here for comparison.

antidepressants have a wide range of potencies in blocking this uptake, suggesting that it is not known how these drugs alleviate depression.

B. CHANGES IN PHARMACODYNAMICS OF ANTIDEPRESSANTS IN THE ELDERLY

Although the pathophysiology and etiology of depression are not understood, evidence supports the hypothesis that β-adrenergic receptors are partly involved in the mechanisms of the therapeutic effect of antidepressants and the pathophysiology of depressive illness. Peripheral β-adrenergic receptors have been reported to become less responsive with normal aging.[11] These aging effects can be independent of the loss of receptors. Similar effects of aging on the receptors in the brain may occur in the elderly. Indeed, age-related loss of noradrenergic neurons has been reported in human brains.[12] With normal aging, noradrenergic transmission in the brain may decrease. Also, monoamine oxidase activity is reported to increase with aging.[13] These findings suggest that not only changes in pharmacokinetic variables, but also changes in sensitivity to drugs or modified pharmacodynamics with aging may be responsible for the different clinical profile of the treatment of depression in the elderly.

C. ONSET OF ACTIVITY

All of the pharmacologic effects, but not the therapeutic effects, of the drugs discussed herein occur shortly after a patient has ingested a dose of the medication. Thus, most of the possible clinical effects, including side effects, occur early in the treatment of patients. However, with chronic administration of the drug, adaptive changes may occur which can cause an adjustment to certain side effects, the development of new side effects, and the onset of therapeutic effects.

Physicians know that antidepressants begin to cause mood-elevating effects after about 1 to 2 weeks after treatment is initiated. If a patient has not received an adequate dosage for at least 6 weeks, the medication has not had an adequate trial. However, we know that the synaptic effects of these drugs occur within hours after being ingested. Because many side effects have the same time course as the synaptic effects of antidepressants, the synaptic effects of these drugs can be related to certain adverse effects and drug-drug interactions.

For patients with severe depression, physicians would like to have a drug whose clinical effect is as fast as its synaptic effects. Rapid onset of activity would be one characteristic of an ideal antidepressant. However, no antidepressant appears to work more rapidly than another, and the time course is generally prolonged.

Methylphenidate and amphetamine are psychostimulants that are sometimes used to treat depression in the elderly. These drugs have less anticholinergic side effects and have shorter time of onset of action. They may be useful for elderly patients with medical illnesses in which typical antidepressants are likely to cause severe side effects.[14] Methylphenidate and amphetamine are effective for the symptoms of psychomotor retardation, but they sometimes exacerbate the agitation, restlessness, anxiety, and confusion associated with this condition. The effect these drugs produce may explain how dopamine possibly contributes to the cause of depression. However, because of the possible addictive and dependency effects, these psychostimulants should not be the drugs of first choice in treating depression.

IV. PHARMACOKINETICS OF ANTIDEPRESSANTS IN THE ELDERLY

Many types of physiologic changes that occur with aging affect the pharmacokinetics of antidepressants. Indeed, pharmacokinetic variables in the elderly are markedly different from those in younger patients. These variables include absorption, distribution, metabolism, and excretion.

A. CHANGES OF PHARMACOKINETIC VARIABLES IN THE ELDERLY

1. Absorption

Decreased motility of the gastrointestinal tract, decreased blood flow in the bowel, and increased gastric pH generally occur in the elderly. A drug that has anticholinergic properties (as discussed below) may decrease intestinal motility and delay the rate at which it and co-administered drugs are absorbed.

2. Drug Distribution

An increase in the mass of adipose tissue and a decrease in lean body mass relative to total body weight are generally found in elderly patients. Therefore, lipid-soluble antidepressants (tricyclic antidepressants), and anxiolytics (benzodiazepines) become more extensively distributed in the elderly. The changes in the volume of distribution do not affect the steady-state plasma concentration of the drug. However, the increased volume of distribution prolongs the elimination half-life of the drug without a change in drug clearance.

Plasma levels of albumin are decreased in the elderly and the concentration of α_1-acid glycoprotein is increased.[15] Albumin and α_1-acid glycoprotein are the main proteins involved in the binding of tricyclic antidepressants. Drugs that bind extensively with binding proteins may be affected by changes in protein binding capacity. However, the changes in plasma concentration of these drugs are reported to be small; thus, changes in plasma levels of binding protein may have little clinical effect.

3. Drug Metabolism

The variable decreases in systemic clearance of the drugs that are due to age-related changes in drug metabolism have been demonstrated in many studies.[16] Administered drugs are transformed by two distinct metabolic (biotransformation) pathways.

One pathway is a reaction that involves oxidation, reduction, or hydrolytic processes (phase I reactions). The anti-inflammatory antipyrine has been widely used as a general marker of hepatic drug oxidation. More than 95% of the metabolism of this compound is by hepatic microsomal monooxygenase enzymes (cytochrome P450 systems). One group has demonstrated that the half-life of antipyrine is prolonged about 45% in the elderly, because of decreased plasma clearance.[17] However, others have reported that the effect of aging on plasma clearance is smaller than that of smoking and interindividual variability.[18]

10-Hydroxynortriptyline, a major active metabolite of nortriptyline, may be affected more by aging than the parent drug.[19,20] It is likely that the active hydroxylated metabolite of other tricyclic antidepressants is affected similarly by physiologic changes in the elderly. It has not been demonstrated experimentally, but the selective changes in the activity of cytocrome P450 with aging may be responsible for these effects.

The other pathway is a conjugation (phase II) reaction that includes glucuronidation, sulfation, methylation, acylation, and mercaptan formation. For many of the antidepressant drugs, hydroxylation and conjugation with glucuronic acid are important metabolic pathways.[21] The decreases in liver mass, cardiac output, and hepatic blood flow in the elderly may affect the metabolism of antidepressants. The decrease in liver mass and volume in the elderly may explain decreased elimination of low-extraction drugs.[22] Also, decreased liver blood flow may account for the decrease in systemic clearance of high-extraction drugs in the elderly. However, conjugation reactions are generally unaffected by the aging process.

4. Drug Excretion and Renal Function

Decreases in cardiac output, renal blood flow, and renal glomeruli function and changes in membrane permeability affect the excretion and reabsorption of antidepressants in the kidney. The glomerular filtration rate (GFR) is reduced 35% in the elderly in comparison with that in young subjects.[23]

Changes in volume of distribution in combination with decreasing renal function with aging prolong the elimination half-life of antidepressants, thus increasing the risk of toxicity. To prevent an adverse drug reaction, the dose of certain drugs must be adjusted in elderly patients. Lithium salt, an antimanic drug often used to prevent recurrence of manic-depressive episodes, has a narrow therapeutic window so that adjustment of the dose is especially important for this drug. Renal clearance of 2-hydroxydesipramine, a metabolite of desipramine, is decreased in the elderly.[24] Creatinine clearance is a general indicator of renal function.

B. CLEARANCE AND ELIMINATION HALF-LIFE

Changes in the plasma concentration of an antidepressant or prolonged elimination half-life may affect not only the therapeutic property of the drug, but also the incidence of adverse drug reactions. These changes should be considered when treating depression in the elderly. The effects of an antidepressant ultimately depend on the concentration of the drug at the site of action.

Drug clearance is an independent variable that depends on hepatic metabolism (biotransformation) and renal excretion. Usually, antidepressants are used for a specific period of time as multiple oral dose medication, and the steady-state plasma concentration of the drug depends directly on dosage rate and inversely on drug clearance. Thus, when drug clearance decreases, the steady-state plasma concentration of that drug will increase at any given dosage rate.

Antidepressants can be rank-ordered according to their elimination half-lives (Table 11.4).[10] It is important to know that these data are derived largely from studies on healthy, young, adult men. Also, active metabolites, which are known to exist for most of these compounds, are not discussed herein. Ideally, both the parent compound and the active metabolite should have an intermediate half-life about 24 hr. This is an important issue in regard to fluoxetine, whose active metabolite norfluoxetine has a half-life of 7 to 15 d.[25]

TABLE 11.4.
Elimination Half-Lives of Antidepressants

Antidepressants	Elimination half-lives (hr)
Fluoxetine	87
Protriptyline	78
Maprotiline	43
Nortriptyline	36
Imipramine	28
Sertraline	26
Clomipramine	23
Paroxetine	21
Amitriptyline	21
Desipramine	21
Fluvoxamine	19
Doxepin	17
Bupropion	15
Trimipramine	13
Amoxapine	8
Venlafaxine	3.6
Trazodone	6.5
Nefazodone	3

From a theoretical standpoint, antidepressants with a half-life between 17 and 36 hr can be dosed once per day to maintain a good steady-state level. Drugs with a shorter half-life need to be dosed more frequently, and those with longer half-life can be dosed less than once daily. Simplifying the dosage regimen is important in achieving good drug compliance in elderly patients.

The effects of age on single-dose kinetics and multiple-dose kinetics for some antidepressants has been studied.[26,27] However, the interpretation of the results in the elderly is often complicated by the presence of other chronically administered drugs and by the disease state itself.

Pharmacokinetics of monoamine oxidase inhibitors are not well defined. The elimination half-life of these drugs may be as short as 1 to 3 hr. However, their duration of action is much longer, because the effect of the presently available drugs in the U.S. is due to irreversible inhibition of the enzyme.

C. THERAPEUTIC BLOOD CONCENTRATION

Studies of steady-state plasma concentrations of antidepressants have shown that concentrations of these drugs are higher in elderly than in younger patients at the same doses. Furthermore, interindividual variability is greater among the elderly.[26] If a therapeutic blood level were defined, physicians could tailor the dose to achieve therapeutic effects and to avoid adverse effects. The American Psychiatric Association Task Force on the Use of Laboratory Tests in Psychiatry concluded that measurements of the plasma levels of imipramine, desipramine, and nortriptyline are useful clinically in certain cases.[28] However, this conclusion was not made on the basis of data obtained from elderly patients. The optimal therapeutic ranges for other antidepressants and their active metabolite have not been established. Nonetheless, therapeutic drug monitoring is the standard of care to avoid toxic effects, especially when treating depression in the elderly.

V. SIDE EFFECTS AND PHARMACODYNAMIC DRUG INTERACTIONS OF ANTIDEPRESSANTS

Some physicians may withhold antidepressant medication in the elderly because of their potential risks for major adverse reactions. However, the response to treatment with antidepressants in elderly patients with depression is generally good. The risks of not treating the condition are usually greater than the potential risks of adverse drug reactions. In addition, newer second-generation drugs are less likely to cause the more serious side effects in the elderly patient.

The choice of prescribing one antidepressant instead of another is usually based on the side effect profiles. To minimize the side effects of antidepressant treatment, the initial dose should be lower (about 50% of the young adult dose) than that for younger subjects. The dosages should be increased gradually until a good therapeutic effect or unacceptable adverse drug reaction occurs. The safety of antidepressant therapy will be enhanced by close monitoring of the treatment by medical staff and by educating of patients and their families about the drug. Side effects and drug interactions of antidepressants that are particularly problematic in the elderly are listed in Table 11.5.

Most of the side effects and certain drug interactions of antidepressants can be explained by their synaptic effects. The three most important synaptic effects of antidepressants are the blockade of neurotransmitter (norepinephrine, serotonin, and dopamine) uptake, the blockade of receptors for specific neurotransmitters, and the inhibition of monoamine oxidase. The most clinically relevant receptor blockade is at histamine H_1, muscarinic acetylcholine, α_1-adrenergic, and dopamine D_2 receptors. Some of these synaptic effects may be required for the therapeutic effects of antidepressants. If this is true, then antidepressants can never be devoid of certain adverse effects caused by interactions of these drugs with neurotransmitters and their receptors.

The newer, second-generation antidepressants are weaker than the older compounds at blocking neurotransmitter receptors.[29] This pharmacology makes these drugs closer to the

TABLE 11.5.
Pharmacological Properties of Antidepressants and Their Possible Clinical Consequences

Property	Possible clinical consequences
Blockade of norepinephrine uptake at nerve endings	Tremors Tachycardia Erectile and ejaculatory dysfunction Blockade of the antihypertensive effects of guanethidine and guanadrel Augmentation of pressor effects of sympathomimetic amines
Blockade of serotonin uptake at nerve endings	Gastrointestinal disturbances Increase or decrease in anxiety (dose dependent) Sexual dysfunction Extrapyramidal side effects Interactions with L-tryptophan, monoamine oxidase inhibitors, and fenfluramine
Blockade of dopamine uptake at nerve endings	Psychomotor activation Antiparkinsonian effect Aggravation of psychosis
Blockade of histamine H_1 receptors	Potentiation of central depressant drugs Sedation, drowsiness Weight gain Hypotension
Blockade of muscarinic receptors	Blurred vision Dry mouth Sinus tachycardia Constipation Urinary retention Memory dysfunction
Blockade of α_1-adrenergic receptors	Potentiation of the antihypertensive effect of prazosin, terazosin, doxazosin, and labetalol Postural hypotension, dizziness Reflex tachycardia
Blockade of dopamine D_2 receptors	Extrapyramidal movement disorders Endocrine changes Sexual dysfunction (males)

"ideal antidepressant" — one that has no side effects. Support for the relationship between some of these synaptic effects of antidepressants and adverse effects comes from a multicenter trial that compared sertraline with amitriptyline.[30]

A. FROM BLOCKADE OF UPTAKE OF NEUROTRANSMITTERS

Blockade of the uptake of norepinephrine, serotonin, and dopamine at synapses by antidepressants can explain certain adverse effects and drug-drug interactions (Table 11.5). For example, the blockade of serotonin uptake is likely the cause of the gastrointestinal side effects seen more commonly with the SSRIs.[30] It is also the cause of a serious drug interaction called the "*serotonergic syndrome*". Most often, this occurs when a monoamine oxidase inhibitor is used in combination with an antidepressant that blocks serotonin uptake.[31]

When a patient who is taking an antidepressant that potently blocks uptake of norepinephrine (Table 11.3) needs a local anesthetic, a local anesthetic without epinephrine is preferred, if possible. Otherwise, anesthetics with epinephrine may induce hypertension. Psychostimulants such as methylphenidate and amphetamine alone or in combination with antidepressants that potently block uptake of norepinephrine can induce hypertension, tachycardia, and arrhythmias.

Rare effects of fluoxetine that include extrapyramidal side effects have been reported anecdotally.[32] These extrapyramidal side effects, which have also been reported for sertraline,[33] are not due to blockade of dopamine receptors, because these drugs are very weak at this binding site.[9,29] These side effects likely involve serotonin, because blockade of serotonin uptake is the most potent property of fluoxetine and sertraline. Animal studies suggest that fluoxetine can inhibit dopaminergic neurons that end in the corpus striatum and nucleus accumbens, but this is a point of controversy.[34,35]

Adverse interactions between L-tryptophan, the precursor of serotonin, and fluoxetine have been reported.[36] An interaction between fluoxetine and fenfluramine, an orally administered anorectic drug that increases synaptic levels of serotonin, has been predicted but not observed.[37]

B. FROM BLOCKADE OF CERTAIN NEUROTRANSMITTER RECEPTORS

1. Blockade of Histamine H_1 Receptors

Histamine H_1 receptor antagonism is probably responsible for the side effects of sedation and drowsiness. In addition to orthostatic hypotension, sedation can be another troublesome side effect for elderly patients. However, sedation may be a wanted effect in patients who are agitated as well as depressed. This property may also be responsible for weight gain and postural hypotension.

Trazodone frequently causes sedation and drowsiness. However, its low affinity for the histamine H_1 receptor suggests that this drug causes these side effects by other mechanisms.[29] However, trazodone reaches high concentrations in plasma (which is related to brain levels). As a result, trazodone causes significant blockade of histamine H_1 receptors and thereby causes sedation and drowsiness.[38,39]

2. Blockade of Muscarinic Receptors

One of the most potent effects of antidepressants, especially for the tricyclic antidepressants, is at the muscarinic acetylcholine receptor. Muscarinic receptor blockade by antidepressants can be responsible for several adverse effects, which can be especially severe in the elderly. Monoamine oxidase inhibitors have no direct effects on muscarinic receptors.

Muscarinic receptors are the predominant type of cholinergic receptor in the brain and are involved with memory, learning, and other functions.[40] Toxic effects of central muscarinic receptor blockade, which occur more frequently in the elderly, include acute confusion, delirium, disorientation, hallucination, delusion, and memory dysfunction.

The peripheral anticholinergic effects include blurred vision, dry mouth, urinary hesitancy or retention (which may cause eventual ascending urinary tract infection), severe constipation (even paralytic ileus), and acute glaucoma. Also, antimuscarinic effects can cause tachycardia, and antidepressants that potently block these receptors (e.g., amitriptyline) should be used with caution in patients with a history of ischemic heart disease.

Antidepressants have a broad range of affinities for human muscarinic receptors.[29] The most potent is amitriptyline. The SSRI paroxetine is unique among the newer compounds for having appreciable antimuscarinic potency, similar to that for imipramine.[29] Studies with cloned human muscarinic receptors show that paroxetine has greatest affinity for the m3 subtype of this receptor,[41] which is found predominantly in the brain, glandular tissue, and smooth muscle. In general, antidepressants vary little in their affinities for the five subtypes of the human muscarinic receptor. The relatively high affinity of the new antidepressant paroxetine for these receptors distinguishes it from the other newer, second-generation compounds. Also, it may explain the common complaint of dry mouth and constipation reported in some published clinical trials with paroxetine.[42] Clinicians need to be especially careful in the choice of medication for elderly patients to avoid or to minimize these antimuscarinic effects of antidepressants.

Drugs that have anticholinergic properties or hypotensive effects exacerbate the adverse effects of antidepressants. For elderly patients whose condition requires the co-administration of these drugs with antidepressants, those that have low anticholinergic and low hypotensive effects are preferred.

3. Blockade of α_1-Adrenoceptors

The property of blocking α_1-adrenoceptors likely leads to postural hypotension.[29] In the elderly, dizziness from orthostatic hypotension is a common symptom due to normal physiologic changes with aging.[43] Moreover, orthostatic hypotension is the most common serious cardiovascular adverse reaction of tricyclic antidepressants.[44] A sudden decrease in blood pressure may induce brain ischemia (even stroke) or cardiac ischemia. However, loss of consciousness and falls are more common effects in the elderly. Together with the sedative side effects, orthostatic hypotension may lead to accidental injury or death in elderly patients. Standing and supine blood pressure should be monitored before and after initiating treatment with tricyclic antidepressants and monoamine oxidase inhibitors in elderly patients. The newer second-generation antidepressants are much less likely to cause these problems.

This α_1-adrenoceptor blocking property of antidepressants can also result in the potentiation of the antihypertensive drugs that are potent α_1-antagonists (e.g., prazosin and terazosin). Antidepressants with potent α_1-adrenoceptor antagonistic property[29] are likely to have their effects clinically. Although some reports suggest that the tricyclic antidepressants doxepin and nortriptyline cause less orthostatic hypotension[45,46] than others of this class, the newer second-generation drugs are even less likely to do so.

4. Blockade of Dopamine D_2, α_2-Adrenergic, and Serotoninergic Receptors

The elderly are particularly susceptible to the side effects resulting from blockade of dopamine D_2 receptors in brain. These side effects include the so-called extrapyramidal movement disorders as well as endocrine changes. In general, antidepressants are weak competitive antagonists of dopamine D_2 receptors.[9,29] The most potent compound, amoxapine, is a demethylated derivative of the neuroleptic loxapine. It is likely that this *in vitro* activity of amoxapine explains its extrapyramidal side effects and its ability to increase prolactin levels in patients.[47,48] Because amoxapine blocks dopamine receptors, physicians are using it to treat psychotic depression. This drug is not recommended for depression in the absence of psychosis.

Amoxapine and trimipramine have no real differences in affinity for dopamine D_2 receptors. However, side effects due to this blockade have not been reported for trimipramine. One possible explanation for this difference may be that trimipramine, unlike amoxapine, has relatively potent effects on muscarinic receptors. This property can reverse the side effects caused by blocking dopamine receptors. Of interest, researchers have suggested that trimipramine may be an atypical neuroleptic.[49]

Antidepressants also block α_2 adrenoceptors, and 5-HT_{1A} and HT_{2A} serotonin receptors.[29,50] In general, antidepressants are weak blockers of these receptors. The exceptions are trazodone and nefazodone, which have a relatively potent effect at these three receptors. Potent blockade of these serotonin receptors may explain why trazodone, despite its ability to block serotonin uptake, can be used in combination with monoamine oxidase inhibitors without causing the *serotonergic syndrome*.[51]

C. FROM MISCELLANEOUS MECHANISMS

Tricyclic antidepressants affect cardiac action potentials and delay conduction through the His-Purkinje system, similar to class IA antiarrhythmic agents.[52] This property accounts for the serious risk of cardiotoxicity (heart block) associated with tricyclic antidepressants and contributes to the narrow therapeutic index of these drugs. Thus, tricyclic antidepressants should be avoided in patients with known conduction abnormalities. Furthermore, electrocardiography should be considered for elderly patients before and during treatment for depression. This effect on the conduction system of the heart is a major pharmacologic distinction between the older, tricyclic compounds and the newer, second-generation compounds. Trazodone, one of the atypical antidepressants, has few reported effects on cardiac conduction. After an overdose with trazodone, patients rarely die, but may do so as a result of seizures rather than from cardiovascular events.[53,54]

Monoamine oxidase inhibitors are sometimes prescribed for depression in the elderly. These drugs rarely cause effects on cardiac rhythm and contractility. Most commonly, these drugs cause postural hypotension. On the other hand, ingestion of foodstuffs containing tyramine (e.g., aged cheeses) by a patient on a monoamine oxidase inhibitor can cause a hypertensive crisis. This hypertension may occur more frequently in elderly than in younger patients, because cardiovascular systems of the elderly are already compromised by age. Sympathomimetic drugs in combination with monoamine oxidase inhibitors may also elevate blood pressure.

In combination with tricyclic antidepressants, lithium may be used for the treatment of manic-depressive illness. Lithium may induce sinus node abnormalities and serious disturbances of conduction.[55]

At higher dosages, maprotiline causes seizures, which limits its use in all patients, including the elderly.[56]

VI. PHARMACOKINETIC DRUG INTERACTIONS

Drug interactions for antidepressants can be divided into two groups: pharmacokinetic and pharmacodynamic. Pharmacokinetic interactions occur when one drug affects the metabolism or protein binding of another drug. Pharmacodynamic interactions occur when one drug affects the mechanism of action of another drug. We have mentioned some potential pharmacodynamic drug interactions of antidepressants, which relate to their synaptic effects. These are among the more than 40 documented drug interactions for commonly used antidepressants.[57] The prevalence of chronic physical illness and associated use of medications increases with age. For the elderly the consequence of polypharmacy is substantial. Three or more prescription drugs are taken by 85% of elderly patients,[4] and about 70% take over-the-counter drugs without discussing them with their physicians.[58] Therefore, drug interactions are common among elderly patients.

For example, antiulcer drugs (i.e., histamine H_2 receptor blockers such as cimetidine and ranitidine) can change the ionization of antidepressants. In addition, these drugs can delay gastric emptying time and the absorption of drugs administered orally.

However, one of the most significant pharmacokinetic interactions of antidepressants with other drugs is at the level of the cytochrome P450 system. The inhibition of cytochrome P450 2D6 enzyme by the SSRI fluoxetine and its metabolite norfluoxetine is now well established.[59,60] This enzyme is involved with the aromatic 2-hydroxylation of imipramine and the biotransformation of many other drugs. Inhibition of cytochrome P450 2D6 likely underlies the numerous reports of increased plasma levels of other drugs used in combination with fluoxetine.

Initially, newer SSRIs were thought to be less likely to cause these problems. However, *in vitro* studies and clinical reports suggest differences among these newer drugs. From these *in vitro* studies can be derived the following rank-order of potency for inhibition of cytochrome P450 2D6 enzyme: paroxetine > fluoxetine > sertraline >> fluvoxamine > clomipramine > venlafaxine. Among these SSRIs, fluvoxamine is the most potent at inhibiting cytochrome P450 1A2,[61] which is involved with the N-demethylation of imipramine and other compounds. Fluvoxamine is considerably more potent at inhibiting cytochrome P450 1A2 than cytochrome P450 2D6.[61]

The interactions of the newer compounds are not completely known, especially in elderly patients, but with the expanded use of these drugs more information will become available.

VII. TOXICITY IN OVERDOSE

Because of the potential risk of suicide, adverse drug reactions and toxicity in overdose are important factors to consider when choosing an antidepressant for an elderly patient. The toxicity of antidepressants in overdose is listed in Table 11.6. The newer compounds appear to be safer drugs, although little is known about their use in the elderly. Except for monoamine oxidase inhibitors, antidepressants with low affinity for cholinergic and adrenergic receptors appear to have lower toxicity in overdose.

TABLE 11.6.
Toxicity in Overdose

Antidepressants	Toxicity in Overdose
Monoamine oxidase inhibitors	High
Classic tricyclic antidepressants	Very high
Amoxapine	Very high
Maprotiline	Very high
Trazodone	Low
Bupropion	Low
Fluoxetine	Low
Sertraline	Low
Paroxetine	Low
Venlafaxine	Low
Nefazodone	Low

VIII. SUMMARY

The population of elderly people is growing rapidly and the incidence of depression increases with age. Elderly patients are generally more susceptible than younger patients to side effects, including adverse drug reactions. In this chapter, we have reviewed the pharmacodynamics and pharmacokinetics of antidepressants in the elderly. The second-generation compounds offer clear advantages over the tricyclic antidepressants. However, they are not without some problems. Information presented here should help physicians select the appropriate antidepressant for an elderly patient to avoid or minimize certain adverse effects and drug-drug interactions.

REFERENCES

1. *Diagnostic and Statistical Manual of Mental Disorders (Third Edition — Revised)*, American Psychiatric Association, Washington, D.C., 1987.
2. **Judd, L. L., Braff, D. L., Britton, K. T., Risch, C., Gillin, C., and Grant, I.,** Psychiatry and medicine, in *Harrison's Principles of Internal Medicine*, Wilson, J. D., Braunwald, E., Isselbacher, K. J., Petersdorf, R. G., Martin, J. B., Fauci, A. S., and Root, R. K., Eds., McGraw-Hill, New York, 1991, chap. 368.
3. **Brown, W. A.,** Effect of aging on DST Results, *Am. J. Psychiatry*, 139, 1376, 1982.
4. **Jenike, M. A.,** Handbook of Geriatric Psychopharmacology, John Wright PSG Publishing, Littleton, 1985.
5. **Cunha, U. V.,** Antidepressants: their uses in nonpsychiatric disorders of aging, *Geriatrics*, 41, 63, 1986.
6. **Evans, L., Kenardy, J., Schneider, P., and Hoey, H.,** Effect of a selective serotonin uptake inhibitor in agoraphobia with panic attacks — a double-blind comparison of zimelidine, imipramine and placebo, *Acta Psychiatr. Scand.*, 73, 49, 1986.

7. **Murphy, D. L., Zohar, J., Benkelfat, C., Pato, M. T., Pigott, T. A., and Insel, T. R.,** Obsessive-compulsive disorder as a 5-HT subsystem-related behavioral disorder, *Br. J. Psychiatry*, 155, 15, 1989.
8. **Sulser, F.,** Mode of action of antidepressant drugs, *J. Cl. Psychiatry*, 5, 14, 1983.
9. **Richelson, E.,** Antidepressants and brain neurochemistry, *Mayo Clin. Proc.*, 65, 1227, 1990.
10. **Richelson, E.,** Pharmacology of antidepressants — characteristics of the ideal drug, *Mayo Clin. Proc.*, 69, 1069, 1994.
11. **Halper, J. P., Mann, J. J., Weksler, M. E., Bilezikian, J. P., Sweeney, J. A., Brown, R. P., and T., G.,** Beta adrenergic receptors and cyclic AMP levels in intact human lymphocytes: effects of age and gender, *Life Sci.*, 35, 855, 1984.
12. **Mann, J. J. and Arango, V.,** CNS adrenergic receptors and beta blockade [Review], *Postgrad. Med.*, 135, 1988.
13. **Gottfries, C. G., Adolfsson, R., Aquilonius, S. M., Carlsson, A., Eckernas, S. A., Nordberg, A., Oreland, L., Svennerholm, L., Wiberg, A., and Winblad, B.,** Biochemical changes in dementia disorders of Alzheimer type (AD/SDAT), *Neurobiol. Aging*, 4, 261, 1983.
14. **Brown, A. S. and Gershon, S.,** Dopamine and depression, *J. Neural Transm. Gen. Sect.*, 91, 75, 1993.
15. **Wallace, S. M. and Verbeeck, R. K.,** Plasma protein binding of drugs in the elderly, *Clin. Pharmacokinetics*, 12, 41, 1987.
16. **Greenblatt, D. J., Sellers, E. M., and Shader, R. I.,** Drug therapy: drug disposition in old age, *N. Engl. J. Med.*, 306, 1081, 1982.
17. **O'Malley, K., Crooks, J., Duke, E., and Stevenson, I. H.,** Effect of age and sex on human drug metabolism, *Br. Med. J.*, 3, 607, 1971.
18. **Vestal, R. E., Norris, A. H., Tobin, J. D., Cohen, B. H., Shock, N. W., and Andres, R.,** Antipyrine metabolism in man: influence of age, alcohol, caffeine, and smoking, *Clin. Pharmacol. Ther.*, 18, 425, 1975.
19. **Young, R. C., Dhar, A. K., Kutt, H., and Alexopoulos, G. S.,** Isomers of 10-hydroxynortriptyline in geriatric depression, *Ther. Drug Monit.*, 10, 164, 1988.
20. **Schneider, L. S., Cooper, T. B., Suckow, R. F., Lyness, S. A., Haugen, C., Palmer, R., and Sloane, R. B.,** Relationship of hydroxynortriptyline to nortriptyline concentration and creatinine clearance in depressed elderly outpatients, *J. Clin. Psychopharmacol.*, 10, 333, 1990.
21. **Gram, L. F.,** Metabolism of tricyclic antidepressants. A review, *Dan. Med. Bull.*, 21, 218, 1974.
22. **Woodhouse, K. W. and James, O. F.,** Hepatic drug metabolism and ageing, *Br. Med. Bull.*, 46, 22, 1990.
23. **Rowe, J. W., Andres, R., Tobin, J. D., Norris, A. H., and Shock, N. W.,** The effect of age on creatinine clearance in men: a cross-sectional and longitudinal study, *J. Gerontol.*, 31, 155, 1976.
24. **Kitanaka, I., Ross, R. J., Cutler, N. R., Zavadil, A. P. D., and Potter, W. Z.,** Altered hydroxydesipramine concentrations in elderly depressed patients, *Clin. Pharmacol. Ther.*, 31, 51, 1982.
25. **Bergstrom, R. F., Beasley, C. M., Levy, N. B., Blumenfield, M., and Lemberger, L.,** The effects of renal and hepatic disease on the pharmacokinetics, renal tolerance, and risk benefit profile of fluoxetine, *Int. Clin. Psychopharmacol.*, 8, 261, 1993.
26. **Norman, T. R.,** Pharmacokinetic aspects of antidepressant treatment in the elderly, *Progr. Neuro-Psychopharmacol. Biol. Psychiatry*, 17, 329, 1993.
27. **von Moltke, L. L., Greenblatt, D. J., and Shader, R. I.,** Clinical pharmacokinetics of antidepressants in the elderly. Therapeutic implications, *Clin. Pharmacokinetics*, 24, 141, 1993.
28. Tricyclic antidepressants — blood level measurements and clinical outcome: an APA Task Force report, Task Force on the Use of Laboratory Tests in Psychiatry, *Am. J. Psychiatry*, 142, 155, 1985.
29. **Cusack, B., Nelson, A., and Richelson, E.,** Binding of antidepressants to human brain receptors — focus on newer generation compounds, *Psychopharmacology*, 114, 559, 1994.
30. **Reimherr, F. W., Chouinard, G., Cohn, C. K., Cole, J. O., Itil, T. M., LaPierre, Y. D., Masco, H. L., and Mendels, J.,** Antidepressant efficacy of sertraline: a double-blind, placebo- and amitriptyline-controlled multicenter comparison study in outpatients with major depression, *J. Clin. Psychiatry*, 51, 18, 1991.
31. **Beasley, C. M., Masica, D. N., Heiligenstein, J. H., Wheadon, D. E., and Zerbe, R. L.,** Possible monoamine oxidase inhibitor serotonin uptake inhibitor interaction — fluoxetine clinical data and preclinical findings, *J. Clin. Psychopharmacol.*, 13, 312, 1993.
32. **Bouchard, R. H., Pourcher, E., and Vincent, P.,** Fluoxetine and extrapyramidal side effects, *Am. J. Psychiatry*, 146, 1352, 1989.
33. **Shihabuddin, L. and Rapport, D.,** Sertraline and extrapyramidal side effects, *Am. J. Psychiatry*, 151, 288, 1994.
34. **Gardier, A. M., Lepoul, E., Trouvin, J. H., Chanut, E., Dessalles, M. C., and Jacquot, C.,** Changes in dopamine metabolism in rat forebrain regions after cessation of long-term fluoxetine treatment — relationship with brain concentrations of fluoxetine and norfluoxetine, *Life Sci.*, 54, 51, 1994.
35. **Baldessarini, R., Marsh, E. R., and Kula, N. S.,** Interactions of fluoxetine with metabolism of dopamine and serotonin in rat brain regions, *Brain Res.*, 579, 152, 1992.
36. **Caccia, S., Fong, M. H., Garattini, S., and Zanini, M. G.,** Plasma concentrations of trazodone and 1-(3-chlorophenyl) piperazine in man after a single oral dose of trazodone, *J. Pharm. Pharmacol.*, 34, 605, 1982.

37. **Abernethy, D. R., Greenblatt, D. J., and Shader, R. I.,** Plasma levels of trazodone: methodology and applications, *Pharmacology*, 28, 42, 1984.
38. **Richelson, E.,** Muscarinic receptors: molecular biology and neuropsychopharmacology, in *Treatment of Dementias*, Meyer, E., Ed., Plenum Press, New York, 1992, 3.
39. **Stanton, T., Bolden-Watson, C., Cusack, B., and Richelson, E.,** Antagonism of the 5 cloned human muscarinic cholinergic receptors expressed in CHO-K1 cells by antidepressants and antihistaminics, *Biochem. Pharmacol.*, 45, 2352, 1993.
40. **Boyer, W. F. and Blumhardt, C. L.,** The safety profile of paroxetine, *J. Clin. Psychiatry*, 53, 61, 1992.
41. **Caird, F. I., Andrews, G. R., and Kennedy, R. D.,** Effect of posture on blood pressure in the elderly, *Br. Heart J.*, 35, 527, 1973.
42. **Glassman, A. H. and Bigger, J. T., Jr.,** Cardiovascular effects of therapeutic doses of tricyclic antidepressants. A review, *Arch. Gen. Psychiatry*, 38, 815, 1981.
43. **Neshkes, R. E., Gerner, R., Jarvik, L. F., Mintz, J., Joseph, J., Linde, S., Aldrich, J., Connolly, M. E., Rosen, R., and Hill, M.,** Orthostatic effect of imipramine and doxepin in depressed geriatric outpatients, *J. Clin. Psychopharmacol.*, 5, 102, 1985.
44. **Roose, S. P., Glassman, A. H., Siris, S. G., Walsh, B. T., Bruno, R. L., and Wright, L. B.,** Comparison of imipramine- and nortriptyline-induced orthostatic hypotension: a meaningful difference, *J. Clin. Psychopharmacol.*, 1, 316, 1981.
45. **Steele, T. E.,** Adverse reactions suggesting amoxapine-induced dopamine blockade, *Am. J. Psychiatry*, 139, 1500, 1982.
46. **Cooper, D. S., Gelenberg, A. J., Wojcik, J. C., Saxe, V. C., Ridgway, E. C., and Maloof, F.,** The effect of amoxapine and imipramine on serum prolactin levels, *Arch. Intern. Med.*, 141, 1023, 1981.
47. **Eikmeier, G., Berger, M., Lodemann, E., Muszynski, K., Kaumeier, S., and Gastpar, M.,** Trimipramine — an atypical neuroleptic?, *Int. Clin. Psychopharmacol.*, 6, 147, 1991.
48. **Richelson, E. and Nelson, A.,** Antagonism by antidepressants of neurotransmitter receptors of normal human brain in vitro, *J. Pharmacol. Exp. Ther.*, 230, 94, 1984.
49. **Nierenberg, A. A. and Keck, P. E.,** Management of monoamine oxidase inhibitor-associated insomnia with trazodone, *J. Clin. Psychopharmacol.*, 9, 42, 1989.
50. **Glassman, A. H. and Preud'homme, X. A.,** Review of the cardiovascular effects of heterocyclic antidepressants, *J. Clin. Psychiatry*, 54, 16, 1993.
51. **Hames, T. K., Burgess, C. D., and George, C. F.,** Hemodynamic responses of trazodone and imipramine, *Clin. Pharmacol. Ther.*, 32, 497, 1982.
52. **Glassman, A. H.,** The newer antidepressant drugs and their cardiovascular effects, *Psychopharmacol. Bull.*, 20, 272, 1984.
53. **Montalescot, G., Levy, Y., Farge, D., Brochard, L., Fantin, B., Arnoux, C., and Hatt, P. Y.,** Lithium causing a serious sinus-node dysfunction at therapeutic doses, *Clin. Cardiol.*, 7, 617, 1984.
54. **Grüter, W. and Poldinger, W.,** Maprotiline, *Mod. Probl. Pharmacopsychiatry*, 18, 17, 1982.
55. **Perry, P. J., Alexander, B., and Liskow, B. I.,** Psychotropic drug handbook, Harvey Whitney Books, Cincinnati, 1991.
56. **Lamy, P. P.,** Drug interactions and the elderly — a new perspective, *Drug Intell. Clin. Pharmacol.*, 14, 513, 1980.
57. **Crewe, H. K., Lennard, M. S., Tucker, G. T., Woods, F. R., and Haddock, R. E.,** The effect of selective serotonin uptake inhibitors on cytochrome-p4502d6 (CYP2d6) activity in human liver microsomes, *Br. J. Clin. Pharmacol.*, 34, 262, 1992.
58. **Otton, S. V., Wu, D., Joffe, R. T., Cheung, S. W., and Sellers, E. M.,** Inhibition by fluoxetine of cytochrome-P450 2D6 activity, *Clin. Pharmacol. Ther.*, 53, 401, 1993.
59. **Brosen, K., Skjelbo, E., Rasmussen, B. B., Poulsen, H. E., and Loft, S.,** Fluvoxamine is a potent inhibitor of cytochrome-p4501a2, *Biochem. Pharmacol.*, 45, 1211, 1993.
60. **Steiner, W. and R., F.,** Toxic reaction following the combined administration of fluoxetine and L tryptophan: five case reports, *Biol. Psychiatry*, 21, 1067, 1986.
61. **Hollander, E., DeCaria, C. M., Schneier, F. R., Schneier, H. A., Liebowitz, M. R., and Klein, D. F.,** Fenfluramine augmentation of serotonin uptake blockade antiobsessional treatment, *J. Clin. Psychiatry*, 51, 119, 1990.

Chapter 12

NOOTROPICS AND AGENTS FOR TREATING ALZHEIMER'S DISEASE

Jair C. Soares and Samual Gershon

CONTENTS

0-8493-8306-4/96/$0.00+$.50

I. INTRODUCTION

It has been more than 80 years since Alois Alzheimer first described the degenerative brain disorder that later would have his name.[1] Individuals with Alzheimer's disease (AD) develop a syndrome of acquired intellectual deterioration, which manifests as memory loss accompanied by a variety of other cognitive impairments, such as visuospatial dysfunction, dysphasia, and problems with abstraction, calculation, and concentration.

Dementia has been defined as a clinical syndrome characterized by memory loss and impairment in higher cortical functions, which interferes with daily living activities and social functioning.[2] In the U.S., community surveys indicated that as much as 6.2% of the population over age 65 and up to 47.2% of those over 85 have dementia.[3] Most demented individuals (up to 80%) are thought to have AD. Hagnell et al.[4] suggested an annual incidence rate of 0.7% for men and 0.5% for women, aged 70 to 79 years, and 1.9 and 2.5% for over 80 years of age. Prevalence of dementia increases with age, due to rising incidence with age. As the proportion of elderly people in the population has been increasing, dementia is gradually becoming a great challenge for public health systems worldwide.

AD is characterized histopathologically by the formation of senile plaques, which are collections of granular material, including degenerating neurites and glia, around a core of amyloid material and neurofibrillary tangles (NFT). The nature of these abnormalities has been the object of intense research efforts over the past decade.

The sequence of pathologic processes in AD is currently under discussion: AD could begin with synaptic loss and deposition of amyloid β-protein following the neurodegeneration or, on the contrary, plaques, NFT, Lewy bodies, infarcts, and lacunae would induce neuronal loss and dementia.

Specific symptom clusters require treatment in AD patients, such as agitation, anxiety, insomnia, depression, and delusions. These symptoms are extremely important in the overall treatment of the disorder, since they are common and cause significant comorbidity. Another approach for treatment is aimed at improving cognition. The majority of trials in AD over the past 3 decades have targeted this aspect of the disorder.

If treatments for preventing, curing, or retarding the cognitive deficits caused by AD become available, this would certainly be of great importance to an elderly population that will increase even more in the future, and also will become a major issue in health care policy planning.

II. DIAGNOSIS

A. CLASSIFICATION OF COGNITIVE DEFICITS

Cognitive impairment can be either congenital, as in mental retardation, or acquired during life. There are many types of acquired cognitive disorder. Some involve acute loss of cognitive skills, such as intoxication, delirium, or depression with cognitive deficit, and others are more chronic, such as dementias, amnestic syndrome, and other brain syndromes. Age-associated cognitive deficits (AACD) involve the dementias and cognitive deficits of normal aging. It is a very controversial issue to what extent cognitive decline would be part of the normal process of aging.[5] Amaducci et al.,[6] in a review of this literature, conclude that "benign forgetfullness" probably represents an early stage of AD in a high percentage of cases.

B. DSM-IV CRITERIA

Standard diagnostic criteria are of great assistance for research on dementia. They help to assure that different investigators are studying the same disorder. Accurate diagnosis of specific dementias is difficult to obtain during a patient's life. Definitive diagnosis must be obtained from neuropathological confirmation at autopsy or biopsy. Thus, both clinicians and researchers must rely on a clinical diagnosis only. Then, the diagnosis of the syndrome of dementia is much more practical than diagnosing specific diseases, since it is defined only in terms of clinical features.

Among the most accepted diagnostic criteria are those published by the American Psychiatric Association in their Diagnostic and Statistical Manual of Mental Disorders. These criteria had a recent major revision in 1987 (DSM IIIR),[2] and a new revision recently became effective (DSM IV).[7] The new DSM IV criteria for diagnosis of dementias are listed below.

DSM IV criteria-Dementias

Dementia of the Alzheimer Type

A. The development of multiple cognitive deficits manifested by both:

(1) memory impairment (inability to learn new information and to recall previously learned information)

(2) at least one of the following cognitive disturbances:

(a) aphasia (language disturbance)

(b) apraxia (inability to carry out motor activities despite intact motor function)

(c) agnosia (failure to recognize or identify objects despite intact sensory function)

(d) disturbance in executive functioning (i.e., planning, organizing, sequencing, abstracting)

B. The course is characterized by gradual onset and continuing cognitive decline.

C. The cognitive deficits cause significant impairment in social or occupational functioning and represent a significant decline from a previous level of functioning.

D. The cognitive deficits in A are not due to any of the following:

(1) central nervous system conditions that cause progressive deficits in memory and cognition (e.g., cerebrovascular disease, Parkinson's disease, Huntington's disease, subdural hematoma, normal pressure hydrocephalus)

(2) systemic conditions that are known to cause dementia (e.g., hypothyroidism, vitamin B12 or folic acid deficiency, niacin deficiency, hypercalcemia, neurosyphilis, HIV infection)

(3)Substance-induced conditions

E. The deficits do not occur exclusively during the course of Delirium.

F. Not better accounted for by another Axis I disorder (e.g., Major Depressive Disorder, Schizophrenia).

Vascular Dementia

Same criteria for dementia reported above, but with focal neurologic signs and symptoms (e.g., exaggeration of deep tendon reflexes, extensor plantar response, pseudobulbar palsy, gait abnormalities, weakness of an extremity) or laboratory evidence indicative of cerebral vascular disease (e.g., multiple infarctions involving cortex and underlying white matter) that are judged to be etiologically related to the disturbance

Dementia Due to Other Medical Conditions

There is evidence from history, physical examination, or laboratory findings of one of the following conditions, that is judged to be etiologically related to the disturbance: HIV disease, head trauma, Parkinson's Disease, Huntington's Disease, Pick's Disease, Creutzfeldt-Jakob Disease, other general medical conditions including normal pressure hydrocephalus, hypothyroidism, brain tumor, vitamin B12 deficiency.

Substance-Induced Persisting Dementia

There is evidence from the history, physical examination, or laboratory findings of substance use (e.g., drugs of abuse, medication, toxin exposure) judged to be etiologically related to the disturbance.

Dementia Due to Multiple Etiologies

Evidence from the history, physical examination, or laboratory tests that the disturbance has more than one etiology (e.g., head trauma plus chronic alcohol use, Dementia of the Alzheimer's Type, with the subsequent development of Vascular Dementia)

Dementia Not Otherwise Specified

Cognitive Disorder Not Otherwise Specified

C. DIFFERENTIAL DIAGNOSIS

The differential diagnosis of a suspected case of memory impairment should include various neuropsychiatric conditions, including delirium, mental retardation, amnestic syndrome, other organic brain disorders, functional psychiatric disorders, diminished cognitive capacity (early dementia), subjective change, age-associated memory impairment (AAMI), and dementia.[8]

Age-related cognitive disorders can be divided into five types: AAMI, pseudodementias, secondary dementias, vascular dementias, and primary dementias.[9] AAMI may be part of an increased normal aging process or may be an early phase of dementia.[5] Pseudodementia is

TABLE 12.1.
Differential Diagnosis of Suspected Memory Impairment

Mental retardation
Delirium
Amnestic syndrome and other circumscribed neuropsychological disorders
Other organic brain disorder
Functional psychiatric disorder
Diminished cognitive capacity (early dementia)
Subjective change
Age-associated memory impairment (AAMI)
Dementia

Extracted from: Erkinjuntti et al. Diagnostic assessments and criteria for memory disorders in clinical drug trials, in *Guidelines for Drug Trials in Memory Disorders*, N. Canal et al., Eds., Raven Press, New York, 1993. With permission.

the cognitive impairment attributable to other psychiatric disorders, such as depression or delirium. Secondary dementias are those cognitive impairments due to somatic diseases that affect the brain, like neuroendocrine diseases or hypovitaminoses. Vascular dementias and Alzheimer's dementia are the two most important primary dementias.

Primary degenerative dementias are the most frequent disorders causing the syndrome of dementia. This group includes diseases whose etiology or pathogenesis is assumed to be within the brain itself, evidenced by an atrophic process or a metabolic dysfunction. Among the dementias, differential diagnoses to be considered include AD, Pick's disease, normal pressure hydrocephalus, multi-infarct dementia, Lewy body disease, frontobasal degeneration, subcortical gliosis, alcoholic dementia, dementia associated with depression and AAMI.

TABLE 12.2.
Differential Diagnosis of Primary Degenerative Dementia

Dementia associated with depression
Normal pressure hydrocephalus
Multi-infarct dementia
Alcoholic dementia
Frontobasal degeneration
Subcortical gliosis
Alzheimer's disease
Pick's disease
Lewy body disease
Age-associated memory impairment

AD used to be classified as a presenile dementia as distinguished from the more common senile dementia of the elderly. Tomlinson et al.,[10] in their pathological studies of elderly demented patients, found neuropathological characteristics of AD in most of these cases, while a smaller proportion had multiple infarcts. After that, the term senile dementia of the Alzheimer type became increasingly established, but it was still distinguished from presenile AD. Katzman[11] had an important role in promoting a unitary concept of AD, referring to both presenile and senile cases under the same name. Currently, AD is commonly used to refer to all cases, irrespective of age at onset.

III. DRUGS FOR COGNITION ENHANCEMENT — HISTORICAL BACKGROUND

An enormous number of drug trials in AD have been published over the past several years. Several drugs have been tried in an attempt to improve memory and cognitive function, to alter the course of the disease, or to modify behavioral symptoms associated with AD, such as delusions, agitation, insomnia, and depression.

There is some evidence that memory training and drug treatment have a complementary effect on cognitive functions, and that they could potentiate each other, suggesting a role for these techniques in the treatment of AACD.[12]

Most of the drugs being investigated for AD are proposed to improve cognitive functions by enhancing neurotransmission. This group includes cholinomimetics, other neurotransmitter agonists, neuropeptides, and nootropics. Treatments aimed at changing the course of AD have been proposed based on current hypotheses for the etiology of the disease. They include chelation agents, hormone therapy, nerve growth factor (NGF), and neuronal transplantation. Finally, treatments designed to control behavioral abnormalities include antipsychotic agents, minor tranquilizers, and antidepressant drugs. In this chapter, we will limit the scope of our review to the treatments proposed to enhance cognition in these patients.

A. HYPERBARIC OXYGEN

Increased cerebral oxygenation was proposed to treat AD patients, because it was thought that cerebral vascular disease was related to the disorder. Jacobs et al.,[13] in an uncontrolled study, described benefits after 15 d of intermittent exposure to 100% oxygen at 2.5 atm, two times a day, in sessions of 1.5 hr each. This study was followed by a controlled study,[14] under the same conditions as the original one, which showed no advantage in cognitive performance, cerebral blood flow, or EEG. Goldfarb et al.[15] also failed to find benefits with this therapy.

B. VASODILATORS

The use of vasodilators for the treatment of dementia was originally based on the assumption that a narrowing of the brain vessels caused decreased cerebral blood flow. Two distinct types of vasodilators were studied, pure pharmacological vasodilators and those which also stimulate cerebral metabolism. The first class of agents included papaverine, cyclandelate, cinarizine, ixosuprine, and carbonic anhydrase inhibitors. Papaverine was shown to increase cerebral blood flow, and some studies reported cognitive improvement with this drug over placebo.[16–19] None of the other pure vasodilators have shown long-term clinical improvement. Yesavage et al.,[20] in a review of this literature, found two-thirds of the studies showing some evidence of improvement, but only one claimed clinically significant improvement. The second type of vasodilators, dihydroergotoxin mesylate (Hydergine) and naftidrofuryl, act presumably by increasing central nervous system (CNS) metabolism. Hydergine increases intracellular cyclic adenosine monophosphate (cAMP), and naftidrofuryl increases relative adenosine triphosphate stores. The studies done with these agents failed to find a definitive improvement in cognition.[21–37] Dementia caused by vascular diseases was later considered to be the result of infarctions rather than chronic hypoxia, and then there was little rationale for using vasodilators to try to enhance cognition.

C. ANTICOAGULANTS

The anticoagulants theoretically would be of value for multi-infarct dementia by preventing thrombotic processes. Agents such as bishydroxycoumarin and warfarin sodium have been investigated, but the studies performed did not demonstrate benefits of these agents as cognitive enhancers.[38,39]

D. PSYCHOSTIMULANTS

Psychostimulants have effects of arousal and mood elevation. They were used as mood elevators and as attention enhancers. This class of drug was investigated after findings of decreased adrenergic activity and increase in monoamine oxidase B (MAO B) in AD patients. The agents that were investigated include procaine hydrochloride, dextroamphetamine, methylphenidate, pentylenetetrazol, pipradol, and pemoline.

Dextroamphetamine, in normal subjects, was found to produce paradoxical drowsiness and decreased brain activity in 65% of subjects.[40] Of the three controlled studies done with methylphenidate,[41–43] only one found clinical improvement. For pentylenetetrazol, the great majority of studies did not show clear positive results.[44] For pipradol, one controlled study showed it to be better than placebo after 3 weeks of administration, but not thereafter on weeks 4 through 9.[45] For pemoline, the investigations done were generally negative.[46,47]

E. NOOTROPICS

The "metabolic enhancers" or nootropics do not interact directly with any specific neurotransmitter system. Preclinical research suggested that metabolic enhancers (nootropics) may improve cognitive functions, including vigilance, acquisition, and memory.[48] The main agents in this class include piracetam, oxiracetam, and newer agents, like BMY 21502.

Piracetam is a cyclic derivative of GABA that does not have GABAergic effects. The results of preclinical research were promising,[49,50] but the results of clinical trials were discouraging. It was reported to improve memory in nondemented elderly subjects,[51] but in demented patients the results have been conflicting.[52,53] A recent double-blind, placebo-controlled trial in 33 early probable AD patients, with high doses over 1 year, suggested that this agent might slow the progression of cognitive deterioration in these patients.[54]

Several studies examined the efficacy of piracetam combined with choline[55] or lecithin[55–60] for treatment of AD patients, but the results of these studies were disappointing.

Oxiracetam has been found to be at least two to five times more active than piracetam in improving learning and memory in both normal and cerebrally impaired animals.[61] Initial clinical trials in elderly patients with organic brain syndrome showed oxiracetam to be superior to placebo[62] and provetam[63] in decreasing symptomatology. Compared to piracetam, it seems to offer some advantages.[64] More recent clinical trials conducted in patients with primary degenerative dementia and multi-infarct dementia suggested that oxiracetam might be useful for dementia patients, producing improvement in some measures of cognitive performance,[65–68] but the studies done in AD patients[69–73] did not find evidence of effectiveness. Therefore, the efficacy of oxiracetam for this indication is not adequately defined.

Pramiracetam has also been tested in AD patients, but to date there is no consistent evidence of a beneficial effect.[74,75]

Aniracetam is another nootropic which underwent investigation. The initial trials on AD did not find any evidence of effectiveness,[76,77] and a more recent trial[78] suggested that it can improve psychobehavioral measures in AD patients.

F. NEUROPEPTIDES

ACTH and vasopressin were reported to influence the maintenance of conditioned avoidance responses in animals.[79] Findings of reduced concentrations of somatostatin, vasopressin, substance P, corticotropin releasing factor, neuropeptide Y, galanin, and neurotensin, and normal concentrations of cholecystokinin and vasoactive intestinal polypeptide in post-mortem brain tissue of AD patients have been reported.[80]

The use of GABA agonists, like 4,5,6,7-tetrahydroisoxazolo(5,4-c)pyridin-3-ol, was studied by Mohr et al.[81] in a double blind study, which did not find any clinically significant change in cognition. Clinical trials done with lysine vasopressin and the vasopressin-related peptides 1-desamino-8-D-arginine vasopressin and desglycinamide arginine vasopressin failed to identify consistent improvement in memory.[82–87] The somatostatin analog L363,586 did not show significant improvement in cognition in AD patients.[88] Thyrotropin releasing hormone has been proposed to increase cholinergic function in AD, but in the one trial showing improvement in semantic memory, the effects on arousal and mood were more impressive than the effects on cognition.[89]

ACTH components 4-9 and 4-10 have been investigated. Studies on ACTH 4-9 showed improvements in ratings of depression, anxiety, and sociability, but little effect on memory deficits.[90] A recent study in a small sample of AD patients showed activating properties of ACTH 4-9, and no significant effects on cognition.[91] Miller et al.[92] reported a study of a synthetic ACTH 4-9 analog (Org 2766), using doses twice those reported in previous studies, and did not find a positive effect on cognition in AD patients. The studies done on ACTH 4-10 also failed to show clear benefits on cognition or memory.[93–95] An ACTH analog that has been investigated is HOE 427. This compound has been found to have good tolerability, to have significant effects in mood and attention, but not clearly beneficial effects on cognition.[96]

Somatostatin replacement therapy, with the synthetic analog octreotide, was tested in a double-blind placebo-controlled trial in AD patients, without any findings suggestive of benefits in either neuropsychological or cerebral metabolic measures.[97]

G. CHOLINOMIMETICS

The findings of decreased choline acetyltransferase in the brains of AD patients and a loss of cholinergic neurons in the ventral forebrain stimulated investigations on drugs that could enhance cholinergic transmission.

Choline was initially studied, but the majority of the studies were discouraging.[98] Lecithin, a natural dietary source of acetylcholine (ACh), had an initial open trial showing positive results,[99] but several subsequent studies were negative.[100–104]

Arecoline, a natural alkaloid, was shown to improve serial learning in normal volunteers,[105] but studies with intravenous administration of arecoline to AD patients did not find significant effects in cognition,[106,107] except for a recent small controlled trial in eight AD patients, which showed evidence of significant improvements of verbal memory during intravenous administration for a 2-week period.[108]

RS-86, a long-acting cholinergic agonist, was given orally to AD patients, but no clinically significant improvement was reported.[109–112]

Bethanechol, an ACh analog, has been tested in intracerebral administration, since it does not penetrate the blood-brain barrier, but the results have been disappointing.[113–117]

Davis et al.[118] studied the effect of oxotremorine, a synthetic cholinergic agonist, in AD patients. They did not find evidence of significant effects on cognition, and the medication had to be discontinued in most of the patients due to significant side effects.

Newhouse et al.[119] studied the effect of intravenous administration of nicotine bitartrate to non-smoking AD patients in a single-blind study, and found that it decreased the rate of intrusion errors, but higher doses caused significant side-effects, limiting the therapeutic potential of this drug. Another trial with this agent showed improvement in attention and information processing in AD patients, but no significant effects in short-term memory.[120]

Molloy and Cape[121] conducted a double-blind, placebo-controlled trial with oral administration of pyridostigmine in AD patients, and did not find any evidence of significant improvement in cognitive function.

Physostigmine, a tertiary amine which acts by inhibiting acetylcholinesterase (AChE), initially was found to have positive results in AD patients in infusion studies,[122,123] but the studies done with oral physostigmine were not encouraging.[124–128] Two recent studies in primary degenerative dementia and senile and presenile AD, testing oral physostigmine in double-blind, placebo-controlled designs, did not find significant cognitive changes associated with physostigmine.[129,130] Two other recent studies raised the possibility that a subgroup of AD patients might benefit from long-term physostigmine therapy, which could decrease the rate of cognitive deterioration.[131,132] A combination strategy with oral physostigmine and yohimbine, an α_2 pre- and post-synaptic adrenergic receptor antagonist, was tested in AD patients under double-blind, placebo-controlled conditions, and no evidence of significant cognitive improvement was found.[133]

H. OPIATE ANTAGONISTS

Opiate antagonists were found to increase learning and memory in animal models.[134] Since then, opiate antagonists have been investigated as potential agents for the treatment of cognitive dysfunction. Initial trials with intravenous administration of naloxone (opioid antagonist) in AD patients produced positive results,[135] but subsequent studies did not confirm these findings.[136,137] Two other trials failed to demonstrate significant benefits on cognition of intravenous naloxone.[138,139] Another opiate antagonist, naltrexone, in oral administration failed to demonstrate significant clinical improvement in cognition in AD patients.[140,141]

I. HORMONES

The incidence of AD is slightly higher in women than in men above 50 years of age.[142] There are data suggesting that the administration of estrogen to ovariectomized rats increases choline acetyltransferase activity, and it was proposed that estrogen replacement therapy might prevent AD.[143]

Some clinical trials with administration of estrogen to "organic brain syndrome" and demented patients reported benefits in cognition,[143–145] but there also have been negative trials.[146] Nonetheless, the cognitive changes detected in the above trials are difficult to separate from effects on attention and mood. Lifshitz and Kline,[147] administering estrogens for 15 months to elderly men in a psychogeriatric unit, found increased mortality in the estrogen group.

K. MONOAMINERGIC DRUGS

Post-mortem studies have found decreased concentrations of noradrenaline and dopamine-β-hydroxylase, as well as extensive neuronal loss in the locus ceruleus, in brains of AD patients.[148,149] Decreased D_2 dopamine receptors and dopamine levels have also been reported in these patients.[150,151] Patients with AD have also been found to have decreased concentrations of 5-HIAA on autopsy[152] and low levels in the cerebrospinal fluid.[153]

Drugs that stimulate catecholamine function seem to improve cognitive performance, but their action on memory appears mainly to be related to changes in arousal and concentration.

L-Dopa treatment has been tested in patients with AD. Out of three double-blind studies,[154–156] only one showed benefits.

The α_2-adrenoreceptor agonists clonidine and guanfacine were found to improve memory in aged monkeys,[157] but clinical trials with these agents in AD patients did not show significant benefits.[158–160]

5-Hydroxytryptamine (5-HT) reuptake blockers, such as citalopram, alaproclate, and zimeldine, are also among the agents studied as possible cognition enhancers. The initial studies with these drugs have not been promising.[161–163] Three more recent studies with citalopram failed to find evidence of benefits on cognition, but found evidence of improvement in behavioral symptoms, such as mood, irritability, anxiety, and restlessness.[164–166] A more recent double-blind, placebo-controlled trial with fluvoxamine (150 mg/d) in 46 patients with primary degenerative dementia or multi-infarct dementia, for 6 weeks, also failed to find any evidence of benefit on cognition or behavior.[167]

Meta-chlorophenylpiperazine, a 5-HT agonist, was administered to moderate to severe AD patients, in a 16-d, double-blind, placebo-controlled trial, and it was found to increase anergy and depressive symptoms, without any significant change in cognition.[168]

IV. NEW DEVELOPMENTS IN AD PHARMACOTHERAPY

A. CHOLINERGIC AGENTS

In AD and several other dementias, dysfunction in cholinergic basal forebrain neurons correlates with the severity of cognitive impairment, and this led to the development of strategies aimed at enhancing the activity in this system. Post-mortem neuropathologic and biochemical analyses have confirmed that AD is associated with abnormalities of the cholinergic system. Davies and Maloney,[169] in an examination of autopsy AD brain tissue, found decreased choline acetyltransferase, which is the enzyme responsible for the conversion of choline to ACh, in the amygdala, hippocampus, and cortex. Whitehouse et al.[170] reported a selective degeneration of the neurons in the nucleus basalis of Meynert, an area rich in cholinergic innervation. The approaches currently tested to increase cholinergic transmission are listed below.

1. AchE Inhibitors

THA (9-amino-1,2,3,4-tetrahydroacridine) is a synthetic AChE inhibitor that crosses the blood-brain barrier. It is a potent AChE inhibitor, and also has actions in different systems: inhibits AChE, is a partial antagonist of morphine, and inhibits cyclic AMP phosphodiesterase. It is also postulated to selectively block K channels and inhibit Na channel inactivation, down-regulate type 1 muscarinic receptors, alter phosphorylation, and stimulate cholinergic firing, and at high doses blocks pre- and post-synaptic muscarinic and nicotinic receptors.

TABLE 12.3.
Chemical Structure of THA

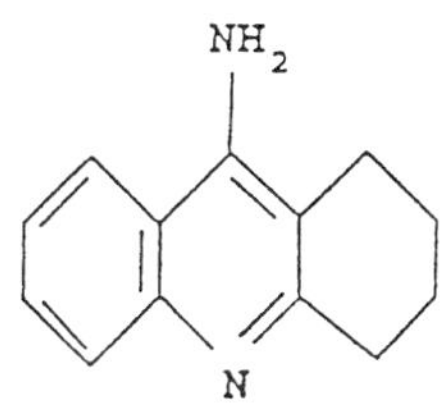

Extracted from Thornton, J. E. and Gershon, S., The history of THA, in *Current Research in Alzheimer Therapy*, E. Giaconini and R. Becker, Eds., Taylor & Francis, New York, 1988. With permission.

TABLE 12.4.
Pharmacologic Actions of 1,2,3,4-Tetrahydro-5-Aminoacridine (THA)

Established actions

Inhibits acetylcholinesterase (AChE)
Partially antagonizes morphine
Inhibition of cyclic AMP phosphodiesterase

Likely actions

Down-regulation of type 1 muscarinic receptors
Selective blockade of K channels
Inhibition of Na channel inactivation
Cholinergic firing stimulation
Interference with protein phosphorylation
Blockade of pre- and postsynaptic muscarinic and nicotinic receptors (at high doses)

The results of clinical trials on the administration of THA in humans have been conflicting. Summers et al.,[171] in an uncontrolled study, administered THA intravenously to 12 patients, and cognitive improvement was noted in 75%. Kaye[172] failed to find any significant difference between THA and placebo on tests of memory and cognition, but found positive results in patients receiving both lecithin and THA. Summers et al.[173] found significant clinical benefits from THA plus lecithin in the long-term treatment of AD, but the design and methodology of this study received severe criticism.

The "enriched sample" strategy has been proposed as a way to identify a subgroup of patients that may benefit from treatment with a particular drug, even if the majority of patients do not. The basic rationale is to pretest patients with the drug, select those that seem to respond favorably, and randomize them into a subsequent double-blind, placebo-controlled, parallel-groups test phase to assess effectiveness. Nonetheless, although this strategy deserves future consideration, there are several pending questions, concerning carryover effect, possible rebound or withdrawal effects, limitations on generalizability of results, and ineffectiveness, since most of the individuals initially enrolled are not actually randomized for the trial. Some studies of THA have employed this "enrichment design" strategy, in which THA was begun at a low dose and increased to a maximum tolerated dose.

Chatellier and Lacomblez[174] studied 67 patients with a diagnosis of probable AD, treated with a mean daily dose of 114 mg of THA plus 1200 mg of lecithin, in which patients had a 4-week active treatment period and a 4-week control period, and no significant improvement in clinical symptoms of AD was noted. However, 15% of the patients developed hepatotoxicity from THA. Davies et al.,[175] administered THA over a 3-month course, in a double-blind, placebo-controlled, crossover study of ten patients, and found a trend towards deteriorating memory scores in all except one of the subjects. Gauthier et al.[176] studied 52 AD patients in an uncontrolled study in which 38 were able to reach a dose of THA of 100 mg/d, 8 received lower doses because of side-effects, and 6 dropped out of the study. After 4 weeks of treatment, Mini-Mental State Examination and Rapid Disability Rating Scale II scores were significantly increased, and these effects reversed with discontinuation of THA.

Molloy et al.,[177] in a randomized, double-blind crossover trial of 34 AD patients, with three treatment periods, each consisting of 3 weeks of active drug therapy and 3 weeks of placebo, using doses from 50 to 100 mg of THA daily, found significant toxic effects (liver toxicity and gastrointestinal side effects), and no clinically significant effects in cognition, functional status, or behavior. Davis et al.[178] studied 215 patients who improved on THA during a preliminary crossover phase to determine responsiveness and the best dose of THA, out of 632 eligible patients with probable AD. Then, these 215 patients were randomly assigned to placebo or their best dose of THA (10 or 20 mg four times daily), in a 6-week, double-blind trial. At the end of the 6-week trial, treatment with THA resulted in a statistically significant reduction in the decline of cognitive function, but not large enough to be detected by measures of global assessment of patients. Eagger et al.[179] reported a randomized, double-blind, placebo-controlled crossover study of 65 probable AD patients during two 13-week treatment periods, separated by a 4-week washout, using THA doses of up to 150 mg/d. They found significant effects of THA within the first 2 to 4 weeks of treatment, reaching the maximum effect in 4 to 6 weeks. The effect was maintained for the rest of the treatment period, and after withdrawal, worsening to a "point worse than one would expect" was not detected on three of four cognitive tests or in any of the outcome measures used. Farlow et al.,[180] in a 12-week, double-blind, placebo-controlled, parallel-group study of 486 patients with probable AD, using doses from 20 to 80 mg a day of THA, found clinically significant effects. Liver toxicity was found to be easily detected by weekly determinations of alanine aminotransferase and was reversible on discontinuation of medication. Minthon et al.,[181] in a recent double-blind crossover trial of THA, lecithin, and placebo in 17 patients with AD, with treatment periods of 6 weeks each and washout periods of 2 weeks, using daily doses of THA of 20 mg/d, did not find any evidence of THA alone or in combination with lecithin to be better than placebo. Knapp et al.,[182] in a recent, large, 30-week, double-blind, placebo-controlled parallel group trial involving 663 mild to moderate AD patients, found significant improvement in all three outcome measures in the group that received 160 mg/d. This study enrolled initially 663 patients, but only 263 could complete the 30-week trial. The main reasons for withdrawal from the protocol were adverse reactions (74%), lack of compliance (5%), lack of efficacy (5%), and other reasons, such as caregiver request, use of nonpermitted concurrent medication, and medication dispensing errors (16%). Of the patients randomized to the 160 mg/d group, only 28% (67/239) could remain in the study until the end of the 30-week period, and the major reasons for withdrawing from the trial in this group were elevation of liver enzymes more than three times the upper limit of normal, in about half of the patients who withdrew, and cholinergic adverse effects, including nausea and vomiting. Thus, it seems that for the patients that can tolerate the higher doses of THA (160 mg/d), this drug may result in more consistently identified benefits on cognition.

TABLE 12.5.
Double-Blind Trials with THA

Author	Sample	Dosage	Methods	Outcome
Chatellier et al.[174]	67 prob.[a] AD	THA mean dose = 114 mg daily, lecithin = 1200 mg daily	Two 4-week periods, one with active treatment and one control period	No significant differences
Fitten et al.[183]	10 prob. AD	THA dose up to 250 mg qd, lecithin = 30 g qd	Randomly assigned to best dose of THA + lecithin or placebo for 1 week, then 1 week THA free and 1 week on other treatment	No significant effects
Gauthier et al.[176]	52 prob. AD	THA up to 100 mg/d lecithin = 4.7 g/d	8-week titration, then two sequential THA or placebo periods, 8-week each	No significant effects
Eagger et al.[185]	89 prob. AD	THA up to 150 mg/d 10.8 g lecithin/d	Active or placebo treatment for 13 weeks, 4-week washout, and crossover to other treatment	Significant benefits of treatment, in mild to moderate AD patients
Eagger et al.[179]	65 prob. AD	THA up to 150 mg qd, plus lecithin (dose not stated)	Two 13-week periods, 4-week washout, placebo-controlled crossover study	Significant benefits with THA
Molloy et al.[177]	34 prob. AD	THA 50 to 100 mg qd	Randomized, multiple crossover	No clinically significant effects
Weinstein et al.[184]	12 prob. AD	THA = 100 mg qd, lecithin = 10 g/d	12-week, placebo controlled	No significant effects
Davis et al.[178]	215 prob. AD	THA = 10 or 20 mg 4 times/day	Enriched sample, determined best dose, 6-week trial	No differences in global scores, but significantly lower cognitive decline with THA
Farlow et al.[180]	468 prob. AD	THA up to 80 mg qd	12-week, placebo-controlled, parallel-group study	Clinically significant improvement with THA
Minthon et al.[181]	17 prob. AD	THA = 20 mg daily, lecithin = 4 g daily	Crossover design, three periods of 6 week on THA + lecithin, THA + placebo, placebo + placebo	No significant clinical effects
Knapp et al.[182]	663 prob. AD	THA up to 160 mg qd	30-week, placebo-controlled, parallel group	263 completed the 30-week period, significant improvement in patients who tolerated 160 mg/d

[a] prob. = probable.

A problem for the administration of THA is the high incidence of side effects. A large multicenter trial of THA had to be temporarily discontinued because of the development of hepatotoxicity in approximately one third of the patients. The most common adverse effect of THA is an increase in serum alanine aminotransferase, which occurs in almost 50% of patients. About 25% have increases three times the upper normal limit. These elevations generally occur in 4 to 12 weeks after the first dose, and in most cases return to normal within 4 to 6 weeks after stopping the drug. Ames et al.[186] reported a study of 14 patients receiving 100 to 200 mg of THA daily, and 5 of these patients developed persistent elevations in serum aminotransferase. Three patients were found to have focal necrosis and one was found to have granulomatous hepatitis at liver biopsy. Hammel et al.[187] reported a case of a patient who had his THA dose increased from 25 to 100 mg daily in 5 d, and developed jaundice and hepatocellular necrosis on biopsy. In both reports, hepatic function came back to normal within a few weeks after the drug was stopped. Other side effects that have been related to THA include nausea, vomiting, diarrhea, ataxia, myalgia, and headache.

Knapp et al.[182] reported that 54% of 479 THA-treated patients in a large trial involving 663 AD patients, receiving doses of THA up to 160 mg/d had increase of at least one ALT value during a 30-week trial, and that in 29% of these patients the increase was at least three times the upper normal limit. Of all clinically significant ALT elevations, 90% occurred within the first 12 weeks of treatment, and in all cases it resolved with discontinuation of the drug. Watkins et al.,[188] studying the hepatotoxic effects of THA in six multicenter trials using doses between 20 and 160 mg/d, reported occurrence of ALT increase in at least one occasion in 49% of the patients, with levels greater than three times the upper normal limit in 25% of the cases. In all cases, discontinuation of THA completely reversed the ALT alterations, and no deaths related to hepatotoxicity occurred. In these trials, the liver enzymes were monitored weekly. Nonetheless, the authors did not report the incidence of hepatotoxic side effects by the different dose ranges used, particularly in the higher-dose groups, which are the doses that might have more clear benefits on cognition.

THA recently gained a lot of attention in the scientific community and in the lay press after it was approved by the FDA for use as a cognition enhancer. The bulk of evidence available does not permit absolute conclusions about its effectiveness for the treatment of these disorders, but suggests that it might be useful for some mild to moderate AD patients, particularly if used in higher doses. THA seems to improve or slow the decline in various tests of cognitive function for some patients with mild to moderate AD, but the studies done so far do not show conclusive evidence of substantial functional improvement. The recent findings of Knapp et al.[182] that in higher doses it would produce more consistent benefits on cognition, still wait further replication in other trials. Additionally, the safety of THA for large groups of AD patients, including patients with systemic disease, is still unknown.[189]

THA approved labeling will require weekly monitoring of ALT/SGPT for at least the first 18 weeks of therapy, with the possibility of decreasing to every 3 months then, if the same dose is maintained. If the dose is increased, resumption of weekly monitoring is then necessary for a minimum of 6 weeks for each time that the dose is increased. Thus, many patients with mild enzyme elevation will be able to safely take the drug on a reduced dosage, or when on a lower dose after a drug-free period. Recommended initial dosage is 40 mg daily, in four divided doses, increasing to 80, 120, and 160 mg daily in patients who tolerate this. It is marketed as Cognex, by Warner-Lambert.

Velnacrine maleate, 9-amino-1,2,3,4,-tetrahydroacridine-1-ol maleate, a derivative of THA, was reported to have memory-enhancing effects in rats.[190] It was found to have good oral bioavailability and to be well tolerated in young and elderly volunteers.[191,192] Cutler et al.[193] suggested a dose of 225 mg/d as probably safe for trials in AD patients. In this study, patients receiving 300 or 450 mg/d had significant side effects, including seizures, nausea, vomiting, abdominal cramps, diarrhea, dizziness, and syncope. Ebmeier et al.[194] found that a single dose of 75 mg/d of velnacrine was able to increase word recognition memory in AD patients, and that it was also associated with an increase of cerebral blood flow to higher frontal regions, particularly on the left side, as measured by ^{99m}Tc-exametazime SPECT.

Galanthamine, a tertiary amine which is an AChE inhibitor, has been used in small open trials with promising preliminary results.[195,196] A small open trial in 18 possible AD patients, using 30 mg/d, did not show any evidence of significant change in neuropsychological measures.[197]

E2020, (R,S)-1-benzyl-4-((5,6-dimethoxy-1-indanon)-2-yl) methylpiperidine hydrocloride, is a new AChE inhibitor which was found to be well tolerated in humans in initial studies,[198] but trials on AD patients have not been reported yet.

2. Acetyl-L-Carnitine

Acetyl-L-Carnitine is the acetyl-ester of carnitine. Historically, it was thought to be a cholinergic agent, as it promoted synthesis and release of ACh in animal experiments, but more recent evidence suggested that it may act on other neurotransmitter systems as well. Calvani et al.[199] suggested that it should be considered a neuroprotective agent, considering its actions as an antioxidizing agent, membrane stabilizing function, influence on mitochondrial energy supply, and cholinergic transmission enhancement.

Bonnavita[200] administered acetyl-L-carnitine to 40 dementia patients, who were given either 300 mg of acetyl-L-carnitine per day or placebo, during 40 d. The group on acetyl-L-carnitine showed significant improvement from baseline on all eight mental status measures, and on four of five clinical rating measures, and the placebo group did not have significant improvement. Rai et al.[201] conducted a double-blind, placebo-controlled trial with 1 g of acetyl-L-carnitine in 36 AD patients, and found a trend to benefit of this drug on some features of AD, particularly on short-term memory. Spagnoli et al.,[202] in a double-blind, placebo-controlled trial, followed 130 AD patients treated with 2 g of acetyl-L-carnitine, and found a statistically significant slower rate of cognitive deterioration after 1 year in the acetyl-L-carnitine group. Sano et al.,[203] in a recent double-blind, placebo-controlled trial involving 30 mild to moderate AD patients treated with 2.5 g/d of acetyl-L-carnitine for 3 months, followed by 3 g/d for another 3 months, found that this drug significantly retarded the deterioration in some cognitive functions in these patients, suggesting that it might be useful, and emphasizing the need for a large study of this agent.

3. Cholinergic Agonists

RS-86 (2-ethyl-8-methyl-2,8 diazaspirol(4,5)-decane-1,3 dione hydrobromide), a direct post-synaptic muscarinic cholinergic receptor agonist, failed to show consistent benefit in cognitive performance.[204]

2-Dimethylaminoethanol (Deanol), which increases CNS ACh concentrations, was not shown to have any significant effect on cognition, but was found to decrease behavioral symptoms associated with AD, such as anxiety, depression, and irritability.[205]

4. ACh-Releasing Agents

4-Aminopyridine (4AP) and ***3,4 diaminopyridine*** (DAP) increase intraneuronal calcium through their action on voltage-regulated calcium channels, resulting in prolonged action potentials and increased release of ACh.[206] Wessenling et al.[207] conducted a small clinical trial with 4AP on 14 patients, in a double-blind, randomized, crossover design, and reported a significant improvement on tests of memory, perception, and cognition, but subjects also developed increased agitation and nervousness during treatment. Davidson et al.[208] failed to find significant cognitive improvement with this agent. DAP is much more potent than 4AP, but clinical trials with this agent have not been reported.

DuP 996, 3,3-bis(4-pyridinylmethyl-1-phenylindolin-2-one), has similar properties to 4AP. It enhances the release of ACh and other neurotransmitters, such as dopamine and serotonin. It was shown to improve learning in animal models.[209,210] In human volunteers, it was found to be well tolerated and to induce electroencephalographic changes suggestive of beneficial effects.[211] However, data of its effectiveness in AD patients did not show it to be effective, and it was dropped from further study.

B. MAO B INHIBITORS

L-Deprenyl is a selective MAO-B inhibitor when given in low doses (10 mg/d). It also interferes with the conversion of inactive substrates to free radicals, and retards the production of free radicals. Tariot et al.[212] administered L-deprenyl, in doses of 10 to 40 mg a day, and placebo, in a double-blind serial design, and found a significant improvement in memory and learning with the low dose (10 mg/d). Schneider et al.[213] conducted a small, 4-week open trial with 14 patients with probable AD, receiving low dose of L-deprenyl (10 mg/d), and found evidence that it might be helpful for behavior and cognition. Piccinin et al.[214] reported benefits on cognition of L-deprenyl 10 mg/d administered to 20 AD patients in 3 and 6 months, in a double-blind crossover, placebo-controlled design. Finali et al.,[215] in a 6-month, double-blind, crossover, placebo-controlled study of 29 AD patients, found beneficial effects of L-deprenyl 10 mg/d on cognition. Mangoni et al.[216] studied 119 AD patients in a double-blind, placebo-controlled study using 10 mg/d of L-deprenyl, for a period of 3 months, and found that the drug improved cognitive function and decreased behavior abnormalities, despite having good tolerability in this dose, suggesting that L-deprenyl might be a useful agent for this condition. Agnoli et al.[217] reported a double-blind, placebo-controlled trial with 5 mg twice a day of L-deprenyl on a small sample (n = 10) of mild to moderate AD patients, and found that in 2 months the patients treated with L-deprenyl showed improvement in cognition, and no changes in SPECT ^{99}TcHMPAO measures of CBF, while the placebo group showed worsening in cognition and further reduction in parietal lobe CBF. Burke et al.[218] reported the initial results of a double-blind, placebo-controlled trial with 5 mg/d of L-deprenyl on 39 AD patients, and found that in 2 months no improvement in behavior or cognition was detected. Strategies combining L-deprenyl with AChE inhibitors, like physostigmine or THA, have been suggested to be useful in initial studies.[219,220] The possibility that L-deprenyl interferes with the progression of the disease certainly merits further investigation in longer clinical trials.

Milacemide is a MAO B inhibitor and a prodrug for glycine, and has been tested in AD patients as a possible cognition enhancer, but the results were discouraging.[221,222]

C. NEW NOOTROPICS

BMY-21502 is a nootropic agent whose mechanism of action is unknown, but animal studies have shown that it does not alter cholinergic, monoaminergic, amino acid, or peptidergic receptor systems, and does not have an effect on calcium channels. Animal studies have shown that this compound can enhance long-term potentiation, promote the survival of neuron-like PC-12 cells *in vitro*, reverse age-related deficits in glucose utilization in the hippocampus, enhance the acquisition of new learning in animals with experimental lesions in the nucleus basalis, and protect memory from insults caused by electroconvulsive shock or scopolamine in animal models. Preclinical toxicological studies have shown increases in liver function tests, cholesterol, and triglycerides.[223] This agent has undergone some preliminary clinical trials with inconclusive results.

D. NERVE GROWTH FACTORS

The discovery of NGF in 1964 by Levi-Montalcini[224] initiated the study of nerve differentiation. After it was known that NGF had a trophic effect on CNS cholinergic neurons, it was hypothesized that a lack of NGF could be responsible for AD.[225,226] This hypothesis was supported by evidence indicating a beneficial role of NGF for degenerating neurons, and by NGF-induced hypertrophy in AD.[227–231] If such approaches prove to be useful, they may provide means to stop the cognitive decline in AD, rather than just attempting to remedy the biochemical deficits resulting from neuronal death. One potential difficulty in these developments is the fact that they do not pass the blood-brain barrier, making difficult the development of viable delivery strategies for these agents. Thus, much hope is placed on the development of this kind of strategy.

E. GANGLIOSIDES

Gangliosides are responsible for giving stability to the plasma membrane, are involved in the maturation and plasticity of neurons, and have neurotrophic effects. GM1 ganglioside was found to be reduced in brains of AD patients.[232]

There are only limited data supporting the idea that systemic administration of GM1 results in significantly increased brain levels of the ganglioside,[233] and the initial treatment attempts with this agent were given intrathecally. Most recently, Svennerholm et al.[234] reported relatively high and constant plasma levels after subcutaneous administration of 100 mg daily of GM1 in AD patients. Ala et al.[235] did not find significant benefits in mild to moderate AD patients, in a 24-week, double-blind, placebo-controlled study with 100 mg of GM1 daily intramuscular for 12 weeks. Flicker et al.,[236] in a double-blind, placebo-controlled study of 12 probable AD patients, also failed to find any significant effects on cognition of GM1 100 mg/d intramuscularly.

F. PHOSPHATIDYLSERINE

Phosphatidylserine (PS) is produced from purified bovine cerebral cortex, and has been found to prevent or reverse age-related neurochemical changes in the brains of aged animals. It is assumed to interfere with the fluidity and functional state of the neuronal membrane.

PS causes structural neuronal changes, rather than the transient metabolic changes produced by most of the components used for treatment of AD. The clinical studies performed with this component showed improvement in some measures, but many of the studies had methodological deficiencies.[237–246] A more recent study yielded promising results,[247] and another one suggested that it might be beneficial for patients with less severe cognitive impairment in the early stages of AD.[248]

G. CALCIUM CHANNEL BLOCKERS

These agents were found to reduce the tone of the cerebral vasculature in animals, and to prevent or limit cerebrovascular spasms and maintain brain tissue viability by limiting calcium overload.[249,250] It was also reported to help to maintain cerebral blood flow and preserve memory following neuronal trauma.[251]

Nimodipine was reported to improve the acquisition of conditioned reflexes in rabbits[252] and to have a positive effect in memory and learning in aged rats.[253] Tollefson[254] administered nimodipine in a randomized, double-blind, placebo-controlled, multicenter, 12-week trial of 227 patients with AD. The patients received 90 mg or 180 mg of nimodipine a day, and the group who received 90 mg/d showed statistically significant slowing in cognitive decline, suggesting that it can prevent further deterioration in these patients. This effect was not observed with the 180-mg dose. One possibility to explain the selective effect at the lower dose is that calcium levels too low or too high may have adverse actions on neural growth and functioning. Two other large, multicenter, double-blind, placebo-controlled trials with this agent showed also that at doses of 90 mg/d this drug is well tolerated, and both studies found significant improvement on measures of behavior and cognition, suggesting that this agent may be beneficial in the treatment of AD patients.[255,256]

H. ACE (ANGIOTENSIN CONVERTING ENZYME) INHIBITORS

There is evidence that ACE inhibitors may facilitate cholinergic function and improve cognitive performance in animals. Angiotensin II was found to reduce ACh release from the rat and human cortex via angiotensin II receptors.[257] In animal models, angiotensin had a negative effect on cognition,[258] while captopril was found to benefit cognitive functions.[259] Patients treated for hypertension with the ACE inhibitor captopril have subjective and objective benefits in cognitive functions, when compared to groups of patients treated with other antihypertensive drugs.[260] Additionally, ACE activity was found to be increased in various areas of AD patient brains in comparison to normal controls.[261] A recent 15-week, double-blind, placebo-controlled clinical trial with cenarapril, an ACE inhibitor, on AD patients did not show significant effects on cognition.[262] Thus, despite initial evidence suggesting that these agents could be helpful for the treatment of AD, the human studies failed to show clear evidence of benefits on cognition.

I. XANTHINE DERIVATIVES

Saletu et al.[263] reported a double-blind, placebo-controlled, multicenter trial of a new xanthine derivative, denbufylline, on 96 mild to moderate AD and MID patients, and found significant effects on psychometric measures compared to placebo. Both AD and MID patients showed similar therapeutic benefit. Propentofylline is another agent in this class undergoing investigation, and a recent double-blind, placebo-controlled trial failed to find evidence of significant effects on psychometric measures on mild dementia patients.[264]

J. ALUMINUM CHELATION THERAPY

Since an increased concentration of aluminum has been found in the NFT in the brains of AD patients, it was hypothesized that aluminum could have a role in AD.[265] It has been postulated that aluminum appears in the NFT after neuronal damage occurs.[266]

McLachlan et al.[267] reported a 2-year, single-blind trial with desferrioxamine intramuscularly in 48 AD patients, and found that it resulted in a 50% reduction in the average rate of cognitive deterioration. Since this agent is frequently associated with potentially severe toxicity and needs to be used intramuscularly, other forms of effective oral aluminum chelation therapy should be developed.

K. NEURAL TRANSPLANT

The use of exogenous neuronal transplants in brain holds promise. In animals, these transplants were shown to reconnect with host cells, produce neurotransmitters, and remain viable. Improved learning and memory were observed in animals with experimentally damaged cholinergic basal forebrain after cholinergic nerve cell transplants.

Advances in molecular biology are making possible the creation of cells with genes that produce specific replacement substances, which could then be transplanted. Thus, specific cell populations can be introduced into brain tissue to produce substances to counteract the disease process.

The use of these strategies is in an early stage of evaluation. Studies on rodent models of learning and memory dysfunctions have been promising, and investigations on nonhuman primates have been conducted. As pointed out by Gash et al.,[268] the safety and effectiveness of this strategy in treating neurodegenerative disorders can only be determined using animal models with a nervous system closely resembling that of humans.

L. D-CYCLOSERINE

D-Cycloserine (D-4-amino-3-isoxazolidone) has been in clinical use as an antibiotic for some years, but recently its neuropharmacological effects became recognized. Based on its effect on learning in animals[269] and its partial agonist effects at the glycine site,[270–272] it has been proposed as a strategy in the treatment of AD cognitive deficits.[273] Nonetheless, clinical trials in humans with this agent for this indication have not been promising.

M. ANTI-INFLAMMATORY THERAPY

Anti-inflammatory agents have been recently hypothesized as possibly affecting the progression of AD. A recent case-control study of AD twin patients reported a significant negative association between occurrence of AD with use of anti-inflammatories, suggesting that these agents may prevent or delay the onset of AD symptoms.[274] Rogers et al.[275] reported the results of a 6-month, double-blind, placebo-controlled trial with indomethacin in mild to moderate AD patients, when they found that the drug significantly decreased the rate of cognitive decline compared to the placebo group.

Thus, initial promising results with these agents await further testing in larger multicenter trials.

V. PERSPECTIVES

A. GLUTAMATERGIC TRANSMISSION (N-METHYL-D-ASPARTATE [NMDA] RECEPTORS)

Excitatory amino acids have been shown to interfere with long-term potentiation (LTP), which is an electrophysiologic process thought to be of fundamental importance in the formation of memory and learning processes. The induction of LTP could be facilitated by promoting the activation of NMDA synaptic receptors. The cortical pyramidal neurons probably are the most important area for cortico-cortical associative connections, and glutamate has been suggested to be their main neurotransmitter.

A loss of intracortical connectivity secondary to the death of pyramidal neuron could theoretically explain part of the symptoms of AD. Lesions very similar to the NFT of AD may be produced by excitatory amino acid-mediated excitotoxicity, and NMDA-receptor blockers have been shown to provide significant protection against ischemic and excitatory amino acid-mediated cortical lesions.[276,277]

Glutamatergic augmentation and receptor blockade have been suggested as possible approaches for the treatment of AD.[278] Augmentation of glutamatergic transmission could facilitate memory and learning through enhancement of intracortical connections, and glutamatergic blockade could prevent the excitatory amino acid excitotoxicity.

B. MEMBRANE FLUIDITY

Structural and functional alterations in cell membranes of AD, in neural and nonneural tissues, have been observed. Zubenko et al.[279] found an increase in fluidity of platelet membranes in AD patients, as measured by a decrease in the fluorescence anisotrophy of 1,6-diphenyl/1,3,5 hexatriene in labeled membranes. Increased platelet membrane fluidity was also found to correlate with dementia severity[280,281] and to identify a subgroup of patients with distinct clinical features, with earlier onset of symptoms, more rapid course, and family history of dementia.[282,283] The identification of these potential biological markers makes the identification of subgroups of patients possible, so that more specific treatment strategies may be used.

C. TAU PROTEINS

Flament et al.[284] reported production of abnormal tau proteins in AD. In another study, Flament et al.[285] reported two abnormal tau variants (tau 64 and 69), exclusively in brain areas with neurofibrillary tangles and senile plaques, suggesting that they would be specific markers of neuronal degeneration in AD. It is possible that abnormal tau proteins precede other changes in AD, being important in the search for the mechanism of neurofibrillary degeneration.

D. β-AMYLOID

The brains of AD patients are characterized by the deposition of β-amyloid peptide, a self-aggregating protein of 42 to 43 amino acids. This protein is formed of 4-kDa polypeptide (A4), which derives from larger precursor proteins (APP or BPP). These precursors are transmembrane glycoproteins, and their function in intact cells is unknown.

Patients with Down's syndrome were found to have a duplication of chromosome 21 and an extra copy of the β-amyloid gene, suggesting that the β-amyloid deposits of Down's individuals might develop because of an overexpression of the β-peptide gene. It has been hypothesized that this gene might be the same as the Alzheimer gene. The amyloid gene is relatively close to the locus for familial AD, on chromosome 21, but amyloid gene duplication has not been confirmed in AD patients.

The amyloid deposit might have an important role in the pathogenesis of AD, and it is reasonable to suspect that secretion of the amyloid protein is likely to produce membrane damage. One very interesting hypothesis about amyloid formation is related to the proteolytic cleavage of the membrane, with the possibility that a membrane injury could be a primary event in the pathological course of the disease.

Therapies aimed at influencing β-amyloid formation have been proposed; however, the worthiness of this approach is still questionable due to our poor knowledge of the relevance of this process to AD pathogenesis. Protease inhibitors have been hypothesized as potential agents for treatment of AD.

The elucidation of the process of formation of β-amyloid could hold promise for therapeutic intervention that might slow the progression of the disease.

E. APOLIPOPROTEIN E

Apolipoprotein E (Apo E) is a protein involved in cholesterol transport. Apo E is deposited with β-amyloid in senile plaques and binds to β-amyloid *in vitro*. In humans, the three variants of the gene that encode Apo E are termed E2, E3, and E4. The Apo E gene is located in chromosome 19. E3 is the most commonly inherited form of apolipoprotein in the population.

Recent research done on these proteins in AD patients found E3 not to be present in the late onset form of AD, with the E4 variant being present instead. The risk of late-onset AD was found to increase in individuals with more than two copies of E4.[286] A recent independent investigation confirmed the findings of a marked increase in Apo E E4 allele frequency in AD patients compared to controls,[287] and another independent study confirmed the association between late-onset AD and increased presence of the E4 allele, indicating an association with the 19q13.2 chromosome region containing the Apo E gene locus.[288] The identification of a clear biological marker brings promise of significant developments in this field.

VI. CONCLUSIONS

Despite the body of theoretical support for the use of cholinomimetic and monoaminergic agents in the treatment of AD, these strategies so far have produced only modest results. Cowburn et al.[289] reviewed the evidence that AD involves multiple neurotransmitter systems, and suggested that approaches to AD therapy aimed at a single transmitter replacement will probably be of limited usefulness. Although it is clear that a single transmitter deficit model for the pathophysiology of AD is not defendable, strategies consisting of neurotransmitter replacement may still be beneficial for certain aspects of the disease, in its early stages, as recent studies seem to suggest.[180,182] As suggested by Levy,[290] until we understand better the process that originates the pathological abnormalities found in AD it seems unrealistic to expect definitive treatments for this condition.

The recent data on THA suggests that cholinergic strategies might have a palliative effect in AD patients, particularly if this drug is used in higher doses, but it seems that the great majority of patients (around two thirds) will not tolerate the medication in the doses that could produce more consistent improvement in cognition. Additionally, the need for close monitoring of liver enzymes is a factor that makes the treatment even more expensive. Nonetheless, in the context of no availability of other alternatives for the treatment of these patients, and given the extreme consequences of AD for the patient and the family, even a small chance of temporary improvement might be worthwhile.

Whitehouse[291] classified the approaches to AD treatment into short, intermediate, and long-term strategies. The short-term neurotransmitter replacement strategies are probably limited because the degenerative dementias affect multiple neurotransmitter systems, and by the inability of a drug administered systemically to replace the functioning of an entire population of nerve cells. The promise of more significant and long-lasting effects could result from intermediate or long-term approaches aimed at enhancing viability or preventing neuronal death. Nonetheless, these approaches would depend on a better understanding of the pathophysiology of AD. The treatment and prevention of AD may become possible if the genetic and environmental interactions that cause the disease are identified.

One of the priorities in studying AD is the search for markers that could be used for early diagnosis, as well as markers which could identify patients who would respond to different treatment strategies. Unfortunately, until this point, biological, neurophysiologic, and imaging findings have not yet revealed anything sufficiently specific or detectable early enough to be of value for this purpose. The recent developments with Apo E findings bring the exciting possibility of more substantial developments in this area.

The development of better animal models, more effective mechanisms for rapid preclinical testing of new compounds, and further basic research in this area will certainly be decisive factors influencing developments in this field.

REFERENCES

1. **Alzheimer, A.,** A characteristic disease of the cerebral cortex, in *The Early Story of Alzheimer's Disease*, Bick, K. B., Amaducci, L., and Pepeu, G., Eds., Raven Press, New York, 1987, chap. 1.
2. **American Psychiatric Association,** *Diagnostic and Statistical Manual of Mental Disorders*, 3rd ed., revised, American Psychiatric Association, Washington, D.C., 1987.
3. **Evans, D. A., Funkenstein, H., Albert, M. S. et al.**, Prevalence of Alzheimer's disease in a community population of older persons higher than previously reported, *J. Am. Med. Assoc.*, 262, 2561, 1989.
4. **Hagnell, O., Lanke, J., Rorsman, B. et al.,** Current trends in the incidence of senile and multi-infarct dementia, *Arch. Psych. Neurol. Sci.*, 233, 423, 1983.
5. **Crook, T., Bartus, R. T., Ferris, S. H. et al.,** Age-associated memory impairment: proposed diagnostic criteria and measures of clinical change. Report of a National Institute of Mental Health Work Group, *Dev. Neuropsychol.*, 2, 261, 1986.
6. **Amaducci, L., Lippi, A., Bracco, L., and Falcini, M.,** Definition and classification of age-related cognitive dysfunctions, in *Treatment of Age-Related Cognitive Dysfunction: Pharmacological and Clinical Evaluation*, Recagni, G. and Mendlewicz, J., Eds., S. Karger, Basel, 1992, pp 86.
7. **Task Force on DSMIV, DSMIV draft criteria,** American Psychiatric Association, 1993, pp. F:1.
8. **Erkinjuntii, T., Sulkava, R., and Hachinski, V. C.,** Diagnostic assessments and criteria for memory disorders in clinical drug trials, in *Guidelines for Drug Trials in Memory Disorders*, Canal, N., Hachinski, V. C., McKhann, G. et al., Eds., Raven Press, New York, 1993, chap. 21.
9. **Gottfries, C. G.,** Reappraisal of current therapy in the treatment of age-related cognitive disorders, in *Treatment of Age-Related Cognitive Dysfunction: Pharmacological and Clinical Evaluation*, Racagni, G. and Mendlewicz, J., Eds., S. Karger, Basel, 1992, pp 121.
10. **Tomlinson, B. E., Blessed, G., and Roth, M.,** Observations on the brains of demented old people, *J. Neurol. Sci.*, 11, 205, 1970.
11. **Katzman, R.,** The prevalence and malignancy of Alzheimer's disease. A major killer, *Arch. Neurol.*, 33, 217, 1976.

12. **Debert, W.,** Interaction between cognitive and pharmacological treatment in age-related cognitive impairment, in *Treatment of Age-Related Cognitive Dysfunction: Pharmacological and Clinical Evaluation*, Racagni, G. and Mendlewics, J., Eds., S. Karger, Basel, 1992, pp 130.
13. **Jacobs, E. A., Winter, P. M., Alvis, M. J. et al.,** Hyperoxygenation effects on cognitive functioning in the aged, *N. Engl. J. Med.*, 281, 753, 1969.
14. **Raskin, A., Gershon, S., Crook, T. et al.,** The effects of hyperbaric and normobaric oxygen on cognitive impairment in the elderly, *Psychopharmacol. Bull.*, 13, 45, 1977.
15. **Goldfarb, A., Hochstadt, N., Jacobsen, J. et al.,** Hyperbaric oxygen treatment of organic mental syndrome in aged persons, *J. Gerontol.*, 27, 212, 1972.
16. **Stern, F. H.,** Management of chronic brain syndrome secondary to cerebral arteriosclerosis with special reference to papaverine hydrochloride, *J. Am. Geriatr. Soc.*, 18, 507, 1970.
17. **Ritter, R. H., Nail, H. R., Tatum, P. et al.,** The effect of papaverine in patients with cerebral arteriosclerosis, *Clin. Med.*, 18, 18, 1971.
18. **McQuillan, L. M., Lopec, C. A., and Vibal, J. R.,** Evaluation of EEG and clinical changes associated with Pavabid therapy in chronic brain syndrome, *Curr. Ther. Res.*, 16, 49, 1974.
19. **Branconnier, R. J. and Cole, J. O.,** Effects of chronic papaverine administration on mild senile organic brain syndrome, *J. Am. Geriatr. Soc.*, 22, 458, 1977.
20. **Yesavage, J. A., Tinklenberg, J. R., Hollister, L. E. et al.,** Vasodilators in senile dementias: a review of the literature, *Arch. Gen. Psychiatry*, 36(2), 220, 1979.
21. **Fontaine, L., Brand, M., Chabert, J. et al.,** Cerebral pharmacology of a new vasodilatory drug, naftidrofuryl, *Bull. Chem. Thermodyn.*, 6, 463, 1968.
22. **Gerin, J.,** Symptomatic treatment of cerebrovascular insufficiency with hydergine, *Curr. Ther. Res.*, 11, 539, 1969.
23. **Triboletti, F. and Ferri, H.,** Hydergine for treatment of symptoms of cerebrovascular insufficiency, *Curr. Ther. Res.*, 11, 609, 1969.
24. **Ditch, M., Kelly, F. J., and Resnick, O.,** An ergot preparation (hydergine) in the treatment of cerebrovascular disorders in the geriatric patient; double-blind study, *J. Am. Geriatr. Soc.*, 19, 208, 1971.
25. **Jennings, W. G.,** An ergot alkaloid preparation (hydergine) versus placebo for the treatment of symptoms of cerebrovascular insufficiency: double-blind study, *J. Am. Geriatr. Soc.*, 20, 407, 1972.
26. **Judge, T. G. and Urquihart, A.,** Naftidrofuryl — a double-blind crossover study in the elderly, *Curr. Med. Res. Opin.*, 1, 168, 1972.
27. **Rao, D. B. and Norris, J. R.,** A double-blind investigation of hydergine in the treatment of cerebrovascular insufficiency in the elderly, *Johns Hopkins Med J.*, 130, 317, 1972.
28. **McConnachie, R. W.,** A clinical trial comparing "hydergine" with placebo in the treatment of cerebrovascular insufficiency in elderly patients, *Curr. Med. Res. Opin.*, 1, 463, 1973.
29. **Rehman, S. A.,** Two trials comparing "hydergine" with placebo in the treatment of patients suffering from cerebrovascular insufficiency, *Curr. Med. Res. Opin.*, 1, 456, 1973.
30. **Banen, D. M.,** An ergot preparation (hydergine) for relief of symptoms of cerebrovascular insufficiency, *J. Am. Geriatr. Soc.*, 20, 22, 1974.
31. **Gerin, J.,** Double-blind trial of naftidrofuryl in the treatment of cerebral arteriosclerosis, *Br. J. Clin. Pract.*, 28, 177, 1974.
32. **Thibault, A.,** A double-blind evaluation of "hydergine" and placebo in the treatment of patients with organic brain syndrome and cerebral arteriosclerosis in a nursing home, *Curr. Med. Res. Opin.*, 2, 482, 1974.
33. **Hughes, J., Williams, J., and Currier, A.,** An ergot alkaloid preparation (hydergine) in the treatment of dementia: critical review of literature, *J. Am. Geriatr.*, 24, 490, 1975.
34. **Brodie, N. H.,** A double-blind trial of naftidrofuryl in treating confused elderly patients in general practice, *Practitioner*, 218, 274, 1977.
35. **McDonald, R.,** Hydergine: a review of 26 clinical studies, *Neuropsychopharmacology*, 12, 407, 1979.
36. **Hollister, L., and Yesavage, J.,** Ergoloid mesylates for senile dementias: unanswered questions, *Ann. Intern. Med.*, 100, 894, 1984.
37. **Thompson, T. L., Filley, C. M., Mitchelli, W. D. et al.,** Lack of efficacy of hydergine in patients with Alzheimer's disease, *N. Engl. J. Med.*, 323, 445, 1990.
38. **Walsh, A. C. and Walsh, B. M.,** Senile and presenile dementia: further observations on the benefits of dicumalol psychotherapy regimen, *J. Am. Geriatr. Soc.*, 20, 127, 1972.
39. **Walsh, A. C., Walsh, B. M., and Maloney, C.,** Senile-presenile dementia: follow-up data on an effective psychotherapy-anticoagulant regimen, *J. Am. Geriatr. Soc.*, 26, 467, 1978.
40. **Tecce, J. J. and Cole, J. O.,** Amphetamine effects in man: paradoxical drowsiness and lowered electrical brain activity, *Science*, 85, 451, 1974.
41. **Gilbert, J. G., Ponnelly, K. J., Zimmer, L. E. et al.,** Effect of magnesium pemoline and methylphenidate on memory improvement and mood in normal aging subjects, *Int. J. Aging Hum. Dev.*, 4(1), 35,,1973.
42. **Crook, T., Ferris, S., Sathananthan, G. et al.,** The effect of methylphenidate on test performance in the cognitively impaired aged, *Psychopharmacology*, 52, 251, 1977.

43. **Kaplitz, S. E.**, Withdrawn, apathetic geriatric patients responsive to methylphenidate, *J. Am. Geriatr. Soc.*, 23, 271, 1975.
44. **Lehman, H. E. and Ban, T. A.**, Central nervous system stimulants and anabolic substances in geropsychiatric therapy, in *Aging: Genesis and Treatment of Psychologic Disorders in the Elderly*, Vol. 2, Gershon, S. and Raskin, A., Eds., Raven Press, New York, 1975, pp 179.
45. **Turek, I., Kurland, A. A., Ota, K. Y. et al.**, Effects of pipradol hydrochloride on geriatric patients, *J. Am. Geriatr. Soc.*, 17, 408, 1969.
46. **Eisdorfer, C., Conner, J. F., and Wilkie, F. L.**, The effect of magnesium pemoline on cognition and behavior, *J. Gerontol.*, 23, 283, 1968.
47. **Ban, T. A.**, *Psychopharmacology for the Aged*, S. Karger, Basel, 1980.
48. **Saletu, B. and Grunberger, J.**, Cerebral hypoxic hypoxidosis, neurophysiological, psychometric and pharmacotherapeutic aspects, *Adv. Biol. Psychiatr.*, 13, 146, 1983.
49. **Wolthius, O. L.**, Behavioral effects of etiracetam in rats, *Pharmacol. Biochem. Behav.*, 15, 247, 1981.
50. **Vincent, G., Verderese, A., and Gamya, E.**, The effects of duiracetam (Ro 13-5057) on the enhancement and protection of memory, *Ann. N.Y. Acad. Sci.*, 444, 489, 1985.
51. **Mindus, P., Cronhom, B., Levander, S. E. et al.**, Piracetam-induced improvement of mental performance: a controlled study on normally aging individuals, *Acta Psychiatr. Scand.*, 54, 150, 1976.
52. **Chouinard, G., Annable, L., Ross-Chouinard, A. et al.**, A double-blind, placebo-controlled study of piracetam in elderly psychiatric patients, *Psychopharmacol. Bull.*, 17(1), 129, 1981.
53. **Stegnick, A.**, The clinical use of piracetam, a new nootropic drug, *Arzneim-Forsch-Drug Res.*, 22, 975, 1972.
54. **Croisile, B., Trillet, M., Fondarai, J. et al.**, Long-term and high dose piracetam treatment of Alzheimer's disease, *Neurology*, 43, 301, 1993.
55. **Friedman, E., Sherman, K. A., Ferris, S. H. et al.**, Clinical response to choline plus piracetam in senile dementia: relation to red-cell choline levels, *N. Engl. J. Med.*, 304, 1490, 1981.
56. **Davidson, M., Mohs, R. C., Hollander, E. et al.**, Lecithin and piracetam in patients with Alzheimer's disease, *Biol. Psychiatry*, 22, 112, 1987.
57. **Ferris, S. H., Reisberg, B., Crook, T. et al.**, Pharmacological treatment of senile dementia: choline, L-dopa, piracetam and choline plus piracetam, in *Alzheimer's Disease: a Report of Progress*, Corkin, S., Davis, K. L., Growdon, J. H. et al., Eds., Raven Press, New York, 1982, pp 475.
58. **Growdon, J. H., Corkin, S., Huff, F. J. et al.**, Piracetam combined with lecithin in the treatment of Alzheimer's disease, *Neurobiol. Aging*, 7, 269, 1986.
59. **Pomara, N., Block, R., Moore, N. et al.**, Combined piracetam and cholinergic precursor treatment for primary degenerative dementia, *IRCS Med. Sci.*, 12, 388, 1984.
60. **Smith, R. C., Vroulis, G., Hohnson, R. et al.**, Comparison of therapeutic response to long-term treatment with lecithin versus piracetam plus lecithin in patients with Alzheimer's disease, *Psychopharmacol. Bull.*, 20, 542, 1984.
61. **Banfi, S. and Dorigotti, L.**, Experimental behavioural studies with oxiracetam on different type of chronic cerebral impairment, *Clin. Neuropharmacol.*, 7 (Suppl. 1), 768, 1984.
62. **Saletu, B., Linzmayer, L., Grunberg, J., and Pietschmann, H.**, Double-blind, placebo-controlled, clinical, psychometric and neurophysiological investigations with oxiracetam in the organic brain syndrome of late life, *Neuropsychobiology*, 13, 44, 1985.
63. **Ferrero, E.**, Controlled clinical trial of oxiracetam in the treatment of chronic cerebrovascular diseases in the elderly, *Curr. Ther. Res.*, 36, 298, 1984.
64. **Turan, M., Mehon-Gopi, N., Bosak, M., and Songar, A.**, The effects of oxiracetam (ISF 2522) in patients with organic brain syndrome (a double-blind controlled study with Piracetam), *Drug Dev. Res.*, 2, 447, 1982.
65. **Dysken, M. W., Katz, R., Stallone, F. et al.**, Oxiracetam in the treatment of multi-infarct dementia and primary degenerative dementia, *J. Neuropsychiatry*, 1(3), 249, 1989.
66. **Maina, G., Fiori, L., Torta, R. et al.**, Oxiracetam in the treatment of primary degenerative and multi-infarct dementia: a double-blind, placebo-controlled study, *Neuropsychobiology*, 21, 141, 1989.
67. **Bottini, G., Vallar, G., Cappa, S. et al.**, Oxiracetam in dementia: a double-blind, placebo-controlled study, *Acta Neurol. Scand.*, 86, 237, 1992.
68. **Villardita, C., Grioli, S., Lomeo, C. et al.**, Clinical studies with oxiracetam in patients with dementia of Alzheimer type and multi-infarct dementia of mild to moderate degree, *Neuropsychobiology*, 25, 24, 1992.
69. **Itil, T. M., Gopi, N., and Menon, G. N.**, The effects of oxiracetam (ISF 2522) in patients with organic brain syndrome (a double-blind controlled study with piracetam), *Drug Dev. Res.*, 2, 447, 1982.
70. **Itil, T. M., Menon, G. N., Songar, A. et al.**, CNS pharmacology and clinical therapeutical effects of oxiracetam, *Clin. Neuropharmacol.*, 9 (Suppl. 3), 670, 1986.
71. **Moglia, A., Sinforiani, E., Zandrini, C. et al.**, Activity of oxiracetam in patients with organic brain syndrome: a neuropsychological study, *Clin. Neuropharmacol.*, 9 (Suppl. 3), 573, 1986.
72. **Villardita, C., Parini, J., Grioli, S. et al.**, Clinical and neuropsychological investigations on oxiracetam in patients with mild to moderate dementia, *Clin. Neuropharmacol.*, 9 (Suppl. 14), 301, 1986.

73. **Green, R. C., Goldstein, F. C., Auchus, A. P. et al.,** Treatment trial of oxiracetam in Alzheimer's disease, *Arch. Neurol.*, 49, 1135, 1992.
74. **Branconnier, R. J., Cole, J. O., Dessain, E. C. et al.,** The therapeutic efficacy of piracetam in Alzheimer's disease: preliminary observations, *Psychopharmacol. Bull.*, 19, 726, 1983.
75. **Claus, J. J., Ludwig, C., Mohr, E. et al.,** Nootropic drugs in Alzheimer's disease: symptomatic treatment with pramiracetam, *Neurology*, 41, 570, 1991.
76. **Mizuki, Y., Yamada, M., Kato, I. et al.,** Effects of aniracetam, a nootropic drug, in senile dementia — a preliminary report, *Kurume Med. J.*, 31, 135, 1984.
77. **Sourander, L. B., Portin, R., Molsa, P. et al.,** Senile dementia of Alzheimer's type treated with aniracetam, *Psychopharmacology*, 91, 90, 1987.
78. **Senin, U., Abate, G., Fieschi, C. et al.,** Aniracetam (Ro 13-5057) in the treatment of senile dementia of Alzheimer type (SDAT): results of a placebo controlled multicentre clinical study, *Eur. Neuropsychopharmacol.*, 1, 511, 1991.
79. **De Wied, D.,** The importance of vasopressin in memory, *Trends Neurosci.*, 7, 62, 1984.
80. **Gottfries, C. G.,** Reappraisal of current therapy in the treatment of age-related cognitive disorders, in *Treatment of Age-Related Cognitive Dysfunction: Pharmacological and Clinical Evaluation*, Recagni, G. and Mendlewicz, J., Eds., S. Karger, Basel, 1992, 121.
81. **Mohr, E., Bruno, G., Foster, N. et al.,** GABA-agonist therapy for Alzheimer's disease, *Clin. Neuropharmacol.*, 9(3), 257, 1986.
82. **Chase, T. N., Durso, R., Fedio, P. et al.,** Vasopressin treatment of cognitive deficits in Alzheimer's disease, in *Aging*, Vol. 19, Corkin, S., Ed., Raven Press, New York, 1982, 457.
83. **Tamminga, C. A., Durso, R., Fedio, P. et al.,** Vasopressin studies in Alzheimer's disease, *Psychopharmacol. Bull.*, 18, 48, 1982.
84. **Tinklenberg, J. R., Pigache, R., Berger, P. A. et al.,** Desglycinamide-9-arginine-8-vasopressin (DGAVP, Organon 5667) in cognitively impaired patients, *Psychopharmacol. Bull.*, 18, 202, 1982.
85. **Ferris, S.,** Neuropeptides in the treatment of Alzheimer's disease, in *Alzheimer's Disease: the Standard Reference*, Reisberg, B., Ed., The Free Press, New York, 1983, 369.
86. **Peabody, C. A., Davies, H., Berger, P. A. et al.,** Desamine-D-arginine-vasopressin (DDAVP) in Alzheimer's disease, *Neurobiol. Aging*, 7, 301, 1986.
87. **Wolters, E. C., Reikkinen, P., Lowenthal, A. et al.,** DGAVP (Org 5667) in early Alzheimer's disease patients: an international double-blind, placebo-controlled multicenter trial, *Neurology*, 40, 1099, 1990.
88. **Cutler, N., Haxby, J., Narang, P. et al.,** Evaluation of an analogue of somatostatin (L363,586) in Alzheimer's disease, *N. Engl. J. Med.*, 312, 725, 1985.
89. **Mellow, A. M., Sunderland, T., Cohen, R. M. et al.,** Acute effects on high-dose thyrotropin releasing hormone infusions in Alzheimer's disease, *Psychopharmacology*, 98, 403, 1989.
90. **Dornbush, R. L., Shapiro, B., and Freedman, A. M.,** Effects of an ACTH short chain neuropeptide in man, *Am. J. Psychiatry*, 138, 962, 1981.
91. **Heuser, I., Heuser-Link, M., Gotthardt, U. et al.,** Behavioral effects of a synthetic corticotropin 4-9 analog in patients with depression and patients with Alzheimer's disease, *J. Clin. Psychopharmacol.*, 13, 171, 1993.
92. **Miller, T. P., Fong, K., and Tinklenberg, J. R.,** An ACTH 4-9 analog (Org 2766) and cognitive performance: high-dose efficacy and safety in dementia of the Alzheimer's type, *Biol. Psychiatry*, 33, 307, 1993.
93. **Dornbush, R. L. and Volavka, J.,** ACTH 4-10: a study of toxicological and behavioral effects in an aging sample, *Neuropsychobiology*, 2, 350, 1976.
94. **Ferris, H., Sathananthan, G., Gershon, S. et al.,** Cognitive effects of ACTH 4-10 in the elderly, *Pharmacol. Biochem. Behav.*, 5(1), 73, 1976.
95. **Branconier, R. J., Cole, J. O., and Gardos, G.,** ACTH 4-10 in the amelioration of neuropsychological symptomatology associated with senile organic brain syndrome, *Psychopharmacology*, 61, 161, 1979.
96. **Siegfried, K. R.,** First clinical impressions with an ACTH analog (HOE 427) in the treatment of Alzheimer's disease, *Ann. N.Y. Acad. Sci.*, 640, 280, 1991.
97. **Mouradian, M. M., Blin, J., Giuffra, M. et al.,** Somatostatin replacement therapy for Alzheimer dementia, *Ann. Neurol.*, 30, 610, 1991.
98. **Vogel-Scibilia, S. and Gershon, S.,** An update on cognitive enhancers for the elderly, *New Trends Clin. Neuropharmacol.*, 3(4), 207, 1989.
99. **Etienne, P., Gauthiers, S., Dastoor, D. et al.,** Lecithin in Alzheimer's disease, *Lancet*, 2(8101), 1206, 1978.
100. **Domino, E. F., Minor, L., Duff, I. F. et al.,** Effects of oral lecithin on blood choline levels and memory tests in geriatric volunteers, in *Alzheimer's Disease: A Report of Progress* (Aging, Vol. 19), Corkin, S. et al., Eds., Raven Press, New York, 1982, pp. 393.
101. **Brinkman, S. D., Smith, R. C., Meyer, J. S. et al.,** Lecithin and memory training in suspected alzheimer's disease, *J. Gerontol.*, 37, 4, 1982.
102. **Dysken, M. W., Foval, P., Harris, C. M. et al.,** Lecithin administration in patients with primary degenerative dementia and in normal volunteers, in *Alzheimer's Disease: A Report of Progress* (Aging, Vol. 19), Corkin, S. et al., Eds., Raven Press, New York, 1982, pp. 385.

103. **Heyman, A., Logue, P., Wilkinson, W. et al.**, Lecithin therapy of Alzheimer's disease: a preliminary report, in *Alzheimer's Disease. A Report of Progress* (Aging, Vol. 19), Corkin, S. et al., Eds., Raven Press, New York, 1982.
104. **Wettstein, A.**, No effect from the double-blind trial of physostigmine and lecithin in Alzheimer's disease, *Ann. Neurol.*, 13(2), 210, 1983.
105. **Sitaram, N., Weingartner, H., and Gillin, J. C.**, Human serial learning: enhancement with arecoline and impairment with schopolamine correlated with performance on placebo, *Science*, 201, 274, 1978.
106. **Christie, J. E., Shering, A., Ferguson, J. et al.**, Physostigmine and arecoline: effects of intravenous infusions in Alzheimer's presenile dementia, *Br. J. Psychiatry*, 138, 46, 1981.
107. **Tariot, P. N., Cohen, R. M., Welkowitz, J. A. et al.**, Multiple-dose arecoline infusions in Alzheimer's disease, *Arch. Gen. Psychiatry*, 45, 901, 1988.
108. **Raffaele, K. C., Berardi, A., Asthana, S. et al.**, Effects of long-term continuous infusion of the muscarinic cholinergic agonist arecoline on verbal memory in dementia of the Alzheimer type, 27(3), 315, 1991.
109. **Wettstein, A. and Spiegal, R.**, Clinical studies with the cholinergic drug RS-86 in Alzheimer's disease (AD) and senile dementia of Alzheimer type (SDAT), *Psychopharmacology*, 84, 572, 1984.
110. **Bruno, G., Mohr, E., Gillespie, M. et al.**, RS-86 therapy of Alzheimer's disease, *Arch. Neurol.*, 43, 659, 1985.
111. **Hollander, E., Davidson, M., Mohs, R. C. et al.**, RS 86 in the treatment of Alzheimer's disease: cognitive and biological effects, *Biol. Psychiatry*, 22, 1067, 1987.
112. **Mouradian, M. M., Mohr, E., Williams, A. J. et al.**, No response to high-dose muscarinic agonist therapy in Alzheimer's disease, *Neurology*, 38, 606, 1988.
113. **Harbaugh, R. E.**, Intracerebroventricular bethanechloride administration in Alzheimer's disease. Preliminary results of a double blind study, *J. Neurotransm.*, 24 (Suppl.), 271, 1987.
114. **Penn, R. D., Martin, E. M., Wilson, R. S. et al.**, Intraventricular bethanechol infusion of Alzheimer's disease: results of double blind and escalating dose trials, *Neurology*, 38, 219, 1988.
115. **Wilson, R. S. and Martin, E. M.**, New intrathecal drugs in Alzheimer's disease and psychometric testing, *Ann. N.Y. Acad. Sci.*, 531, 180, 1988.
116. **Harbaugh, R. E., Reeder, T. M., Senter, H. J. et al.**, Intracerebroventricular bethanechol chloride infusion in Alzheimer's disease — results of a collaborative double-blind study, *J. Neurosurg.*, 71, 481, 1989.
117. **Read, S. L., Frazee, J., Shapira, J. et al.**, Intracerebroventricular bethanechol for Alzheimer's disease. Variable dose-related responses, *Arch. Neurol.*, 47, 1025, 1990.
118. **Davis, K. L., Hollander, E., Davidson, M. et al.**, Induction of depression with oxotremorine in Alzheimer's disease patients, *Am. J. Psychiatry*, 144, 468, 1987.
119. **Newhouse, P. A., Sunderland, T., Tariot, P. N. et al.**, Intravenous nicotine in Alzheimer's disease: a pilot study, *Psychopharmacology*, 95, 171, 1988.
120. **Sahakian, B., Jones, G., Levy, R. et al.**, The effects of nicotine on attention, information processing, and short-term memory in patients with dementia of the Alzheimer type, *Br. J. Psychiatry*, 154, 797, 1989.
121. **Molloy, D. W. and Cape, R. D. T.**, Acute effects of oral pyridostigmine on memory and cognitive function in SDAT, *Neurobiol. Aging*, 10, 199, 1989.
122. **Davis, K. L., Mohs, R. C., Davis, B. M. et al.**, Human memory and the effects of physostigmine and choline chloride, *Psychopharmacol. Bull.*, 16(4), 27, 1980.
123. **Christie, J. E., Shering, A., Ferguson, J. et al.**, Physostigmine and arecoline: effects of intravenous infusions in Alzheimer's presenile dementia, *Br. J. Psychiatry*, 138, 46, 1981.
124. **Bajada**, A trial of choline chloride and physostigmine in Alzheimer's dementia, in *Alzheimer's Disease: A Report of Progress in Research* (Aging, Vol. 19), Corkin, S. et al., Eds., Raven Press, New York, 1982, pp. 427.
125. **Wettstein, A.**, No effect from double-blind trial of physostigmine and lecithin in Alzheimer disease, *Ann. Neurol.*, 13, 210, 1983.
126. **Schmechel, D., Schmitt, F., Horner, J. et al.**, Lack of effect of oral physostigmine and lecithin in patients with probable Alzheimer's disease, *Neurology*, 34 (Suppl. 1), 280, 1984.
127. **Mitchel, A., Drachman, D. A., O'Donnell, B. et al.**, Oral physostigmine in Alzheimer's disease, *Neurology*, 36 (Suppl. 1), 295, 1986.
128. **Stern, Y., Sano, M. and Mayeux, R.**, Effects of oral physostigmine in Alzheimer's disease, *Ann. Neurol.*, 22, 306, 1987.
129. **Jenike, M. A., Albert, M. S., Baer, L. et al.**, Oral physostigmine for primary degenerative dementia: a double blind placebo-controlled inpatient trial, *J. Geriatr. Psychiatry Neurol.*, 3, 13, 1990.
130. **Jenike, M. A., Albert, M. S., Heller, H. et al.**, Oral physostigmine treatment for patients with presenile and senile dementia of Alzheimer's type: a double blind placebo-controlled trial, *J. Clin. Psychiatry*, 51, 3, 1990.
131. **Jenike, M. A., Albert, M. S., and Baer, L.**, Oral physostigmine as treatment for dementia of Alzheimer's type: a long-term outpatient trial, *Alzheimer's Dis. Assoc. Disord.*, 4, 226, 1990.
132. **Harrell, L. E., Jope, R. S., Falgout, J. et al.**, Biological and neuropharmacological characterization of physostigmine responders and nonresponders in Alzheimer's disease, *J. Am. Geriatr. Soc.*, 38, 113, 1990.
133. **Bierer, L. M., Aisen, P. S., Davidson, M. et al.**, A pilot study of oral physostigmine plus yohimbine in patients with Alzheimer disease, *Alzheimer Dis. Assoc. Disord.*, 7(2), 98, 1993.

134. **Izquierdo, I.**, Effect of Beta-endorphin and naloxone on acquisition, memory and retrieval of shuttle avoidance and habituation learning in rats, *Psychopharmacology*, 69, 111, 1980.
135. **Reisberg, B., Ferris, S. H., Anand, R. et al.,** Effects of naloxone in senile dementia: a double-blind trial, *N. Engl. J. Med.*, 308, 721, 1983.
136. **Panella, J. J., Jr. and Blass, J. P.,** Lack of clinical benefit from naloxone in a dementia day hospital, *Ann. Neurol.*, 15, 308, 1984.
137. **Steiger, W. A., Mendelson, M., Jenkins, T. et al.,** Effects of naloxone in treatment of senile dementia, *J. Am. Geriat. Soc.*, 33(2), 155, 1985.
138. **Tariot, P. N., Sunderland, T., Murphy, D. L. et al.,** Design and interpretation of opiate antagonist trials in dementia, *Progr. Neuro-Psychopharmacol. Biol. Psychiatry*, 10, 611, 1986.
139. **Henderson, V. W., Roberts, E., Wimer, C. et al.,** Multicenter trial of naloxone in Alzheimer's disease, *Ann. Neurol.*, 25, 404, 1989.
140. **Serby, M., Resnick, R., Jordan, B. et al.,** Naltrexone and Alzheimer's disease, *Progr. Neuro-Psychopharmacol. Biol. Psychiatry*, 10, 587, 1986.
141. **Pomara, N., Stanley, M., Rhiew, H. B. et al.,** Loss of the cortisol response to naltrexone in Alzheimer's disease, *Biol. Psychiatry*, 23, 726, 1988.
142. **Jorm, A., Korten, A., and Henderson, A.,** The prevalence of dementia: a quantitative integration of the literature, *Acta Psychiatr. Scand.*, 76, 465, 1987
143. **Fillet, H., Weinreb, H., Cholst, I. et al.,** Observations in a preliminary open trial of estradiol therapy for senile dementia — Alzheimer's type, *Psychoneuroendocrinology*, 11, 337, 1986.
144. **Michael, C. M., Kanto, H. I., and Shore, H.,** Further psychometric evaluation of older women. The effect of estrogen administration, *J. Gerontol.*, 25, 337, 1970.
145. **Honjo, H., Ogino, Y., Naitoh, K. et al.,** In vivo effects by estone sulfate on the central nervous system-senile dementia (Alzheimer's type), *J. Steroid Biochem.*, 34, 511, 1989.
146. **Weiss, B. L.,** Failure of nalmefene and estrogen to improve memory in Alzheimer's disease, *Am. J. Psychiatry*, 144, 386, 1987.
147. **Lifshitz, K. and Kline, N. S.,** Use of estrogen in the treatment of psychosis with cerebral arteriosclerosis, *JAMA*, 176, 501, 1961.
148. **Bondareff, W., Mountjoy, C. Q., and Roth, M.,** Loss of neurons of origin of the adrenergic projection to cerebral cortex (nucleus locus coeruleus) in senile dementia, *Neurology*, 32, 164, 1982.
149. **Rossor, M. and Iversen, L. L.,** Non-cholinergic neurotransmitter abnormalities in Alzheimer's disease, *Br. Med. Bull.*, 42, 70, 1986.
150. **Riederer, P. and Jellinger, K.,** Morphological and biochemical changes in the aging brain: pathophysiological and possible therapeutic consequences, *Exp. Brain Res.*, 5 (Suppl.), 158, 1982.
151. **Gottfries, C. G., Adolfsson, R., Aquilonius, S. M. et al.,** Biochemical changes in dementia disorders of the Alzheimer type (AD/SDAT), *Neurobiol. Aging*, 4, 261, 1983.
152. **Arai, H., Kosaka, K., and Ijzuka, R.,** Changes of biogenic amines and their metabolites in post-mortem brains from patients with Alzheimer's type dementia, *J. Neurochem.*, 43, 388, 1984.
153. **Gottfries, C. G., Ujailquist, U., Ponten, E. et al.,** Cerebrospinal fluid pH and monoamine and glucolytic metabolites in Alzheimer's disease, *Br. J. Psychiatry*, 124, 280, 1974.
154. **Adolfsson, R., Brane, G., Bucht, G. et al.,** in *Alzheimer's Disease: A Report of Progress in Research*, Corkin, K. L., Davis, J. H., Growdon, J. H. et al., Eds., Raven Press, New York, 1982, pp. 469.
155. **Ferris, S. H., Reisberg, B., Crook, T. et al.,** Pharmacologic treatment of senile dementia: choline, L-dopa, piracetam and choline plus piracetam, in *Alzheimer's Disease: A Report of Progress*, Corkin, S., Davis, K. L., Growdon, J. H. et al., Eds., Raven Press, New York, 1982, 475.
156. **Jellinger, K., Flament, H., Riederer, P. et al.,** Levodopa in the treatment of (pre)senile dementia, *Ageing Dev.*, 14, 253, 1980.
157. **Arnstein, A. F. T., Cai, J. X., and Goldman-Rakic, P. S.,** The alpha-2 adrenergic agnoist guanfacine improves memory in aged monkeys without sedative or hypotensive side effects: evidence for alpha-2 receptor subtypes, *J. Neurosci.*, 8, 4287, 1988.
158. **Mohr, E., Schlegel, J., Fabbrini, G. et al.,** Clonidine treatment of Alzheimer's disease, *Arch. Neurol.*, 46, 376, 1989.
159. **Schlegel, J., Mohr, E., Williams, J. et al.,** Guanfacine treatment of Alzheimer's disease, *Clin. Neuropharmacol.*, 12, 124, 1989.
160. **Crook, T., Wilner, E., Rothwell, A. et al.,** Noradrenergic intervention in Alzheimer's disease, *Psychopharmacol. Bull.*, 28(1), 67, 1992.
161. **Bergmann, I. Brane, G., Gottfries, C. G. et al.,** Alaproclate: a pharmacokinetic and biochemical study in patients with dementia of Alzheimer's type, *Psychopharmacology*, 80, 279, 1983.
162. **Cutler, N. R., Haxby, J., Kay, A. D. et al.,** Evaluation of zimelidine in Alzheimer's disease: cognitive and biochemical measures, *Arch. Neurol.*, 42, 744, 1985.
163. **Dehlin, O., Hedenrud, B., Jansson, P. et al.,** A double-blind comparison of alaproclate and placebo in the treatment of patients with senile dementia, *Acta Psychiatr. Scand.*, 71, 190, 1985.

164. **Nyth, A. L. and Gottfries, C. G.,** The clinical efficacy of citalopram in treatment of emotional disturbances in dementia disorders — a nordic multicentre study, *Br. J. Psychiatry*, 157, 894, 1990.
165. **Gottfries, C. G., Karlsson, I., and Nyth, A. L.,** Treatment of depression in elderly patients with and without dementia disorders, *Int. Clin. Psychopharmacol.*, 6 (Suppl. 5), 55, 1992.
166. **Gottfries, C. G. and Nyth, A. L.,** Effect of citalopram, a selective 5-HT reuptake blocker, in emotionally disturbed patients with dementia, *Ann. N.Y. Acad. Sci.*, 640, 276, 1991.
167. **Olafsson, K., Jorgensen, S., Jensen, H. V. et al.,** Fluvoxamine in the treatment of demented elderly patients: a double-blind, placebo-controlled study, *Acta Psychiatr. Scand.*, 85, 453, 1992.
168. **Lawlor, B. A., Sunderland, T., Mellow, A. M. et al.,** A pilot placebo-controlled study of chronic m-CPP administration in Alzheimer's disease, *Biol. Psychiatry*, 30, 140, 1991.
169. **Davies, P. and Maloney, A. J.,** Selective loss of central cholinergic neurons in Alzheimer's disease, *Lancet*, 2, 1403, 1976.
170. **Whitehouse, P. J., Price, D. L., Struble, R. G. et al.,** Alzheimer's disease and senile dementia: loss of neurons in the basal forebrain, *Science*, 215, 1237, 1982.
171. **Summers, W. K., Viesselman, J. O., Marsh, G. M. et al.,** Use of THA in treatment of Alzheimer-like dementia; pilot study in twelve patients, *Biol. Psychiatry*, 16, 145, 1981.
172. **Kaye, W. H.,** Modest facilitation of memory in dementia with combined lecithin and anticholinesterase treatment, *Biol. Psychiatry*, 17, 275, 1982.
173. **Summers, W. K., Majovski, L. V., Marsh, G. M. et al.,** Oral tetrahydroaminoacridine in long-term treatment of senile dementia of the Alzheimer type, *N. Engl. J. Med.*, 315, 1241, 1986.
174. **Chatellier, G. and Lacomblez, L.,** Tacrine (tetrahydroaminoacridine; THA) and lecithin in senile dementia of the Alzheimer type: a multicentre trial, *BMJ*, 300, 495, 1990.
175. **Davies, B., Andrewes, D., Stargatt, R. et al.,** Tacrine in Alzheimer's disease, *Lancet*, 2, 163, 1989.
176. **Gauthier, S., Bouchard, R., Lamontagne, A. et al.,** Tetrahydroaminoacridine-lecithin combination treatment in patients with intermediate-stage Alzheimer's disease — results of a Canadian double-blind, crossover, multicenter study, *N. Engl. J. Med.*, 322, 1272, 1990.
177. **Molloy, D. W., Guyatt, G. H., Wilson, D. B. et al.,** Effect of tetrahydroaminoacridine on cognition, function and behavior in Alzheimer's disease, *Can. Med. Assoc. J.*, 144(1), 1991.
178. **Davis, K. L., Thal, L. J., Gamzu, E. R. et al.,** A double-blind, placebo-controlled multicenter study of tacrine for Alzheimer's disease, *N. Engl. J. Med.*, 327, 1253, 1992.
179. **Eagger, S., Morant, N., Levy, R. et al.,** Tacrine in Alzheimer's disease — time course of changes in cognitive function and practice effects, *Br. J. Psychiatry*, 160, 36, 1992.
180. **Farlow, M., Gracon, S., Hershey, L. A. et al.,** A controlled trial of tacrine in Alzheimer's disease, 268, 2523, 1992.
181. **Minthon, L., Gustafson, L., Dalfelt, G. et al.,** Oral tetrahydroaminoacridine treatment of Alzheimer's disease evaluated clinically and by regional cerebral blood flow and EEG, *Dementia*, 4, 32, 1993.
182. **Knapp, M. J., Knopman, D. S., Solomon, P. R. et al.,** A 30-week randomized controlled trial of high-dose tacrine in patients with Alzheimer's disease, *JAMA*, 271(13), 985, 1994.
183. **Fitten, L. J., Perryman, K. M., Gross, P. L. et al.,** Treatment of Alzheimer's disease with short- and long-term oral THA and lecithin: a double-blind study, *Am. J. Psychiatry*, 147(2), 239, 1990.
184. **Weinstein, H. C., Teunisse, S., and van Gool, W. A.,** Tetrahydroaminoacridine and lecithin in the treatment of Alzheimer's disease — effect on cognition, functioning in daily life, behavioural disturbances and burden experienced by the carers, *J. Neurol.*, 238, 34, 1991.
185. **Eagger, S. A., Levy, R., and Sahakian, B. J.,** Tacrine in Alzheimer's disease, *Lancet*, 337, 989, 1991.
186. **Ames, D. J., Bhathal, P. S., Davies, B. M. et al.,** Heterogeneity of adverse hepatic reactions to tetrahydroaminoacridine, *Aust. N.Z. J. Med.*, 20, 193, 1990.
187. **Hammel, P., Larrey, D., Bernuau, J. et al.,** Acute hepatitis after tetrahydroaminoacridine administration for Alzheimer's disease, *J. Clin. Gastroenterol.*, 12, 329, 1990.
188. **Watkins, P. B., Zimmerman, H. J., Knapp, M. J. et al.,** Hepatotoxic effects of tacrine administration in patients with Alzheimer's disease, *JAMA*, 271(13), 992, 1994.
189. **Winker, M. A.,** Tacrine for Alzheimer's disease — which patient, what dose?, *JAMA*, 271(13), 1023, 1994.
190. **Murphy, M. F., Hardiman, S. T., Nash, R. J. et al.,** Evaluation of HP 029 (velnacrine maleate) in Alzheimer's disease, Ann. N.Y. Acad. Sci., 640, 253, 1991.
191. **Puri, K., Hsu, R. S., Ho, I. et al.,** Single dose safety, tolerance, and pharmacokinetics of HP 029 in healthy young men: a potential Alzheimer's agent, *J. Clin. Pharmacol.*, 29, 278, 1989.
192. **Fielding, S., Cornfeldt, M. L., Szewczak, M. R. et al.,** HP-029, a new drug for the treatment of Alzheimer's disease: its pharmacological profile, presented at the Fourth World Conference on Clinical Pharmacology and Therapeutics, Berlin (West), July 28 to 30, 1989.
193. **Cutler, N. R., Murphy, M. F., Nash, R. J. et al.,** Clinical safety, tolerance, and plasma levels of the oral anticholinesterase 1,2,3,4-tetrahydro-9-aminoacridin-1-oL-maleate (HP 029) in Alzheimer's disease: preliminary findings, *J. Clin. Pharmacol.*, 30, 556, 1990.

194. **Ebmeier, K. P., Hunter, R., Curran, S. M. et al.,** Effects of single dose of the acetylcholinesterase inhibitor velnacrine on recognition memory and regional cerebral blood flow in Alzheimer's disease, *Psychopharmacology*, 108, 103, 1992.
195. **Dal-Bianco et al.,** AD — Therapie durch cholinesterasehemmung, presented at the 19th Central European Neurobiol Symposium-CNS, Vienna, June 29 to July 1st, 1989.
196. **Rainer, M., Mark, T. H., and Haushofer, A.,** Galanthaminum hydrobromicum in treatment of senile dementia (Alzheimer's disease), presented at the Fourth World Conference on Clinical Pharmacology and Therapeutics, Berlin (West), July 28 to 30, 1989.
197. **Dal-Bianco, P., Maly, J., Wober, C. et al.,** Galanthamine treatment in Alzheimer's disease, *J. Neural Transm.*, 33 (Suppl.), 59, 1991.
198. **Mihara, M., Ohnishi, A., Tomono, Y. et al.,** Pharmacokinetics of E2020, a new compound for Alzheimer's disease, in healthy male volunteers, *Int. J. Clin. Pharmacol., Ther. Toxicol.*, 31(5), 233, 1993.
199. **Calvani, M., Carta, A., Caruso, G. et al.,** Action of acetyl-L-carnitine in neurodegeneration and Alzheimer's disease, *Ann. N.Y. Acad. Sci.*, 663, 483, 1992.
200. **Bonnavita, E.,** Study of the efficacy and the stability of L-acetyl-carnitine therapy in the senile brain, *Int. J. Clin. Pharmacol. Ther. Toxicol.*, 23, 511, 1986.
201. **Rai, G., Wright, G., Scott, L. et al.,** Double-blind, placebo controlled study of acetyl-L-carnitine in patients with Alzheimer's dementia, *Curr. Med. Res. Opin.*, 11(10), 638, 1990.
202. **Spagnoli, A., Lucca, U., Menasce, G. et al.,** Long-term acetyl-L-carnitine treatment in Alzheimer's disease, *Neurology*, 41, 1726, 1991.
203. **Sano, M., Bell, K., Cote, L. et al.,** Double-blind parallel design pilot study of acetyl levocarnitine in patients with Alzheimer's disease, *Arch. Neurol.*, 49, 1137, 1992.
204. **Bruno, G., Mohr, E., Gillespie, M. et al.,** Muscarinic agonist therapy of Alzheimer's disease, *Arch. Neurol.*, 43, 659, 1986.
205. **Ferris, S. H., Sathananthan, G., Gershon, S. et al.,** Senile dementia: treatment with deanol, *J. Am. Geriatr. Soc.*, 25, 241, 1977.
206. **Drachman, D. A. and Swearer, J. M.,** The therapy of Alzheimer's disease, in *Controlled Clinical Trials in Neurologic Disease*, Foster, R. and Schoenberg, B., Eds., Kluwer Academic Publishers, Norwell, MA, 1989, 113.
207. **Wessenling, H., Agoston, S., Van Dan, G. et al.,** Effects of 4-aminopyridine in elderly patients with Alzheimer's disease, *N. Engl. J. Med.*, 310, 988, 1984.
208. **Davidson, M., Zemishland, Z., Mohs, R. et al.,** 4-Aminopyridine in the treatment of Alzheimer's disease, *Biol. Psychiatry*, 23, 485, 1988.
209. **Cook, L., Nickolson, V. J., Steinfels, G. F. et al.,** Cognition enhancement by the acetyl-choline releaser DuP 996, *Drug Dev. Res.*, 19, 301, 1990.
210. **Nickolson, V. J., Tam, W. S., Meyers, M. J. et al.,** DuP 996 (3,3-bis(4-pjyridinylmethyl)-1-phenylindolin-2-one) enhances the stimulus-induced release of acetylcholine from rat brain in vitro and in vivo, *Drug Dev. Res.*, 19, 285, 1990.
211. **Saletu, B., Darragh, A., Salmon, P. et al.,** EEG brain mapping in evaluating the time-course of the central action of DUP 996 — a new acetylcholine releasing drug, *Br. J. Clin. Pharmacol.*, 28, 1, 1989.
212. **Tariot, P. N., Sunderland, T., Weingartner, H. et al.,** Cognitive effects of L-deprenyl in Alzheimer's disease, *Psychopharmacology*, 91, 489, 1987.
213. **Schneider, L. S., Pollock, V. E., Zemansky, M. F. et al.,** A pilot study of low-dose L-deprenyl in Alzheimer's disease, *J. Geriatr. Psychiatry Neurol.*, 4, 143, 1991.
214. **Piccinin, G. L., Finali, G., and Piccirilli, M.,** Neuropsychological effects of L-deprenyl in Alzheimer's type dementia, *Clin. Neuropharmacol.*, 13(2), 147, 1990.
215. **Finali, G., Piccirilli, M., Oliani, C. et al.,** L-Deprenyl therapy improves verbal memory in amnesic Alzheimer patients, *Clin. Neuropharmacol.*, 14(6), 523, 1991.
216. **Mangoni, A., Grassi, M. P., Grattola, L. et al.,** Effects of a MAO-B inhibitor in the treatment of Alzheimer's disease, *Eur. Neurol.*, 31, 100, 1991.
217. **Agnoli, A., Fabbrini, G., Fioravanti, M. et al.,** CBF and cognitive evaluation of Alzheimer type patients before and after IMAO-B treatment: a pilot study, *Eur. Neuropsychopharmacol.*, 2, 31, 1992.
218. **Burke, W. J., Ranno, A. E., Roccaforte, W. H. et al.,** L-deprenyl in the treatment of mild dementia of the Alzheimer type: preliminary results, *J. Am. Geriatr. Soc.*, 41, 367, 1993.
219. **Sunderland, T., Molchan, S., Lawlor, B. et al.,** A strategy of "combination chemotherapy" in Alzheimer's disease: rationale and preliminary results with physostigmine plus deprenyl, *Int. Psychogeriatr.*, 4 (Suppl. 2), 1992.
220. **Schneider, L. S., Olin, J. T., and Pawluczyk, S.,** A double-blind crossover pilot study of L-deprenyl (selegiline) combined with cholinesterase inhibitor in Alzheimer's disease, *Am. J. Psychiatry*, 150, 321, 1993.
221. **Dysken, M. W., Mendels, J., LeWitt, P. et al.,** Milacemide: a placebo-controlled study in senile dementia of the Alzheimer type, *J. Am. Geriatr. Soc.*, 40, 503, 1992.

222. **Cutler, N. R., Fakouhi, D., Smith, W. T. et al.,** Evaluation of multiple doses of milacemide in the treatment of senile dementia of the Alzheimer's type, *J. Geriatr. Psychiatry Neurol.*, 6, 115, 1993.
223. **Mattson, R. J.,** Investigator brochure: BMY 21502, psychogeriatric agent, Bristol-Myers Company, Wallingford, 1988, 1.
224. **Levi-Montalcini, R.,** The nerve growth factor, *Ann. N.Y. Acad. Sci.*, 113, 149, 1964.
225. **Hefti, F.,** Alzheimer's disease caused by a lack of nerve growth factor?, *Ann. Neurol.*, 13, 109, 1983.
226. **Hefti, F. and Weiner, W. J.,** Nerve growth factor and Alzheimer's disease, *Ann. Neurol.*, 20, 275, 1986.
227. **Hagg, T., Hanthorpe, M., Vahlsing, H. C. et al.,** Delayed treatment with nerve growth factor reverses the apparent loss of cholinergic neurons after acute brain damage, *Exp. Neurol.*, 101, 303, 1988.
228. **Williams, L. R., Varon, S., Peterson, G. M. et al.,** Continuous infusion of nerve growth factor prevents vasal forebrain neuronal death after fimbria fornix transection, *Proc. Natl. Acad. Sci. U.S.A.*, 83, 9231, 1986.
229. **Hoffman, D., Wahlber, L., and Aebischer, P.,** NGF released from a polymer matrix prevents loss of ChAT expression in basal forebrain neurons following a fimbria-fornix lesion, *Soc. Neurosci. Abstr.*, 16, 477, 1990.
230. **Corsi, P. and Coyle, J. T.,** Nerve growth factor corrects developmental impairments of basal forebrain cholinergic neurons in the trisomy 16 mouse, *Proc. Natl. Acad. Sci. U.S.A.*, 88, 1793, 1991.
231. **Hefti, F. and Schneider, L. S.,** Nerve growth factor and Alzheimer's disease, *Clin. Neuropharm.*, 14, S62, 1991.
232. **Gottfries, C. G., Adolfsson, R., Aquilonius, S. M. et al.,** Biochemical changes in dementia disorders of Alzheimer type (AD/SDAT), *Neurobiol. Aging*, 4, 261, 1983.
233. **Bellato, P., Milan, F., and Toffano, G.,** Disposition of exogenous tritium-labelled GM1 monosialoganglioside in the rat, *Clin. Trials J.*, 26, 39, 1989.
234. **Svennerholm, L., Gottfries, C. G., Blennow, K. et al.,** Parenteral administration of GM1 ganglioside to presenile Alzheimer patients, *Acta Neurol. Scand.*, 81, 48, 1990.
235. **Ala, T., Romero, S., Knight, F. et al.,** GM-1 treatment of Alzheimer's disease — a pilot study of safety and efficacy, *Arch. Neurol.*, 47, 1126, 1990.
236. **Flicker, C., Ferris, S. H., Kalkstein, D. et al.,** A double-blind, placebo-controlled crossover study of ganglioside GM1 treatment of Alzheimer's disease, *Am. J. Psychiatry*, 151, 126, 1994.
237. **Satzger, W., Bove, D., Gerko, S. et al.,** Preliminary results of a six-month double-blind crossover study of phosphatidylserine vs. placebo in patients with early senile dementia of Alzheimer's type, *Psychopharmacology*, 96 (Suppl.), 301, 1988.
238. **Amaducci, L. and the SMID Group**, Phosphatidylserine in the treatment of Alzheimer's disease: results of a multi-center study, *Psychopharmacol. Bull.*, 24, 130, 1988.
239. **Delwaide, P. J., Gyselynek-Mambourg, A. M., Hurlet, A. et al.,** Double blind randomized controlled study of phosphatidylserine in senile demented patients, *Acta Neurol. Scand.*, 73, 136, 1986.
240. **Palmieri, G., Palmieri, R., Inzoli, M. R. et al.,** Double-blind controlled trial of phosphatidylserine in patients with senile mental deterioration, *Clin. Trials J.*, 24(1), 73, 1987.
241. **Villartita, C., Grioli, S., Salmeri, G. et al.,** Multicenter clinical trial of brain phosphatidylserine in elderly patients with intellectual deterioration, *Clin. Trials J.*, 24(1), 84, 1987.
242. **Puca, F. M., Savarese, M. A., and Mirervini, M. G.,** Exploratory trial of phosphatidylserine efficacy in mildly demented patients, *Clin. Trials J.*, 24(1), 94, 1987.
243. **Granata, Q. and Michelle, J. D.,** Phosphatidylserine in elderly patients, *Clin. Trials J.*, 24(1), 99, 1987.
244. **Allegro, L., Favaretto, V., and Zilliotto, G.,** Oral phosphatidylserine in elderly patients with cognitive deterioration: an open study, *Clin. Trials J.*, 24(1), 104, 1987.
245. **Caffarra, P. and Santamaria, V.,** The effects of phosphatidylserine in patients with mild cognitive decline: an open trial, *Clin. Trials J.*, 24(1), 109, 1987.
246. **Sinforiani, E., Agostinis, C., Merlo, P. et al.,** Cognitive decline in aging brain: therapeutic approach with phosphatidylserine, *Clin. Trials J.*, 24(1), 115, 1987.
247. **Engel, R. R., Satzger, W., Gunther, W. et al.,** Double-blind cross-over study of phosphatidylserine vs. placebo in patients with early dementia of Alzheimer's type, *Eur. Neuropsychopharmacol.*, 2, 149, 1992.
248. **Crook, T., Petrie, W., Wells, C. et al.,** Effects of phosphatidylserine in Alzheimer's disease, *Psychopharmacol. Bull.*, 28(1), 61, 1992.
249. **LeVere, T. E., Brugler, T., Sandin, M. et al.,** Recovery of function after brain damage: facilitation by the calcium entry blocker nimodipine, *Behav. Neurosci.*, 103(3), 561, 1989.
250. **Harris, R. J., Branston, W. M., Symon, L. et al.,** Cerebral ischemia and calcium, *Stroke*, 13, 759, 1982.
251. **Betz, E., Deck, K., and Hoffmeister, F.,** Therapeutic effects of nimodipine, in *Nimodipine: Pharmacological and Clinical Properties*, Schattauer, Verlag, Stuttgart, 1985.
252. **Deyo, R. A., Straube, K. T., and Disterhoft, J. F.,** Nimodipine facilitates associative learning in aging rabbits, *Science*, 243, 809, 1989.
253. **Schuurman, T. and Traber, J.,** Old rats as an animal model for senile dementia: behavioral effects of nimodipine, in *Diagnosis and Treatment of Senile Dementia*, Bergener, M. and Reisberg, B., Eds., Springer-Verlag, Berlin, 1989, 295.

254. **Tollefson, G. D.,** Short-term effects of the calcium channel blocker nimodipine (Bay-e-9736) in the management of primary degenerative dementia, *Biol. Psychiatry*, 27, 1133, 1990.
255. **Ban, T. A., Morey, L., Aguglia, E. et al.,** Nimodipine in the treatment of old age dementias, *Prog. Neuro-Psychopharmacol. Biol. Psychiatry*, 14, 525, 1990.
256. **Parnetti, L., Senin, U., Carosi, M. et al.,** Mental deterioration in old age: results of two multicenter, clinical trials with nimodipine, *Clin. Ther.*, 15(2), 394, 1993.
257. **Barnes, J. M., Barnes, N. M., Costall, B. et al.,** Angiotensin II inhibits the release of (^{3}H) acetylcholine from rat entohinal cortex in vitro, *Brain Res.*, 491, 136, 1989.
258. **Morgan, J. M. and Routtenberg, A.,** Angiotensin injected into the neostriatum after learning disrupts retenditon performance, *Science*, 196, 87, 1977.
259. **Mondadori, C. and Etienne, P.,** Nootropic effects of ACE inhibitors in mice, *Psychopharmacology*, 100, 301, 1990.
260. **Croog, S. H., Sudilovsky, A., Levine, S. et al.,** Work performance, absenteeism and antihypertensive medications, *J. Hypertens.*, 5 (Suppl. 1), 47, 1987.
261. **Arregui, A., Perry, E. K., Rossor, M. et al.,** Angiotensin converting enzyme in Alzheimer's disease: increased activity in caudate nucleus and cortical areas, *J. Neurochem.*, 38, 1490, 1982.
262. **Sudilovsky, A., Cutler, R., Sramek, J. J. et al.,** A pilot clinical trial of the angiotensin-converting enzyme inhibitor ceranapril in Alzheimer disease, *Alzheimer Dis. Assoc. Disord.*, 7(2), 105, 1993.
263. **Saletu, B., Anderer, P., Fischhof, P. K. et al.,** EEG mapping and psychopharmacological studies with denbufylline in SDAT and MID, *Biol. Psychiatry*, 32, 668, 1992.
264. **Saletu, B., Moller, H. J., Grunberger, J. et al.,** Propentofylline in adult-onset cognitive disorders: double-blind, placebo-controlled, clinical, psychometric and brain mapping studies, *Neuropsychobiology*, 24, 173, 1990.
265. **DeBoni, V., Gapper, D., and McLachlan, D.,** Biochemical aspect of SDAT and aluminum as a neurotoxic agent, in *Strategies for the Development of an Effective Treatment for Senile Dementia*, Crook, T. and Gershon, S., Eds., Mark Powley Associates, New Canaan, CT, 1986, 196.
266. **Markeslery, W., Ehman, W., Hossian, T. et al.,** Instrumental neuron activation analysis of brain aluminum in Alzheimer's disease and aging, *Ann. Neurol.*, 10, 511, 1981.
267. **McLachlan, D. R. C., Dalton, A. J., Kruck, T. P. A. et al.,** Intramuscular desferrioxamine in patients with Alzheimer's disease, *Lancet*, 337, 1304, 1991.
268. **Gash, D. M., Notter, M. F. D., and Kordower, J. H.,** Cognitive dysfunctions and neural implants, in *Treatment Development Strategies for Alzheimer's Disease*, Crook, T., Bartus, R. T., Ferris, S. et al., Eds., Mark Powley Associates, Madison, CT, 1986, chap. 25.
269. **Monahan, J. B., Handelmann, G. E., Hood, W. F. et al.,** d-Cycloserine, a positive modulator of the N-methyl-d-aspartate receptor, enhances performance of learning task in rats, *Pharmacol. Biochem. Behav.*, 34, 649, 1989.
270. **Hood, W. F., Compton, R. P., and Monahan, J. B.,** d-Cycloserine: a ligand for the N-methyl-d-aspartate coupled glycine receptor has partial agonist characteristics, *Neurosci. Lett.*, 98, 91, 1989.
271. **Henderson, G., Hohnson, J. W., and Ascher, P.,** Competitive antagonists and partial agonists at the glycine modulatory site of the mouse N-methyl-d-aspartate receptor, *J. Physiol.*, 430, 189, 1990.
272. **Watson, G. B., Bolanowski, M. A., Baganoff, M. P. et al.,** d-Cycloserine acts as partial agonist in the glycine modulatory site of the NMDA receptor expressed in *Xenopus oocytes*, *Brain Res.*, 510, 158, 1990.
273. **Chessell, I. P., Procter, A. W., Francis, P. T. et al.,** d-Cycloserine, a putative cognitive enhancer, facilitates activation of the N-methyl-d-aspartate receptor-ionophore complex in Alzheimer brain, *Brain Res.*, 565, 345, 1991.
274. **Breitner, J. C. S., Gau, B. A., Welsh, K. A. et al.,** Inverse association of anti-inflammatory treatments and Alzheimer's disease: initial results of a xo-twin control study, *Neurology*, 44, 227, 1994.
275. **Rogers, J., Kirby, L. C., Hempelman, S. R. et al.,** Clinical trial of indomethacin in Alzheimer's disease, *Neurology*, 43, 1609, 1993.
276. **Greenamyre, J. T. and Young, A. B.,** Review: excitatory amino acids and Alzheimer's disease, *Neurobiol. Aging*, 10, 593, 1989.
277. **Palmer, A. M. and Gershon, S.,** Is the neuronal basis of Alzheimer's disease cholinergic or glutamatergic?, *FASEB J.*, 4, 2745, 1990.
278. **Davidson, M. and Stern, R. G.,** The treatment of cognitive impairment in Alzheimer's disease: beyond the cholinergic approach, *Psychiatr. Clin. North Am.*, 14(2), 461, 1991.
279. **Zubenko, G. S., Cohen, B. M., Growden, J. et al.,** Cell membrane abnormality in Alzheimer's disease, *Lancet*, ii, 235, 1984.
280. **Zubenko, G. S., Cohen, B. M., Reynolds, C. F. et al.,** Platelet membrane fluidity in Alzheimer's disease and major depression, *Am. J. Psychiatry*, 144, 860, 1987.
281. **Zubenko, G. S., Cohen, B. M., Reynolds, C. F. et al.,** Clinical subtypes of Alzheimer's disease identified by platelet membrane fluidity, *Progr. Neuro-Psychopharmacol. Biol. Psychiatry*, 11, 683, 1987.

282. **Zubenko, G. S. and Teply, I.,** Longitudinal study of platelet membrane fluidity in Alzheimer's disease, *Biol. Psychiatry*, 24, 918, 1988.
283. **Zubenko, G. S., Cohen, B. M., Boller, F. et al.,** Platelet membrane abnormality in Alzheimer's disease, *Ann. Neurol.*, 22, 237, 1987.
284. **Flament, S. and Delacourte, A.,** Abnormal tau species are produced during Alzheimer's disease neurodegenerating process, *FEBS Lett.*, 247(2), 213, 1989.
285. **Flament, S., Delacourte, A., Hernon, B. et al.,** Characterization of two pathological tau proteins, variants in Alzheimer's brain cortices, *J. Neurol. Sci.*, 92(2–3), 133, 1989.
286. **Saunders, A. M., Strittmatter, W. J., Schmechel, D. et al.,** Association of apolipoprotein E allele E4 with late-onset familial and sporadic Alzheimer's disease, *Neurology*, 43, 1467, 1993.
287. **Peacock, M. L. and Fink, J. K.,** ApoE E4 allelic association with Alzheimer's disease: independent confirmation using denaturing gradient gel electrophoresis, *Neurology*, 44, 339, 1994.
288. **Brousseau, T., Legrain, S., Berr, C. et al.,** Confirmation of the E4 allele of the apolipoprotein E gene as a risk factor for late-onset Alzheimer's disease, *Neurology*, 44, 342, 1994.
289. **Cowburn, R. F., Hardy, J. A., and Roberts, P. J.,** Neurotransmitter deficits in Alzheimer's disease, in *Alzheimer's Disease: Towards an Understanding of the Aetiology and Pathogenesis*, Davies, D. C., Ed., John Libbey & Co. Ltd., 1989.
290. **Levy, R.,** Are drugs targeted at Alzheimer's disease useful?, *BMJ*, 300, 1131, 1990.
291. **Whitehouse, P. J.,** Treatment of Alzheimer disease, *Alzheimer Dis. Assoc. Disord.*, 5 (Suppl. 1), S32, 1991.

Chapter 13

AGENTS USED IN ANEMIA AND COAGULATION DISORDERS OF THE ELDERLY

Walter Fried

CONTENTS

I. INTRODUCTION

The diagnosis of anemia is established when the blood hemoglobin concentration and/or the hematocrit fall below the normal values for the laboratory in which they are determined. The norms for these parameters are dependent on the altitude of the region and on the gender of the patient; they are usually not adjusted for age.

Erythrocytes are enucleate cells that cannot synthesize proteins. As they age, their enzymatic functions decline and changes occur in their membrane structure. As a result, new antigens are exposed on the cell surface, which are recognized by the macrophages and result in phagocytosis of the senescent cells. The life span of the erythrocyte is 120 d; consequently, preservation of a normal red cell mass requires a daily turnover of 0.8%. Anemia ensues when either the red blood cell (RBC) life span is excessively shortened or the production of erythrocytes is impaired.

The RBC life span is decreased by defects in their hemoglobin, enzymes, or membrane proteins; or by extra-erythrocytic lesions that involve the spleen, microvasculature, heart valves, or plasma components. Hemolytic anemias result from uncompensated reductions of

0-8493-8306-4/96/$0.00+$.50

the erythrocyte life span. Hypoproliferative anemias, which occur more commonly in patients of all ages, are caused by rate-limiting defects in the production of erythrocytes. The following section of this chapter will review the regulatory mechanisms that determine the rate of erythropoiesis and how they are affected by aging; the impact of age-related changes in erythropoiesis on the blood counts of elderly persons; and the role of recombinant human erythropoietin (rHuEpo) in the management of various anemias.

III. FACTORS INVOLVED IN THE REGULATION OF THE RATE OF ERYTHROPOIESIS

A. PROGENITOR CELLS

Pluripotential stem cells[1–3] capable of commitment and differentiation along the lymphocytic, myelocytic, monocytic, erythrocytic, and megakaryocytic cell lines are present in the circulating blood and bone marrow of all mammals. All but a small fraction of these cells are in G_0, or noncycling phase, during steady-state conditions. Migration of circulating stem cells into the extrasinusoidal marrow areas is regulated by the interaction of specific adhesion molecules, expressed on their surface, with others on the endothelial cell membrane.[4] Once in the hematopoietic microenvironment, they become fixed into special niches by interactions between lectins on their surface and those on fixed stromal cells; and also by interactions between receptors on their membrane with cell-bound ligands, such as the stem cell factor.[5] After fixation in favorable sites, the stem cells undergo commitment in an undirected stochastic manner.[6] The earliest committed erythroid progenitors are the burst-forming unit-erythroid (BFU-E).[7]

As BFU-E mature, they express receptors for a variety of growth factors (stem cell factor, interleukin-3 [IL-3], granulocyte monocyte colony-stimulating factor [GM-CSF] and insulin-like growth factor). Interaction with these factors is required for maturation to proceed.[7] Erythropoietin (Epo) receptors[8] first become detectable on the surface of intermediate BFU-E and increase in density as the cells mature into colony-forming units-erythroid (CFU-E), which express the maximum number of Epo receptors.[9] Most CFU-E, the primary target cells for Epo, are in cell cycle. CFU-E are not identifiable on routine microscopic examination of bone marrow aspirates or biopsies. However, they are only one or two cell divisions away from being transformed into proerythroblasts, the earliest recognizable erythroid precursor.

B. ERYTHROPOIETIN (EPO)

Epo is a glycoprotein with a molecular weight of 35,000 Da.[10] During fetal life it is produced predominantly by the liver.[11] Shortly after birth, Epo production shifts to the kidney.[12] However, in anephric patients a small, but significant, amount of Epo can be produced by the liver.[13] The site of renal Epo production is a specialized peritubular endothelial cell, found predominantly in the cortex.[14] Conditions that stimulate Epo production are accompanied by an increase in the number of Epo-producing cells. Epo production in the liver occurs in hepatocytes, located in centrilobular areas.[15] Unlike renal Epo production, stimuli increase the amount of Epo produced per hepatocyte, without increasing the number of Epo-producing cells.The rate of Epo production in both the kidney[16] and the liver[17] is primarily a function of the ratio of the O_2 demand: O_2 supply at the site of production. However, a variety of other factors modulate the rate of Epo production. These include hormones that affect the rate of O_2 utilization;[18] the status of protein nutrition;[19] androgenic steroids, which increase Epo production;[20] inflammatory cytokines, such as tumor necrosis factor (TNF), and IL-1,[21,22] which decrease Epo production; prostaglandins;[23,24] prolactin;[25] cobaltous chloride;[26] and the functional integrity of the erythron.[27,28] The latter is a manifestation of an important, but poorly understood mechanism that fine tunes the rate of erythropoiesis. Some of these conditions affect either renal or hepatic Epo production, whereas others affect both.

Epo exerts its effects by interaction with specific receptors,[29] found predominantly on late BFU-E and CFU-E, but which are also present, in low concentration, on megakaryocytes[30] and on some endothelial cells.[31] Interaction of Epo with receptors on late BFU-E increases their proliferating fraction and, consequently, the size of the Epo target cell population.[32] Interaction of Epo with receptors on CFU-E inhibits apoptosis[33] and thereby permits them to undergo terminal maturation. The rate of erythropoiesis is determined by the serum Epo titer and by the number of functional CFU-E, provided that the supply of nutrients needed for terminal maturation is adequate.

C. TERMINAL MATURATION OF ERYTHROCYTES

Terminal maturation refers to the process that results in the transformation of CFU-E into mature erythrocytes. During terminal maturation, the cell must synthesize sufficient hemoglobin to produce an optimal mean cell hemoglobin concentration, while simultaneously undergoing approximately four terminal cell divisions. The rates of hemoglobin and DNA synthesis are not determined by Epo. They proceed at predetermined velocities, unless limited by the availability of iron, vitamin B_{12}, and folic acid. Conditions that limit the rate of hemoglobin synthesis often result in microcytic anemias, whereas those that impede DNA synthesis result in macrocytic anemias.

The most common anemias of humans are caused by defects in the terminal maturation of erythrocytes, particularly those that limit hemoglobin synthesis. The rate of hemoglobin synthesis is most commonly limited by the supply of iron-saturated transferrin to its specific receptor on the erythroid precursors. Normally, the daily rate of RBC production approximates that of RBC destruction. Consequently, by recycling all of the iron that is extracted from the hemoglobin of senescent erythrocytes, the macrophages provide all but 1 or 2 mg of the iron requirements of adults. The additional 1 or 2 mg of iron is readily supplied by dietary sources. Iron deficiency develops when the delivery of iron to the erythron becomes the limiting factor that determines the rate of erythropoiesis. Iron deficiency can be actual or functional. In both, the serum iron and the transferrin saturation are decreased. Actual iron deficiency is characterized by low serum ferritin and absent iron stores, whereas in functional iron deficiency these parameters are normal, indicating that the amount of storage iron is adequate. The defect is in the ability to mobilize storage iron rapidly enough to satisfy the needs of the erythron.

Actual iron deficiency in adults is almost always caused by blood loss. The anemia of chronic disease has previously been considered to be a classic example of functional iron deficiency, although new information indicates that its pathogenesis is complex. In this condition, the ability of the macrophages to mobilize iron is impaired, presumably due to the actions of the inflammatory cytokines, IL-1, IL-6, tumor necrosis factor (TNF), and/or interferon. Another cause of functional iron deficiency was recently uncovered during clinical trials of rHuEpo in patients with chronic renal failure. A significant percentage of patients enrolled in these studies initially responded to rHuEpo, but later developed hypoferremia and ceased to respond, even though their iron stores remained ample.[34] The apparent interpretation is that rHuEpo increases daily RBC production to a rate that substantially exceeds that of RBC destruction. To satisfy the iron requirements of the hyperactive erythron, iron must be supplied in excess of the amounts that are deposited into the stores daily. A modest amount of extra iron is provided by an increase in the absorption of dietary iron that occurs in response to an increase in the rate of erythropoiesis.[35,36] The remainder must be derived from the storage pool. When iron is initially deposited into the stores, it is incorporated into ferritin, from which it is readily released. However, the longer iron remains in this form, the more likely it is to be transformed into a more stable storage form, from which it is less readily mobilized.[37] Accordingly, once the readily mobilizable iron is depleted, the serum iron and the transferrin saturation decline, the rate of erythropoiesis slows, but the serum ferritin remains normal or increased.

After iron-transferrin reacts with its receptor on the erythroid precursor, the complex is internalized and the iron is delivered to the mitochondria, where heme is synthesized. The newly synthesized heme molecules are released into the cytosol, where they attach to globin molecules, being synthesized on ribosomes. Hemoglobin is then formed by the polymerization of four globin molecules. Defects in mitochondrial heme synthesis and defects in globin synthesis result in sideroblastic anemias and thalassemia, respectively.

Macrocytic anemias are caused by faulty DNA synthesis during the terminal maturation process. The most common cause of macrocytic anemia, in persons of all ages, is an insufficient supply of folic acid or vitamin B_{12}, which results in a decreased rate of endogenous thymidine synthesis. Other less common causes of macrocytic anemia include drugs that either interfere with DNA synthesis, replication, or repair; drugs that interfere with folic acid absorption and/or metabolism; liver disease; myelodysplastic syndromes; and congenital defects of purine metabolism.

III. EFFECTS OF AGING ON ERYTHROPOIESIS

Our understanding of the effect of aging on the regulation of erythropoiesis is derived largely from animal experiments. The hematopoietic stem cell is not capable of undergoing an infinite number of divisions, as evidenced by a decline in the proliferative capacity of murine marrow-derived stem cells after repeated passages through lethally irradiated mice.[38] However, because only a small fraction of multipotential stem cells are in cell cycle, the proliferative capacity of murine pluripotential stem cells does not decline significantly during the life span of the animal.[39,40] Very old, but healthy, mice and humans have only a slight decrease in their mean blood hemoglobin concentration and hematocrit, which in the case of humans becomes significant, but not of importance, after age 75.[41] This suggests that the erythron of very old persons functions normally under basal steady-state conditions. However, its response to stressful conditions becomes less vigorous with age. The recovery of the blood hemoglobin concentration of aged mice made severely anemic by phlebotomy is slower than in young animals,[42,43] and its rise in aged mice exposed to chronic hypoxia is slower than in young mice.[44] These differences are not attributable to decreased Epo production, since the ability to produce Epo does not change, demonstrably, with age.[45] The effect of aging on serum Epo titers in humans has not yet been thoroughly studied. In one study,[46] patients over the age of 70 with normocytic anemias were observed to have mean serum Epo levels that were lower than those of comparably anemic younger persons. In this study, similar differences were not observed in patients with microcytic and macrocytic anemias. In contrast, Nafziger et al.[47] found that aged persons with iron deficiency anemia had lower serum Epo titers than comparably anemic young persons. These inconsistencies suggest that the observed decreases are not due directly to the effects of age on the site of Epo production. It is more likely that they reflect the effects of concomitant conditions, such as malnutrition, undiagnosed infections, and alterations in renal function, which are more prevalent in the aged.

Elderly persons have a larger plasma volume than their younger counterparts,[48] which may contribute to the mild, but significant, decrease in the blood hemoglobin concentration and hematocrit observed as persons age. The iliac crest bone marrow becomes hypocellular as persons age; this does not necessarily mean, though, that total hematopoietic cellularity declines. Lipschitz et al.[49] studied the total marrow cellularity of elderly patients by a radioisotopic method and found that the marrow of healthy persons, over 70 years of age, had significantly fewer CFU-E, but not BFU-E, than did younger healthy controls. They concluded that the uncommitted and early committed progenitor cell populations remain intact, but alterations in the late maturation phase of erythropoiesis in elderly persons diminished their erythroid reserve.

The erythrocytes of elderly rats and humans are subtly different than those of their younger counterparts.[50] The erythrocyte life span of aged rats is slightly, but significantly shortened, as measured by the survival of Cr^{51}-labeled erythrocytes. The shortened RBC life span of old rats is the result of both intra- and extra-erythrocytic changes. The blood of healthy elderly persons contains more low-density red cells and slightly more reticulocytes than does that of young persons. These differences are not large and their significance is uncertain. They suggest that the percentage of young erythrocytes is increased in elderly persons, which implies a moderately decreased RBC life span. Other changes in the red cells of healthy aged individuals include alterations in the composition of membrane protein, decrease in membrane protein phosphorylation, increase in the rate of band 3 degradation due to increased Calpain activation, and an increase in membrane-bound IgG.

IV. ANEMIA IN THE AGED

The results of cross-sectional surveys of large populations indicate that the mean blood hemoglobin concentration of octogenarians is slightly, but significantly, lower than that of the younger members of the population. To determine whether or not this is directly due to the aging process, Nilsson-Ehle et a1.[41] measured the blood hemoglobin concentrations and the hematocrits of a healthy group of men and women, sequentially, at ages 71, 75, and 81 years. Those who developed illnesses during this 10-year period were excluded from the reference group. They found that the blood hemoglobin concentration of men dropped from a mean of 15.5 to 14.6 g/dL, and that of the women in the study dropped from a mean of 14.1 to 13.6 g/dL. These differences were significant, but the values remained within the normal range of most laboratories.

Epidemiologic surveys of large populations[51–53] have detected an increased incidence of anemia amongst the elderly (ages 70 and above), which is more marked in males than in females. In some studies, as many as 30% of the elderly males were anemic.[54] In most cases, the anemia resulted from definable disorders which also occur in younger persons, albeit in lower incidence. The most common anemias in the elderly are caused by a reduced availability of iron due to actual or functional iron deficiency. Other anemias that occur relatively frequently in the aged population include nutritional anemias, pernicious anemia, and those associated with myelodysplasia and neoplastic disorders.

Lipschitz et a1.[49] and Mansouri and Lipschitz[54] observed that a substantial number of elderly persons have mild normocytic anemias, for which no specific etiology is identified after intense diagnostic investigations. They noted that mild neutropenia was not uncommon in this group. Additionally, they demonstrated that this cohort of patients had a reduced total marrow cellularity and fewer myeloid progenitors than did the healthy nonanemic elderly and younger members of the study population.[49] The marrows of these patients contained a decreased number of CFU-E, but a normal number of BFU-E. Although it is tempting to attribute this mild, unexplained normocytic anemia and neutropenia to a specific "anemia of senescence", the authors were careful to point out that it is risky to do so because the various possible causes of marrow dysfunction in the elderly are divers, complicated, and can often not be distinguished at presentation. The incidence of unexplained anemias was reported to be significantly lower in affluent populations.[55] This suggests that the "anemia of senescence" may be the result of nutritional deficiencies or undiagnosed infectious and inflammatory conditions, which are prevalent in impoverished populations. Whether or not an anemia of senescence exists, persons older than 75 years of age often have mild anemias for which a cause cannot readily be determined. Even if the World Health Organization's criteria for anemia are used (a blood hemoglobin concentration below 13 g/dL for men and below 12 g/dL for women), the incidence of anemia in the elderly is substantial and many of these have no definable cause. Therefore, common sense and good clinical judgment must be the guide to physicians in determining the extent of the workup to which mildly anemic elderly patients should be subjected.

V. THERAPY WITH RECOMBINANT HUMAN EPO (rHuEpo)

A. GENERAL PRINCIPLES

The diagnosis and therapy of anemias in elderly patients is based on the same principles that apply to those of younger ones; in general, the response to therapy is comparable.

After identifying the cause of the anemia, specific therapy for the anemia and/or for the underlying cause should be instituted. In patients with anemias for which there is no specific therapy, the risk to benefit ratio for correcting the anemia should be determined by assessing the severity of the symptoms that are directly attributable to the anemia and the risks, costs, and likelihood that the therapy will be successful. The choice of therapies available to this group of patients consists primarily of blood transfusions or rHuEpo. The adverse effects of transfusion therapy in elderly anemic persons[56] include:

(1) the risk of precipitating congestive heart failure

(2) sensitization to blood group antigens

(3) the risk of acquiring blood-borne viral infections (this has been markedly reduced in recent years by the improved ability to identify antigens of the causative agents)

(4) the deposition of excess iron in the reticuloendothelial system and subsequently in the hepatocytes (since this process causes tissue damage only after patients are transfused frequently for years, it is not likely to be an important cause of morbidity in elderly persons)

(5) the potential, but not definitely established immunosuppressive effects of transfusion, which may adversely effect the outcome of therapy in patients with neoplastic disorders and

(6) the inconveniences of transfusion therapy

For these reasons, rHuEpo is the treatment of choice for patients with anemias that are likely to respond in a predictable manner to doses of rHuEpo that are financially practical. The remainder of this article will be devoted to the discussion of rHuEpo therapy and its effectiveness in the management of various anemias.

Commercially available rHuEpo, produced by Chinese hamster ovary cells,[57] is virtually identical to naturally produced Epo extracted from the urine of patients with aplastic anemia.[58] It became available for human use about 10 years ago, and the first clinical trials of its use in patients with chronic renal failure were reported in 1986.[59,60] Since then, the results of its use in patients of various ages, with a variety of anemias have been published. However, the data do not indicate whether or not elderly persons respond to rHuEpo differently than their younger counterparts.

The sites and mechanism of clearance of Epo are still not clearly designated in either humans or in experimental animals. Less than 10% of Epo injected intravenously into rats is excreted in the urine,[61] and no differences have been observed in the rate of clearance of Epo from the plasma of uremic as compared to nonuremic persons. Whereas desialated Epo is rapidly cleared by the liver,[62] there are no definitive data that demonstrate that the plasma clearance rate of Epo is prolonged in humans or in experimental animals with impaired hepatic function. One study in totally hepatectomized dogs demonstrated that the liver does not significantly affect the rate of clearance of Epo from the plasma.[63] A variety of observations indicate that plasma Epo levels are higher in experimental animals[27] and humans[64,65] with marrow failure than in comparably anemic ones with an intact erythron. This has fostered the hypothesis that interaction of Epo with its cellular receptor and the subsequent internalization of the complex is the primary mechanism for clearing Epo from the plasma. However, this is doubtful, since there are few Epo receptors present on its primary target cell, the CFU-E, and the clearance of Epo from the plasma of mice[28,66,67] is unaffected by damaging the hematopoietic system. In support of the hypothesis, one study[68] in patients with myelodysplastic syndrome demonstrated a prolonged plasma clearance of rHuEpo when compared to that reported elsewhere for patients with chronic renal failure and nonanemic persons.

rHuEpo is usually administered three times weekly by either the intravenous or subcutaneous route. In general, rHuEpo injected subcutaneously is more effective than that injected intravenously in comparable doses.[69,70] The $T_{1/2}$ for the plasma clearance of intravenously administered rHuEpo is in the range of 5 to 7 hr[71–73] and is unaffected by hemodialysis. In some studies, the $T_{1/2}$ was reported to have declined after ten or more doses had been administered,[72] whereas in others no change occurred after repeated doses.[73] Subcutaneously administered rHuEpo is absorbed at a $T_{1/2}$ of about 8.5 hr, reaches a maximum plasma titer in about 18 hr, and is cleared from the plasma at a $T_{1/2}$ of about 17 hr.[69,71] The distribution space of intravenously injected rHuEpo is somewhat larger than the plasma volume (60 to 70 mL/kg).

rHuEpo is well tolerated. Less than 5% of patients report mild muscular aches and "flu-like" symptoms, which rarely require interruption of therapy.[74] Antibodies to rHuEpo have not yet been observed. To date, no serious adverse reactions have been reported that are attributable to rHuEpo, per se. The adverse effects that have been observed are ascribed to the response to Epo, i.e., the increase in the rate of erythropoiesis and consequent increase in the hematocrit, the whole blood viscosity, and the rate of iron utilization. These effects, which include exacerbation of hypertension and epileptic seizures in patients with renal failure who respond most briskly to the administration of rHuEpo, and whose altered intrarenal blood circulation is particularly sensitive to increases in the hematocrit.

The most common and predictably successful use of rHuEpo is in patients with the anemia of renal failure. In this group of patients, with damage to the site of Epo production, rHuEpo constitutes specific replacement therapy.

B. THE ANEMIA OF CHRONIC RENAL FAILURE

The anemia of chronic renal failure[75] is a normocytic anemia associated with a normal or near-normal reticulocyte index (which is low for the level of the blood hemoglobin concentration) and a modestly shortened RBC survival. The anemia varies in severity from one individual to another. However, in any individual patient, the anemia becomes progressively more severe as uremia progresses and usually plateaus when the patient develops end-stage renal failure. The anemia of chronic renal failure is caused primarily by the inability of the damaged kidneys to produce sufficient Epo. The serum Epo titer, in patients with chronic renal failure, is almost invariably lower than that of comparably anemic patients with normal renal function.[76,77] Therapy with rHuEpo is indicated and nearly always successful in treating the anemia of patients with chronic renal failure, whether they are on hemodialysis, peritoneal dialysis, or not yet on dialysis.[70] The goal of therapy is to increase the hematocrit to between 32 and 38% and maintain it at that level without transfusions. To achieve this, rHuEpo is injected, either subcutaneously or intravenously, three times weekly in doses that must be individualized and vary from 50 to 100 mg/kg per dose.[74] Rarely, higher doses are required.

Since rHuEpo represents replacement therapy, it should be effective in virtually all patients with the anemia of chronic renal failure. Accordingly, if patients fail to respond, or if their response is curtailed before the target hematocrit is reached, then a search for complicating factors should be initiated. Patients with chronic renal failure are subject to a variety of disorders that increase the severity of the anemia, and may cause it to be resistant to rHuEpo therapy.[78] The most common of these conditions are actual and functional iron deficiency. Uremic patients are predisposed to excess blood loss due to sequestration of erythrocytes on the dialysis membranes and to gastrointestinal blood loss. The latter is commonly caused by the combination of uremic gastroenteritis and platelet dysfunction.[34] Patients with chronic renal failure are prone to develop functional iron deficiency, because of an increased incidence of infectious or inflammatory disorders, which impair the ability of macrophages to mobilize storage iron. Functional iron deficiency also develops, not infrequently, when the rate of erythropoiesis is accelerated by rHuEpo and the readily mobilizable iron stores have been exhausted.[34,74] To detect both functional and actual iron deficiency, in a timely manner it is advisable to determine the serum ferritin, the serum iron, and the total iron binding capacity (TIBC) prior to initiating therapy, and to correct the underlying conditions, if possible. It is also recommended that these parameters be monitored at monthly intervals during therapy. A fall in the serum iron and the ratio of the serum iron to TIBC, while the serum ferritin is still normal or supernormal, suggests the onset of functional iron deficiency. The administration of parenteral iron should alleviate this condition and prevent an interruption in the response to rHuEpo.

Other conditions that cause resistance to rHuEpo therapy include hyperparathyroidism, aluminum toxicity, and a variety of hemolytic anemias.

As mentioned previously, there are no serious side effects attributable to rHuEpo, per se. The side effects that occur are usually sequelae of the response to Epo. The most frequently observed adverse effect in patients with renal failure is the development of hypertension or the exacerbation of pre-existing hypertension. This occurs most commonly while the hematocrit is rising and particularly when it is rising rapidly. Hypertension which occurs during rHuEpo therapy is usually controlled by medications and rarely requires termination of therapy. Other complications of rHuEpo therapy include epileptic seizures. These do not occur more frequently in patients on rHuEpo therapy than in those that are not, but they do occur often during the first few weeks of therapy while the hematocrit is rising rapidly. This coincides with the period when hypertension is most likely to intensify, and the two events may be related. Other potential problems, such as increased thrombotic events and decreased efficiency of hemodialysis, due to the increased hematocrit, have not been demonstrated to occur more frequently in patients on rHuEpo therapy. Correction of the anemia of renal failure results in an increased sense of well-being and an increased exercise tolerance.[79]

rHuEpo is both safe and effective in increasing the hematocrit and relieving the anemia-dependent symptoms of patients with renal failure. A recent study[80] attempted to determine the cost of rHuEpo therapy relative to that of transfusion therapy. These comparisons are admittedly crude because many assumptions are needed to assess the true cost of transfusion therapy. The authors determined that the annual cost of transfusion therapy for patients with renal failure was $4,630.00, as compared to $6,178.00 for rHuEpo. They concluded that the benefits of rHuEpo therapy justified the increased cost of therapy.

Although the response of patients with renal failure to rHuEpo therapy was predictable, from our knowledge of the pathogenesis of the anemia and from the results of studies on the use of Epo to treat the anemia of uremic rats[81] and sheep,[82] the response of patients with anemias other than those due to renal failure is less predictable.

C. THE ANEMIA OF RHEUMATOID ARTHRITIS

The anemia of rheumatoid arthritis is considered to be a classic example of the anemia of chronic disease. The classic concept of the pathogenesis of this anemia is that it results from an impaired reutilization of iron derived from senescent erythrocytes.[83] Accordingly, it represents an example of functional iron deficiency. As such, one would predict that it would not be responsive to rHuEpo. However, the serum Epo levels of patients with the anemia of rheumatoid arthritis have been shown by some,[84–86] but not all observers,[87] to be lower than those of comparably anemic patients with iron deficiency. For this reason, and because of the high prevalence of the anemia of chronic disease it was selected for one of the earliest clinical trials of rHuEpo.[88] Patients with rheumatoid arthritis with hematocrits of 30% or less were randomized to receive doses of 0, 50, 100, or 150 mU/kg per dose of rHuEpo thrice weekly for 8 weeks. Afterwards, those that did not achieve an increase of their hematocrits of at least five percentage points were entered into an open phase study. In this phase, the dose of rHuEpo was increased by 50 mU/kg per dose until the hematocrit increased by the targeted amount. Very few patients responded during the initial closed phase of the study, but all eventually responded during the open phase. However, responses occurred only when doses of 300 to 600 mU/kg were reached. The conclusion from this study was that the anemia of rheumatoid arthritis is relatively refractory to rHuEpo, in replacement doses, but is responsive to large doses. The expense of very high-dose therapy is not warranted to increase the hematocrit of most patients with rheumatoid arthritis, since the anemia is usually not severe, is seldom progressive, and improves as the activity of the systemic disease subsides. Its use should be restricted to special circumstances, such as short-term therapy designed to increase the preoperative hematocrit of patients who are scheduled to undergo major elective surgical procedures, such as joint replacements. The response of patients with the anemia of rheumatoid arthritis to high-dose rHuEpo therapy has, however, led to a very productive re-examination of the pathogenesis of the anemia of chronic disease, particularly to an increased understanding of the effect of the inflammatory cytokines on the production of Epo and the response to it.[89]

D. THE ANEMIA OF CANCER

The anemia of cancer is a complex condition caused, in part, by the same factors that give rise to the anemia of chronic disease (functional iron deficiency and relatively low serum Epo titers). However, other factors frequently and variably contribute to the pathogenesis of the anemia and consequently to its severity. These include: (1) the effects of chemotherapy on the Epo target cells and Epo production (the latter is pertinent in patients receiving chemotherapy regimens that include platinum compounds) and (2) the effects of the tumor, per se, on the hematopoietic progenitors and on the hematopoietic microenvironment. Several groups[90–92] have reported their results with the use of rHuEpo to treat the anemia of cancer, myeloma, chronic leukemias, and lymphoma. All have observed responses to doses of 150 to 300 mU/kg, given three times per week. In one study,[92] over 150 patients were classified into three groups: those on no chemotherapy, those on chemotherapy with regimens that did not include cis-platinum, and those on chemotherapy regimens that included cis-platinum. Administration of 150 mU/kg of rHuEpo, thrice weekly, was observed to increase the hematocrit and the general sense of well-being of patients with mild to moderate anemias in all three groups. It also increased the hematocrit and decreased the transfusion requirements of some patients that were more severely anemic and transfusion dependent. However, responses to therapy were less predictable in this latter group, regardless of whether or not they were receiving chemotherapy. Perhaps a greater number of responses would have been observed if even higher doses were used, but this might have made therapy too expensive to be a practical alternative to transfusion therapy.

According to the hypothesis that the rate of erythropoiesis is determined by the serum Epo titer and the size and functional integrity of the CFU-E population, one would predict that anemias associated with a reduced CFU-E population would only respond to large doses of rHuEpo, and the effective dose would be inversely proportional to the size of the CFU-E population. Data derived from experiments in irradiated mice support this prediction.[93] The anemias in this category include: some patients with malignancies, particularly those with substantial marrow involvement and those that are receiving intensive myelosuppressive therapy, and patients with aplastic anemia, myelodysplastic syndromes, and myelofibrosis.

E. THE ANEMIA ASSOCIATED WITH HIV INFECTION, TREATED WITH AZT

AZT is an antiviral agent that is frequently used in patients infected with the human immunodeficiency virus (HIV). AZT is a myelosuppressive agent, as is HIV in some patients. AZT therapy is frequently complicated by severe transfusion-dependant anemia. A multicenter trial of high-dose rHuEpo therapy in HIV-infected patients receiving AZT[94] demonstrated success in alleviating the anemia and reducing the transfusion requirements of a subset of patients that had pretreatment serum Epo levels below 500 mU/mL. Since very high serum Epo levels occur most frequently in patients with damage to the erythroid progenitor cell compartment, this suggests that rHuEpo therapy is most likely to be effective in those with residual erythron function.

F. APLASTIC ANEMIA AND MYELODYSPLASTIC SYNDROMES

The efficacy of rHuEpo therapy in ameliorating the anemia of patients with aplastic anemia[95,96] and of patients with myelodysplasia[97,98] has been studied. In general, large doses of rHuEpo are used, and responses are observed in 25 to 30% of patients. Unfortunately, it is not yet possible to predict which patients will respond. Consequently, many third-party payers do not approve reimbursement for this expensive therapy. Generally, patients with very high pretreatment serum Epo levels (greater than 500 mU/mL) are unlikely to respond to rHuEpo in doses that have been used to date. A noteworthy report by Negron et al.[99] found that the anemias of patients with myelodysplastic syndromes that received both rHuEpo and the granulocyte CSF (G-CSF) responded twice as frequently as did those that received only rHuEpo. This suggests that in patients with anemias caused by progenitor cell dysfunction, combination growth factor therapy may become an option in the future.

G. NONANEMIC PATIENTS UNDERGOING REPEATED PHLEBOTOMIES

rHuEpo effectively increases the rate of erythropoiesis in nonanemic persons. Accordingly, by using rHuEpo as an adjunct to phlebotomy programs, patients have been able to increase the yield of blood to be used for autologous transfusions[100,101] and the amount that can be withdrawn for therapy of iron overload states.[102]

VI. SUMMARY

With advancing age, changes occur in the hematopoietic system that manifest themselves in subtle declines in the hematocrits of elderly persons.

From the results of studies in experimental animals, and to a lesser extent in humans, it appears that the ability of the erythron to compensate for injury is reduced in the aged. Anemia is more prevalent in the elderly, but usually results from specific disorders that also occur in younger persons. The existence of an anemia of senescence that is primarily caused by the effects of aging on hematopoiesis, has been postulated; however, the available data are still too circumstantial to support the existence of such an entity with any degree of certainty. Until recently, anemias for which no specific therapy was available were treated by transfusion of RBCs. Now, rHuEpo offers a safer, more convenient option for patients with some types of anemia. It has become the treatment of choice for patients with the anemia of chronic renal failure, for which it represents replacement therapy and is, consequently, almost always effective in relatively low doses (50 to 150 mU/kg). It is also effective in treating many patients with moderately severe anemias, associated with malignancies, albeit in higher doses (150 to 300mU/kg). Most patients with anemia, secondary to rheumatoid arthritis and other inflammatory conditions, respond to high-dose therapy (300 to 600 mU/kg), although it is indicated only in a few special circumstances in this group. In these conditions, it is noteworthy that endogenous Epo production is relatively decreased. There remains, a large group of patients with severe anemias in whom rHuEpo therapy is sometimes very beneficial. However, because of the high cost of this therapy, its relatively infrequent effectiveness, and the inability to accurately predict who will respond, most insurers are unwilling to pay for it. It is in this group, which includes patients with severe transfusion-dependent anemias associated with malignancies, myelodysplastic syndromes, and aplastic anemia, that research into methods to more accurately identify responders will result in major benefits in the future. To date, we assume that elderly persons respond to rHuEpo as well as their younger counterparts. There is a need to gather more specific information to determine if this assumption is correct.

The clinical use of rHuEpo has initiated the era of hematopoietic growth factor therapy, which is rapidly expanding. As new growth factors are discovered and made available for human use, particularly those that affect the primitive hematopoietic progenitors, it may be possible to treat patients that are now refractory to therapy with rHuEpo alone with combinations of growth factors that stimulate the primitive erythroid progenitors to produce more Epo-responsive cells.

REFERENCES

1. **Lajtha, L. G.,** Hematopoietic stem cells, *Br. J. Haematol.*, 29, 529, 1975.
2. **Till, J. E. and McCulloh, E. A.,** A direct measure of the radiation sensitivity of normal mouse cells, *Radiat. Res.*, 14, 213, 1961.
3. **Orlic, D. and Bodine, D. M.,** What defines a pluripotential hematopoietic sem cell (PHSC) — will the real PHSC please stand up!, *Blood*, 84, 3991, 1994.
4. **Teixido, J., Hemler, M. E., Greenberger, J. S., and Anklesaria, P.,** Role of β_1 and β_2 integrins in the adhesion of human $CD34^+$ stem cells to bone marrow stroma, *J. Clin. Invest.*, 90, 358, 1992.
5. **Kodama, H., Makoto, N., Shumpei, N., Satomi, N., and Shin-Ichi, N.,** Involvement of the c-Kit receptor in the adhesion of hematopoietic stem cells to stromal cells, *Exp. Hematol.*, 22, 978, 1994.
6. **Leary, A. G., Ogawa, M., Strauss, L. C., and Givin C.,** Single cell origin of multilineage colonies in culture, *J. Clin. Invest.*, 74, 2193, 1984.
7. **Krantz, S. B.,** Erythropoietin, *Blood*, 77, 419, 1991.
8. **Sawyer, S. T., Krantz, S. B., and Goldwasser E.,** Binding and receptor mediated endocytosis of erythropoietin in Friend virus-infected erythroid cells, *J. Biol. Chem.*, 262, 5554, 1987.
9. **Wickerema A., Krantz S. B., Winkelman, J. C., and Bondurant, M. C.,** Differentiation and erythropoietin receptor gene expression in human erythroid progenitor cells, *Blood*, 80, 1940, 1992.
10. **Miyake, T., Kung, C. K. H., and Goldwasser, E.,** Purification of human erythropoietin, *J. Biol. Chem.*, 252, 5558, 1977.
11. **Zanjani, E. D., Foster, J., Burlington, H., Mann, L. J., and Wasserman, L. R.,** Liver as the primary site of erythropoietin formation in the fetus, *J. Lab. Clin. Med.*, 89, 640, 1977.
12. **Zanjani, E. D., Ascensao, J. L., McGlave, P. B., Banisadre, M., and Ash, A. L.,** Studies on the liver to kidney switch of erythropoietin production, *J. Clin. Invest.*, 67, 1183, 1981.
13. **Naets, J. P. and Wittek M.,** Presence of erythropoietin in the anephric patient, *Blood*, 31, 249, 1968.
14. **Koury, S. T., Koury, M. J., Bondurant, M. C., Caro, J., and Graber, S. E.,** Quantitation of erythropoietin-producing cells in kidneys of mice by in situ hybridization: correlation with hematocrit, renal erythropoietin mRNA, and serum erythropoietin concentration, *Blood*, 74, 645, 1989.
15. **Koury, S. T., Bondurant, M. C., and Koury, M. J.,** Localization of cells producing erythropoietin in murine liver by in situ hybridization, *Blood*, 77, 2497, 1991.
16. **Fried, W., Plzak, L. F., Jacobson, L. O., and Goldwasser, E.,** Studies on erythropoiesis. III. Factors controlling erythropoietin production, *Pro. Soc. Biol. Med.*, 94, 237, 1957.
17. **Fried, W., Kilbridge, T., Krantz, S., McDonald, T. P., Lange, R. D.,** Studies on extrarenal erythropoietin, *J. Lab. Clin. Med.*, 73, 244, 1969.
18. **Evans, E. S., Rosenberg, L. L., and Simpson, M. E.,** Erythropoietic response to calorigenic hormones, *Endocrinology*, 68, 517, 1961.
19. **Reissman, K. R.,** Protein metabolism and erythropoiesis. II. Erythropoietin formation and erythroid responsiveness in protein-deprived rats, *Blood*, 23, 146, 1964.
20. **Gurney, C. W., Fried, W., and Fessler, A.,** Erythropoietic effect of androgens, in *Hematopoietic Cellular Proliferation*, Stohlman, F., Ed., Grune & Stratton, New York, 1970, 133.

21. **Jelkmann, W., Pagel, H., Wolff, M., and Fandrey, J.,** Monokines inhibiting erythropoietin production in human hepatoma cultures and in isolated perfused rat kidneys, *Life Sci.*, 50, 301, 1992.
22. **Faquin, W. C., Schneider, T. J., and Goldberg, M. A.,** Effect of inflammatory cytokines on hypoxia induced erythropoietin production, *Blood*, 79, 1987, 1992.
23. **Fisher, J. W.,** Prostaglandins and kidney erythropoietin production, *Nephron*, 25, 53, 1980.
24. **Fried, W., Morley, C., Barone-Varelas, J., Bindani, A., and Prancan, A.,** Effects of indomethacin and of prostaglandins on extrarenal erythropoietin production in rates, *J. Lab. Clin. Med.*, 111, 184, 1988.
25. **Jepson, J. H. and Lowenstein, L.,** Effect of prolactin on erythropoiesis in the mouse, *Blood*, 24, 726, 1964.
26. **Goldwasser, E., Jacobson, L. O., Fried, W., and Plzak, L. F.,** Studies on erythropoiesis. V. The effect of cobalt on the production of erythropoietin, *Blood*, 13, 55, 1958.
27. **Stohlman, F. and Brecher, G.,** Humoral regulation of erythropoiesis V. Relationship of plasma erythropoietin level to bone marrow activity, *Proc. Soc. Exp. Biol. Med.*, 100, 40, 1959.
28. **Fried, W., Knospe, W. H., and Trobaugh, F. E., Jr.,** Regulation of plasma erythropoietin levels in mice with impaired responsiveness to erythropoietin, *J. Lab. Clin. Med.*, 78, 449, 1971.
29. **Youssoufian, H., Longmore, G., Neumann, D., Yoshimura, A., and Lodish, H. F.,** Structure, function and activation of the erythropoietin receptor, *Blood*, 81, 223, 1993.
30. **Fraser, J. K., Tan, A. S., Lin, F. K., and Berridge, M. V.,** Expression of specific high-affinity binding sites for erythropoietin on rat and mouse megakaryocytes, *Exp. Hematol.*, 17, 10, 1989.
31. **Anagnostou, A., Lee, E. S., Kessimian, N., Levinson, R., and Steiner, M.,** Erythropoietin has a mitogenic and positive chemotactic effect on endothelial cells, *Proc. Natl. Acad. Sci. U.S.A.*, 85, 5978, 1990.
32. **Umemura, T., Papayannoupoulou, T., and Stamatoyannopoulos, G.,** The mechanism of expansion of late erythroid progenitors during erythroid regeneration: target cells and effects of erythropoietin and interleukin-3, *Blood*, 73, 1993, 1989.
33. **Koury, M. J.,** Programmed cell death, *Exp. Hematol.*, 20, 391, 1992.
34. **Adamson, J. W.,** The relationship of erythropoietin and iron metabolism to red blood cell production in humans, *Semin. Oncol.*, 21, No. 2, Suppl. 3, 9, 1994.
35. **Finch, C.,** Regulators of iron balance in humans, *Blood*, 84, 1697, 1994.
36. **Skikne, B. S. and Cook, J. D.,** Effect of enhanced erythropoiesis on iron absorption, *J. Lab. Clin. Med.*, 120, 746, 1992.
37. **Schade, S. G. and Fried, W.,** The utilization of senescent red cell and hemolysate iron for erythropoiesis, *Proc. Soc. Exp. Biol. Med.*, 151, 78, 1976.
38. **Siminoviteh, L., Till, J. E., and McCulloch, E. A.,** Decline in colony forming ability of marrow cells subjected to serial transplantation into irradiated mice, *J Cell Comp Physiol*, 64, 23, 1964.
39. **Harrison, D. E.,** Proliferative capacity of erythropoietic stem cell lines and aging, A*n overview mechanism of aging and development*, 9, 409, 1979.
40. **Hellman, S., Botnick, L. E., Hannon, E. C., and Vignvello, R. M.,** Proliferative capacity of murine hematopoietic stem cells, *Proc. Natl. Acad. Sci. U.S.A.*, 75, 490, 1978.
41. **Nilsson-Ehle, H., Jagenburg, R., Landahl, S., Svanborg, A., and Westin, J.,** Decline of blood hemoglobin in the aged: a longitudinal study of an urban Swedish population from age 70 to 81, *Br. J. Haematol.*, 71, 437, 1989.
42. **Boggs, D. R. and Patrene, K. D.,** Hematopoiesis and aging. III. Anemia and blunted erythropoietic response to hemorrhage in aged mice, *Am. J. Hematol.*, 19, 327, 1985.
43. **Tyan, L. M.,** Old mice: marrow response to bleeding or endotoxin, *Proc. Soc. Exp. Biol. Med.*, 169, 295, 1982.
44. **Williams, L. H., Udupa, K. B., and Lipshitz, D. A.,** Evaluation of the effect of age on hematopoiesis in C57BL/6 mice, *Exp. Hematol.*, 14, 827, 1986.
45. **Powers, J. S., Krantz, S. B., Collins, J. C., et al.,** Erythropoietin response to anemia as a function of age, *J. Am. Geriatr. Soc.*, 39, 30, 1991.
46. **Chapman, C., Sebastian, J. P., Carpenter, M. A., Kendall, R. A., O'Brien, A. E. et al.,** Reduced erythropoietin response to anemia in elderly patients with normocytic anemia, *Eur. J. Haematol.*, 49, 119, 1992.
47. **Nafziger, J., Pailla, L., Luciasm, L., Andreux, J. P., Olivier, S. J., and Casadevall, N.,** Decreased erythropoietin responsiveness to iron deficient anemia in the elderly, *Am. J. Hematol.*, 43, 172, 1993.
48. **Piomeli, S., Nathan, D. G., and Cummin, T. F.,** The relationship of total red cell volume to total body water in octogenarian males, *Blood*, 19, 89, 1962.
49. **Lipschitz, D. A., Udupa, K. B., and Thompson, L. O.,** Effect of age on hematopoiesis in man, *Blood*, 63, 502, 1986.
50. **Kosower, N. S.,** Altered properties of erythrocytes in the aged, *Am. J. Hematol.*, 42, 241, 1993.
51. **Nilsson-Ehle, R., Jagenburg, S., Landahl, A., Svanborg, A., and Westin, J.,** Hematological abnormalities and reference intervals in the elderly, *Acta Med. Scand.*, 224, 594, 1988.
52. **Inelman, E. M., Alessio, M. D., Gatto, M. R. A., Baggio, M. B., Jimenez, G., and Bizzotto, M. G.,** Descriptive analysis of the prevalence of anemia in a randomly selected sample of elderly people living at home: some results of an Italian multicentric study, *Aging Clin. Exp. Res.*, 6, 81, 1994.

53. **Hellman, N. and Rubenstein, L. S.,** Effects of age, sex and smoking on erythrocytes and leukocytes, *Am. J. Clin. Pathol.*, 63, 35, 1975.
54. **Mansouri, A. and Lipschitz, D. A.,** Anemia in the elderly patient, *Med. Clin. North Am.*, 76, 619, 1992.
55. **Parson, P. L., Whitney, J. L., and Kilpatrick, G. S.,** The prevalence of anemia in the elderly, *Practitioner*, 195, 656, 1965.
56. **Klein, H. G.,** Immunologic aspects of blood transfusion, *Semin. Oncol.*, No.2, Suppl. 3, 21, 16, 1994.
57. **Lin, F. K., Suggs, S., Lin, C. H., Browne, J. K., Smalling, R. et al.,** Cloning and expression of the human erythropoietin gene, *Proc. Natl. Acad. Sci. U.S.A.*, 82, 7580, 1985.
58. **Egrie, J. C., Strickland, T. W., Lane, J., Aoki, K., Cohen, A. M. et al.,** Characterization of biological effects of recombinant human erythropoietin, *Immunobiology*, 172, 213, 1986.
59. **Winearls, C. G., Oliver, D. O., Pippard, J. J., Reid, C., Downing, M. R. et al.,** Effect of human erythropoietin derived form recombinant DNA on the anaemia of patients maintained by chronic hemodialysis, *Lancet*, 2, 1175, 1986.
60. **Eschbach, J. W., Egrie, J. C., Downing, M. R., Browne, J. K., and Adamson, J. W.,** Correction of the anemia of end-stage renal disease with recombinant human erythropoietin, *N. Engl. J. Med.*, 316, 73, 1987.
61. **Emanouel, D. S., Goldwasser, E., and Katz, A. I.,** Metabolism of pure human erythropoietin in the rat, *Am. J. Physiol.*, 247, 168, 1984.
62. **Dordal, M. S., Wang, F. F., and Goldwasser, E.,** The role of carbohydrate in erythropoietin action, *Endocrinology*, 116, 2293, 1985.
63. **Kukral, J., Carney, A. L., Ebroon, E., Pollitt, J., Zeineh, R. A. et al.,** The role of the liver and surgical stress in erythropoietin metabolism, *Surg. Forum*, 19, 348, 1968.
64. **Pavlovvic-Kentera, F., Milenkovic, P., Ruvidic, R., Jovanovic, V., and Biljanovic-Paunovic, L.,** Erythropoietin in aplastic anemia, *Blut*, 39, 345, 1979.
65. **Hammond, D., Shore, N., and Movassaghi, N.,** Producion, utilization, and excretion of erythorpoietin. I Chronic anemias. II. Aplastic crisis. III. Erythropoietic effects of normal plasma, *Ann. N.Y. Acad. Sci.*, 149, 516, 1968.
66. **Naets, J. P. and Wittek, M.,** Erythropoietic activity of marrow and disappearance rate of erythropoietin in the rat, *Am. J. Physiol.*, 217, 297, 1969.
67. **Bozzini, C. E.,** Influence of the erythroid activity of the bone marrow on the plasma disappearance of injected erythropoietin in dogs, *Nature (London)*, 209, 1140, 1966.
68. **Bowen, D., Bernhard, E., Neubert, P., Lewis, T., and Jacobs, A.,** The clearance of a single IV bolus of recombinant human erythropoietin from the serum of patients with myelodysplastic syndromes and its effects on erythropoiesis, *Exp. Hematol.*, 19, 613, 1991.
69. **Schoufen, J. P., Voorhorst, G., Helbirg, A. R., Janssen, J. W., Diderich, P. P. N. M., and Op de Hoek, C. T.,** Pharmacokinetics of epoetin in hemadialysis patients after subcutaneous administration: influence of chronic treatment, *Pharm. World Sci.*, 15, 251, 1993.
70. **Eshbach, J. W., Kelly, M. R., Haley, R., Abels, R. I., and Adamson, J. W.,** Treatment of anemia of progressive renal failure with recombinant human erythropoietin, *N. Engl. J. Med.*, 321, 158, 1989.
71. **McMahon, F. G., Vargas, R., Ryan, M., Adesh, K., Jain, A. K. et al.,** Pharmacokinetics and effects of recombinant human erythropoietin after intravenous and subcutaneous injections in healthy volunteers, *Blood*, 76, 1718, 1990.,
72. **Brockmoller, J., Kochling, J., Weber, W., Looby, M., Roots, I., and Neumayer, H. H.,** The pharmacokinetics and pharmacodynamics of recombinant human erythropoietin in hemodialysis patients, *Br. J. Clin. Pharmacol.*, 34, 499, 1992.
73. **Gladziwa, V., Klotz, V., Baumer, K., Zollimyer, R., Mann, H., and Sieberth, H. G.,** Pharmacokinetics of epoetin after long term therapy in patients undergoing hemodialysis and hemofiltration, *Clin. Pharmacol.*, 25, 145, 1993.
74. **Eschbach, J. W., Abdulhadi, M. H., Browne, J. K., Delano, B. G., Downing, M. R. et al.,** Recombinant human erythropoietin in anemic patients with end stage renal failure: results of a phase III multicenter clinical trial, *Ann. Int. Med.*, III, 992, 1989.
75. **Eshbach, J. W. and Adamson, J. W.,** Anemia of end stage renal failure (ESRD), *Kidney Int.*, 28, 11, 1985.
76. **Naets, J. P., Garcia, J. F., Tousaaint, C., Buset, M., and Waks, D.,** Radioimmunoassay of erythropoietin in chronic uraemia or anephric patients, *Scand. J. Haematol.*, 37, 390, 1986.
77. **Pavlovic-Kentera, V., Clemons, G. K., Djukanovic, L., and Biljanovic-Paunovic, L.,** Erythropoietin and anemia in chronic renal failure, *Exp. Hematol.*, 15, 785, 1987.
78. **Fried, W.,** Hematology abnormalities in chronic renal failure, *Sem. Nephrol.*, 1, 176, 1981.
79. **Lundin, P.,** Quality of life: subjective and objective improvements what recombinant human erythropoietin therapy, *Sem. Nephrol.*, 9, 22, 1989.
80. **Denton, T. A., Diamond, G. A., Matloff, J. M., and Gray, R. J.,** Anemia therapy: individual benefit and societal cost, *Semin. Oncol.*, 21, 29, 1994.
81. **Anagnostou, A., Barone, J., Kedo, A., and Fried, W.,** Effect of erythropoietin therapy on the red cell volume of uremic and non-uremic rats, *Br. J. Haematol.*, 37, 85, 1977.

82. **Eschbach, J. W., Mladenovic, J., Garcia, J. F., Wahl, P. W., and Adamson, J. W.,** The anemia of chronic renal failure in sheep: response to erythropoietin-rich plasma in-vivo, *J. Clin. Invest.*, 74, 434, 1984.
83. **Cartwright, G. E. and Lee, G. R.,** The anemia of chronic disorders, *Br J Hem*, 21, 147, 1971.
84. Baer, A. N., Dessypris, E. N., Goldwasser, E., Krantz, S. B., Blunted erythropoietin response to anaemia in rheumatoid arthritis, *Br. J. Haematol.*, 66, 559, 1987.
85. **Ward, H. P., Kurnick, J. E., and Pisarchzyk, M. J.,** Serum level of erythropoietin in anemias associated with chronic infection, malignancy, and primary hematopoietic disease, *J. Clin. Invest.*, 50, 332, 1971.
86. **Hochberg, M. C., Arnold, C. M., Hogans, B. B., and Spivak, J. L.,** Serum immunoreactive erythropoietin in rheumatoid arthritis: impaired response to anaemia, *Arthritis Rheum.*, 31, 1318, 1988.
87. **Erslev, A. J., Wilson, J., and Caro, J.,** Erythropoietin titers in anemic non-uremic patients, *J. Lab. Clin. Med.*, 109, 429, 1987.
88. **Pincus, T., Olsen, N. J., Russel, I. J., Eolfe, F., Harms, R. E. et al.,** Multicenter study of recombinant human erythropoietin in correction of anemia in rheumatoid arthritis, *Am. J. Med.*, 89, 161, 1990.
89. **Krantz, S. B.,** Pathogenesis and treatment of the anemia of chronic disease, *Am. J. Med. Sci.*, 307, 353, 1994.
90. **Ludwig, H. L., Fritz, E., Kotzmann, H., Hocker, P., Gisslinger, H., and Barnas, U.,** Erythropoietin treatment of anemia associated with multiple myeloma, *N. Engl. J. Med.*, 322, 1693, 1990.
91. **Spivak, J. L.,** Recombinant human erythropoietin and the anemia of cancer, *Blood*, 84, 997, 1994.
92. **Henry, D. H. and Abels, R. I.,** Recombinant human erythropoietin in the treatment of cancer and chemotherapy induced anemia: results of double-blind and open label follow-up studies, *Semin. Oncol.*, 21, No. 2, Suppl. 3, 21, 1994.
93. **Kilbridge, T. and Fried, W.,** Response of mice with a decreased number of hematopoietic stem cells to doses of erythropoietin, *J. Lab. Clin. Med.*, 72, 85, 1968.
94. **Henry, D. H., Beal, G. M., Benson, C. A., Cary, J., Cone, L. A. et al.,** Recombinant human erythropoietin in the treatment of anemia associated with human immunodeficiency virus (HIV) infection and zidovudine therapy, *Ann. Int. Med.*, 117, 739, 1992.
95. **Bessho, M., Jinnai, I., Matsuda, A., Saito, M., and Kunitake, H.,** Improvement of anemia by recombinant erythropoietin in patients with myelodysplastic syndrome and aplastic anemia, *Int. J. Cell. Clon.*, 8, 445, 1990.
96. **Stebler, C. Tichelli, A., Dazzi, H., Gratwolh, R., Nissen, C., and Speck, B.,** High dose recombinant human erythropoietin for treatment of anemia in myelodysplastic syndromes and paroxysmal nocturnal hemoglobinuria: a pilot study, *Exp. Hematol.*, 18, 1204, 1990.
97. **Kurtzrock, R., Talpaz, M., Estey, E., O'Brien, S., and Gutterman, J. V.,** Erythropoietin treatment in patients with myelodysplastic syndrome and anemia, *Leukemia*, 5, 985, 1991.
98. **Stein, R. S., Abels, R. I., and Krantz, S. B.,** Pharmacologic doses of recombinant human erythropoietin in the treatment of myelodysplastic syndromes, *Blood*, 78, 1658, 1991.
99. **Negrin, R. S., Stein, R., Vardiman, J., Doherty, K., Cornwell, J., Krantz, S., and Greenberg, P.,** Treatment of the anemia of myelodysplastic syndromes using recombinant human granulocyte colony stimulating factor in combination with erythropoietin, *Blood*, 82, 737, 1993.
100. **Goodnough, L. T., Price, T. H., Friedman, K. D., Johnston, M., Ciavarella, D. et al.,** A phase III trial of recombinant human erythropoietin therapy in non anemic orthopedic patients subjected to aggressive removal of blood for autologous use: dose, response, toxicity, and efficancy, *Transfusion*, 34, 66, 1994.
101. **Abraham, P. A., Halstenson, C. E., Macres, M. M., Opsahl, J. A., Rank, B. H. et al.,** Epoetin enhances erythropoiesis in normal men undergoing repeated phlebotomies, *Clin. Pharmacol. Ther.*, 52, 205, 1992.
102. **McCarthy, J. T., Johnson, W. J., Nixon, D. E., Jenson, B. M., and Moyer, T. P.,** Transfusional iron overload in patients undergoing dialysis: treatment with erythropoietin and phlebotomy, *J. Lab. Clin. Med.*, 114, 193, 1989.

Chapter 14

AGENTS USED IN COAGULATION DISORDERS OF THE ELDERLY

J. Bruce Miller

CONTENTS

I. INTRODUCTION

There has been increasing recognition of the importance of advancing age as a definite risk factor for the development of thromboembolic disease and that the practice of avoidance of anticoagulation in the elderly on the basis of age alone is unwarranted. Many excellent review articles on anticoagulation have been published recently.[1–11] This review will concern the use of heparin and warfarin with special attention to the benefits and risks of these agents in the elderly. Antiplatelet and thrombolytic agents will not be covered, although thrombolytic therapy should always be considered in elderly patients with massive thrombosis who have no contraindications to their use.[12,13] Improvements in laboratory monitoring of anticoagulation and in nomogram dosing of heparin in order to achieve more rapid therapeutic anticoagulation will be discussed. Conversely, lower-dose warfarin regimens have been shown to be as effective as previous higher-dose regimens and are associated with less bleeding. This

0-8493-8306-4/96/$0.00+$.50

makes warfarin use safer, particularly in the elderly with nonrheumatic atrial fibrillation (AF), a setting in which warfarin is probably still underused.

II. HEPARIN

A. STRUCTURE AND MECHANISM OF ACTION

Unfractionated heparin is a mixture of negatively charged glycosaminoglycans made up of alternating D-glycosamine and uronic acid residues.[2–4,8–11] The major anticoagulant properties of heparin are due to a unique pentasaccharide that has a high affinity for antithrombin III (AT III), but only one third of heparin molecules contain this. Binding of heparin to AT III greatly accelerates its irreversible binding to and inactivation of the coagulation enzymes of thrombin, Factor X_a and Factor IX_a, as well as XI_a and XII_a. Heparin then can dissociate and bind to other AT III molecules. Thrombin is the most sensitive factor to this inhibition. A single molecule of heparin must be able to bind to and span AT III and thrombin to form a neutralizing ternary complex. For this to occur, a heparin species of a minimum of 18 residues in length is required.

Unfractionated heparin is heterogenous in molecular size (average MW 15,000 Da, range 5 to 30,000 Da), which is in large part responsible for its complex pharmacokinetics and unpredictable dose-response curve. Only one third of heparin molecules bind to AT III, and both the anticoagulant properties and clearance are influenced by the heparin chain length. Following parenteral administration, heparin recovery is reduced because of its binding to platelets, vascular endothelial cells, and plasma proteins.

Fractionated low-molecular weight heparin (LMWH) is prepared by controlled chemical or enzymatic depolymerization.[14,15] LMWH preparations are relatively homogenous in size (average molecular weight of 4 to 5000 Da with a range of 2 to 8000 Da). Because of the minimum length of 18 residues needed for heparin to accelerate the inactivities of thrombin by AT III, LMWH inhibits F. X_a much more than thrombin. The much lower degree of binding of LMWH to platelets, endothelial cells, and plasma proteins results in excellent bioavailability and a prolonged half-life, resulting in a more predictable dose response and reduced frequency of administration.

B. MONITORING AND ADMINISTRATION

The anticoagulant effects of unfractionated heparin are usually monitored by the activated partial thromboplastin time (aPTT), which is sensitive to heparin effect on predominantly thrombin, but also F. X_a and F. IX_a. It has been shown that commercially produced aPTT reagents vary in their responsiveness to heparin effect. For many of these reagents, a therapeutic effect is achieved by an aPTT of 1.5 to 2.5 times control value (the therapeutic range). With a very sensitive reagent, the therapeutic range is higher than 1.5 to 2.5, and for an insensitive one, lower. It is recommended that a therapeutic range for each aPTT reagent be determined using as reference protamine titration heparin levels of 0.2 to 0.4 u/mL or F. X_a inhibitor levels of 0.3 to 0.7 u/mL.[16]

The model of heparin use in initial treatment of an established deep vein thrombosis (DVT) will be used in this discussion. Heparin is administered parenterally, either subcutaneously or intravenously. The therapeutic threshold of heparin anticoagulation is defined by an aPTT of equal to or greater than 1.5 times the control value. The pivotal importance of rapidly achieving this target degree of anticoagulation has strong support. The relative risk of recurrent venous thromboembolism was found to be 15 times higher in patients treated with heparin, but with aPTT response below the lower limit (1.5 times control) of the prescribed range for 24 hr or more from the start of therapy than in those patients with aPTT response at or above the lower limit.[17] In this study, there was a superior rapid achievement of therapeutic threshold of the aPTT response in those patients treated with continuous intravenous infusion of heparin compared to those given intermittent subcutaneous heparin.

However, in those patients receiving subcutaneous heparin who did achieve early therapeutic aPTTs, the treatment success was equal to that in patients treated with continuous infusion of intravenous heparin. A European meta-analysis of the use of subcutaneous or continuous infusion of intravenous heparin as initial treatment for DVT demonstrated that subcutaneous heparin was at least as effective and safe as continuous heparin.[18] Intermittent intravenous bolus heparin has been associated with more bleeding complications than continuous infusion administration, but this may have been due to the higher total doses of heparin given in intermittent intravenous regimens.[4] Most patients hospitalized in the U.S. for established DVT are treated with a continuous infusion of intravenous standard heparin.

The recognition of the importance of rapidly achieving therapeutic threshold aPTT values has led to the study of aPTT-driven nomograms which have been compared to a standard regimen. The results of the use of a nomogram on aPTT measurements and therapeutic outcomes were compared in one study with a historical control group using a "standard" regimen, namely 5000 u i.v. initial bolus followed by 1000 u/hr continuous infusion.[19] The proportion of patients achieving a therapeutic aPTT at 24 and 48 hr after starting heparin was 66 and 81% in the nomogram group as compared with 37 and 58% in the control group. The use of this standardized heparin nomogram reduced periods of both under- and overanti-coagulation.

A more recent study refined this approach by comparing a body weight-based nomogram with a "standard 5000 and 1000" nomogram.[20] In the weight-based heparin nomogram group, who were managed by staff nurses using the nomogram directions, 97% of patients exceeded the therapeutic threshold (>1.5 times control) within 24 hr compared to 77% with the standard regimen. Only one major bleeding event occurred (in the standard arm) and recurrent venus thromboembolism was more frequent in the standard arm, with a relative risk of 5.0. The weight-based nomogram was considered to be safe and superior to a treatment approach based on standard practice. Verification of the value of this body weight-based heparin nomogram as administered by pharmacist-nurse teams is ongoing.

While the aPTT has generally been useful to predict heparin antithrombotic failure, in at least one study there has been no relationship between supratherapeutic aPTT response to heparin and the occurrence of bleeding complications.[21] The use of intuitive (and often subtherapeutic) determination of heparin doses that interfere with the rapid achievement of therapeutic aPTT because of the fear of bleeding is to be avoided. Rapid response to supra-therapeutic aPTTs as dictated by available nomograms while achieving a therapeutic aPTT as soon as possible is a clear goal in the optimal use of heparin.

LMWH, because of its excellent bioavailability and long half-life, can be administered by intermittent subcutaneous injection once or twice daily. Since LMWHs have little if any effect on thrombin activity and the aPTT, F. X_a assays are needed for measurement of the therapeutic effect. The reliability of this assay in determining therapeutic effects and especially in predicting bleeding from anticoagulation is controversial.

C. COMPLICATIONS OF HEPARIN

1. Bleeding

The major complication of heparin anticoagulation is bleeding.[5] Bleeding is detrimental not only because it decreases the net benefit of anticoagulation, but its potential occurrence also leads to the avoidance of anticoagulation especially in the elderly and in populations with newer indications. Bleeding has been defined as major if it was intracranial or retro-peritoneal, if it led directly to death, or if it resulted in hospitalization or transfusion. All other bleeding is classified as minor. The most serious site of bleeding is intracranial, which comprises only 2% of bleeding episodes, but is 10 to 70% fatal. The most common sites are in the gastrointestinal (GI) and genitourinary (GU) tracts, but bleeding is also seen in surgical wounds, areas of tissue trauma, and in the retroperitoneal space. The incidence of major bleeding during a treatment course for venous thromboembolism with heparin is approximately

5%. The average daily risk of fatal, major, and minor bleeding during heparin is 0.05, 0.8, and 2.0%, respectively. This rate is considered to be twice that expected without the use of heparin.

There have been many studies to determine high bleeding risk factors, the results of which are not uniform.[22–24] Most studies that have examined the effect of age have found an independently increased risk of bleeding with advanced age. Prolonged duration of heparin therapy increases major bleeding risk, although the highest risk was found to occur on day 3 in one study. The total dose of heparin has been found to be a risk factor independent of aPTT effect, especially in patients with low BSA. Although a markedly elevated aPTT(>3 × control) has been associated with increased risk, the aPTT is neither a sensitive nor specific predictor of heparin-associated bleeding. It has been estimated that at least half of bleeding during heparin is simply due to the use of anticoagulation without an underlying condition. Several comorbid conditions have been risk factors: serious cardiac disease (acute myocardial infarction, congestive heart failure), renal failure, liver failure (especially that worsening during therapy), major alcoholism, poor performance status or poor overall condition including cancer or anemia with hematocrit less than 30% without recent bleeding, recent surgery or trauma, and concomitant use of antiplatelet (particularly aspirin) or thrombolytic drugs. Female gender has not been a uniform high-risk factor. These factors can be used to identify high-risk patients, but bleeding risk cannot be considered alone without considering the potential benefit from anticoagulation therapy.

D. HEPARIN-INDUCED THROMBOCYTOPENIA (HIT)

This is one of the most serious types of drug-induced thrombocytopenia.[25] From 1 to 5% of patients treated with heparin (three times greater with bovine than porcine) become thrombocytopenic, although only a 40% drop from baseline and not absolute thrombocytopenia is necessary for the diagnosis of this condition. It rarely occurs before day 4, but usually by day 14 of heparin therapy. An IgG antibody develops after exposure to heparin which its presence binds to platelets, causing platelet aggregation and thrombotic rather than bleeding manifestations. With subsequent exposure to heparin, thrombocytopenia may occur much more quickly, even in only 1 to 2 d. HIT occurs most after higher-dose therapeutic IV heparin, but can occur with lower dose prophylaxis, heparin flushes for maintenance of intravascular catheters, and even from heparin-impregnated catheters. Approximately 10% of patients with HIT will have thrombotic complications, most often arterial "white clots" often involving major limbs or other peripheral arteries following procedural trauma or with underlying pathology. This may result in gangrene and eventual amputation. Myocardial infarcts and thrombotic strokes as well as less commonly venous thrombosis may be seen. Heparin-induced skin necrosis is related to this complication. The generally available diagnostic tool for this condition is platelet aggregation studies to detect heparin-induced *in vitro* aggregation, and this is a specific, but not sensitive assay. HIT must be considered in any patient with a decreasing platelet count while exposed to heparin. Discontinuation of all heparin exposure if at all possible, alternative methods of anticoagulation if needed, and appropriate management of thrombotic episodes are methods of management. HIT is also associated with the use of LMWH, with one study detecting a 2% incidence of HIT with LMWH as compared to 3% with standard heparin.

III. WARFARIN

A. MECHANISM OF ACTION

Warfarin induces an anticoagulant effect by interfering with the cyclic conversion of vitamin K and its 2,3 epoxide (vitamin K epoxide).[1,6] Vitamin K is needed for the post-translational modification through γ-carboxylation of specific N-terminal glutamic acid residues of the vitamin K-dependent coagulation proteins (Factors II, VII, IX, and X and proteins

C and S) to form γ-carboxylglutamate (Gla). This carboxylation takes place through a vitamin K-dependent carboxylase enzyme and requires the reduced form of vitamin K (vitamin KH_2), molecular oxygen, and carbon dioxide. Gla residues are formed and vitamin K is oxidized to vitamin K epoxide. This is cycled back to vitamin K by vitamin K epoxide reductase, and vitamin K is then reduced by vitamin K reductase. By inhibiting vitamin K epoxide reductase and possibly vitamin K reductase, warfarin leads to the accumulation of vitamin K epoxide in liver and plasma and depletion of vitamin KH_2, decreasing γ-carboxylation of vitamin K-dependent proteins and impairing their biological function in blood clotting. The presence of Gla residues allows calcium binding and conformational changes in vitamin K-dependent proteins that are needed for binding to their cofactors on negatively charged phospholipid surfaces. Vitamin K-dependent coagulation proteins normally contain 10 to 13 Gla residues, all in their N-termini. Prothrombin molecules with 9 Gla residues have 70% of normal activity, while those with only 6 Gla residues have only 2%. Although the prothrombin time result begins to rise as active F. VII is depleted (having a short half-life of 4 to 6 hr), the full therapeutic effect of warfarin is not seen until prothrombin itself (half-life of 60 hr) is sufficiently decreased, which usually takes four or more days.

B. PHARMACOLOGY

Warfarin is a 4-OH coumarin compound, which is the most commonly used oral anticoagulant in North America.[1,6] It is highly water soluble and is rapidly absorbed from the GI tract after an oral dose. Peak absorption occurs in 60 to 90 min, and it should probably be taken on an empty stomach.

Warfarin is a racemic mixture of approximately equal amounts of two stereoisomers, the R and S forms. The R isomer has a longer half-life, a lower potency, and a different metabolism (excreted in the urine) compared to the S isomer (excreted in the bile). Both are highly protein bound, and only the free fraction is pharmacologically active. The average half-life of the racemic mixture is 35 to 40 hr. Warfarin accumulates rapidly in the liver, primarily in the microsomes. Dose response to warfarin varies between different subjects and in the same person over time, due principally to variability in warfarin half-life, due to changes in warfarin metabolism due to disease or the effect of other drugs.

C. INITIAL DOSING AND MONITORING

The practice of high loading doses of warfarin is now avoided, since it can lead to bleeding due to the rapid fall of F. VII (half-life of only 6 hr), whereas it produces no faster a decrease in the longer-lived factors (Factor X, 36 hr; prothrombin, 60 hr). If the need for anticoagulation is not urgent, warfarin can be started at an average maintenance dose of 5 mg daily in order to achieve a steady state at 5 to 6 d. If the need for anticoagulation is immediate, heparin is administered, and the first two daily doses of warfarin are 10 mg each, which achieves a therapeutic effect in 4 to 5 d, at which time the heparin can be stopped. A rapid response in the first 2 to 3 d implies a slow metabolism of warfarin and that maintenance doses will be low. The goal of warfarin maintenance therapy is simplicity without losing effectiveness, especially in patients who are likely to be elderly and receiving many other medications. The use of a single tablet strength (normally 5 mg) with fractions or multiples thereof, make up the dosages assigned to days of the week. If necessary, cumulative weekly doses should be adjusted by 10 to 20%, spreading the dose change over the entire week.

The laboratory test most often used to monitor warfarin anticoagulation is the one-stage prothrombin time (PT), in which citrated plasma is mixed with calcium and tissue thromboplastin to activate the tissue factor pathway of coagulation. The result is highly dependent on the reagent (tissue thromboplastin consisting of tissue factor and phospholipid) used. In response to a decrease in vitamin K-dependent coagulation factors, the PT will rise to a greater degree when the higher-sensitivity human brain thromboplastin is the testing reagent compared with rabbit brain thromboplastin. An important disparity existed between the dose needed for a therapeutic PT in the U.S. compared with other countries. It occurred when the major U.S. manufacturer of tissue thromboplastin changed from human brain to rabbit brain source. The PT can vary as much as 3 sec when a single blood sample is tested in different laboratories with different tissue thromboplastins. In order to standardize laboratory monitoring of warfarin anticoagulation effects, the International Normalized Ratio (INR) was devised.[26] The INR is defined as the ratio of the patient's PT over control PT taken to the power of the International Sensitivity Index (ISI). The ISI represents the slope of a regression line from the log plot of the reference thromboplastin PTs (in seconds) compared with the PTs obtained with the thromboplastin being tested. The more sensitive the thromboplastin, the lower the ISI value. The international reference thromboplastin has by definition an ISI of 1.0. The ISI for most thromboplastins used in the U.S. is 1.9 to 2.6, and the generally recommended therapeutic INR of 2.0 to 3.0 roughly corresponds to a PT ratio of 1.3 to 1.5. The use of lower doses of warfarin to achieve this corrected laboratory test range has resulted in less bleeding associated with warfarin therapy in the U.S. without loss of effectiveness.[27] Tissue thromboplastins of low ISI (high sensitivity) are needed to effectively monitor low-dose warfarin regimens that will be discussed below.

D. MANAGEMENT OF WARFARIN OVERDOSE

The management of excessive warfarin anticoagulation depends on the degree of elevation of the INR and the actual presence or absence of bleeding or high risk of bleeding. If the INR is only moderately elevated (up to 6) and there is no bleeding, discontinuation of warfarin will result in partial resumption of synthesis of new, active clotting factors by the liver, although this may take 48 hr to reach a significant level. However, after intravenous administration of vitamin K, active factor synthesis begins within hours and may normalize within 24 hr. Hence, if the INR is 6 to 10, intravenous vitamin K is the optimal therapy. The dose of vitamin K given influences the duration of active factor synthesis, but not the maximal rate.[1,2] Therefore, small intravenous doses of vitamin K (1 to 2 mg, given at 1 mg/min to prevent hypotension) are preferable if anticoagulation is to be continued. If the INR is still too high after 12 to 24 hr, a second intravenous dose can be given. If the INR is 10 to 20 and the patient is not bleeding, a higher dose of vitamin K (3 to 5 mg) is given intravenously, and the INR is checked every 6 to 12 hr. Larger doses of vitamin K may cause warfarin resistance that may persist for weeks and make heparin anticoagulation necessary during this period. With the occurrence of bleeding (especially if life threatening) in the setting of warfarin overdose, fresh frozen plasma will immediately correct the INR when 4 to 6 units (15 mL/kg) are infused in order to raise the low factor levels to 30 to 40%. Since the half-life of F. VII is short (6 hr), the prolonged INR and bleeding risk will recur within 24 hr if no vitamin K is given.

E. FACTORS AFFECTING WARFARIN ANTICOAGULANT RESPONSE

The level of anticoagulant effect of a given dose of warfarin is affected by numerous factors. The effect of advancing age both on the response to warfarin and the risk of bleeding associated with oral anticoagulation is controversial. Several studies have shown that warfarin dosage requirements are lowered in the aged, but the cause of this is still uncertain. Initially, it was felt that a higher rate of anticoagulation complications seen in the elderly was simply a reflection of the greater medication use and higher number of comorbid conditions rather than age itself. Gurwitz et al.[28,29] detected an abnormally high warfarin response and a decrease in mean daily dose of warfarin with advancing age. The exaggerated warfarin response persisted after controlling for relevant clinical variables in a multivariate model. Although an increased sensitivity due to a change in vitamin K epoxide reductase or in its affinity for warfarin has been postulated in the elderly, there is no clear evidence that warfarin pharmacokinetics are altered with advancing age.[30] An age-related decrease in warfarin clearance appears to be present. Isaacs et al.[31] studied prophylactic anticoagulation after hip fractures in the elderly. Elderly patients needed significantly lower doses of warfarin, and this was not solely due to polypharmacy or an increased number of comorbid conditions. Older age was not associated with increased incidence of overall bleeding complications. The increased sensitivity to warfarin in the elderly has also been postulated to be due to decreased vitamin K levels in this population,[32] and the finding of greater postoperative hemoglobin decrease in those patients admitted from institutional care noted by Isaacs et al.[31] may reflect the importance of nutritional status and vitamin K levels in the elderly.

White et al.[33] again demonstrated the effect of advancing age on warfarin response in a study of the rate of change in the INR after the temporary discontinuation of warfarin, simulating a preoperative situation. The INR decreased exponentially, although with a wide intersubject variation in the rate of decrease. Advanced age was associated with a slower rate of decrease. For each 10 years increase in age, the rate of decline in INR decreased by 7%. This was consistent with prior studies showing that older persons eliminate warfarin more slowly than younger ones. It was recommended that an INR of less than 1.5 be verified before surgery, especially in patients at increased risk for bleeding or in the elderly. To ensure the entire population of patients would achieve this INR, 4.8 d of warfarin discontinuation would be required. Alternatively, patients could be given low doses of vitamin K and heparin anticoagulation prior to surgery.

Many reports have described the effects of diet and other drugs on warfarin dose response, but many of these have involved small numbers of subjects and are often not well substantiated. Recent reviews have carefully judged the strength of evidence for individual factors.[1,34] Several drugs potentiated warfarin by inhibiting its metabolic clearance and raising plasma warfarin levels or by interfering either with the synthesis of vitamin K-dependent factors or other pathways of coagulation. Strong support was found in the literature for warfarin potentiation by antibiotics, including trimethoprim-sulfamethoxazole, erythromycin (unknown mechanism), fluconazole, isoniazid, metronidazole, and miconazole. Although many broad-spectrum antibiotics appear to play a role in potentiating warfarin by contributing to vitamin K deficiency through elimination of intestinal bacterial flora, a clinical effect is seen only in those patients who are not eating or are on vitamin K-deficient diets, and the importance of the contribution of intestinal bacteria to vitamin K supplies is very controversial.[35] Strong literature support exists for warfarin potentiation by many cardiac drugs (especially amiodarone, clofibrate, propafenone, propranolol, sulfinpyrazone), phenylbutazone, piroxicam, alcohol, cimetidine, and omeprazole. Plasma warfarin levels are lowered and the anticoagulant effect inhibited by drugs that prevent absorption (cholestyramine) or accelerate metabolic clearance by increasing the activity of hepatic mixed oxidases. Such drugs include griseofulvin, rifampin, nafcillin, barbiturates, carbamazepine, chlordiazepoxide, and sucralfate. Warfarin inhibition is also seen with foods high in vitamin K content (especially green leafy vegetables) and large amounts of avocado.[34]

In summary, there is ample evidence of increased sensitivity to warfarin anticoagulation in elderly patients that is independent of their greater number of potentially complicating drugs and comorbid conditions. However, with adequate monitoring of their INR and careful consideration of causes of increased risk of bleeding complications, including review of concomitant medications, the potential benefit of anticoagulant therapy should always be considered strongly before assuming contraindication to such therapy by increased bleeding risk, per se, in the elderly.

F. COMPLICATIONS OF WARFARIN THERAPY

Bleeding is the most common complication of warfarin anticoagulation. The overall risk of major bleeding on long-term anticoagulation is 1 to 8%.[1–3,5] The cumulative incidence of fatal hemorrhage at 1 and 3 years is 1 and 2%, respectively. The average annual frequencies of fatal, major, and overall (major plus minor) bleeding during warfarin therapy in one study were 0.6, 3.0, and 9.6%, respectively.[5] This was estimated to be five times the risk of bleeding expected without warfarin. Bleeding risk has correlated with the intensity of anticoagulation therapy in most studies. An INR of 4.5 or greater is associated with increased bleeding, and an INR range of 2.0 to 3.0 is recommended for most warfarin indications. Major risk factors also include the patient's underlying medical disorders and the concomitant use of aspirin.

Increased risk of bleeding from warfarin has been linked with increasing age, with a relative risk of 3.2 in patients greater than 65 years.[36,38] This has been shown to be an independent factor by some investigators, possibly reflecting increased vascular vulnerability. But this remains controversial and is not found universally.[37,39] Other bleeding risk factors include uncontrolled hypertension, history of cerebrovascular disease or GI bleeding, AF, recent surgery, and serious coexisting conditions such as hepatic and renal failure and unexplained anemia. Patients can be stratified on the basis of risk factors.[36] Bleeding risk is highest within the first year of anticoagulation (5 to 10% major bleeding episodes). Importantly, the risk is ten times higher during the first month of therapy than the risk after the first year of treatment.

The most common sites of bleeding are GI, soft tissue, and genitourinary (GU). Intracranial hemorrhage is the most serious site, and more than 5% of patients on anticoagulation for cerebrovascular disease will suffer this. In particular, subdural hematomas have been associated with advanced age and excessive anticoagulation level.[40]

The results of workup of anticoagulation-associated bleeding have been reported extensively. In one study, 12% of patients on anticoagulation were found to have occult (GI) bleeding compared to the finding of 3% in a control group not on anticoagulation. The PT in these anticoagulant patients with occult bleeding were not significantly different from those without bleeding. Most patients in this series who underwent evaluation had previously undiagnosed lesions detected.[41] Wilcox and Truss[42] evaluated patients with GI bleeding on warfarin and found that the majority (80%) with upper GI bleeding had underlying ulcer disease, but that only half of those with lower GI bleeding had detectable lesions. However, the inability to find a definitive lesion in this group carried a good prognosis. Bleeding that occurs when the INR was less than 3.0 was frequently associated with an occult GI or GU lesion (40 to 50% of cases), hence full workup is warranted.[43,44] Even if the INR is supratherapeutic, up to 30% of bleeding patients on warfarin will have an underlying lesion.[44] Major bleeding was no more likely to occur with underlying pathology than was occult bleeding. The mean PT rose sharply at the time of bleeding in patients without important lesions compared to those with them.[44] New, previously unknown lesions (including nine cancers) were discovered in 20/59 cases (34%) with GI or GU bleeding, but only in 2/71 (3%) patients with other bleeding sites.

Risks for bleeding are not absolute contraindications to warfarin anticoagulation, and judgment is needed to assess the net benefit from antithrombotic therapy. Careful patient analysis, modifying risk factors, and frequent monitoring especially early in the course of anticoagulation will improve the outcome of warfarin therapy.

The most important nonhemorrhagic complication of warfarin is skin necrosis.[1–3] This uncommon entity usually occurs on the third to eighth day of warfarin therapy and is caused by extensive thrombosis of capillaries and venules within subcutaneous fat, especially over the breasts, thighs, and buttocks. There is an association of this complication with protein C and less commonly protein S deficiency, but it can also occur without these deficiencies. After administration of warfarin, protein C (especially if initially low) falls rapidly to very low levels before commensurate decreases in the other vitamin K-dependent coagulation factors. This results in an excess of procoagulant activity, and a hypercoagulable state ensues. The cost effectiveness of screening for protein C deficiency or placing all patients on heparin before warfarin is doubtful. Low initial doses of warfarin as well as early recognition of this complication with prompt treatment including discontinuation of warfarin, vitamin K administration, and heparin therapy are needed.[1–3]

G. FUTURE IMPROVEMENTS IN WARFARIN THERAPY

Computerized programs for the management of warfarin therapy have been developed, and in one study they provided significantly better control for patients in higher INR ranges (3.0 to 4.5) who were undertreated by medical staff nearly half the time.[45] Improvements in overall outcome of warfarin therapy by the use of these programs is yet to be proven.

A whole-blood PT monitor which is portable and hand-held has been developed, and its results have been shown to be accurate and equivalent to standard PT.[46] Blood is obtained by a finger stick, and test results are available within minutes, including calculation of the INR. This instrument has the potential to simplify INR monitoring, and in two studies its home use by patients resulted in improved anticoagulation control compared with those receiving standard management.[47,48]

Patient education and warfarin management are now often provided by dedicated anticoagulation centers which may provide better therapeutic control, reduce bleeding complications, and be more cost effective than traditional models of care.[49] These centers are often directed by nurses or pharmacists and may employ the portable whole-blood PT monitor described above.

New laboratory tests have been developed that have the potential sensitivity to detect minimal warfarin-induced anticoagulation effects. Levels of the prothrombin activation fragment F_{1+2} reflect prothrombin activation *in vivo*, and decreases (by about 50%) in F_{1+2} correlate well with a target INR of 1.3 to 1.6 in a series of patients receiving low-dose warfarin.[50,51] This low INR range could otherwise only be detected in a PT assay using a highly sensitive thromboplastin reagent (ISI of 1.3). This F_{1+2} assay can be used to tailor the dose of warfarin to an individual patient's level of hypercoagulability. Finally, antigen assays for native and decarboxylated prothrombin have proven as good or better than PT in monitoring warfarin therapy and predicting bleeding.[52] Several other laboratory assays have the potential to improve warfarin monitoring, especially in low-dose regimens.[53]

The dose intensity of warfarin for many indications has been adjusted downward steadily in recent years. The downward adjustment of the PT ratio to 1.3 to 1.5 was initially suggested, and the use of an INR range of 2.0 to 3.0, especially using more sensitive thromboplastin reagents, decreased the occurrence of all types of bleeding from 22 to 4% with no increase in the incidence (2%) of venous thromboembolism.[1,54] The use of low-dose warfarin (INR 1.7 to 2.5) has become standard for treating many clinical conditions.[53,55–57] Very low-dose warfarin (1 mg/d) prevented thrombosis of central venous catheters and also reduced thromboembolism in patients receiving chemotherapy for metastatic breast cancer, maintaining an INR of 1.3 to 1.9 without inducing any bleeding complications.[58,59] If these low-dose regimens prove successful and applicable to both general practice and more of the clinical entities requiring oral anticoagulation, the bleeding complications of warfarin therapy may be significantly decreased.

IV. SPECIFIC INDICATIONS FOR ANTICOAGULATION

A. PROPHYLAXIS OF VENOUS THROMBOEMBOLIC DISEASE

Prophylaxis is the most effective overall management for venous thromboembolic disease, and its wider use could greatly reduce the occurrence of this complication.[60–62] Prophylaxis benefits both surgical and immobilized medical patients and has been shown to be underused, particularly in nonteaching hospitals.[63] Major risks for venous thrombosis have been clearly identified.[60,61] Surgery, especially orthopedic procedures involving the lower extremities with lengthy convalescence at bed rest, is a high risk. Other risk factors apply to both surgical and hospitalized medical patients. Risk increases exponentially with age, most significantly above age 40 years. Cancer increases the risk depending on type, and chemotherapy raises the risk even more. Stroke, paralysis, and prolonged immobilization of any cause may raise the risk to as high as 50%. Myocardial infarction, congestive heart failure, and obesity as well as a previous episode of venous thromboembolic disease are increased risk factors. Moderate-risk patients without high bleeding risk benefit from low-dose heparin. High-risk orthopedic surgery patients have been shown to suffer a calf DVT rate of about 50%, proximal DVT in 20% or more, and pulmonary emboli in 5 to 10% of cases. Effective prophylaxis has resulted from low-dose warfarin, LMWH, and adjusted dose heparin.

Several LMWHs have been shown to be superior to placebo in preventing postoperative DVT, especially after orthopedic surgery. Only one LMWH has been approved for use in the U.S. Several studies have demonstrated LMWHs to be as good as the best other prophylaxis agents, and early reports claimed to find less bleeding than with standard heparin.[64] Hull et al.[65] reported a reduction, albeit small, in DVT with the use of LMWH compared to warfarin prophylaxis after hip or knee implantation, but this was offset by increased bleeding (incidence of major bleeding of 1.2% for warfarin compared to 2.8% in the LMWH arm). Spiro et al.[66] showed that higher-dose enoxaparin regimens were more effective in prophylaxis after hip replacement surgery than lower doses and were as effective as the best drug treatments previously reported. However, the incidence of bleeding was higher with the higher-dose regimens, with major hemorrhage in 4 to 5% of patients on high doses, with operative site bleeding seen particularly. Both the simplicity of administering LMWH in one or two subcutaneous doses daily and the cost saving due both to laboratory monitoring being unnecessary and to its outpatient use make LMWH attractive as a prophylaxis of choice. However, the considerably higher drug cost of LMWH in the U.S. and the small, but real increase in bleeding confuses the issue. Continued careful study of LMWH is needed both in this clinical setting and in wider applications that are now being addressed.[67]

B. Treatment of Established Venous Thromboembolism

Immediate anticoagulation is indicated with either adjusted dose subcutaneous heparin or continuous infusion intravenous heparin, with dosing for the latter determined optimally by weight-adjusted aPTT-driven nomograms, with the important goal of achieving a therapeutic aPTT of 1.5 times control as early as possible during the first 24 hr and maintaining a therapeutic range of 1.5 to 2.5.[9,17] Heparin is continued for 5 to 10 d and warfarin is overlapped by 3 to 5 d. If the DVT is uncomplicated, warfarin is begun on day 1 and only 5 d of heparin may be needed, shortening hospitalization and possibly decreasing the incidence of heparin-induced thrombocytopenia.[68] If a pulmonary embolus or iliofemoral thrombosis is present, a longer period of heparin therapy may be indicated. An INR of 2.0 to 3.0 using warfarin anticoagulation is maintained for at least 3 months.

C. Stroke Prevention in Atrial Fibrillation

Prospective studies have proven nonrheumatic AF as a common cause of stroke, increasing in incidence and clinical importance with age. The Framingham study documented that the occurrence of stroke in patients with AF increases fivefold with advancing age, from 6.7% at 50 to 59 years to 36.2% at 80 to 89 years.[69] Meta-analysis of six randomized clinical trials revealed an overall reduction of 64% in relative risk of stroke among patients treated with warfarin as compared to placebo.[70]

In patients with nonrheumatic AF less than 60 years of age and who have no other risk factors ("lone AF"), there is no increased risk for stroke. However, in nonrheumatic AF patients over age 60 or who have additional risk factors, warfarin is strongly recommended.[70–76] In patients with higher bleeding risk, aspirin may be used. The value of warfarin remains unclear in patients over 75 years of age who are at higher risk for bleeding. Maintenance of lower INR ranges (2.0 to 3.0 or even lower at 1.5 to 2.7) may make advanced age a less critical factor. Physician survey has documented persisting hesitation to use oral anticoagulants for the prevention of stroke in the elderly with AF.[77] When used, it was most often after an ischemic episode (transient ischemic attack or cerebrovascular accident) had occurred or in patients with mitral valve disease. Withholding anticoagulation based on age alone places patients at undue risk for severely disabling thromboembolic complications.

V. SUMMARY

Recent improvements in laboratory monitoring and in dosing regimens for both heparin and warfarin have increased the effectiveness and, particularly in the case of warfarin, the safety of these agents. The use of aPTT-driven dosing nomograms for heparin achieves therapeutic level anticoagulation more rapidly with fewer recurrent venous thromboembolism episodes, but no increase in bleeding. Risk assessment for bleeding from both heparin and warfarin is necessary, with advanced age probably being an independent risk factor for both agents. However, anticoagulation should not be avoided on the basis of age alone without considering other risks and the potential benefits in each individual. Bleeding must be watched for carefully during anticoagulation, and evaluation of unexplained bleeding, especially GI and GU (even with supratherapeutic aPTT or INR), is often worthwhile, discovering previously unknown lesions in from one third up to one half of patients. Venous thromboembolism prophylaxis in high-risk surgical and medical patients is effective and probably underused. The convenience and effectiveness of LMWHs in this prophylactic setting has been proven, but the increased incidence of bleeding with their use is a concern, and low-dose heparin or, in high-risk patients, low-dose warfarin, remain options.

Improved laboratory monitoring of warfarin therapy using the INR as well as lower dosing regimens have provided effective oral anticoagulation with less danger of bleeding. Recognition that the elderly require lower doses of warfarin with increasing age as well as a careful assessment of the effects of concomitant drug therapy and comorbid medical conditions will maximize the safe use of this agent. Better warfarin control with portable wholeblood INR monitors, dedicated anticoagulation centers, and the use of improved INRs with highly sensitive thromboplastin reagents or newer assays of warfarin anticoagulant effect will again improve safety and laboratory control at the low- and very low-dose warfarin regimens recently begun in use. The high risk of stroke in the elderly with nonrheumatic AF and the effectiveness and safety of low-dose warfarin in this setting seem to be the epitome of the goal of careful identification of clinical settings that will benefit from anticoagulation as well as effective and safe anticoagulation regimens for the elderly. The many recent clinical trials supporting the use of warfarin to prevent stroke in AF will hopefully lead to an appropriately increased use of anticoagulation in this setting.

REFERENCES

1. **Hirsh, J.,** Oral anticoagulant drugs, *N. Engl. J. Med.*, 324, 1865, 1991.
2. **Guidry, J. R., Raschke, R. A., and Morkunas, A. R.,** Anticoagulants and thrombolytics: risks and benefits, *Crit. Care Clin.*, 7, 533, 1991.
3. **Berkman, S. A,** Current concepts in anticoagulation, *Hosp. Pract.*, 187, 1992.
4. **Hirsh, J., Dalen, J. E., Deykin, D., and Poller, L.,** Heparin: mechanism of action, pharmacokinetics, dosing considerations, monitoring, efficacy, and safety, *Chest*, 102 (Suppl. 4), 337S, 1992.
5. **Levine, M. N., Hirsh, J., Landefeld, S., and Raskob, G.,** Hemorrhagic complications of anticoagulant treatment, *Chest*, 102 (Suppl. 4), 352S, 1992.
6. **Hirsh, J., Dalen, J. E., Deykin, D., and Poller, L.,** Oral anticoagulants: mechanism of action, clinical effectiveness, and optimal therapeutic range, *Chest*, 102 (Suppl. 4), 312S, 1992.
7. **Ansell, J. E.,** Oral anticoagulant therapy — 50 years later, *Arch. Intern. Med.*, 153, 586, 1993.
8. **Merli, G. J.,** Old and new agents in the treatment of thromboembolic disease, *Hem/Onc Ann.*, 1, 113, 1993.
9. **Weinmann, E. E., and Salzman, E. W.,** Deep-vein thrombosis. *N. Engl. J. Med.*, 331, 1630, 1994.

10. **Becker, R. C. and Ansell, J.,** Antithrombotic therapy: an abbreviated reference for clinicians, *Arch. Intern. Med.*, 155, 149, 1995.
11. **Litin, S. C. and Gastineau, D. A.,** Current concepts in anticoagulant therapy, *Mayo Clin. Proc.*, 70, 266, 1995.
12. **Sasahara, A. A., St. Martin, C. C., Henkin, J., and Barker, W. M.,** Approach to the patient with venous thromboembolism: treatment with thrombolytic agents, *Hem/Onc Clin. North Am.*, 6, 1141, 1992.
13. **Meneveau, N., Bassand, J. P., Schiele, F., Bouras, Y., Anguenot, T., Bernard, Y., and Schultz, R.,** Safety of thrombolytic therapy in elderly patients with massive pulmonary embolism, *J. Am. Coll. Cardiol.*, 22, 1075, 1993.
14. **Verstraete, M.,** Pharmacotherapeutic aspects of unfractionated and low molecular weight heparins, *Drugs*, 40, 498, 1990.
15. **Hirsh, J. and Levine, M. N.,** Low molecular weight heparin, *Blood*, 79, 1, 1992.
16. **Brill-Edwards, P., Ginsberg, J. S., Johnston, M., and Hirsh, J.,** Establishing a therapeutic range for heparin therapy, *Ann. Intern. Med.*, 119, 104, 1993.
17. **Hull, R. D., Raskob, G. E., Hirsh, J., Jay, R. M. et al.,** Continuous intravenous heparin compared with intermittent subcutaneous heparin in the initial treatment of proximal-vein thrombosis, *N. Engl. J. Med.*, 315, 1109, 1986.
18. **Hommes, D. W., Bura, A., Mazzolai, L., Buller, H. R., and tenCate, J. W.,** Subcutaneous heparin compared with continuous intravenous heparin in the initial treatment of deep vein thrombosis: a meta-analysis, *Ann. Intern. Med.*, 116, 279, 1992.
19. **Cruickshank, M. K., Levine, M. N., Hirsh, J., Roberts, R., and Siguenza, M.,** A standard heparin nomogram for the management of heparin therapy, *Arch. Intern. Med.*, 151, 333, 1991.
20. **Raschke, R. A., Reilly, B. M., Guidry, J. R., Fontana, J. R., and Srinivas, S.,** The weight-based heparin dosing nomogram compared with a "standard care" nomogram, *Ann. Intern. Med.*, 119, 874, 1993.
21. **Hull, R. A., Raskob, G. E., Rosenbloom, P., Lemaire, J. et al.,** Optimal therapeutic level of heparin therapy in patients with venous thrombosis, *Arch. Intern. Med.*, 152, 1589, 1992.
22. **Walker, A. M. and Jick, H.,** Predictors of bleeding during heparin therapy, *JAMA*, 244, 1209, 1980.
23. **Nieuwenhuis, H. K., Albada, J., Banga, J. D., and Sixma, J. J.,** Identification of risk factors for bleeding during treatment of acute venous thromboembolism with heparin or low molecular weight heparin, *Blood*, 78, 2337, 1991.
24. **Landefeld, C. S. and Beyth, R. J.,** Anticoagulant-related bleeding: clinical epidemiology, prediction, and prevention, *Am. J. Med.*, 95, 315, 1993.
25. **Warkentin, J. E. and Kelton, J. G.,** Heparin-induced thrombocytopenia, *Prog. Hemostasis Thromb.*, 10, 1, 1991.
26. **Le, D. T., Weibart, R. T., Sevilla, B. K., Donnelly, K. J., and Rapaport, S. I.,** The international normalized ratio (INR) for monitoring warfarin therapy: reliability and relation to other monitoring methods, *Ann. Intern. Med.*, 120, 552, 1994.
27. **Hull, R., Hirsh, J., Jay, R., Carter, C. et al.,** Different intensities of oral anticoagulant therapy in the treatment of proximal-vein thrombosis, *N. Engl. J. Med.*, 307, 1676, 1982.
28. **Gurwitz, J. H., Avorn, J., Ross-Degnan, P., Choodnovsky, I., and Ansell, J.,** Aging and the anticoagulant response to warfarin therapy, *Ann. Intern. Med.*, 116, 901, 1992.
29. **Gurwitz, J. H. and Avorn, J.,** The ambiguous relation between aging and adverse drug reactions, *Ann. Intern. Med.*, 114, 956, 1991.
30. **Mungall, D. and White, R.,** Aging and warfarin, *Ann. Intern. Med.*, 117, 878, 1992.
31. **Isaacs, C., Paltiel, O., Blake, G., Beaudet, M., Conochie, L., and Leclerc, J.,** Age-associated risks of prophylactic anticoagulation in the setting of hip fracture, *Am. J. Med.*, 96, 487, 1994.
32. **Shepherd, A. M. M., Hewick, D. S., Moreland, T. A., and Stevenson, I. H.,** Age as determinant of sensitivity to warfarin, *Br. J. Clin. Pharmacol.*, 4, 315, 1977.
33. **White, R. H., McKittrick, Hutchison, R., and Twitchell, J.,** Temporary discontinuation of warfarin: changes in the international normalized ratio, *Ann. Intern. Med.*, 122, 40, 1995.
34. **Wells, P. S., Holbrook, A. M., Crowther, N. R., and Hirsh, J.,** Interactions of warfarin with drugs and food, *Ann. Intern. Med.*, 121, 676, 1994.
35. **Lipsky, J. J.,** Nutritional sources of vitamin K, *Mayo Clin. Proc.*, 69, 462, 1994.
36. **Landefeld, C. S., McGuire, E., and Rosenblatt, M. W.,** A bleeding risk index for estimating the probability of major bleeding in hospitalized patients starting anticoagulant therapy, *Am. J. Med.*, 89, 569, 1990.
37. **Launbjerg, K., Egeblad, H., Heaf, J., Nielsen, N. H., Fugleholm, A. M., and Ladefoged, K.,** Bleeding complication to oral anticoagulant therapy: multivariate analysis of 1010 treatment years in 551 outpatients, *J. Intern. Med.*, 229, 351, 1991.
38. **Landefeld, C. S. and Goldman, L.,** Major bleeding in outpatients treated with warfarin: incidence and prediction by factors known at the start of outpatient therapy. *Am. J. Med.*, 87, 144, 1989.
39. **Fihn, S. D., McDonell, M., Martin, D., Henikoff, J. et al.,** Risk factors for complication of chronic anticoagulation, *Ann. Intern. Med.*, 118, 511, 1993.

40. **Hylek, E. M. and Singer, D. E.,** Risk factors for intracranial hemorrhage in outpatients taking warfarin, *Ann. Intern. Med.,* 120, 897, 1994.
41. **Jaffin, B. W., Bliss, C. M., and Lamart, J. T.,** Significance of occult gastrointestinal bleeding during anticoagulation therapy, *Am. J. Med.,* 83, 269, 1987.
42. **Wilcox, C. M. and Truss, C. D.,** Gastrointestinal bleeding in patients receiving long-term anticoagulant therapy, *Am. J. Med.,* 84, 683, 1988.
43. **Schuster, G. A. and Lewis, G. A.,** Clinical significance of hematuria in patients on anticoagulant therapy, *J. Urol.,* 137, 923, 1987.
44. **Landefeld, C. S., Rosenblatt, M. W., and Goldman, L.,** Bleeding in outpatients treated with warfarin: relation to the prothrombin time and important remediable lesions, *Am. J. Med.,* 87, 153, 1989.
45. **Poller, L., Wright, D., and Rowlands, M.,** Prospective comparative study of computer programs used for management of warfarin, *J. Clin. Pathol.,* 46, 299, 1993.
46. **Lucas, F. V., Duncan, A., Jay, R. M. et al.,** A novel whole blood capillary technique for measuring the prothrombin time, *Am. J. Clin. Pathol.,* 88, 442, 1987.
47. **White, R. H., McCurdy, S. A., vonMarensdorff, H., Woodruff, D. E., and Letgoff, L.,** Home prothrombin time monitoring after the initiation of warfarin therapy, *Ann. Intern. Med.,* 111, 730, 1989.
48. **Anderson, D. R., Harrison, L., and Hirsh, J.,** Evaluation of portable prothrombin time monitor for home use by patients who require long-term oral anticoagulant use, *Arch. Intern. Med.,* 153, 1441, 1993.
49. **Garabedian-Ruffalo, S. M., Gray, D. R., Sax, M. J., and Ruffalo, R. L.,** Retrospective evaluation of a pharmacist-managed warfarin anticoagulation clinic, *Am. J. Hosp. Pharm.,* 42, 304, 1985.
50. **Kistler, J. P.,** for the Boston area anticoagulation trial for atrial fibrillation investigators, Effect of low-intensity warfarin anticoagulation on level of activity of the hemostatic system in patients with atrial fibrillation, *Stroke,* 24, 1360, 1993.
51. **Millenson, M. M., Bauer, K. A., Kistler, J. P. et al.,** Monitoring "mini-intensity" anticoagulation with warfarin: comparison of the prothrombin time using a sensitive thromboplastin with prothrombin fragment F_{1+2} levels, *Blood,* 79, 2034, 1992.
52. **Furie, B., Diuguid, C. F., Jacobs, M. et al.,** Randomized prospective trial comparing the native prothrombin antigen with the prothrombin time for monitoring oral anticoagulant therapy, *Blood,* 75, 344, 1990.
53. **Bern, M. M.,** Considerations for using lower doses of warfarin, *Hem/Onc Clin. North Am.,* 6, 1105, 1992.
54. **Hirsh, J. and Levine, M. N.,** The optimal intensity of oral anticoagulant therapy, *JAMA,* 250, 2723, 1987.
55. Boston area anticoagulation trial for atrial fibrillation trial investigators, The effect of low-dose warfarin on the risk of stroke in patients with nonrheumatic atrial fibrillation, *N. Engl. J. Med.,* 323, 1505, 1990.
56. **Turpie, A. G. G., Hirsh, J., Guntensen, J., Nelson, H., and Gent, M.,** Randomized comparison of two intensities of oral anticoagulant therapy after tissue valve replacement, *Lancet,* 1, 1242, 1988.
57. **Albers, G. W., Atwood, J. E., Hirsh, J. et al.,** Stroke prevention in nonvalvular atrial fibrillation, *Ann. Intern. Med.,* 115, 727, 1991.
58. **Bern, M. M., Lokich, J. J., Wallach, S. R. et al.,** Very low doses of warfarin can prevent thrombosis in central venous catheters, *Ann. Intern. Med.,* 112, 423, 1990.
59. **Levine, M., Hirsh, J., Gent, M. et al.,** Very low-dose warfarin reduces thromboembolism in patients with metastatic breast cancer receiving chemotherapy, *Lancet,* 343, 886, 1994.
60. **Clagett, G. P., Anderson, F. A., Levine, M. N., Salzman, E. W., and Whealer, H. B.,** Prevention of venous thromboembolism, *Chest,* 102 (Suppl. 4), 391S, 1992.
61. **Kashyep, A. and Francis, C. W.,** Methods of prophylaxis for deep vein thrombosis and pulmonary embolism, *Hem/Onc Ann.,* 1, 125, 1993.
62. **Halkin, H., Goldberg, J., Modan, M., and Modan, B.,** Reduction of mortality in general medicine in-patients by low dose heparin prophylaxis, *Ann. Intern. Med.,* 96, 561, 1982.
63. **Anderson, F. A., Whealer, H. B., Goldberg, R. J. et al.,** Physician practices in the prevention of venous thromboembolism, *Ann. Intern. Med.,* 115, 591, 1991.
64. **Turpie, A. G. G., Levine, M. N., Hirsh, J. et al.,** A randomized controlled trial of a low molecular weight heparin (enoxaparin) to prevent deep-vein thrombosis in patients undergoing elective hip surgery, *N. Engl. J. Med.,* 315, 925, 1986.
65. **Hull, R., Raskob, G., Pineo, G. et al.,** A comparison of subcutaneous low-molecular-weight heparin with warfarin sodium for prophylaxis against deep-vein thrombosis after hip or knee implantation, *N. Engl. J. Med.,* 329, 1370, 1993.
66. **Spiro, T. E., Johnson G. J., Christie M. J. et al.,** Efficacy and safety of enoxaparin to prevent deep venous thrombosis after hip replacement surgery, *Ann. Intern. Med.,* 121, 81, 1994.
67. **Imperiale, T. F. and Speroff, T.,** A meta-analysis of methods to prevent venous thromboembolism following total hip replacement, *JAMA,* 271, 1780, 1994.
68. **Hull, R. D., Raskob, G. E., Rosenbloom, D. et al.,** Heparin for 5 days as compared with 10 days in the initial treatment of proximal venous thrombosis, *N. Engl. J. Med.,* 322, 1260, 1990.
69. **Wolf, P. A., Abbott, R. P., and Kannel, W. B.,** Atrial fibrillation: a major contributor to stroke in the elderly, *Arch. Intern. Med.,* 147, 1561, 1987.

70. **Barnett, H. J. M., Eliasziw, M., and Meldriam, H. E.,** Drugs and surgery in the prevention of ischemic stroke, *N. Engl. J. Med.*, 332, 238, 1995.
71. **Jahnigen, D. W.,** Atrial fibrillation in the elderly: management update, *Geriatrics*, 45, 26, 1990.
72. **Esekowitz, M. D., Bridgers, S. L., James, K. E. et al.,** Warfarin in the prevention of stroke associated with nonrheumatic atrial fibrillation, *N. Engl. J. Med.*, 327, 1406, 1992.
73. **Matchar, D. B., McCrory, D. C., Barnett, H. J. M., and Feussner, J. R.,** Medical treatment for stroke prevention. *Ann. Intern. Med.,* 121,41, 1994.
74. **Atrial fibrillation investigators,** Risk factors for stroke and efficacy of antithrombotic therapy in atrial fibrillation, *Arch. Intern. Med.,* 154, 1449, 1994.
75. **Albers, G. W.,** Atrial fibrillation and stroke, *Arch. Intern. Med.,* 154, 1443, 1994.
76. **Dunn, M. and Blackburn, T.,** Anticoagulant treatment of atrial fibrillation in the elderly, *Postgrad. Med. J.*, 68 (Suppl. 1), 557, 1992.
77. **Kutner, M., Nixon, G., and Silverstone, F.,** Physician's attitudes toward oral anticoagulant and antiplatelet agents for stroke prevention in elderly patients with atrial fibrillation, *Arch. Intern. Med.,* 151, 1950, 1991.

Chapter 15

ANTIHYPERLIPIDEMIC AGENTS

John M. Morgan

CONTENTS

I. CORONARY HEART DISEASE AND SERUM LIPIDS

Coronary heart disease (CHD) is the leading cause of death in the elderly.[1] Importantly, CHD is also associated with significant morbidity and treatment costs, which are increasing with the aging of the population. For example, by the year 2030, the proportion of the population over the age of 65 years is projected to increase from its current level of 13% to more than 20%.[2] Since the life expectancy of an otherwise healthy 65-year-old individual is

0-8493-8306-4/96/$0.00+$.50

15 years for men and almost 20 years for women,[3] and since two or more years of aggressive medical therapy have been shown to stabilize, slow the progression, or promote the regression of coronary artery plaques,[4] the opportunity for prevention management of CHD in the elderly to reduce CHD events makes good medical and economic sense. Furthermore, because of the high prevalence of CHD in this country, a 1% reduction in CHD mortality represents approximately 4200 fewer CHD deaths per year in the U.S. alone.[5]

The risk factors for the development of CHD have been extensively investigated. The association between CHD and elevated serum lipid levels, in particular low-density lipoprotein (LDL) cholesterol, has been well documented. Thus, in recent years, dietary and pharmacologic interventions aimed at reducing serum LDL cholesterol comprise an important approach to the prevention, deceleration, and treatment of coronary atherosclerosis. The second report of the Expert Panel on Detection, Evaluation, and Treatment of High Blood Cholesterol in Adults (Adult Treatment Panel II) presented compelling scientific data to support their recommendations for the treatment of hypercholesterolemia.[6] As shown in Table 15.1, the recommended treatments and therapeutic goals are based on the CHD risk status of the patient. It is important to note that the Adult Treatment Panel II includes age as a major risk factor for CHD. This is not surprising when one considers that the atherosclerotic process increases with age,[7] with the peak incidence of CHD events observed in men at age 65 and in women at age 75.

TABLE 15.1.
Treatment Decisions and Goals Based on LDL Cholesterol Levels

Risk status	Initiation of dietary therapy	Consideration of drug therapy	LDL cholesterol goals
Without CHD and <2 risk factors[a]	≥160 mg/dL	≥190 mg/dL	<160 mg/dL
Without CHD and ≥2 risk factors[a]	≥130 mg/dL	≥160 mg/dL	<130 mg/dL
With CHD	>100 mg/dL	≥130 mg/dL	≤100 mg/dL

[a] The Adult Treatment Panel II defines risk factors as the following: age (≥45 years for men and ≥55 years for women), a family history of premature CHD, cigarette smoking, hypertension, low levels of HDL cholesterol (<35 mg/dL), and diabetes mellitus. A high level of HDL cholesterol (>60 mg/dL) is a "negative" risk factor. This means that one risk factor is subtracted for a high HDL cholesterol.[6]

The question that was not addressed by the Adult Treatment Panel II is whether the therapeutic approach to the regulation of serum lipids as a means of decreasing CHD risk should be different, or modified, for patients over the age of 65 years. With respect to the primary prevention of CHD, the data are controversial. The risk ratio for CHD mortality vs. total cholesterol actually declines with age,[8] suggesting that there may be less benefit in lowering serum total cholesterol levels in the elderly. However, analysis of the Framingham data indicates that increased serum total cholesterol is a CHD risk factor, and that elevated LDL cholesterol is associated with an increased risk of CHD at all ages through 82 years.[9] High-density lipoprotein (HDL) cholesterol also demonstrates an important inverse relationship to the risk of CHD in the elderly.[10] Furthermore, the attributable risk of cholesterol (i.e., the difference in the absolute rates of CHD between the highest and lowest quartiles) increases with age,[11] suggesting that cholesterol lowering should have an even greater impact on CHD risk in older vs. younger individuals.

With respect to secondary prevention in a patient with clinical evidence of CHD, the data suggest that dietary and/or drug treatment of elevated serum cholesterol is clearly warranted. However, the clinician is faced with difficult decisions in the treatment of the elderly patient. To make these decisions, recommendations based on clinical trials involving middle-aged patients must be tailored for the individual elderly patient based on such considerations as general health status, physiological age vs. chronological age, activity level, quality of life issues, the presence of other CHD risk factors and the ability to control those factors, the importance of dietary intervention vs. the maintenance of adequate nutrition, the attitude of the patient, and the optimal use of drug therapy to maximize benefits while minimizing adverse reactions. In this chapter, the current antihyperlipidemic treatment options will be reviewed in terms of their effects on lipoprotein metabolism and atherogenesis in elderly patients. The special considerations regarding the selection and appropriate use of antihyperlipidemic therapy in elderly patients will be examined.

II. LIPOPROTEINS, ATHEROSCLEROSIS, AND AGING

A. LIPOPROTEINS AND ATHEROSCLEROSIS

Lipoproteins are spherical particles with a core comprised of nonpolar components, such as cholesterol esters and triglycerides. The outer surface of lipoproteins forms a polar interface with plasma and consists of apolipoproteins, phospholipids, and free cholesterol. Based on their densities lipoproteins are classified into five basic groups. The size and density of lipoproteins are largely a function of their triglyceride content. The largest and least dense lipoproteins are chylomicrons, which consist almost entirely of triglycerides. Next in size are the very low-density lipoproteins (VLDL), which are composed primarily of triglycerides, followed by the intermediate-density lipoproteins (IDL), LDL, and HDL, which contain progressively more cholesterol and protein and less triglyceride.

The cholesterol that accumulates in atherosclerotic lesions originates primarily from plasma lipoproteins, including LDL cholesterol. Chronic hypercholesterolemia results in a positive cholesterol balance at the vascular interface, with more cholesterol entering than exiting the arterial wall. This directed cholesterol flux promotes the atherogenic process. Oxidation of LDL in the subendothelial layers of the arterial wall, which can be produced by activated endothelial cells, smooth muscle cells, or macrophages, appears to be a key irreversible event in atherogenesis. Oxidized LDL, which is taken up by macrophages via the acetyl LDL receptor much more rapidly than native LDL, facilitates the accumulation of esterified cholesterol and the formation of foam cells, the earliest cellular lesions observed in atherosclerosis (stary I lesion). Modified forms of other lipoproteins that can be taken up by macrophages via similar scavenger receptors include VLDL, aggregates of LDL, oxidized Lipoprotein(a), complexes of proteoglycans, and probably immune complexes of modified forms of LDL linked to specific autoantibodies.[12] Though much remains unknown about this process, elucidation of the steps involved in the formation of atherosclerotic lesions should promote development of future antihyperlipidemic therapies. These modalities include agents that prevent the oxidation, inhibit the deposition of lipoproteins, especially LDL cholesterol, or stimulate the egress of cholesterol from the vascular wall.

As the atherosclerotic lesion, or fatty streak, develops under an intact layer of endothelial cells, macrophages below this layer may release toxic products, namely superoxide anion and proteolytic enzymes, which can perturb and disrupt the endothelium. The disruption attracts platelets and fibrin and initiates the formation of the more advanced lesion of atherosclerosis, the fibrofatty plaque. Fissures or ulcerations within these plaques can lead to plaque disruption and thrombotic occlusion, which, in turn, can produce the clinical manifestations of a coronary artery disease event.[7]

The apolipoprotein (apo) constituents of lipoproteins have a number of important functions, including the binding and solubilization of lipids and the activation of enzymes. For example, apo A-I, which accounts for more than half the content of HDL, activates the enzyme lecithin-cholesterol acyltransferase (LCAT). Apolipoproteins also function as ligands that recognize and bind to the receptors on the surface of cells that utilize lipids. Hepatocyte receptors recognize apoB-100, the predominant apo of LDL, apoB-48, a constituent of chylomicrons, and apoE, which is a constituent of VLDL and intermediate density lipoproteins (IDL). These receptors are the primary means by which lipoproteins are taken up by the cells. ApoC, which is contained in both chylomicrons and VLDL, activates lipoprotein lipase (LPL) in the capillaries. LPL in turn promotes the catabolism and removal of triglycerides from these lipoproteins. Finally, apo(a) has close homology to plasminogen and may compete with plasminogen for binding to fibrin. The resulting inhibition of thrombolysis may explain why Lipoprotein(a), an LDL-like lipoprotein formed by the covalent linkage of apo(a) and apoB-100, is a lipoprotein risk factor for CHD.[13]

B. LIPOPROTEIN METABOLISM

The endogenous pathway of lipoprotein metabolism,[14] which is illustrated in Figure 15.1, is the primary focus of dietary and drug therapy for the reduction of LDL cholesterol and the noninvasive management of the atherogenic process.

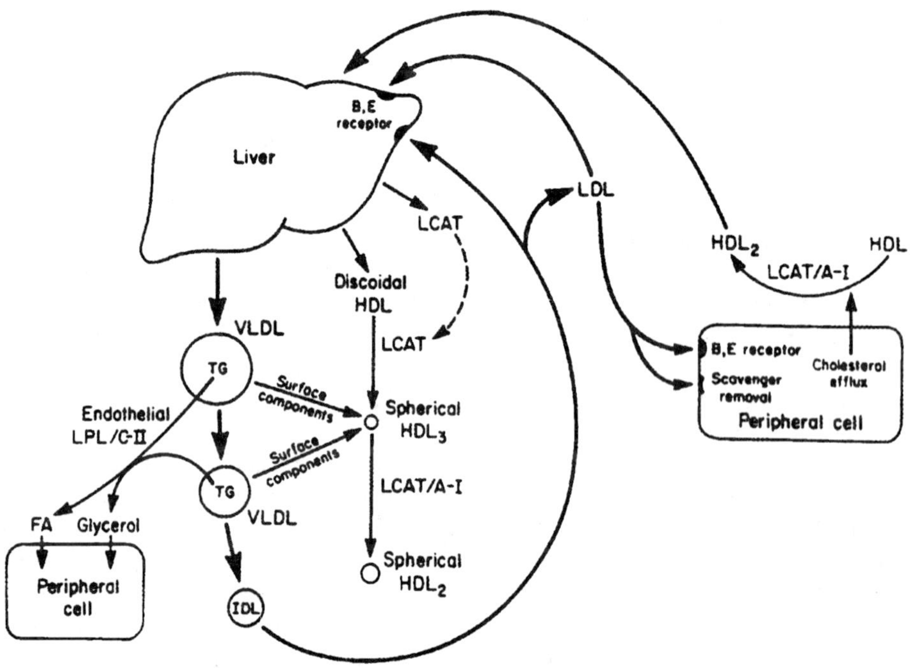

FIGURE 15.1. Endogenous pathway of lipoprotein metabolism. (From Capuzzi, D. M., in *Internal Medicine for Dentistry*, 2nd ed., Kaye, D. and Ross, L. F., Eds., C. V. Mosby, St. Louis, 1989, 1133–1153. With permission.)

1. VLDL Cholesterol

The lipoprotein synthetic pathway begins in hepatic parenchymal cells with the generation of VLDL cholesterol from fatty acids that are mobilized from deposited adipose tissue triglycerides or synthesized *de novo* from carbohydrates. Triglycerides comprise the core and are the major component (55 to 75% by weight) of VLDL, whereas the apo of VLDL particles consist mainly of apoC, apoB, and some apoE. The production of VLDL cholesterol can be stimulated by an increased intake of calories and carbohydrates, excessive intake of alcohol, and elevated circulating levels of insulin. The major antihyperlipidemic drug that probably acts on this step of the pathway is niacin. Niacin may prevent the synthesis of VLDL in the liver and may inhibit the release of VLDL into the circulation.[15,16]

After VLDL is released into the circulation, it is transported to the tissue capillaries, where it undergoes triglyceride removal. This process is catalyzed by apoC-II-activated lipoprotein lipase (LPL/C-II). When compared with young subjects (aged 19 to 28 years), older subjects (aged 40 to 72 years) appear to have reduced lipoprotein lipase activity and delayed clearance of the triglyceride-rich particles (chylomicrons and VLDL) following a high-fat meal.[17] One of the mechanisms by which gemfibrozil and other fibric acid derivatives reduce plasma triglycerides may be the stimulation of triglyceride removal mechanisms and, particularly, LPL activity.[18]

As the triglycerides are progressively removed from VLDL, the surface components (phospholipids, unesterified cholesterol, and apo) of the lipoprotein are transferred to HDL_3 particles. As a result, the VLDL particle is transformed into the more dense, cholesterol-enriched IDL particle. With the removal of the remaining triglycerides as well as all of the apo, except for apoB-100, the IDL is transformed into an LDL particle, which has a core that consists almost exclusively of cholesterol esters and a surface comprised of apoB-100. Although the majority of circulating IDL is rapidly converted to LDL in this manner, IDL can also be removed from the circulation via binding to hepatic apoB/E receptors, which also bind LDL.

2. LDL Cholesterol

Through the lipoprotein metabolic pathway described above and in Figure 15.1, LDL arises as the catabolic end product of VLDL degradation. One of the functions of LDL is to serve as a source of cholesterol for a variety of cells. LDL binds to an LDL receptor that is present on most nucleated cells by receptor-mediated recognition of surface apoB-100. After binding to this receptor, the LDL particle is internalized and incorporated into a lysosome to form an endosome, wherein the LDL is hydrolyzed to amino acids and free cholesterol, which is released into the cytoplasm (Figure 15.2). The increased intracellular cholesterol suppresses the synthesis of LDL receptors on the cell surface, thereby restricting further uptake of LDL by cells, primarily hepatocytes. The free cholesterol also inhibits hydroxymethyl glutaryl CoA reductase (HMG CoA reductase), the rate-limiting enzyme for hepatic cholesterol synthesis. In this manner, intracellular cholesterol balance is maintained. Approximately two thirds of LDL particles are removed from the circulation and catabolized by this mechanism, mainly by the liver (approximately 75%) and to a lesser extent by steroid-producing and other extrahepatic tissues.

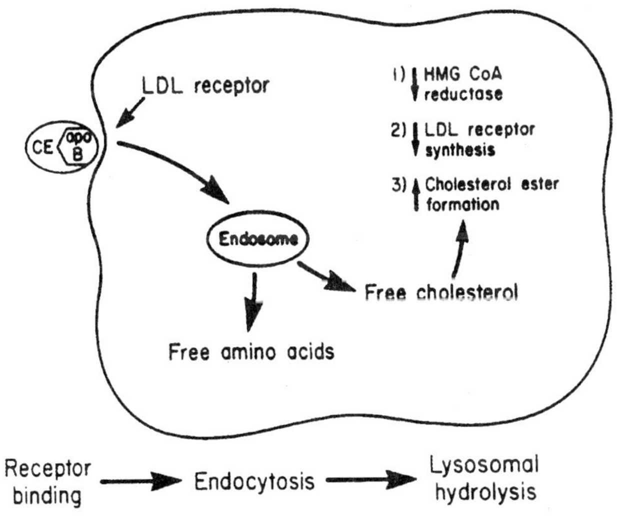

FIGURE 15.2. Formation of intracellular cholesterol from extracellular LDL cholesterol, which enters the cell via LDL receptor binding, and undergoes lysosomal endocytosis followed by hydrolysis to free cholesterol. (From Capuzzi, D. M., in *Internal Medicine for Dentistry*, 2nd ed., Kaye, D. and Ross, L. F., Eds., C. V. Mosby, St. Louis, 1989, 1133–1153. With permission.)

The fractional clearance of LDL cholesterol has been shown to be inversely related to the serum LDL cholesterol level, with reduced clearance at high LDL cholesterol serum levels. However, at serum LDL cholesterol levels of 160 mg/dL and higher, the reduction in fractional clearance begins to level off. As individuals age, the fractional clearance of LDL cholesterol also appears to decrease.[19] This decrease may be related to a reduction in the number of LDL cell surface receptors or a reduction in the activity of these receptors.[20] It is unclear whether the decrease in fractional LDL cholesterol clearance is attributable or due to age-related processes, age-related increases in hepatic fat and cholesterol, or to both factors. An increase in these constituents of nascent lipoproteins would promote the production of VLDL, which would lead to increased production of VLDL remnants and LDL, both of which can mediate inhibition of LDL receptors. The net effect would be an age-associated increase in LDL cholesterol in the serum stemming from diminished removal capacity for circulating LDL.

Increased LDL cholesterol that is not cleared by the receptor-mediated process described above can be removed from the circulation by a receptor-independent or scavenger mechanism. Much is currently unclear about the molecular mechanisms involved. However, this scavenger uptake of LDL has low affinity for native LDL and is poorly regulated and may become pathologically significant as LDL serum levels rise above concentrations that saturate the LDL receptors. Evidence exists that modifications of native LDL, such as oxidation, acetylation, or glycosylation, may stimulate the uptake of circulating LDL by scavenger cells and macrophages even in the arterial wall, thereby increasing the cardiovascular risk associated with a given serum level of LDL cholesterol.

Two major classes of antihyperlipidemic drugs — the bile acid sequestrants and the HMG-CoA reductase inhibitors — act by increasing the number of LDL receptors. Bile acid sequestrants deplete hepatic cholesterol by binding bile acids in the intestine and preventing their enterohepatic reuptake and thereby increasing the removal of hepatic cholesterol by promoting its conversion to bile acids. This removal of hepatic cholesterol stimulates the synthesis of LDL receptors and cholesterol.[21] Because bile acid sequestrants appear to stimulate production of all lipoproteins in a nonselective manner, VLDL production is also increased. The latter can lead to elevated serum triglyceride levels,[22] an increase that may be transient or sustained, depending upon the ability of the liver to reregulate the rate of VLDL production.

3. HDL Cholesterol

An important component of the lipoprotein metabolic pathway is HDL in its various forms. HDL with its lipophilic peptides, especially apoA-I, provides a major mechanism whereby cholesterol is transported among the other lipoproteins from the peripheral tissues and to the liver. HDL generally transports cholesterol in the direction opposite to that of LDL cholesterol, that is, from the cells to either the liver or other lipoproteins, and is considered the major biological determinant for reverse cholesterol transport. Nascent or discoidal HDL is produced in the liver (Figure 15.1). In this form, HDL can accept VLDL surface components (phospholipids and apo) and free cholesterol, the latter originating from peripheral tissues including arterial plaques as well as the liver for removal of this hydrophobic sterol. The free cholesterol in the HDL can be esterified by the apoA-I, the major apoprotein of HDL LCAT enzyme, activated LCAT/A-I. Through this process, discoidal HDL is sequentially transformed into spherical HDL_3 and then to HDL_2. By accepting free cholesterol from peripheral cells, HDL mediates the reverse pathway of cholesterol transport. After the cholesterol is esterified, the HDL delivers the cholesterol esters either directly to the liver or to VLDL, IDL, or LDL particles, before these lipoproteins are transported and catabolized by the liver.

III. CHD AND LIPOPROTEIN METABOLISM IN POSTMENOPAUSAL WOMEN

Premenopausal women have a lower incidence of CHD than age-matched men, but this advantage declines greatly after menopause.[23] Natural menopause without estrogen replacement therapy is associated with a slight increase in total and LDL cholesterol, usually accompanied by a small decrease in HDL cholesterol levels. These changes in serum lipoprotein levels appear to result, at least in part, from a decrease in the fractional catabolic rate for LDL apoB, which is more pronounced in hypercholesterolemic women.[24] In postmenopausal women, LDL also appears to have more cholesterol per particle than does LDL in males. The net effect of these changes is that a postmenopausal woman's risk of CHD is increased more than for men of the same age group.

Estrogen replacement therapy raises serum levels of HDL cholesterol by up to 15% and lowers LDL cholesterol levels by approximately 15%, thereby reversing the changes that begin with menopause. Thus, the unfavorable effects of menopause on lipoprotein levels can be prevented by estrogen replacement therapy.[25] Estrogen therapy also increases serum triglycerides, with significant elevations observed in women with preexisting hypertriglyceridemia.[26] Data from uncontrolled clinical trials predict that postmenopausal women given estrogen replacement will lower their risk of CHD by approximately 50% compared to women who did not receive estrogen.[27] Although the protective effect of estrogen appears to be mediated through an increase in HDL cholesterol levels and, to a lesser extent, a decrease in LDL cholesterol,[28] evidence exists that part of the decreased risk is due to protective changes in the coronary arterial wall. Pending the results of a large prospective multicenter study, it is unknown whether these effects on CHD risks observed for postmenopausal estrogen users can be generalized to this population. Moreover, unopposed estrogen replacement has been associated with an increased risk of endometrial cancer and possibly breast cancer.[29] It is unknown whether or not concomitant progestational treatment offsets these increased potential risks and whether or not it decreases the apparent cardioprotective effects of estrogens.

Until well-controlled clinical trial data are available to determine whether the risk/benefit relationship favors the use of estrogen in postmenopausal women, estrogen replacement cannot be unequivocally recommended for the reduction of CHD risk, and treatment should be individualized. Elderly women who require antihyperlipidemic drug therapy and who have undergone a hysterectomy may be candidates for estrogen replacement therapy as long as they are appropriately apprised of the risk/benefit assessment and have appropriate followup for safety and efficacy endpoints. For postmenopausal women with an intact uterus, co-administration of estrogen and a progestin, which probably minimizes the risk of endometrial cancer, may be considered. However, as shown in Table 15.2, androgenic progestins generally have effects on lipoproteins that are opposite to those of estrogens; thus, co-administration with a progestin, depending upon its androgenicity, may neutralize or attenuate the apparent cardioprotective effect of estrogen alone.[30] As with unopposed estrogen, well-controlled trials of estrogen/progestin combination therapies are needed before this approach is adopted for the treatment of postmenopausal lipoprotein abnormalities, but should be considered judiciously for use particularly in women at high CHD risk. There are no data available on these issues of estrogen replacement therapy in women who underwent natural menopause and present with hyperlipidemia 10 or more years later.

IV. ANTIHYPERLIPIDEMIC THERAPY IN THE ELDERLY

The three major drug classes for the current treatment of lipid abnormalities include the bile acid sequestrants, nicotinic acid, and HMG CoA reductase inhibitors. In addition, two other classes of drugs, fibric acid derivatives and probucol, may be used for hyperlipidemias. Table 15.3 lists the currently available agents, their usual daily doses, and the approximate

TABLE 15.2.
Effects of Estrogen and Progestins on Serum Lipoproteins

Lipid	Estrogen effect	Progestin effect
HDL	Increases	Decreases
Triglyceride	Increases	Decreases
VLDL	Increases	Decreases
LDL	Decreases	Increases

effect of each agent on serum lipoproteins. In selecting antihyperlipidemic treatment for elderly patients, it is important to consider age-related alterations in drug metabolism and elimination, coexisting diseases and conditions, concomitant medication,[31] apparent physiological age, and the presence or absence of overt CHD. Because of these considerations the approach to antihyperlipidemic therapy may be different for older vs. younger individuals.

TABLE 15.3.
Antihyperlipidemic Drugs: Daily Doses and Effects on Serum Lipoproteins

Drugs	Class	Usual dose/day	LDL effect	HDL effect	Triglycerides effect
Cholestyramine	Bile acid sequestrants	4–16 g	↓10–30%	↑3–5%	May increase
Cholestipol	Bile acid sequestrants	5–20 g	↓10–30%	↑3–5%	May increase
Niacin	Nicotinic acid	1–3 g	↓10–25%	↑10–35%	↓10–50%
Sustained-release niacin	Nicotinic acid	1–2 g	↓10–25%	↑10–35%	↓10–50%
HMG CoA reductase inhibitors	Lovastatin	20–80 mg	↓20–40%	↑6–10%	↓7–12%
	Simvastatin	5–40 mg	↓24–40%	↑7–12%	↓10–19%
	Pravastatin	10–40 mg	↓22–34%	↑7–12%	↓15–24%
	Fluvastatin	20–80 mg	↓22–34%	↑Small	↓Small
Fibric acids	Clofibrate	2 g	↓10–15%	↑10–15%	↓20–50%
	Gemfibrozil	1200 mg	↓10–15%	↑10–15%	↓20–50%
	Fenofibrate	300 mg	↓17–29%	↑0–40%	↓38–57%
Probucol		0.5–1 g	↓5–15%	↓20–30%	No significant effect

Note: These values represent ranges of changes from baseline of lipoprotein for a variety of Frederickson classification II–IV, although the majority are for class II patients. The actual change for a given patient will depend on their classification and individual response.

A. BILE ACID SEQUESTRANTS

Bile acid sequestrants, including cholestyramine and colestipol, have been shown to lower serum LDL cholesterol and reduce CHD.[32] These agents lower LDL cholesterol indirectly by binding bile cholesterol in the gastrointestinal tract, thus preventing its reabsorption into the enterohepatic circulation. This action stimulates the conversion of cholesterol into bile acid,[22] which results in a depletion of intrahepatic cholesterol. The lower levels of intrahepatic cholesterol stimulate the production of cholesterol via an increase in the synthesis of LDL receptors.[21] Because older individuals may have increased hepatic levels of cholesterol, this class of drugs would appear to be appropriate for the elderly hyperlipidemic population.

However, elderly patients also may have increased hepatic and serum triglycerides, and bile acid sequestrants may exacerbate the hypertriglyceridemia.[33]

Bile acid sequestrants are generally considered first-line antihyperlipidemic therapy, especially for younger patients, because these agents are not systemically absorbed and chronic administration is not thought to be associated with significant toxicity. The disadvantages of bile acid sequestrants include inconvenience of administration and frequent gastrointestinal complaints. The gastrointestinal side effects, which appear to be dose related, include nausea, abdominal discomfort, indigestion, constipation, impaction, and aggravation of hemorrhoids, which are apt to be a greater problem in the elderly than in earlier years. Among participants in the Lipid Research Clinical Program, there were more colorectal tumors and oral/pharyngeal cancers during the 6-year followup period in cholestyramine-treated patients than in patients who received placebo; however, this difference was not statistically significant, and the intake of bile acid sequestrants was very variable among the individual male subjects in this study.[34] High doses of bile acid sequestrants can also cause steatorrhea and can inhibit absorption of fat-soluble vitamins, such as vitamin K, which can lead to hypoprothrombinemia and bleeding. They may also rarely cause esophageal obstruction, requiring endoscopy. Finally, these agents can inhibit absorption of several drugs, including digoxin, thiazide diuretics, warfarin, tetracycline, thyroxin, phenobarbital, and propranolol.[35,36] For this reason, patients should be instructed to take all concomitant medications at least 1 hr before or 4 hr after bile acid sequestrants. The overall long-term safety for bile acid sequestrants is excellent and low-dose, and carefully staggered regimens may be tailored for individual needs.

Antihyperlipidemic therapy with bile acid sequestrants may be complicated by poor nutritional status, multiple concomitant medications, chronic constipation, and decreased gastrointestinal transient time, all of which are relatively common in older individuals. On the other hand, since bile acid sequestrants are not absorbed, their use is not complicated by age-related changes in drug metabolism. If these agents are used in elderly patients, single doses of cholestyramine or colestipol should be limited to 8 or 10 g, respectively, given beginning in the evening with carefully written instructions. Administration of bile acid sequestrants should begin with low doses, followed by a slow upward dose titration in order to avoid or minimize gastrointestinal side effects. Administering divided smaller doses rather than a single daily dose also may reduce the incidence of gastrointestinal complaints; however, dosing should be limited to a twice-daily schedule to facilitate compliance while maintaining a favorable risk/benefit ratio. Elderly patients receiving bile acid sequestrants should be instructed to increase their intake of fluid and dietary fiber to minimize constipation. Use of a dietary fiber laxative, such as psyllium, can have the added benefits of increasing bowel motility, bowel regularity, and producing a small additional reduction in serum cholesterol.[37] For older individuals who require a relatively modest reduction in LDL cholesterol (<15%) and who do not have hypertriglyceridemia or other contraindications, a bile acid sequestrant, administered at low to moderate doses, appears to be a reasonable choice for first-line antihyperlipidemic therapy.

B. NICOTINIC ACID (NIACIN)

Niacin is another agent that is often selected as first-line antihyperlipidemic therapy because of its ability to lower cholesterol and decrease overall mortality.[24] Niacin has multiple effects on lipoprotein metabolism. It decreases the synthesis and release of VLDL.[15,16] As a result, LDL production is reduced because there is less precursor VLDL available as a substrate for LDL. Evidence also exists that niacin can increase lipoprotein lipase activity,[16] which may counterbalance the reduction in activity of this enzyme that is often seen in older individuals. Thus, niacin treatment decreases LDL cholesterol and triglycerides. Niacin can also lower Lipoprotein(a) by up to 30% and increase HDL cholesterol, although the mechanism of the latter effect is unknown.[38]

It is important to distinguish between the physiological requirement of niacin as a vitamin and its pharmacologic use as an antihyperlipidemic agent. The daily recommended dietary allowance for niacin as a vitamin is only approximately 15 mg, whereas niacin doses required to produce significant effects on lipoproteins generally range from 1000 to 6000 mg/d, administered in divided (usually three times daily) doses. At present, only two immediate-release forms of niacin, Niacor® and Nicolar®, are approved in the U.S. with indications for cholesterol lowering; both are available by prescription. All other marketed niacin formulations, which are available without a prescription for use as vitamin supplements, have not undergone the rigorous product and clinical testing and regulatory review required for marketing these products as antihyperlipidemic agents. Therefore, over-the-counter dosing of niacin, especially without medical supervision, is potentially hazardous.

Niacin has a different dose-response relationship for its effects on HDL cholesterol, LDL cholesterol, and triglycerides (Figure 15.3). Increases in HDL cholesterol tend to predominate at lower niacin doses (1000 mg/d), with maximum increases generally achieved at doses of 2000 mg/d. Reductions in LDL cholesterol are initially observed at doses ranging from 1500 to 2000 mg/d.[39] At doses above 2000 mg/d the dose-response curve begins to plateau, and increases beyond this dose level are associated with less added benefit and an increased frequency of adverse reactions, particularly with chronic dosing. The effect of niacin on serum triglycerides is initially observed at low doses and is fairly consistent over the recommended dose range.

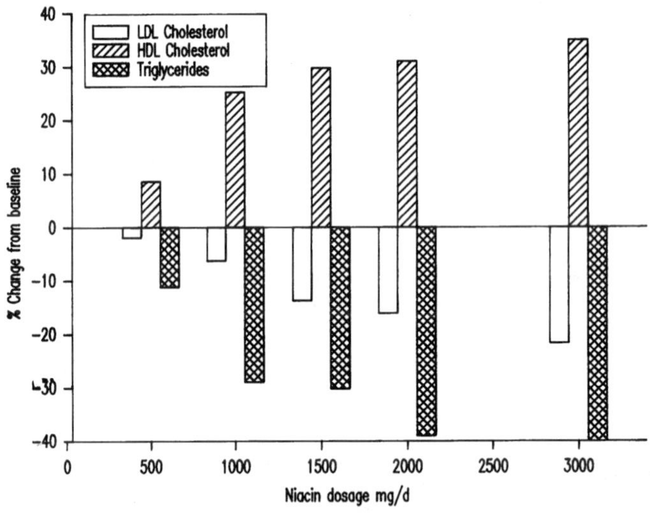

FIGURE 15.3. Effects of various doses of nicotinic acid on serum levels of LDL cholesterol, HDL cholesterol, and triglycerides. (Data adapted from McKenny, J. M., *JAMA*, 271, 672, 1994. With permission.)

With its multiple beneficial effects on lipoproteins, niacin would be an ideal antihyperlipidemic drug except that its use is associated with numerous adverse effects and it requires frequent dosing, which leads to reduced compliance. The most troubling side effect of niacin therapy is flushing, which occurs in almost 50% of patients, particularly on dosing initiation. Flushing can be minimized by initiating therapy with a relatively low dose (100 mg three times daily) followed by a slow upward dose titration at weekly or biweekly intervals; this approach allows the patient to develop a tolerance to the side effects of the medication. This symptom can also be reduced by administration of niacin with meals. Alternatively, since the flushing appears to be prostaglandin mediated, administration of an aspirin tablet (325 mg) approximately 30 to 60 min before each dose also may be effective, but in the elderly the actions of the concomitant aspirin must be carefully weighed and individualized.

Because niacin also has been shown to increase blood glucose, uric acid, and reactivate peptic ulcer disease, its use can exacerbate diabetes mellitus, gout, gastritis, and peptic ulcer disease, respectively. These diseases are common among older individuals. Significant hepatotoxicity also has been reported with niacin administration, but this is usually reversible if it is detected early and the drug is discontinued. For these reasons, it is necessary to monitor serum chemistry parameters (glucose, uric acid, liver function tests) in patients treated with niacin. This monitoring should be performed relatively frequently, especially during dose titration, because the effects of niacin on these parameters appear to be dose related. Niacin may also interact indirectly with antihypertensive medications (e.g., a direct vasodilator) to produce clinically significant hypotension. These vasodilatory effects may be helpful in some patients with occlusive peripheral arterial disease and in hypertensives where the niacin augmentation can be an added benefit.

In the future, the problem of significant flushing and frequent dosing may be alleviated by carefully formulated sustained-release niacin preparations, but at present no sustained-release preparations are specifically approved in the U.S. for cholesterol lowering. Ongoing clinical evaluation of these products indicates that lower doses of the sustained-release niacin formulations produce the same LDL-lowering effects as higher doses of the immediate-release formulations, but the sustained-release products appear to have a less pronounced effect on HDL cholesterol (2% increase, 1000-mg dose) than immediate-release niacin (25% increase, 1000-mg dose) for a given dose level.[39] Although flushing appears to be less common with sustained-released niacin, the incidence of hepatotoxicity is usually higher with sustained-release products. Whether this is due to constant niacin and metabolite blood levels, to absorption of waxy excipients present in many sustained-released preparations or to both is unknown. For both immediate- and sustained-release niacin, the frequency of hepatic toxicities appears to be dose related, with liver function abnormalities generally occurring at lower doses of the sustained-released formulations. In most cases, the hepatic abnormalities are reversible with discontinuation of therapy, but rare cases of fulminant hepatitis have been reported. At present, the relationship between hepatotoxicity and the various niacin preparations remains to be definitively established, and the incidence of hepatic abnormalities is yet to be determined for each of the sustained-release formulations undergoing evaluation. Until these data have been obtained, it is prudent to favor the use of the immediate-release niacin formulations, especially in the elderly. Moreover, the selection of one of the niacin products available by prescription and approved as a lipid-lowering agent will ensure consistency in product quality and bioequivalence, but at a higher cost than the nonprescription, unapproved preparations.

In prescribing any medication for older patients, the clinician also must consider the pharmacokinetics of the agent. Plain nicotinic acid is readily absorbed and then metabolized to two major metabolites — nicotinamide adenine dinucleotide and nicotinuric acid. Approximately 90% of an oral dose is eliminated by the kidney in the form of unchanged nicotinic acid or nicotinuric acid. The predominantly renal elimination pathway of nicotinic acid and its metabolites must be considered when administering niacin to elderly patients with decreased renal function. Unfortunately, no clinical trials have yet been reported demonstrating the use of niacin in elderly patients with renal insufficiency. Finally, there is some evidence that the metabolism of the immediate-release and sustained-release products may differ. Although the metabolic end products are similar, the proportions of the two metabolites may be different for the different formulations.[40] This difference may account, at least in part, for the differences between the immediate- and sustained-release niacin preparations in terms of potency and incidence of adverse effects.

C. HMG CoA REDUCTASE INHIBITORS

HMG CoA reductase inhibitors prevent the production of cholesterol by blocking the rate-limiting step in cholesterol synthesis without causing a complete inhibition of cholesterol formation. The resulting decrease in intracellular cholesterol content stimulates the synthesis of LDL receptors,[18] which promote the clearance of LDL cholesterol. Because serum LDL cholesterol levels may be elevated in older individuals due to age-related downregulation of LDL receptors, HMG CoA reductase inhibitors would seem to be particularly useful for this patient population. Because HMG CoA reductase inhibitors also reduce VLDL via stimulation of hepatic LDL receptor-mediated clearance of VLDL remnants, these agents generally have a modest favorable effect on serum triglyceride levels. Finally, HMG CoA reductase inhibitors may cause small increases (5 to 10%) in HDL cholesterol, but in studies carried out thus far they have not diminished serum Lipoprotein(a) levels.

There are four HMG CoA reductase inhibitors marketed in the U.S. for lipid lowering: lovastatin, simvastatin, pravastatin, and fluvastatin. These agents appear to have similar efficacy, but different potencies with respect to reducing LDL cholesterol. As shown in Figure 15.4, the LDL cholesterol-lowering effect of these agents predominantly occurs at low to moderate doses. Higher doses generally only produce modest incremental LDL cholesterol reductions and are associated with an increased incidence of adverse reactions.

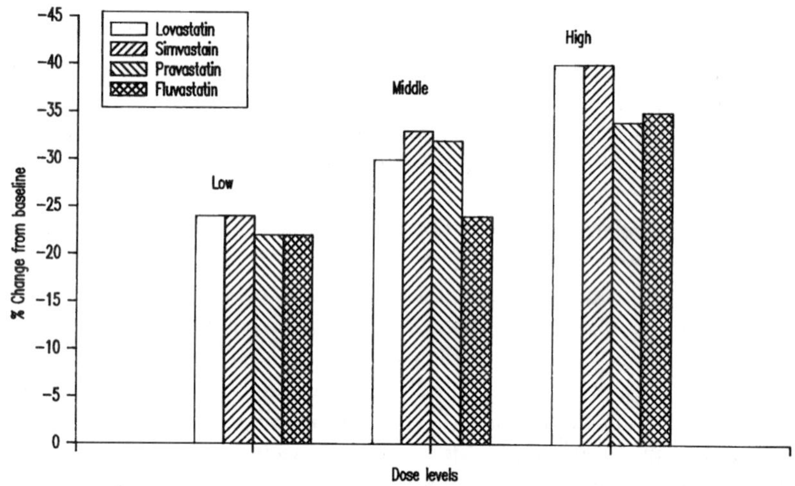

FIGURE 15.4. Effects of low, middle, and high doses of four HMG CoA reductase inhibitors on LDL cholesterol. (Data adapted from the package inserts.)

1. Lovastatin

Lovastatin, which was approved in 1987 as a lipid-lowering agent, was the first HMG CoA reductase inhibitor marketed in the U.S. This agent has enjoyed widespread use because of its demonstrated efficacy and favorable safety profile. Lovastatin is a lipophilic prodrug that is metabolized by the liver to its active metabolites, b-hydroxyacid and the 6-hydroxy derivatives. After oral administration, lovastatin is extracted almost completely during its first pass through the liver, with less than 5% of the parent drug reaching the systemic circulation. It is metabolized by the cytochrome P450 hepatic enzyme system, and the majority of the metabolites are excreted via the intestine, with less than 10% eliminated by the kidneys. The absorption of lovastatin is improved with food, and since the efficacy of once-daily dosing with lovastatin is only slightly less than that seen with twice-daily dosing,[41] the total daily dose is generally administered with the evening meal.

2. Simvastatin

Simvastatin, a congener of lovastatin and the second HMG CoA reductase approved in the U.S., is lipophilic and an inactive prodrug. Simvastatin is twice as potent as lovastatin. Clinical trials have demonstrated that simvastatin is effective and well tolerated in older patients.[42,43]

3. Pravastatin

Pravastatin, which was recently approved in the U.S., differs from lovastatin and simvastatin in that it is an active drug, not a prodrug, and that it is hydrophilic. Because of its hydrophilicity, pravastatin may not readily cross cell membranes and may require an active transport mechanism to be taken up by hepatocytes. However, pravastatin does undergo extensive first-pass metabolism, with approximately 70% of the parent drug eliminated during its initial pass through the liver. Although the bioavailability is further reduced when the drug is taken with food, it does not result in significant pharmacodynamic differences, but pravastatin is generally prescribed for bedtime administration. Pravastatin has also been shown to have similar efficacy in elderly and younger patients, and it is well tolerated by older individuals.[44]

4. Fluvastatin

Fluvastatin, which was approved in the U.S. in 1994, also has significant first-pass clearance and very limited systemic availability. It is extensively metabolized and then excreted in the bile. The bioavailability of fluvastatin is further reduced when it is taken with food; however, a comparison of the bioavailability of fluvastatin administered with either the evening meal or at bedtime revealed no significant difference.[45]

5. Pharmacokinetic Considerations with HMG CoA Reductase Inhibitors

Lovastatin, simvastatin, and fluvastatin are extensively metabolized by the liver; thus, age-related alterations in the pharmacokinetics of these agents are not expected to be a major concern because the hepatic capacity to metabolize these drugs does not appear to diminish significantly as individuals age.[31] However, the cytochrome P450 system, which is responsible for the metabolism of these and other drugs, can be affected by aging as well as the administration of specific inhibitors of this system.[31] Although these changes may be clinically insignificant when HMG CoA reductase inhibitors are administered alone, co-administration with agents that inhibit cytochrome P450 enzymes (e.g., cyclosporine, erythromycin) may increase the frequency and severity of adverse reactions.[46] This mechanism has been proposed to explain the increased incidence of myopathy that is observed when lovastatin is administered with inhibitors of the cytochrome P450 system.

In contrast to the other three HMG CoA reductase inhibitors, approximately 50% of a pravastatin dose is excreted renally. Pharmacokinetic clinical trials have demonstrated diminished renal clearance of the drug in the elderly as compared with younger individuals.[47] Therefore, lower pravastatin doses are recommended for elderly patients (10 to 20 mg) as compared with the maximum 40-mg dose utilized for middle-aged and younger patients, although, with compromised renal function, there is a compensatory increase in the hepatic metabolism and biliary excretion of pravastatin.

6. Safety of HMG CoA Reductase Inhibitors

In addition to effectively lowering LDL cholesterol, HMG CoA reductase inhibitors are generally well tolerated. Reported adverse effects include headache, diarrhea, constipation, flatulence, and abdominal pain. Well-controlled trials have demonstrated that the frequencies of these side effects are generally comparable in patients treated with HMG CoA reductase inhibitors (at their lowest doses) and placebo-treated patients. Although lovastatin administration may be associated with insomnia, which is a common problem in older patients, the Expanded Clinical Evaluation of Lovastatin (EXCEL) trial demonstrated that the incidence of insomnia was similar to that observed with placebo treatment.[48] Lovastatin can be administered in the morning to patients who complain of insomnia, but the drug has been shown to be much more effective when administered in the evening.

HMG CoA reductase inhibitors can also cause liver function abnormalities, with abnormal liver function test results observed in approximately 2% of patients. The EXCEL trial results suggest that elevations in liver function parameters may be dose related, with significant serum transaminase increases (>3 times the upper limits of normal) noted for 0.1% of patients who received either placebo or 20 mg/d of lovastatin, 0.9% of patients who received 40 mg/d, and 1.5% of those administered 80 mg/d.[48] These elevations generally occur after 3 to 12 months of therapy. Therefore, patients receiving these agents should have liver function tests performed prior to the initiation of therapy, every 6 weeks during the first 3 months of treatment, every 8 weeks during months 4 through 12, and every 6 months thereafter. HMG CoA reductase inhibitor treatment should be discontinued, the dose decreased, or another HMG CoA reductase inhibitor tried for patients who demonstrate significant increases in serum transaminase levels. In contrast to fibric acids and other lipid-lowering agents, the HMG CoA reductase inhibitors do not increase lithogenicity of the bile, and they may even decrease calculus formation which is a common problem in the elderly.

Another area of concern with the use of HMG CoA reductase inhibitors is their potential for causing increases in creatine kinase and myopathies, with the development of rhabdomyolysis. These adverse effects have been reported in rare cases when HMG CoA reductase inhibitors are administered alone (although it has not been reported with fluvastatin at the time of its approval), and more commonly when they are co-administered with cyclosporine, gemfibrozil, nicotinic acid (>1000 mg/d), or erythromycin. In general, these drugs should not be used with the HMG CoA reductase inhibitors without very careful consideration of the risks and benefits, especially for the elderly patient. Moreover, creatine kinase should be evaluated for patients who complain of muscle pain or weakness and probably routinely checked even though not generally required. The clinician should also bear in mind that sporadic elevations of creatine kinase that are unrelated to drug therapy are common in individuals, especially after exercise and that a number of patients will show a nonclinically significant increase in creatine kinase on HMG CoA reductase therapy. Thus, modest increases in creatine kinase (<3 times the upper limits of normal) may not require the discontinuation of therapy, but may indicate the need for periodic monitoring. If the creatine kinase is greater than three times the upper limits of normal the drug should be discontinued and the creatine kinase followed regardless of symptoms.

When the HMG CoA reductase inhibitors were first investigated, there was a suggestion that their use was associated with an increased incidence of cataracts. Although this finding has not been confirmed in well-controlled clinical trials, it may be prudent to perform baseline and yearly ophthalmologic examinations of elderly patients, as they are more prone than younger individuals to develop cataracts.

At present, further investigations are underway of HMG CoA reductase inhibitor therapy in elderly hyperlipidemic patients. This class of drug has the potential to be the first-line therapy in older patients as these agents have beneficial effects on lipoproteins and excellent safety profiles and ease of administration and tolerability. In addition, HMG CoA reductase inhibitors do not increase the incidence of cholelithiasis. Although the safety profile of these agents with chronic use remains to be determined, any toxicities that may be associated with long-term use may be less of an issue for the older patient, particularly in patients with CHD.

D. FIBRIC ACID DERIVATIVES

The fibric acid derivatives have their major lipid-lowering effect on triglycerides usually due to increases in serum triglyceride removal. This effect may be mediated by increases in LPL activity and, to a lesser extent, inhibition of VLDL synthesis. However, the mechanism of action appears to vary among drugs in this class. Fibric acid derivatives also cause a partial inhibition of cholesterol and bile acid synthesis and promote the secretion of cholesterol into bile.[18] Use of this class of hyperlipidemic agent appears to be a rational choice for elderly patients, since the fibric acid derivatives may counter age-related decreases in LPL activity. In addition, these drugs lower serum VLDL levels by 50 to 75% and increase HDL cholesterol by 10 to 15%, depending on the triglyceride levels. However, the fibric acid derivatives have variable effects on LDL cholesterol, generally producing only modest reductions (5 to 10%) or slight increases in serum levels of this lipoprotein. Thus, fibric acid derivatives are primarily used for the prevention of pancreatitis in patients with hypertriglyceridemia secondary to decrease in LPL activity and for primary prevention of CHD in patients with combined hyperlipidemias (i.e., elevated triglycerides and LDL cholesterol and low HDL cholesterol).

In the U.S., clofibrate, gemfibrozil, and fenofibrate are the fibric acid derivatives approved for antihyperlipidemic therapy. The use of clofibrate, which has been shown to reduce cardiovascular events, has decreased since a World Health Organization study found an increased incidence of all-cause mortality among patients treated with this agent.[49] Reevaluation of these data suggest that such may not be the case, and the study was designed to treat hypercholesterolemic patients at fixed doses and exclude patients with high triglycerides. Because of these potential risks, clofibrate is rarely used in the U.S. today. Gemfibrozil, the most commonly used fibric acid derivative, is metabolized by oxidation followed by glucuronide conjugation, with the glucuronidated metabolites excreted in the urine. In the Helsinki Heart Study, gemfibrozil treatment reduced cardiovascular morbidity and mortality in patients being treated for primary prevention with elevated serum cholesterol and triglycerides, and low HDL cholesterol levels.[50] However, preliminary analysis of post-trial followup results suggested that gemfibrozil may increase overall mortality, although no explanation has been identified and it remains an open question. Fenofibrate, a recently approved fibric acid derivative, has been reported to have an enhanced LDL-lowering effect as compared with other agents of this class and is more potent than clofibrate or gemfibrozil.[51]

The fibric acid derivatives are generally well tolerated and have a long safety record. The most frequent adverse effects are gastrointestinal complaints — nausea, abdominal pain, and diarrhea — which occur in 3 to 5% of treated patients. Less common adverse effects include rash, eosinophilia, muscle tenderness, anemia, leukopenia, elevated liver function tests, and rare cases of myositis. The myopathy is more frequently reported when gemfibrozil is given in combination with other lipid-lowering agents. Fibric acid derivatives can also increase bile lithogenicity, leading to an increased incidence or aggravation of cholelithiasis.[18] This can be especially problematic in the elderly, since cholecystectomies are associated with significant morbidity and mortality in this group of patients. It should also be noted that fibric acid derivatives can potentiate the effects of warfarin and may require dose adjustment of the warfarin, which is commonly administered to older patients.

E. PROBUCOL

Probucol is approved in the U.S. for the treatment of hypercholesterolemia. Although this agent lowers LDL cholesterol by about 15%, the main interest in probucol is its potential use for CHD treatment because of its ability to inhibit the oxidation and tissue disposition of LDL cholesterol.[52] However, as no clinical data are available to support the hypothesis that inhibition of LDL cholesterol oxidation can reduce the incidence of CHD, well-controlled clinical trials are needed to examine the effect of probucol on CHD. It is also important to note that probucol lowers HDL cholesterol, an effect which is worrisome and not beneficial with respect to treating CHD. Probucol also has been reported to cause regression of xanthomas in patients with severe hypercholesterolemia.

Probucol is generally well tolerated, but its use can be associated with a variety of mild adverse effects that tend to disappear with continued therapy. The most commonly reported side effects include abdominal discomfort, diarrhea, nausea, and headache. Probucol can also prolong the QT interval, and rare serious ventricular arrhythmias have been reported. This agent should not be administered to patients with ventricular irritability, prolonged QT intervals, or those taking drugs that prolong the QT interval. In addition, electrocardiographic monitoring should be performed before and periodically during probucol treatment. Because probucol is a lipophilic compound, it accumulates in adipose tissue, from which it is slowly eliminated. This deposition in adipose tissue may be clinically important in elderly patients who have an increase in the ratio of fat to lean body mass. At present, use of probucol should be restricted to patients who are unable to tolerate or have failed to respond to other cholesterol-lowering drugs.

F. COMBINATION ANTIHYPERLIPIDEMIC THERAPY

Because the Adult Treatment Panel II guidelines recommend more aggressive treatment for the secondary prevention of CHD, the use of combination antihyperlipidemic therapy can be expected to become increasingly useful and more common. To achieve the target therapeutic goals displayed in Table 15.1, serum LDL cholesterol levels often must be reduced by 50% or more. This degree of lipid lowering can rarely be achieved with single-agent therapy. In contrast, by combining agents with different mechanisms of action, additive or synergistic effects on serum lipids may be achieved to increase efficacy (Table 15.4), to increase safety, and to decrease cost. The most useful combination regimens include a bile acid sequestrant and a HMG CoA reductase inhibitor or nicotinic acid. These regimens are effective because bile acid sequestrants stimulate hepatic cholesterol synthesis, which can be blocked or inhibited by the HMG CoA reductase inhibitor. Niacin can inhibit the release of VLDL cholesterol and enhance its degradation. Moreover, since bile acid sequestrants are not absorbed, they have limited systemic toxicity and a low potential for drug-drug interactions. Bile acid sequestrants or niacin also can be administered in combination with fibric acid derivatives to treat combined hyperlipidemias; however, the bile acid sequestrants tend to antagonize the triglyceride-lowering effects of the fibric acid derivatives.

TABLE 15.4.
LDL Reduction Associated with Combination Therapies[53]

Combination with bile acid sequestrant	Percent reduction in LDL cholesterol
HMG CoA reductase inhibitors	52–54%
Nicotinic acid	32–55%
Fenofibrate	36–41%

From Illingworth, R. D., *Clin. Chem.*, 34, B123, 1988. With permission.

Combination regimens involving HMG CoA reductase inhibitors and either nicotinic acid or fibric acid derivatives also have been shown to lower LDL cholesterol by approximately 50%. Unfortunately, these regimens can produce increased toxicity, mainly rhabdomyolysis associated with acute renal failure, particularly in the case of gemfibrozil. For this reason, such combinations are considered to have a poor risk/benefit ratio and generally cannot be recommended. A combination regimen consisting of an HMG CoA reductase inhibitor and nicotinic acid, at a low dose (<1000 mg) that is effective for increasing HDL cholesterol, appears less likely to produce myopathy, and has a reasonable safety profile.

Another advantage of combination therapy is that lower doses of the two agents used in combination may produce reductions in LDL cholesterol that are greater than those possible with high doses of the individual agents. A combination regimen that includes low doses of lovastatin and a bile acid sequestrant rather than a single high dose of lovastatin may be a more reasonable and safe treatment approach.

The use of combination antihyperlipidemic therapy in the elderly requires careful consideration of the primary goal in treating the lipoprotein abnormality as well as the type and number of concomitant medications used by the patient. The frequency and severity of adverse reactions and the potential for drug-drug interactions increase significantly with each new drug added to an older person's treatment regimen.[31] Most importantly, their alertness and need to take these combination medications requires patient education and written instructions.

V. STRATEGY FOR TREATING THE ELDERLY HYPERLIPIDEMIC PATIENT

The Adult Treatment Panel II established the framework for the evaluation of patients with elevated serum cholesterol and the target treatment goals for young, middle-aged, and elderly adults. In all these patient groups, it is important to remember that a comprehensive approach to treatment must attempt to correct the modifiable cardiovascular risk factors, such as smoking, hypertension, high-fat diet, exercise, and obesity. Although the impact of these risk factors on CHD may decrease with age, many of these risk factors are very common in elderly patients, and their correction or treatment can benefit this population.[54] Therefore, the initial treatment for elevated LDL cholesterol is the implementation of the American Heart Association Step I Diet, low fat (<30% of calories from total fat and <10% from saturated fat), and a low dietary cholesterol (<300 mg/d) program calorically designed to achieve and maintain ideal body weight. This diet should offer no risk to older individuals if they maintain a balanced diet and if their nutritional needs are being met with vitamin and mineral supplements. Patients should be maintained on this diet for at least 6 weeks before lipid level evaluations are performed. Two serum lipid determinations, separated by a 1- to 2-week interval, are required to adequately assess the effects of the diet. Patients treated for primary prevention of CHD may be maintained on the diet for a longer period of time before considering drug therapy, whereas patients being treated for secondary prevention may require earlier drug treatment, depending on their overall cardiovascular risk and attitude toward treatment.

Figure 15.5 outlines a useful approach to antihyperlipidemic drug therapy in the elderly. The strategy is designed to optimize benefits while minimizing the risk and, hopefully, the costs of treatment for patients who require modest, moderate, or marked LDL cholesterol reduction.

A. LDL CHOLESTEROL TARGET REDUCTION OF <15%

Any of the hyperlipidemic agents are likely to be effective for elderly patients who require a modest (<15%) reduction in serum LDL cholesterol; thus, patient-specific factors should guide therapy selection. For example, a bile acid sequestrant would be a reasonable choice for patients with serum triglyceride levels below 200 mg/dL, especially if they are not receiving multiple concomitant medications and/or do not have significant gastrointestinal problems. Alternatively, a low dose of an HMG CoA reductase inhibitor may improve compliance in this group of patients, because this low-dose regimen is easily taken, well tolerated, and associated with minimal toxicity. For patients with significant elevated serum triglycerides (>400 mg/dL) and low HDL cholesterol (<35 mg/dL), a fibric acid derivative would be a good candidate for initial therapy, especially for primary CHD prevention. Finally, niacin should be considered for elderly patients with elevated Lipoprotein(a) and who have significant CHD.

B. LDL CHOLESTEROL TARGET REDUCTION OF 15 TO 25%

Therapy with a low (and then increasing to a moderate dose, if required) dose of an HMG CoA reductase inhibitor should be considered for older patients who require a 15 to 25% reduction in LDL cholesterol and normal triglycerides. If a moderate dose of an HMG CoA reductase inhibitors are unable to achieve the desired LDL decreases, the addition of a bile

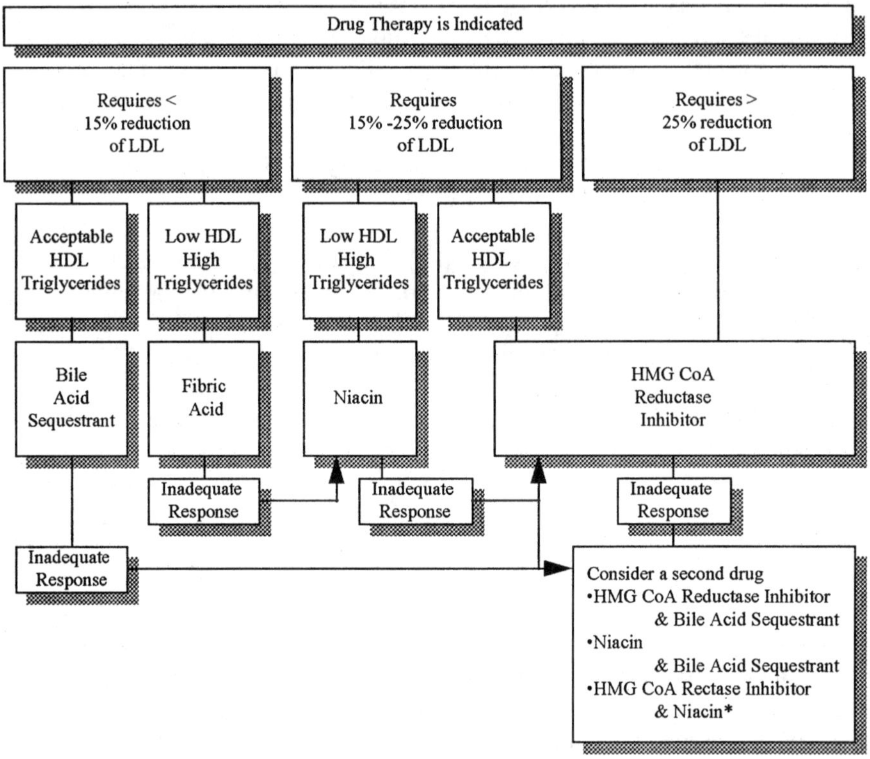

FIGURE 15.5. Treatment approach for achieving modest (15%), moderate (15 to 25%), and marked (>25%) reductions in LDL cholesterol in elderly hyperlipidemic patients. *Possible increased risk of myopathy and hepatitis.

acid sequestrant at a low dose may demonstrate a more favorable risk/benefit ratio, rather than increasing the HMG CoA reductase to its maximum dose, especially for older patients.

For patients with moderate elevations in LDL cholesterol, low HDL cholesterol, and elevated triglycerides, niacin treatment should be initially tried to achieve the LDL cholesterol goals. This will usually require a minimum dose of 2000 mg of the immediate-release form of niacin. If this does not achieve the desired goal and the patient tolerates this dose, a bile acid sequestrant at a low dose can be added to the regimen. Initiating gemfibrozil or niacin first may prevent the increase in triglycerides that can be associated with bile acid sequestrant therapy. An alternative approach would be to decrease the niacin to less than 1000 mg/d, which should maintain the increase in HDL cholesterol and the reduction of triglycerides, and then add an HMG CoA reductase inhibitor to reduce the LDL cholesterol. The initial choice of drug is individualized, depending upon the patient's condition, risk, tolerance to prior therapies, and attitude.

C. LDL CHOLESTEROL TARGET REDUCTION OF >25%

For elderly patients who require a substantial reduction in LDL cholesterol (>25%), combination therapy will most likely be needed. The primary LDL-lowering component of this regimen will likely require an HMG CoA reductase inhibitor. The patient should be started at a low dose to determine initial response. At this time, one can determine if a moderate dose of a HMG CoA reductase inhibitor will achieve the desired results. If not, it may be more reasonable based upon the risk/benefit ratio to add a second drug. For patients with normal HDL and triglycerides, a low dose of a bile acid sequestrant could be added to the combination. For patients with low HDL or high Lipoprotein(a), niacin at less than 1000 mg in three divided doses would be a better choice. For patients who continue to need further

LDL reduction, their HMG CoA reductase can be increased from a moderate to high dose, or a third drug may need to be considered.

VI. CONCLUSION

The second report of the expert panel on detection, evaluation, and treatment of high blood cholesterol in adults applies to all adults, not just those individuals under the age of 65. But like all recommendations, these guidelines are not treatment directions and they need to be individualized for a given patient. The elderly have a number of common issues to address with regard to drug therapy. These include the patient's overall attitude, projected health and life expectancy, the time required to achieve primary and secondary prevention of CHD through LDL cholesterol lowering, and the potential for altered, age-related changes in the lipoprotein and drug metabolism. In addition, the realization that the elderly are already consuming a significant number of drugs, which increases their risk of drug interactions and adverse experiences, requires careful assessment of their drug regimen and communication with their prescribing physician. All of these factors may change the risk/benefit ratio of treating the elderly, and one needs to consider the patients' quality of life in the exchange for assessed potential benefit on their morbidity and mortality. Given the number of procedures (angioplasty, coronary artery bypass, and noninvasive testing for followup) and cost of these "plumbing" measures, an attempt to identify and contain or reverse any abnormal lipid metabolic process is worth the effort for overall quality of life and productivity for patients and their families, depending on the individual circumstances.

REFERENCES

1. **Leaf, A.,** The aging process: lessons from observations in man, *Nutr. Rev.*, 46, 40, 1988.
2. **Anonymous,** Aging america. They've got to eat, so let them work, *The Economist*, 21, 312, 1989.
3. **Wenger, N. K., O'Rourke, R. A., and Marcus, F. I.,** The care of elderly patients with cardiovascular disease, *Ann. Intern. Med.*, 109, 425, 1988.
4. **Brown, G., Albers, J. J., Fisher, L. D., Schaefer, S. M., Lin, J. T., Kaplan, C., Zhao, X. Q., Bisson, B. D., Fitzpatrick, V. F., and Dodge, H. T.,** Regression of coronary artery disease as a result of intensive lipid-lowering therapy in men with high level of apolipoprotein B, *N. Engl. J. Med.*, 323, 12890, 1990.
5. The cholesterol facts: a summary of the evidence relating dietary fats, serum cholesterol, and coronary heart disease, *Circulation*, 81, 1721, 1990.
6. Second report of the expert panel on detection, evaluation, and treatment of high blood cholesterol in adults (adult treatment panel II), *NIH*, 93–3095, 1993.
7. **Ross, R. and Glomset, J. A.,** The pathogenesis of atherosclerosis (second of two parts), *N. Engl. J. Med.*, 295, 420, 1976.
8. **Jacobsen, S. J., Freedman, D. S., Hoffmann, R. G., Gruchow, H. W., Anderson, A. J., and Barboriak, J. J.,** Cholesterol and coronary artery disease: age as an effect modifier, *J. Clin. Epidemiol.*, 45, 1053, 1992.
9. **Castelli, W. P., Wilson, W. F., Levy, D., and Anderson, K.,** Cardiovascular risk factors in the elderly, *Am. J. Cardiol.*, 63, 12H, 1989.
10. **Kannel, W. B. and Gordon, T.,** Evaluation of cardiovascular risk in the elderly: the Framingham study, *Bull. N.Y. Acad. Med.*, 54, 573, 1978.
11. **Malenka, D. J. and Baron, J. A.,** Cholesterol and coronary heart disease: the importance of patient-specific attributable risks, *Arch. Intern. Med.*, vol. 148, 2247–2252, 1988.
12. **Steinberg, D., Parthasarathy, S., Carew, T. E., Khoo, J. C., and Witztum, J. L.,** Beyond cholesterol: modifications of low-density lipoproteins that increase its atherogenicity, *N. Engl. J. Med.*, 320, 915, 1989.
13. **Scanu, A. M. and Fless, G. M.,** Lipoprotein (a): heterogeneity and biological relevance, *J. Clin. Invest.*, 85, 1709, 1990.
14. **Capuzzi, D. M.,** Disorders of lipoprotein metabolism genetics and metabolism, in *Internal Medicine for Dentistry*, 2nd ed., Kaye, D. and Ross, L. F., Eds., C. V. Mosby, St. Louis, 1989, 1133–1153.
15. **Grundy, S. M., Mok, H. Y. I., Zech, L., and Berman, M.,** Influence of nicotinic acid on metabolism of cholesterol and triglycerides in man, *J. Lipid Res.*, 22, 24, 1981.

16. **Gey, K. F. and Carlson, L. A.,** *Metabolic effects of nicotinic acid and its derivatives*, Hans Huber Publishers, Bern, 1971.
17. **Weintraub, M. S., Eisenberg, S., and Breslow, J. L.,** Dietary fat clearance in normal subjects is regulated by genetic variation in apolipoprotein E, *J. Clin. Invest.*, 80, 1571, 1987.
18. **Grundy, S. M. and Vega, G. L.,** Fibric acids: effects on lipids and lipoprotein metabolism, *Am. J. Med.*, 83, 9, 1987.
19. **Grundy, S. M., Vega, G. L., and Bilheimer, D. W.,** Kinetic mechanisms determining variability in low density lipoprotein levels and rise with age, *Arteriosclerosis*, 5, 623, 1985.
20. **Miller, N. E.,** Why does plasma low density lipoprotein concentration in adults increase with age?, *Lancet*, 1, 263, 1984.
21. **Brown, M. S. and Goldstein, J. L.,** A receptor-mediated pathway for cholesterol homeostasis, *Science*, 232, 34, 1986.
22. **Grundy, S. M., Ahrens, E. H., and Salen, G.,** Interruption of the enterohepatic circulation of bile acids in man: comparative effects of cholestyramine and ileal exclusion on cholesterol metabolism, *J. Lab. Clin. Med.*, 78, 94, 1971.
23. **Kannel, W. B.,** Metabolic risk factors for coronary heart disease in women: perspective from the Framingham Study, *Am. Heart J.*, 114, 413, 1987.
24. **Arca, M., Vega, G. L., and Grundy, S. M.,** Hypercholesterolemia in postmenopausal women: metabolic defects and response to low-dose lovastatin, *JAMA*, 271, 453, 1994.
25. **Matthews, K. A., Meilahn, E., Kuller, L. H., Kelsey, S. F., Caggiula, A. W., and Wing, R. R.,** Menopause and risk factors for coronary heart disease, *N. Engl. J. Med.*, 321, 641, 1989.
26. **Granfone, A., Campos, H., McNamara, J. R., Schaefer, M. M., Lamon-Fava, S., Ordovas, J. M., and Schaefer, E. J.,** Effects of estrogen replacement on plasma lipoproteins and apolipoproteins in postmenopausal, dyslipidemic women, *Metabolism*, 41, 1193, 1992.
27. NIH consensus development panel on triglyceride, high-density lipoprotein, and coronary heart disease, *JAMA*, 269, 505, 1993.
28. **Bush, T. L., Barrett-Connor, E., Cowan, L. D., Criqui, M. H., Wallace, R. B., Suchindran, C. M., Tyroler, H. A., and Rifkind, B. M.,** Cardiovascular mortality and noncontraceptive use of estrogen in women: results from the lipid research clinics program, follow-up study, *Circulation*, 75, 1102, 1987.
29. **Grady, D., Rubin, S. M., Petitti, D. B., Fox, C. S., Black, D., Ettinger, B., Ernster, V. L., and Cummings, S. R.,** Hormone therapy to prevent disease and prolong life in postmenopausal women, *Ann. Intern. Med.*, 117, 1016, 1992.
30. **Hirvonen, E., Malkonen, M., and Manninen, V.,** Effects of different progestogens on lipoproteins during postmenopausal replacement therapy, *N. Engl. J. Med.*, 304, 560, 1981.
31. **Goldberg, P. B. and Roberts, J.,** Pharmacologic basis for developing rational drug regimens for elderly patients, *Med. Clin. North Am.*, 67, 315, 1983.
32. Lipid research clinics coronary primary prevention trial results: reduction in incidence of coronary heart disease, *JAMA*, 251, 351, 1984.
33. **Denke, M. A. and Grundy, S. M.,** Hypercholesterolemia in elderly persons: resolving the treatment dilemma, *Ann. Intern. Med.*, 112, 780, 1990.
34. The lipid research clinics coronary primary prevention trial: results of 6 years of post-trial follow-up, *Arch. Intern. Med.*, 152, 1399, 1992.
35. **Ast, M. and Frishman, W. H.,** Bile acid sequestrants, *J. Clin. Pharmacol.*, 30, 99, 1990.
36. **Illingworth, D. R.,** Lipid-lowering drugs: an overview of indications and optimum therapeutic use, *Drugs*, 33, 259, 1987.
37. **Sprecher, D.L.,** Efficacy of psyllium in reducing serum cholesterol levels in hypercholesterolemic patients on high- or low-fat diets, *Ann. Intern. Med.*, 119, 545, 1993.
38. **Carlson, L. A., Hamsten, A., and Asplund, A.,** Pronounced lowering of serum levels of lipoprotein Lp(a) in hyperlipidaemic subjects treated with nicotinic acid, *J. Intern. Med.*, 226, 271, 1989.
39. **McKenny, J. M.,** A comparison of the efficacy and toxic effects of sustained- versus immediate-release niacin in hypercholesterolemic patients, *JAMA*, 271, 672, 1994.
40. **Stern, R. H., Freeman, D., and Spence, J. D.,** Differences in metabolism of time-release and unmodified nicotinic acid: explanation of the differences in hypolipidemic action?, *Metab. Clin. Exp.*, 41, 879, 1992.
41. **Illingworth, D. R.,** Comparative efficacy of once versus twice daily mevinolin in the therapy of familial hypercholesterolemia, *Clin. Pharmacol. Ther.*, 40, 338, 1986.
42. **Bach, L. A., Cooper, M. E., O'Brien, R. C., and Jerums, G.,** The use of simvastatin, an HMG CoA reductase inhibitor, in older patients with hypercholesterolemia and atherosclerosis, *J. Am. Geriatr. Soc.*, 38, 10, 1990.
43. **Kuhn, P., Darioli, R., Bovet, P., Bercher, L., and Brunner, H. R.,** Dose-dependent lipid-lowering effects of simvastatin (MK-733) in the elderly, *Curr. Ther. Res.*, 46, 381, 1989.
44. **Mellies, M. J., DeVault, A. R., Kassler-Taub, K., McGovern, M. E., and Pan, H. Y.,** Pravastatin experience in elderly and non-elderly patients, *Atherosclerosis*, 101, 97, 1993.

45. **Smith, H. T., Jokubaitis, L. A., Troendle, A. J., Hwang, D. S., and Robinson, W. T.,** Pharmacokinetics of fluvastatin and specific drug interactions, *Am. J. Hypertension*, 6, 375S, 1993.
46. **Mantell, G., Burke, M. T., and Staggers, J.,** Extended clinical safety profile of lovastatin, *Am. J. Cardiol.*, 66, 11B, 1990.
47. **Pan, H., Funke, P., Waclawski, A., and Willard, D.,** Comparative pharmacokinetics of pravastatin, an HMG CoA reductase inhibitor, in healthy elderly and young male subjects, *J. Clin. Pharmacol.*, 29, 848, 1989.
48. **Bradford, R. H., Shear, C. L., Chremos, A. N., Dujovne, C., Downton, M., Franklin, F. A., Gould, A. L., Hesney, M., Higgins, J., Hurley, D. P., Langendorfer, A., Nash, D. T., Poo, J. L., and Schnaper, H.,** Expanded clinical evaluation of lovastatin (EXCEL) study results, *Arch. Intern. Med.*, 151, 43, 1991.
49. Committee of Principle Investigators, World Health Organization, W.H.O. cooperative trial on primary prevention of ischaemic heart disease using clofibrate to lower serum cholesterol: mortality follow-up, *Lancet*, 2, 379, 1980.
50. Helsinki heart study: primary-prevention trial with gemfibrozil in middle-aged men with dyslipidemia, *N. Engl. J. Med.*, 317, 1237, 1987.
51. **Blanc, G. F.,** Efficacy and tolerance of fenofibrate: a ten-year experience, *Drugs Affecting Lipid Metabolism*, Springer-Verlag, Berlin, 1987, 309.
52. **Steinberg, D.,** Studies on the mechanism of action of probucol, *Am. J. Cardiol.*, 57, 16H, 1986.
53. **Illingworth, R. D.,** Drug therapy of hypercholesterolemia, *Clin. Chem.*, 34, B123, 1988.
54. **Kannel, W. B.,** Nutrition and the occurrence and prevention of cardiovascular disease in the elderly, *Nutr. Rev.*, 46, 68, 1988.

Chapter 16

USE OF ANTIBACTERIAL AGENTS IN THE ELDERLY

Anthony J. Piraino

CONTENTS

0-8493-8306-4/96/$0.00+$.50

I. INTRODUCTION

Antimicrobials are among the most commonly used drugs in the elderly population. It has been estimated, for example, that 43% of all elderly patients are prescribed antibiotics which rank second, behind cardiovascular medications, as the therapeutic agents most widely employed in this age group.[1] Compared to young adults, infections are more common and frequently are more severe in elders. The frequency and severity of infections can be attributed to aging itself as well as to the higher incidence of serious illnesses in the aged. Another possible cause for a higher frequency and increased severity of infections in the elderly is their impaired immune response. Cellular immunity which is responsible for destroying virus-infected cells and protecting people against fungi, parasites, and some bacteria is impaired in the elderly who exhibit increased anergy and decreased lymphocyte production in response to antigen stimulation. The decline in humoral immune function observed in the elderly results in the decreased clinical response to immunization frequently experienced by patients in this age group against infections such as influenza and pneumococcal pneumonia. In one study of 300 healthy elderly patients, anergy was associated with a twofold higher incidence of pneumonia and a twofold higher mortality. The mortality associated with pneumococcal septicemia is 1.5 times higher in the elderly (25% mortality) compared to children and adolescents (10% mortality).[2] In fact, elderly patients have a greater mortality risk from septicemia of all etiologies, underscoring the need to treat infections in the elderly in an effective and timely fashion. Besides these specific changes, it has been suggested that the elderly may experience a generalized impairment of immune function secondary to the stress which is associated with worries over declining health, the loss of function, or the death of spouse and/or friends.[2]

Having accepted the prompt detection and treatment of infectious diseases in the elderly as a worthwhile goal, it is important to point out that the diagnosis of infectious processes is more challenging in elderly patients compared to their younger counterparts. In the elderly, complaints are frequently less specific and findings associated with infections less focal than in younger adults. The presentation of pneumonia, for example, may be a change in mental status with or without a fever. Other nonspecific complaints which are often associated with infection include loss of appetite, confusion, falls, incontinence, and social withdrawal. Consequently, health care providers and others responsible for the care of the elderly should maintain a high index of suspicion regarding changes in functional capacity as well as deterioration in health status as possible harbingers of infection in this population.

The sources of infection in the elderly are also somewhat different compared to the adult population. Because of a higher incidence of urinary disorders and the use of transurethral catheters, elderly patients have more frequent urinary tract infections and are subsequently at higher risk for Gram-negative sepsis from this source. Urinary pathogens account for from 30 to 50% of all bacteremias and cases of sepsis in elderly patients.[3–7]

Bacterial pneumonia is one of the most important infectious diseases experienced by the elderly. The incidence of community-acquired bacterial pneumonia in older persons is 20 to 40 per 1000 per year, while in the acute care setting the incidence of hospital-acquired bacterial pneumonia in elders has been calculated at 8.6 per 1000 admissions per year. The incidence of such infections for elderly patients (>65 years) is at least double that of younger adults (ages 18 to 50 years). The statistics for nursing home patients are higher yet with 70 to 115 elderly persons per 1000 per year experiencing a bacterial pneumonia infection.[8] In fact, in nursing home residents pneumonia, urinary tract infections, and infected decubitus ulcers account for 80% of the bacteremias experienced.[9]

The significant increase in the incidence of bacterial pneumonia and other infections associated with hospitalization and institutional living in the elderly illustrates the increased risk of infectious diseases presented by these environments. The emergence of methicillin-resistant *Staphylococcus aureus* and *S. epidermidis* in addition to Gram-negative antibiotic-resistant aerobic bacteria (for example, *Pseudomonas*, *Serratia*, and *Acinetobacter* species) has increased the mortality associated with nosocomial infections for the elderly and further complicated their treatment in the acute care setting.

The treatment of infections in the elderly is also more complex because adverse reactions and drug interactions frequently occur. The use of drugs which present specific risks for the kidney, like amphotericin B and aminoglycosides, is more difficult in the elderly because of the age-related decrease in renal function. Similarly, ototoxicity may limit the use of drugs like vancomycin and the aminoglycosides in the already hearing-impaired elderly patient. The elderly are also more likely to experience other factors which place them at increased risk for complications of drug therapy. These include:

1. More frequent hospitalization.
2. Institutional (nursing home) residence.
3. Increased incidence of chronic degenerative disease, pulmonary disease, stroke, diabetes.
4. Immunocompromise and decreased resistance to infection due to aging of the immune system.
5. Loss of effectiveness of barriers to microbial invasion.
6. Use of immunosuppressive drugs, e.g., corticosteroids, cancer chemotherapy.
7. Use of drugs which inhibit cough reflex and which can predispose to aspiration and to pulmonary infections.
8. Use of drugs which impair mental status.
9. Normal aging processes which decrease host defenses. These effects include: decreased gastric acidity, decreased cough reflex, and decreased skin integrity, as summarized in Table 16.1.

TABLE 16.1.
Local Defects in Host Antimicrobial Defense in the Elderly

Organ system	Physiologic change	Alteration in host defense
Respiratory system	↓ Compliance and ↓ lung elastic recoil	Diminished effectiveness of cough
	Unknown	Decreased mucociliary clearance
	Alteration in consciousness or defect in upper airway	Diminished aspiration reflex
Skin	↓Vasculature	↓ Healing
	↓ Release of mediators of inflammatory response	↓ Inflammation
	↓ In thickness of stratum corneum	↓ Barrier against bacterial penetration
Gastrointestinal tract	↓ Gastric acid production	Loss of gastric acid barrier, ↓ motility
Genitourinary tract	Prostatic hypertrophy ↓ Bladder tone	Urinary stasis

From Rose, R. M. and Besdine, R. W., Infectious disease, in *Health and Disease in Old Age*, 1st ed., J. W. Rowe et al., Eds., Little, Brown, Boston, 1982, chap. 20. With permission.

II. ANTIMICROBIAL AGENTS

A. β-LACTAM ANTIBIOTICS

- Penicillins
- Carbapenems
- Cephalosporins
- Monobactams

β-Lactam antibiotics exert their antimicrobial action by inhibiting bacterial cell wall synthesis. This is accomplished by binding to enzymes necessary to that synthetic process called penicillin-binding proteins (PBPs). The β-lactams are divided into four major categories: penicillins, cephalosporins, monobactams, and carbapenems. All β-lactam antibiotics have a four-membered β-lactam ring which is fused to a five-member thiazolidine ring in the penicillins, and to a six-member dihydrothiazine ring in the cephalosporins. Various substitutions on these rings determine the antimicrobial spectrum of activity as well as the pharmacodynamic and pharmacokinetic properties of the β-lactams. The β-lactam ring itself is essential for the antimicrobial activity of these drugs. The primary antimicrobial action of the β-lactams is inhibition of microbial cell wall synthesis, resulting in the activation of autolytic enzymes within the bacterial cell which cause disruption of the cell wall and eventually cell lysis. The antimicrobial activity of β-lactams depends upon three factors: (1) their membrane-penetrating ability, (2) their avoidance of inactivation by β-lactamases, and (3) their ability to bind and inactivate PBPs. The loss of any of these attributes can result in development of antimicrobial resistance.

1. Penicillins

- Penicillin G
- Penicillin V
- Methicillin

Since their discovery by Alexander Fleming in 1929, the penicillins have become one of the most frequently prescribed drugs in the history of medicine. Originally isolated from a mold of the genus *Penicillium*, the most active of the natural penicillins identified to that time, benzyl penicillin, or Penicillin G, was introduced into clinical use in 1941.

a. Penicillin G

Benzyl penicillin (Penicillin G) is active against a variety of Gram-positive bacteria, including α- and β-hemolytic streptococci and *Streptococcus pneumoniae* and Gram-negative bacteria including *Hemophilus influenzae*, which is somewhat less sensitive, and *Neisseria* species. The most common source of microbial resistance to Penicillin G is the production of a β-lactamase. Many strains of *Staphylococcus* and Gram-negative bacteria exhibit resistance due to the production of penicillinase.

Penicillin G is destroyed by gastric acid, and therefore should be administered by injection. The clearance of this drug is predominantly renal. About 60% is excreted by this route. Only about 10% is eliminated by glomerular filtration; the rest is cleared by active secretion in the proximal tubules, with a small amount being reabsorbed in the collecting system. Hepatic biotransformation to penicilloic acid accounts for the elimination of less than 30% of an administered dose, while biliary excretion accounts for approximately 5%.

Hypersensitivity reactions are common with the penicillins, and sensitization is commonplace, probably as a consequence of the widespread use of this class of drugs. Penicillin hypersensitivity includes four main categories of reactions: anaphylaxis, serum sickness, contact dermatitis, and local reactions. Of these, anaphylaxis and serum sickness are the most serious. Anaphylaxis, although uncommon, is potentially life threatening within minutes after administration, having a mortality of approximately 10%. Serum sickness, which affects approximately 2% of exposed patients, may appear within 7 to 10 d of treatment with penicillin. It manifests as fever, malaise, urticaria, and joint pain. Delayed hypersensitivity may present as maculopapular rash, erythema nodosum, exfoliative dermatitis, or Stevens-Johnson syndrome, the latter two of which are also potentially life threatening.

Other varieties of toxicity associated with penicillins include the following: Jarisch-Herxheimer reaction occurs in approximately 50% of patients treated with Penicillin G for primary syphilis and is characterized by malaise, chills, fever, sore throat, myalgia, headaches, and tachycardia. Interstitial nephritis may develop after 1 week of therapy with daily doses of Penicillin G above 10 million units and is characterized by fever, eosinophilia, rashes, increased blood urea levels, and albuminuria. Other rare side effects, among them hemolytic anemia, pancytopenia, and coagulopathies, have also been reported following penicillin usage. Elderly patients, especially those with reduced renal function who are given large intravenous injections of penicillin for serious infections including pneumococcal meningitis or streptococcal endocarditis, are at increased risk to develop seizures, and should be monitored during the first 72 hours of any required high-dose intravenous penicillin therapy.[10,11]

b. Penicillin V

The poor oral absorption of Penicillin G and its relatively narrow antimicrobial spectrum prompted the search for more versatile antimicrobials. This led to the development of phenoxymethyl penicillin (Penicillin V), which is identical in antimicrobial spectrum and activity to Penicillin G, but is absorbed more predictably following oral administration. Bioavailability of Penicillin V is approximately 50% when administered to fasting patients, less when given with meals. The clinical use and toxicities associated with Penicillin V are identical to those of Penicillin G. Other than absorption, the pharmacokinetics are similar to Penicillin G. The plasma protein binding is about 80%.

Penicillin V was introduced into clinical use in 1953 and became one of the most widely used oral penicillins. Penicillin V is effective in the treatment of infections caused by pneumococci and β-hemolytic streptococci. Adverse experiences associated with the drug are comparable in frequency and qualitatively as with the same doses of Penicillin G.

c. Methicillin

As natural penicillins, both penicillins G and V are somewhat limited in their effectiveness by bacterial resistance due to penicillinases, which are possessed by many microorganisms. Methicillin was the first penicillinase-resistant semisynthetic penicillin to be discovered. However, its instability in acid has limited it to parenteral use. The antimicrobial spectrum is similar to Penicillin G with the following two exceptions: (1) methicillin is active against penicillinase-producing (and consequently Penicillin G-resistant) staphylococci; (2) methicillin is not active against enterococci or Gram-negative organisms. A recent development of concern to the hospitalized elderly is the emergence of methicillin-resistant *Staphylococcus aureus* which develop resistance not as a consequence of bacterial enzyme activity (β-lactamase or penicillinase), but because of differences in the cell wall which result in markedly lower affinity of antibiotics for PBPs. The production of higher concentrations of PBPs and the production of different (novel) PBPs have been observed in the presence of methicillin for some resistant species. Although none of the penicillins are specifically nephrotoxic, allergic interstitial nephritis, which occurs with many antibiotics, is a particular problem with methicillin, and this has essentially ended its widespread clinical use.

d. *Other Penicillinase-Resistant Penicillins*

- Cloxacillin
- Dicloxacillin
- Floxacillin
- Nafcillin
- Oxacillin

The group of penicillinase-resistant antibiotics also includes nafcillin, cloxacillin, oxacillin, dicloxacillin, and floxacillin. Unlike methicillin, nafcillin is acid stable. However, because of poor oral bioavailability (10 to 20%), it should be administered by injection. Oxacillin and nafcillin are currently the preferred agents in this group for parenteral therapy, while cloxacillin and dicloxacillin are the agents of choice for oral therapy. Because of extensive protein binding (greater than 90%), oxacillin, dicloxacillin, cloxacillin, and floxacillin are poorly distributed and penetrate peripheral tissues slowly. This feature limits their use in central nervous system (CNS) infections where achieving therapeutic tissue concentrations in the cerebrospinal fluid is necessary. The clearance of nafcillin is predominantly (60%) hepatic with approximately 8% eliminated via the bile. About 30% of an injected dose is excreted unchanged in the urine. Renal clearance is the primary excretory route for the other penicillinase-resistant antibiotics. Some biotransformation to active and inactive metabolites does take place, but this varies with the level of the parent compounds in the plasma. Under normal circumstances less than 10% of the plasma drug content is accounted for by these metabolites. In marked renal insufficiency, however, metabolites of these drugs constitute up to 50% of the total serum antibiotic content. Consequently, while the half-life of nafcillin increases in renal failure, it rarely exceeds 4 hours.

e. *Aminopenicillins*

- Ampicillin
- Amoxicillin

The aminopenicillins, ampicillin and amoxicillin, have identical antimicrobial spectra. These drugs are effective against Gram-positive pathogens and are more active than Penicillin G against Gram-negative bacilli, including *Escherichia coli*, *Proteus mirabilis*, *Salmonella*, *Shigella*, and *Hemophilus influenzae*. Resistance to these drugs is possessed by β-lactamase-producing microorganisms including penicillinase-producing staphylococci. Also, many strains of *E. coli*, *Salmonella*, *Shigella*, and *H. influenzae* have developed resistance to ampicillin, and this agent is inactive against *Enterobacter* species, *Klebsiella* species, and *Pseudomonas aeruginosa*.

Amoxicillin is well absorbed orally, showing oral bioavailability of 75% compared with 40 to 60% oral bioavailability for ampicillin. Peak serum levels can be two times higher for amoxicillin when similar doses are used. Ampicillin also exhibits approximately 50% lower peak serum levels and slower absorption if taken with food. For both drugs, plasma protein binding is low and both are excreted primarily by the kidney. About 70 to 80% of an orally absorbed dose of amoxicillin is excreted unchanged in the urine within 6 hours of dosing, as compared to 40% for orally administered ampicillin. Urinary excretion following parenteral ampicillin administration is higher (about 90%). Both amoxicillin and ampicillin are cleared by glomerular filtration and tubular secretion; up to 25% of both drugs is biotransformed in the liver, while 2 to 3% is excreted unchanged in the bile. Because of the important contribution of renal excretion to the overall clearance of ampicillin and amoxicillin, their elimination half-lives are significantly prolonged in anuric patients. In some elderly populations the plasma clearance and urinary excretion of ampicillin were significantly reduced when compared to younger subjects.[12] For these reasons, dosing adjustments must be made for diminished renal function as is often the case in many elderly patients.[13] Both ampicillin and amoxicillin are associated with a higher incidence of skin rashes compared with penicillin. The incidence of such rashes is increased when ampicillin and allopurinol are used simultaneously. Because it has better absorption and is less likely to produce diarrhea than ampicillin, amoxicillin is usually the preferred oral dosage form. Otherwise an ampicillin ester should be used.

f. Antipseudomonal Penicillins

- Azlocillin
- Carbenicillin
- Mezlocillin
- Piperacillin
- Ticarcillin

Five β-lactamase-sensitive antimicrobials developed since 1967 have been demonstrated to have a broad spectrum of activity against aerobic, Gram-negative bacilli, including *P. aeruginosa*, as well as aerobic bacteria such as *Escherichia coli*, *Enterobacter*, *Proteus mirabilis*, and *H. influenzae*. Among these agents, which include azlocillin, carbenicillin, mezlocillin, piperacillin, and ticarcillin, the most active are azlocillin, mezlocillin, and piperacillin. All five drugs are hydrolyzed by staphylococcal penicillinase and are therefore inactive against Penicillin G-resistant *staphylococci*. Neither carbenicillin nor ticarcillin are active against *Klebsiella* species, although approximately half of *Klebsiella* isolates are susceptible to the remaining agents in this group. The antibiotic potency of this group of agents against *Pseudomonas aeruginosa* varies from agent to agent. In general, piperacillin has the greatest activity, followed by mezlocillin, azlocillin, ticarcillin, and carbenicillin.

None of these agents are well absorbed orally and consequently must be given parenterally. The only exception is the sodium salt of a carbenicillin ester (carbenicillin indanyl sodium) which, although it has low oral bioavailability (35%), is rapidly absorbed from the gastrointestinal (GI) tract and subsequently converted to carbenicillin. Carbenicillin and ticarcillin are both primarily cleared by the renal route through combined glomerular filtration and tubular secretion. About 80% of an administered dose of ticarcillin and approximately 95% of an administered dose of carbenicillin are excreted unchanged in the urine. Probenecid has been shown to inhibit the tubular secretion of both drugs. The remaining drugs mezlocillin, azlocillin, and piperacillin are also primarily cleared (60 to 70%) by the renal route, and the elimination half-life of all these agents is prolonged in renal failure patients. This is more pronounced for carbenicillin and ticarcillin than for mezlocillin, azlocillin, and piperacillin.

For infections outside the urinary tract in compromised, particularly neutropenic patients, and especially for serious infections attributable to *Pseudomonas* species, these drugs should be combined with an aminoglycoside. For carbenicillin and ticarcillin specifically, and with the other drugs in this class in general, platelet dysfunction causing altered hemostasis has been associated with the use of high doses. Three factors, relatively weak activity of carbenicillin against *P. aeruginosa,* its high sodium content (4.7 meq/g), and the high doses (up to 36 g/d vs. 18 g/d for ticarcillin) of carbenicillin sodium which may be required to treat nonurinary infections attributable to these microorganisms, may produce hypernatremia in patients with renal insufficiency so treated. This sodium load can also present a particular problem for patients with congestive heart failure, including the elderly and others for whom high sodium intake is contraindicated.

2. Combined Therapy Using β-Lactamase Inhibitors

The resistance conferred upon many bacteria by β-lactamases can be overcome by co-administration of a β-lactamase inhibitor with an otherwise susceptible antibiotic. Potassium clavulanate acid is a naturally occurring β-lactamase inhibitor which is available in combination with amoxicillin for oral administration and with ticarcillin for intravenous use. Other β-lactamase inhibitors include sodium sulbactam, which is combined with ampicillin for parenteral administration, and tazobactam, which is combined with piperacillin for parenteral administration. In elderly patients (aged 65 to 85) receiving combined ampicillin-sulbactam therapy, the mean urinary excretion and overall clearance was lower compared to young adults (aged 20 to 40) and middle-aged patients (aged 41 to 64) and is consistent with a prolongation of antimicrobial activity in the elderly compared with younger subjects.[14] While these inhibitors do not change the inherent potency of the β-lactam antibiotics, they can extend the range of microorganisms against which these drugs have activity. Bacteria susceptible to such combination therapy include penicillinase-producing strains of *S. aureus, H. influenzae, E. coli, Proteus, Klebsiella*, and *Bacteroides*, among others. The antibiotic resistance possessed by *Pseudomonas aeruginosa*, however, is not inhibited by either clavulanate or tazobactam, which are ineffective in combination with either piperacillin or ticarcillin in treating infections caused by resistant *P. aeruginosa* strains.

3. Cephalosporins

The first of the cephalosporin antibiotics, cephalothin and cephaloridine, which is no longer marketed, were introduced in 1964. The chemical structure includes a β-lactam ring connected to a six-member dihydrothiazine ring. The subsequent development of cephalosporin antibiotics over the past 30 years has resulted in a classification system based upon "generations". Initially, this classification was intended to convey the time frame of the introduction of these drugs, but now by convention the generation to which a cephalosporin is assigned reflects the spectrum of its antimicrobial activity.

Certain cephalosporins, across generations which have an *N*-methylthiotetrazole side chain, present an increased risk of bleeding diathesis for the elderly, specifically resulting from interference with the vitamin K-dependent clotting factors. The presence of malnutrition, renal insufficiency, and a debilitated physical state all predispose the elderly patient to experience this adverse effect associated with these cephalosporin antibiotics. No cephalosporin is active against *enterococci* or against methicillin-resistant *staphylococci*.

a. First Generation Cephalosporins

- Cefazolin
- Cephalothin
- Cephapirin
- Cephalexin
- Cefadroxil
- Cephadrine

The first-generation cephalosporins include three parenteral agents (cefazolin, cephalothin, and cephapirin) and three agents for oral use (cephalexin, cefadroxil, and cephadrine). These drugs, which were discovered during the 1960s and 1970s, are active against Gram-positive aerobic bacteria (other than enterococci and methicillin-resistant staphylococci) and against *E. coli, Klebsiella* species, and some *Proteus* species. Because first-generation cephalosporins are hydrolyzed by the cephalosporinase-type β-lactamases found in some Gram-negative organisms, their antimicrobial spectra are somewhat narrow. The orally administered first-generation cephalosporins are quite well absorbed in the absence of food, which diminishes the peak serum levels achieved. These agents are cleared unchanged renally with minimal biotransformation and half-lives on the order of 1 hour. Their elimination is prolonged in renal insufficiency, with half-lives approaching 10 to 20 hours in renal failure.

The injectable first-generation cephalosporins, cephalothin and cephapirin, participate in some (30%) biotransformation via deacetylation to metabolites possessing minimal antimicrobial activity. The remaining parent drug is cleared unchanged in the urine. Because of the hepatic clearance exhibited by these two agents, their half-lives are only modestly prolonged in renal failure, from about 30 min to about 2 to 3 hours. Cephazolin, which is cleared almost totally via the kidneys, exhibits much more prolonged elimination in renal failure with a half-life of approximately 24 hours in anuric patients. Adjustment of dosage in patients with renal insufficiency, including the elderly, is recommended for most of these drugs.

Cephalexin, cefadroxil, and cephadrine are commonly used to treat urinary tract infections. These drugs are generally safe and exhibit side effects similar to those of the penicillins. While some patients allergic to penicillins may tolerate cephalosporins, these two classes of drugs are known to produce cross sensitivity to each other in about 10% of patients. This risk may be acceptable depending upon the anticipated clinical benefit, but should never be overlooked since these allergic reactions can manifest themselves as anaphylaxis, serum sickness, and exfoliative dermatitis, among other serious clinical conditions. The injectable first-generation cephalosporins likewise share a high degree of safety. They are mainly employed in community-acquired infections caused by suspected Gram-positive organisms. They provide an alternative to penicillins for treatment of staphylococcal and streptococcal infections and are effective in the therapy of infections caused by susceptible strains of *E. coli, Klebsiella* species, and/or *P. mirabilis*. Because of the longer half-life of cefazolin, it maintains higher serum levels and can be administered less frequently than the other first-generation cephalosporins; it is also well tolerated when given intramuscularly. These factors favor its use in the hospital setting. Its therapeutic applications include prophylaxis for cardiovascular, gastric, biliary, pelvic, and orthopedic surgery, particularly in high-risk patients undergoing such procedures, including the elderly.

b. Second-Generation Cephalosporins

True cephalosporins

- Cefuroxime
- Cefamandole
- Cefonicid
- Cefaclor
- Cefuroxineaxetil
- Cefprozil

Cephamycins

- Cefoxitin
- Cefmetazole
- Cefotetan

Carbacephem

- Loracarbef

The second-generation cephalosporins are actually a conglomerate of three groups of antimicrobial drugs: ***true cephalosporins*** which include parenteral agents (cefuroxime, cefamandole, and cefonicid) and oral drugs (cefaclor, cefuroxineaxetil, and cefprozil), as well as the ***cephamycins***, which include cefoxitin, cefmetazole, and cefotetan, and a single, orally administered ***carbacephem*** (loracarbef).

Cefamandole, the first agent in this classification to be introduced, is moderately resistant to β-lactamase, which confers on this agent and other second-generation cephalosporins activity against a wider spectrum of bacteria than the first-generation cephalosporins.

Cefuroxime is particularly resistant to β-actamase and, together with cefonicid, is highly active against β-lactamase-producing strains of *Hemophilus influenzae*. The second-generation cephalosporins are more potent than their first generation counterparts against *E. coli*, *Klebsiella*, and *P. mirabilis*.

The inclusion of a methoxy group in the β-lactam nucleus of the cephamycins produces a high degree of resistance to β-lactamase, making these agents (cefoxitin, cefmetazole, and cefotetan) very active against anaerobics, particularly β-lactamase-producing *Bacteroides fragilis*.

Among the orally administered agents, cefaclor, cefprozil, and loracarbef all exhibit bioavailability in excess of 90%. Cefuroxime axetil, on the other hand, has very poor oral absorption (50%), which may produce unreliable drug levels. Consequently, this agent should not be employed for serious infection, especially those due to *H. influenzae*. The other second-generation cephalosporins must be administered parenterally. Clearance is primarily renal for all agents except cefotetan, which has some biliary excretion. Cefaclor has also been reported to undergo biotransformation; however, no metabolites have been identified.[15] With the exception of cefonicid and cefotetan, which have half-lives of 3.5 and 4.5 hours, respectively, in healthy young patients, the half-lives of second-generation cephalosporins average approximately 1 hour. In renal failure the elimination half-life is prolonged for all drugs in this class, and dosage adjustment for patients with anuria is necessary. Elderly patients with moderate renal insufficiency have exhibited a reduced ability to eliminate cefaclor. However, due to a short elimination half-life and wide therapeutic index, dosage adjustments are not necessary in these patients.[16] In elderly patients receiving cefonicid, serum half-life was found to be longer than values previously noted in younger patients with similar degrees of renal dysfunction, and a linear correlation was noted between cefonicid clearance and creatinine clearance.[17] Kinetic disposition of cefprozil in the elderly is similar to that in young healthy individuals and renal dysfunction (but not hepatic dysfunction) has been shown to significantly reduce elimination of cefprozil for these reasons. It has been recommended that the cefprozil dosage be reduced by 50% in patients whose creatinine clearance is less than 30 mL/min.[18] Pharmacokinetic studies of cefuroxime acetil in elderly patients have revealed no need for dose adjustment based strictly upon age, however. The pharmacokinetics of cefuroxime axetil was evaluated in 20 sick elderly patients with a mean age of 83.9 years, revealing no accumulation after 5 days of therapy (200 mg every 12 hours). The data suggest that the standard dosage regimen is adequate in the sick elderly patient.[19] Systemic clearance of cefmetazole was found to be significantly lower in elderly than in young volunteers (92.4 vs. 112 mL/min). However, the observed age-related differences of cefmetazole pharmacokinetics are most likely due to differences in renal function between the two age groups. Consequently, the small reduction in cefmetazole elimination in the elderly would not appear to warrant dose adjustment in this population.[20] Healthy geriatric volunteers with normal kidney function who received single 400-mg doses of loracarbef revealed pharmacokinetic parameters (including area under the curve [AUC] and clearance) and pharmacodynamic parameters (safety and efficacy) comparable to healthy nongeriatric adults. Despite the fact that all of these drugs are adequately distributed, only parenteral cefuroxime achieves the concentrations in cerebrospinal fluid necessary to treat meningitis, although there have been therapeutic failures.

In general, these drugs are used to treat community-acquired infections attributable to a mixture of Gram-positive and Gram-negative pathogens. Cefuroxime, in particular, is employed in the therapy of community-acquired pneumonia, urinary tract infections, soft tissue infections, bacteremia, and, as noted above, in the treatment of bacterial meningitis.

Some of the second-generation cephalosporins present specific risks for elderly patients, the debilitated, or otherwise frail patients. Cefotetan and cefamandole can cause a reversible hypoprothrominemia particularly in older patients and those who are vitamin K deficient, which can be corrected with supplemental vitamin K or avoided with prophylactic vitamin K.

Other hematologic reactions are possible as is drug fever and, in the elderly, diarrhea, possibly due to *Clostridium difficile* toxin, which may produce pseudomembranous colitis.

c. Third-Generation Cephalosporins

- Cefotaxime
- Ceftizoxime
- Ceftriaxone
- Cefixime
- Cefpodoxime
- Ceftazidime
- Cefepime
- Cefoperazone

The third-generation cephalosporins are highly resistant to β-lactamases and as a group are highly active against *N. meningitidis, N. gonorrhoeae, Moraxella catarrhalis*, and *H. influenzae*, including β-lactamase-producing strains. Compared to the antipseudomonal penicillins and the second-generation cephalosporins, these drugs have a wider spectrum of activity and greater antimicrobial potency against aerobic, Gram-negative bacteria. In this regard the third-generation cephalosporins can be subclassified on the basis of their activity against *Pseudomonas aeruginosa*. The parenteral agents cefotaxime, ceftizoxime, and ceftriaxone and the oral agents cefixime and cefpodoxime lack clinical activity against *P. aeruginosa*. Ceftazidime and cefepime (both parenteral drugs) possess antipseudomonal activity, the latter two agents being the most potent of this category of drugs in this regard. The activity of the third-generation cephalosporins against anaerobic bacteria is variable, with many strains of *B. fragilis* exhibiting resistance.

Cefpodoxime and cefixime are both approximately 50% bioavailable orally with elimination half-lives ranging from 2.5 to 3.0 hours, respectively. Approximately 50% of administered cefixime is recovered unchanged in the urine. There are no known metabolites. Both these agents are cleared primarily by the renal route and their elimination half-lives are prolonged three- to fourfold in renal failure. An evaluation of multiple-dose cefpodoxime administration to young adults (aged 10 to 60) and elderly individuals (aged greater than 70) revealed the pharmacokinetics in both adult and elderly patients to be comparable with those of healthy volunteers and with each other, with the exception of one elderly patient with severe renal impairment. The authors concluded that dosage adjustment of cefpodoxime proxetil is unnecessary in the elderly unless evidence of severe renal insufficiency exists.[21] Another study of single-dose cefpodoxime pharmacokinetics concluded that the differences between young and elderly subjects were negligible, with the exception of the half-life, which increased by only 14%, from 2.67 to 3 hours. This study likewise recommended that cefpodoxime dosage adjustment is not necessary in the elderly.[22] Of the parenteral agents, ceftriaxone has the longest elimination half-life, which is reported to range from 6 to 9 hours and which increases from one- to twofold in renal failure. In patients with normal renal function, 40 to 65% of an injected dose is recovered unchanged in the urine. The remainder is excreted into the bile, unchanged. Ceftizoxime, ceftazidime, and cefepime are cleared primarily by the renal route. The average area under the curves in elderly patients are about 40% higher than those of other healthy adults, presumably due to age-related decreases in renal function.

Ceftizoxime and ceftazidime have half lives of approximately 2 hours. About 80 to 90% of an injected dose is recovered unchanged from the urine. The clearance of these two agents in renal failure is prolonged approximately tenfold compared to the remaining third-generation cephalosporins. The results of one study recommended ceftazidime dose reduction in the elderly based upon creatinine clearance, which was less than 50 mL/min in one half of the 221 elderly (aged over 65 years) patients surveyed. For these reasons, some investigators have suggested that a twice-daily dosage regimen (as compared with three times daily) for ceftazidime in elderly patients who have normal renal function for their age should be employed based on age-related decreases in renal function and drug elimination.[23] In another study, two geriatric patients developed ceftazidime-induced neurotoxicity that produced confusion, disorientation, agitation, generalized weakness, and myoclonus. In the investigator's opinion, these findings emphasize the importance of adjusting the dosage of ceftazidime in patients with renal insufficiency.[23–25]

The half-life of cefepime increases from about 2 hours to about 14 hours in renal failure patients, whereas cefotaxime, which is normally excreted 85% unchanged in the urine of patients with normal renal function, shows only a modest prolongation of half-life from about 1 hour to about 2.5 hours in patients with renal failure. This is probably due to its modest hepatic metabolism by deacetylation to an active biotransformation product. Two separate studies have found no need for cefepime dose adjustment in elderly patients with normal renal function for their age. The pharmacokinetics of cefepime in infected patients appeared to be unaltered by illness and the steady-state disposition of cefepime was predictable using data derived from single-dose studies in volunteers.[26,27] Cefoperazone is the only third-generation cephalosporin with significant (30 to 50%) hepatic biotransformation. Only 25% of cefoperazone is recovered unchanged from the urine after a single parenteral dose. The reduced dependence of this agent on renal clearance is reflected by a negligible prolongation in half-life, from the normal 2 hours, in renal failure. Compared to healthy young adults, the pharmacokinetics of ceftriaxone were only minimally different in the elderly and in patients with renal or hepatic dysfunction. However, pharmacokinetic analysis from one study in the elderly has revealed significant differences in the concentration vs. time profiles for ceftriaxone compared to that expected based upon data obtained in young adults. Consequently, dosing recommendations for elderly patients receiving this agent and those receiving cefoperazone may require modification.[28] While there is some disagreement in the literature as to whether dosage adjustment is necessary in such patients, it is generally accepted that in severe renal and hepatic insufficiency, blood levels of ceftriaxone should be monitored.

The third-generation cephalosporins are useful in the treatment of hospital-acquired infections, particularly those caused by multidrug-resistant Gram-negative bacilli. When treating *P. aeruginosa* infections, ceftazidime is the preferred agent in this group. The extensive distribution of these agents (with the exception of cefoperazone) into the CNS favors their use in meningitis caused by susceptible pathogens. Cefotaxime and ceftriaxone are frequently employed in such therapy. Ceftazidime is successfully used as empiric, single-drug therapy of febrile patients who are neutropenic. The excretion of some third-generation cephalosporins into the bile can interfere with the balance of normal fecal flora and can cause diarrhea or colitis. This untoward effect is quite common in elderly patients. The hypoprothrombinemia observed mainly in the elderly with some second-generation cephalosporins may also be associated with the use of cefoperazone and ceftizoxime, which share a structural similarity (3-methylthiofetrazole side chain).

4. Monobactams

- Aztreonam

Monobactams are simple antibiotics which lack the fused two-ring structure common to other β-lactam agents. Instead, their activity and β-lactamase resistance is conferred by side chains attached to the β-lactam nucleus. Only one monobactam, Aztrenonam, is currently in clinical use. This antibiotic is effective only against Gram-negative aerobic bacteria because of selective affinity for their PBPs. Its activity against Gram-negative aerobic organisms, including *H. influenzae*, *M. catarrhalis*, *Neisseria meningitidis*, and a variety of enteric Gram-negative species, is comparable to Ceftazidime.

Aztreonam is not absorbed orally and hence is administered only parenterally. Clearance is renal with approximately 70% of an injected dose recovered unchanged in the urine. In patients with normal kidney function the half-life is approximately 2 hours. This increases approximately threefold in renal failure. Renal status is the major determinant of dosing in elderly patients; assessment of creatinine clearance should be performed and appropriate dosing adjustment should be made if needed in such patients. In one study the mean total body clearance of aztreonam was observed to be greater for the younger than the elderly group. The data suggest that lower doses of aztreonam given at less frequent intervals may be appropriate in the elderly population.[29] Aztreonam is used for nosocomial infections caused by susceptible Gram-negative aerobes. In mixed infections, including those of the skin, soft tissues, and lower respiratory tract, other agents which provide Gram-positive coverage (e.g., vancomycin, clindamycin, or nafcillin) should be combined with Aztreonam to provide adequate therapy.

Allergic skin rashes are infrequently (<1%) associated with Aztreonam, and no cross sensitivity of this drug for penicillin-allergic patients has been reported. GI complaints including diarrhea and *C. difficile*-mediated colitis are likewise infrequent comparable to other β-lactam drugs.

5. Carbapenems

- Imipenem

The carbapenems are β-lactam antibiotics with an extremely wide spectrum of antimicrobial activity, in fact, the widest of this class. Among the carbapenems, only one agent, imipenem, is currently available for clinical use, and this drug is effective against virtually all bacteria and almost totally resistant to β-lactamases. The species not covered by imipenem include *Streptococcus faecium*, *Corynebacterium JK*, methicillin-resistant staphylococci, all strains of *P. maltophilia* (one of the few bacteria which produces a β-lactamase capable of hydrolyzing the β-lactam nuclei of imipenem and about half of the known strains of *P. cepacia*.

Imipenem has an unusual pharmacokinetic profile. It is cleared by a combination of biotransformation, glomerular filtration, and tubular secretion. A significant portion of this biotransformation is accomplished by a renal enzyme, dihydropeptidase I. The products of this biotransformation lack any antimicrobial activity, and the extent of an administered dose which undergoes such metabolism varies between 30% for "light metabolizers" and 65% in "heavy metabolizers". In its commercially available dosage form for intravenous injection, imipenem is combined in equal parts with cilastatin, a renal dihydropeptidase inhibitor which has no antimicrobial activity of its own. Throughout its actions, however, imipenem is completely spared from renal metabolism, allowing more of the imipenem to retain its antimicrobial activity. When co-administered together, about 70 to 75% of both imipenem and cilastatin are recovered unchanged from the urine, the remainder of each drug being metabolized. Both imipenem and cilastatin have half lives of about 1 hour in patients with normal renal function. In renal failure patients, the half-life of imipenem increases to about 4 hours, while that of cilastatin increases to about 16 hours. Consequently, the dosage should be adjusted in patients with renal insufficiency, particularly elderly patients who are predisposed to experience seizures with high-dose imipenem therapy (see below).

Imipenem is useful in treating infections caused by most Gram-positive cocci, among them penicillinase-producing staphylococci, streptococci, and pneumococci. Its spectrum of activity includes most *Enterobacteriaceae* and most important anaerobic species, except *Clostridium difficile*. Imipenem is indicated for infections due to mixed aerobic/anaerobic flora and as empiric therapy of serious nosocomial infections.

Both imipenem and cilastatin are very safe drugs. The adverse experiences associated with imipenem resemble those of other β-lactam antibiotics, including GI complications (nausea, vomiting, diarrhea) and hypersensitivity reactions (rashes, drug fever, pruritus, urticaria). CNS findings (seizures) have been observed which often have been associated with the injection of high doses relative to a patient's body size and renal function. This may be an issue of particular concern for elderly patients, especially those with renal insufficiency or a history of seizure disorder.

B. AMINOGLYCOSIDES

- Amikacin
- Gentamicin
- Kanamycin
- Netilmicin
- Tobramycin

Aminoglycosides are used primarily for infections due to Gram-negative bacteria. Streptomycin, the first agent in this group, was introduced in 1944. This group of drugs has a rapid bactericidal action which persists after plasma drug levels fall to subtherapeutic levels. Transport of aminoglycosides into the bacterial cell is a multifaceted process, the first phase of which depends upon aerobic metabolism. Consequently, the aminoglycosides have no activity against anaerobic bacteria or against *Rickettsia* or *Chlamydia* species. Over the past 50 years the aminoglycosides have been successfully employed in the treatment of infections caused by aerobic Gram-negative bacilli. The chief factor limiting their use is toxicity, specifically nephrotoxicity, ototoxicity, and neuromuscular blockade. The advent of newer, less toxic drugs is causing a re-examination of aminoglycoside use, particularly in the elderly, with already compromised hearing and renal function.

As a group, the aminoglycosides are active against Gram-negative bacilli including *Escherichia coli, Enterobacter, Klebsiella, Proteus, Pseudomonas aeruginosa, Salmonella, Serratia*, and *Shigella*, and to a lesser extent Gram-positive bacteria including *Staphylococcus aureus* and some *streptococci*. The unique mechanism of action of aminoglycosides allows their combined use with other antibiotics to achieve synergistic bactericidal effects. Often aminoglycosides are combined with β-lactam antibiotics in this regard. Bacteria develop resistance to aminoglycosides in a number of ways, notably by producing deactivating enzymes, by interference with drug transport into the bacterial cell, and by modification of ribosomal binding sites.

Aminoglycosides are not absorbed orally and are therefore administered intravenously (the preferred route), or by intramuscular injection, the absorption of which is sometimes unpredictable. These drugs distribute well to extracellular fluid and poorly into fat. They likewise do not penetrate well into the cerebrospinal fluid, but distribution into the joints, the pleura, the peritoneum, and the pericardial spaces is good. Aminoglycosides bind aggressively to renal cortical tissue and are concentrated in the urine. They are all cleared renally, predominantly by glomerular filtration, and over 90% of an injected dose is recovered unchanged from the urine within 24 hours. Consequently, dosage adjustment is essential in elderly patients with diminished renal function in whom the half-lives of these drugs increase proportionally to the degree of renal insufficiency. For most aminoglycosides, the half-lives in healthy adults range from 2 to 3 hours. In renal failure, this can increase up to 40-fold. In adults with infections, the half-life of amikacin, for example, was reported to be 3 hours compared with 4 hours in elderly patients in one clinical trial.[30] In another study the investigators recommended a 25% (approximately) reduction in amikacin dosage for elderly patients compared to young adults, when this drug is to be given once daily, and emphasize the need for ongoing monitoring of this regimen.[31]

The main adverse experiences associated with the aminoglycosides involve the kidneys, particularly the proximal tubule cells in which aminoglycosides destroy organelles and microvilli, leading ultimately to cell death. Advanced aminoglycoside toxicity is associated first with nonoliguric and finally oliguric renal failure. The incidence of aminoglycoside-induced nephrotoxicity has been estimated to range from 10 to 25%. Advancing age appears to predispose a patient to experience such toxicity as do concomitant renal disease, debilitation, dehydration, and concurrent exposure to other nephrotoxic drugs or toxins. Monitoring renal function during aminoglycoside therapy is important, particularly in the elderly in whom routine screening tests such as a blood urea nitrogen assay and serum creatinine measurements may not reveal reduced renal drug clearance capacity. In these patients, evaluating the creatinine clearance is an absolute requirement.

Aminoglycoside serum levels are directly correlated with the risk of toxicity, and consequently the measurement of peak and trough plasma levels is essential. For long-term amikacin therapy, trough concentrations greater than 10 μg/mL are associated with toxicity. For long-term therapy with other aminoglycosides trough concentrations should be maintained below 2 μg/mL to minimize the risks of kidney damage, which can be irreversible. Aminoglycoside-induced ototoxicity can be either auditory or vestibular in nature. These toxicities are the consequence of damage to the otic hair cells which is not reversible and which results from peak serum concentrations of amikacin greater than 35 μg/mL and of the other aminoglycosides of greater than 12 μg/mL. The elderly are at increased risk for this toxicity, which may be mistaken for age-related hearing loss, as are patients young and old using other ototoxic drugs.

The clinical utility of the aminoglycosides in elderly patients must be evaluated in the context of their effectiveness, the overall cost of their use (including obligate lab studies), and the risks, particularly ototoxicity and nephrotoxicity, they impose for the patient. These drugs are indicated in the therapy of serious infections and because of their potential toxicity should not be used indiscriminately or when another less toxic drug will suffice. Aminoglycosides provide reliable antimicrobial coverage against a variety of aerobic Gram-negative pathogens and are widely employed in the empiric therapy of suspected nosocomial sepsis caused by Gram-negative bacilli of various etiologies including, for example, complicated urinary tract infections, peritoneal contamination due to bowel perforation, nonvenereal pelvic inflammatory disease, and bacteremias.

Aminoglycosides, when combined with synergistic antimicrobial drugs, are effective against infections due to Gram-positive cocci and *P. aeruginosa*. Empiric aminoglycoside therapy should be based on a number of factors, including the severity and type of infection, the incidence of bacterial resistance to aminoglycosides in the specific clinical setting (hospital, nursing home, etc.), and, as noted above, the overall cost of therapy.

Amikacin, gentamicin, netilmicin, and tobramycin can be considered equivalent in many clinical applications. Among these drugs, gentamicin, because of its low cost, is preferred in most circumstances. Bacterial resistance to kanamycin among Enterobacteriaceae is present in many hospitals, and kanamycin has no activity against *P. aeruginosa*. Because of these limitations, kanamycin is seldom used in serious Gram-negative bacillary infections.

C. MACROLIDES

- Erythromycin

As a class, the macrolide antibiotics have been known since 1952 when the prototype agent of this group, erythromycin, was isolated from the metabolic products of a strain of *Streptomyces erythreus*. Although erythromycin has been in clinical use for over 35 years, there is fresh interest in this agent and class of drugs because of its effectiveness in treating infections caused by *Helicobacter, Legionella, Mycoplasma,* and *Chlamydia*. Macrolides, in general, have been demonstrated to be useful in the treatment of respiratory, skin, soft tissue, genital, and gastrointestinal infections, especially when tetracyclines and β-lactam antibiotics cannot be employed. Erythromycin, however, suffers from some significant limitations. For example, its instability in an acidic environment contributes to both low oral bioavailability and high incidence of GI irritation, nausea, and diarrhea. Erythromycin also has limited effectiveness against *H. influenzae*, a common pathogen in respiratory tract infections.

The macrolides reversibly bind to the "P" site on the 50S ribosomal subunit of the messenger RNA of susceptible organisms inhibiting bacterial protein synthesis. Whether their action is bactericidal or bacteriostatic depends upon the concentrations which the macrolides achieve at the locus of the infection. Chemically, the macrolides are weak bases, all of which contain a macrocyclic lactone ring to which sugars are attached. Substitutions on this ring confer the slight differences in antimicrobial spectrum of activity and efficacy and the significant variations in pharmacokinetic properties which distinguish one macrolide from another.

1. Erythromycin

Erythromycin has been widely used as an alternative to β-lactam antibiotics in the therapy of infections due to Gram-positive bacteria, as well as infections attributed to nonbacterial pathogens including *Mycoplasma* and *Chlamydia* species. This drug, which inhibits bacterial protein synthesis, is very effective against Gram-positive aerobic bacteria, among them *S. epidermidis*, *Streptococcus* species including groups A, B, C, and G *streptococci*, *S. pneumoniae*, *S. viridans*, and *S. aureus*, including β-lactamase-producing strains. Among the Gram-negative aerobic bacteria, erythromycin has activity against *N. meningitidis, H. influenzae, Legionella*, and *Bordetella pertussis*. It is also active against *C. trachomatis*, *Rickettsia, Treponema pallidum*, and many mycobacterial species.

Erythromycin is active against a wide spectrum of Gram-positive anaerobes, although its effectiveness against Gram-negative anaerobes is variable due to bacterial resistance. In general, antimicrobial resistance to erythromycin is an emerging problem, particularly with staphylococci and streptococci. Cross resistance with other macrolide and lincosamide antibiotics has been reported.

As noted above, erythromycin base is acid labile and is irritating to the stomach. To improve absorption and avoid this irritation the oral preparations of erythromycin base are manufactured with a variety of enteric coatings. A variety of erythromycin salts and esters have also been developed to improve the bioavailability and palatability of this drug. These include the salt erythromycin stearate and the ester erythromycin ethyl succinate, both of which are still somewhat acid labile, and propionyl erythromycin ester lauryl sulfate, also called erythromycin estolate. This preparation, which is the salt of an ester, more effectively resists destruction by gastric acid and can be administered without regard to the timing of meals. There are also two soluble salts of erythromycin that can be administered intravenously and an ethyl succinate preparation of erythromycin which can be injected intramuscularly. However, because the dosage is large and the infection painful this route of administration is seldom employed. All the oral preparations are about equally absorbed.

Erythromycin is widely and adequately distributed into all tissues except the CNS. It is concentrated in the liver and spleen. Erythromycin is cleared primarily by hepatic biotransformation and biliary excretion, which produces high drug levels in the feces. About 2.5% of orally administered erythromycin and about 15% of an injected dose is excreted unchanged in the urine. The normal elimination half-life of erythromycin is approximately 1.5 hours. This is prolonged to approximately 5.0 hours in renal failure, and no dosage adjustment is recommended in such patients. Liver dysfunction, however, does result in accumulation of erythromycin. Results of one study indicate that the mean elimination half-life for erythromycin is significantly longer in elderly patients after multiple dosing. The investigator suggests that the hepatic biotransformation of erythromycin is impaired in the elderly, necessitating dosage reduction in this population.[32]

Erythromycin is a safe and effective alternative to β-lactam antibiotics and is particularly valuable for patients who have allergic contraindications precluding the use of penicillins and cephalosporins. It is one of the alternate drugs, along with clindamycin and vancomycin, for endocarditis prophylaxis after oropharyngeal procedures. The most common adverse effects of erythromycin are GI including nausea, vomiting, and diarrhea. Rapid intravenous infusion of concentrated erythromycin solutions frequently produces thrombophlebitis and pain. Intramuscular injections of erythromycin produce severe local pain and, as mentioned above, are seldom used. Reversible sensory-neural hearing loss is sometimes associated with high-dose parenteral erythromycin therapy, and cholestatic hepatitis is an infrequent but serious adverse effect attributed exclusively to erythromycin estolate.

Erythromycin and other macrolides participate in numerous drug interactions, which may have important implications for the elderly as a result of their ability to inhibit hepatic drug metabolism mediated by the cytochrome P450 (microsomal) system. Agents whose pharmacokinetics have been shown to be altered as a consequence of this inhibition include the oral anticoagulants (coumadin, warfarin), theophylline, carbamazepine, cyclosporin, and methylprednisolone. The concurrent use of erythromycin and the nonsedating antihistamines terfinidine or astemizole, which rely on hepatic microsomal biotransformation for their clearance, has resulted in a drug interaction producing life-threatening cardiac arrhythmias (torsade de pointes). Similar interactions have been reported for the newer macrolides (see below). Avoiding such adverse cardiovascular sequellae requires ongoing vigilance, particularly in elderly patients who may be using multiple medications.

Erythromycin is the preferred empiric therapy for atypical pneumonia and for *M. pneumoniae*, *C. pneumoniae*, and *Legionella* infections. It is also a preferred agent for treating chancroid, pertussis, diphtheria, *Chlamydia* infections in pregnant females and children, chronic *C. prostatitis*, and enteritis caused by *Campylobacter* species.

2. Newer Macrolides

- Azithromycin
- Clarithromycin

Two new macrolide antibiotics, azithromycin and clarithromycin, have recently been approved by the Food and Drug Administration for treatment of respiratory tract infection and infections of skin and skin structures. Beyond these indications, azithromycin has also been approved for the treatment of nongonococcal urethritis and cervicitis caused by *Chlamydia trachomatis*. These drugs, which are chemically related to erythromycin, represent the most recent effort to improve upon the bioavailability, potency, spectrum of antimicrobial activity, and drug resistance pattern of erythromycin.

a. Azithromycin

Azithromycin is a semisynthetic macrolide which differs from erythromycin in the addition of a methyl-substituted nitrogen into this lactone ring. Azithromycin is considered an alternative to the first-line therapy of mild to moderate upper and lower respiratory tract infection and infection of the skin and its structures caused by susceptible organisms. In these indications azithromycin is administered orally in a dose of 500 mg on the first day of therapy, followed by 250 mg daily for an additional 4 days of treatment. Used in the treatment of sexually transmitted diseases caused by *C. trachomatis, N. gonorrhoeae*, and *Ureaplasma urealyticum*, azithromycin has been found effective in a single oral dose of 1 g. The manufacturer cautions prescribers that azithromycin should not be used to treat pneumonias considered too severe or patients judged too complicated, e.g., debilitated patients, to manage in the outpatient setting or when there are additional risk factors such as immunodeficiency, which could compromise the patient's ability to respond to therapy.

Azithromycin is well absorbed orally with a bioavailability of about 37%. Food decreases its absorption, so azithromycin should be given at least 1 hour before or 2 hours after meals.

Peak serum levels of 0.41 mg/L are achieved 3 to 4 hours after oral dosing. Aluminum and magnesium-containing antacids reduce peak azithromycin serum levels, but not the extent of azithromycin absorption. The drug is well distributed to tissues, which attain higher concentrations than serum. Azithromycin is cleared primarily via biliary excretion of the parent compound and by hepatic biotransformation. For this reason caution is advised in the use of azithromycin in patients with impaired hepatic function. Only small amounts, about 6%, are excreted unchanged in the urine. The extensive tissue distribution of azithromycin contributes to the low serum concentration this drug achieves. In particular, azithromycin has been reported to concentrate within macrophages and polymorphonuclear leukocytes. Extensive distribution also prolongs the presence of the drug in the organism contributing to a serum elimination half-life reported to average between 50 and 68 hours. The half-life and tissue distribution of azithromycin, pharmacokinetic characteristics which make it suitable for once-a-day dosing, exceed those of erythromycin. These attributes are especially useful in the outpatient treatment of *C. trachomatis* and represent an advantage over tetracycline, erythromycin, and doxycycline which, although just as effective as azithromycin, exhibit less satisfactory compliance with therapy because they must be administered in multidose, multiday regimens. In clinical studies, pharmacokinetic parameters in older volunteers were similar to those of younger individuals during a 5-day course of therapy. Dosage adjustment is unnecessary in older patients with normal renal and hepatic function.[33] Because of its structural similarity to erythromycin, caution should be exercised in combining azithromycin with agents known to interact with other macrolide antibiotics (see page 293).

Azithromycin efficacy against infections of the lower respiratory tract, e.g., acute bronchitis and pneumonia, is comparable to that of amoxicillin, amoxicillin with clavulinic acid, and erythromycin. Against sinusitis, amoxicillin and azithromycin produced similar clinical cure rates. Compared to a 10-day (500 mg B.I.D.) course of cephalexin therapy, a 5-day course of azithromycin (500 mg on day 1 followed by 250 mg times four additional days) was judged to be equally effective in the treatment of skin and soft-tissue infections.

Interestingly, although azithromycin is not indicated for first-line therapy in the immunocompromised patient, this drug is effective in treating disseminated *Mycobacterium avium-intracellulare* complex infections in patients with Acquired Immunodeficiency Syndrome (AIDS). About 75% of evaluable AIDS patients treated with daily doses of 500 mg azithromycin experienced resolution of infection-related symptoms.

b. Clarithromycin

Clarithromycin is a semisynthetic macrolide antibiotic which differs from erythromycin through substitution of a methoxy group for a hydroxy group at position 6 of the macrolide ring. Although its spectrum of antimicrobial activity is similar to erythromycin, this simple, single structural change confers upon clarithromycin a 200 to 400% increase in efficacy, compared to erythromycin, against most staphylococci and streptococci pathogens. The 6-methoxy substitution also avoids the rearrangement of the macrolide ring in the acid environment of the stomach, which contributes to the GI irritation commonly observed with erythromycin.

Like erythromycin and azithromycin, clarithromycin inhibits protein synthesis in susceptible organisms by penetrating the cell wall and binding to 50 S ribosomal subunit inhibiting the translocation of aminoacyl transfer RNA, thus inhibiting polypeptide and protein synthesis.

Clarithromycin is rapidly absorbed from the GI tract after oral administration. The oral bioavailability is about 50 to 55% and is not reduced in the presence of food, although food does delay the formation of the active metabolite of clarithromycin, 14-hydroxy clarithromycin, which is reported to be more active against *H. influenzae* than the parent compound and acts synergistically to increase the potency of the parent compound. Clarithromycin is 65 to 70% bound to plasma proteins. Clarithromycin is well distributed into most tissues except the CNS. At serum concentrations of 2.0 mg/L, clarithromycin achieves levels approximately eight to ten times higher in polymorphonuclear leukocytes. Clarithromycin also concentrates in lung tissue at levels six to ten times those achieved in the serum.

Clarithromycin is cleared primarily by the renal route at a rate which approximates the glomerular filtration rate. The major biotransformation product, 14-hydroxy clarithromycin, accounts for 10 to 15% of the urinary excretion. Like other macrolides, clarithromycin is also partially biotransformed to an N-desmethyl metabolite. Only small amounts are excreted via bile and feces. Clarithromycin metabolism appears to be saturable at higher concentrations, inasmuch as the half-life of the parent compound increases from 4 hours after a single 250-mg dose to 11 hours after administration of 1200 mg. The half-life of the 14-hydroxyl metabolite increases similarly with increased dosage. This prolonged half-life allows clarithromycin to be administered twice a day.

Compared to erythromycin, clarithromycin has a similar spectrum of activity, but is more effective against *S. aureus*, *Streptococcus pyogenes*, and *S. pneumoniae*. These differences may be attributable to the pharmacokinetic profile of clarithromycin. Its ability to concentrate in pulmonary tissues and polymorphonuclear leukocytes would appear to favor its efficacy in *S. aureus* respiratory infections. Clarithromycin is FDA approved for acute exacerbations of chronic bronchitis caused by susceptible strains of *H. influenzae*, *Moraxella catarrhalis*, and *Streptococcus pneumoniae*. Clarithromycin is also indicated for the treatment of pharyngitis and tonsillitis caused by *S. pyogenes* as well as pneumonia caused by *Mycoplasma pneumoniae* or *S. pneumoniae*. The other FDA-approved indications of clarithromycin include the treatment of acute maxillary sinusitis caused by *S. pneumoniae* and infections of skin and skin structure infections caused by *S. aureus* and *S. pyogenes*.

Use of clarithromycin in patients with renal impairment (creatinine clearance less than 30 mL/min) results in higher peak plasma concentrations and prolonged half-life compared with patients having creatinine clearance greater than 80 mL/min, although the manufacturer makes no specific recommendations on the extent of dose reductions in this population, nor are there specific dose reductions recommended based solely on age in normal dosing situations (see below). On the other hand, if renal function is normal no dosage reduction is needed in patients with hepatic impairment according to the manufacturer. The higher peak serum concentrations and area under the curve observed in elderly patients parallel age-related decreases in renal function. Adjustments in clarithromycin dosing regimens, therefore, may not be necessary solely on the basis of age.[34] Elderly patients did not experience an increased incidence of adverse events than younger patients during clinical trials involving normal dosing regimens and in normal doses. However, in high doses (2000 mg/d) clarithromycin use was associated with an increase in adverse reactions for elderly patients (mean age 70 years) having reduced creatinine clearances.[35]

Both azithromycin and clarithromycin cause reversible elevations in liver enzymes (SGOT, SGPT, GGT, alkaline phosphatase). Reversible asymptomatic elevation of aminotransferases and GGT were observed in one study in which the rate of appearance of these elevations was slightly lower for azithromycin (5.2%) than for erythromycin (6.8%).

Few documented drug-drug interactions have been reported with either azithromycin or clarithromycin. Because of its structural similarity to erythromycin, however, vigilance is recommended when using clarithromycin together with drugs known to interact with erythromycin (see page 293). Carbamazepine blood levels increased following single-dose administration of clarithromycin, and clarithromycin may be associated with increased serum theophylline concentrations when theophylline is used concurrently in higher therapeutic concentrations.

D. TETRACYCLINES

- Tetracycline

- Oxytetracycline
- Demeclocycline
- Methacycline
- Doxycycline
- Minocycline

The tetracyclines are a group of six structurally similar antibiotics which have been developed over the last 40 years and which share similar antimicrobial spectra. Pharmacokinetically, substitution on the fused, four-ring "tetracyclic" structure confers different onsets and durations of action to this group of compounds. In this regard tetracycline and oxytetracycline have been designated short-acting drugs, demeclocycline and methacycline have been designated intermediate-acting compounds, and doxycycline and minocycline, which are also available for intravenous use, have been identified as long-acting agents.

Tetracyclines produce only bacteriostatic effects. They interfere with bacterial protein synthesis by preventing attachment of transfer RNA to the messenger RNA complex at the 30S ribosomal subunit. Selective toxicity is dose related and appears to depend in part upon the active (energy-dependent) uptake of drug into bacterial, but not mammalian cells. At higher concentrations the tetracyclines inhibit mammalian protein synthesis to some extent. Differences in potency parallel the pharmacokinetic distinctions among these drugs. In this regard, tetracycline and oxytetracycline are considered the least potent compared to doxycycline and minocycline (agents with the greatest lipophilic characteristics) which are the most potent compounds in this group. In general, despite these differences, the tetracyclines as a group share a common antimicrobial spectrum including Gram-positive, Gram-negative anaerobic and aerobic organisms, as well as *Chlamydia* species, *Mycoplasma* species, *Rickettsiae* spirochetes and selected protozoa.

Susceptible organisms include many strains of Gram-positive cocci including *S. viridans* and *S. pyogenes* (group A), *S. agalactiae* (group B), and the anaerobic streptococci. Activity, however, is variable against *S. aureus* and *S. pneumoniae*, as well as most strains of enterococci, since many of these pathogens have developed resistance. Consequently, the tetracyclines are not usually employed in the therapy of streptococcal infections.

Tetracyclines have activity against and are employed as alternative therapy for penicillin-sensitive individuals infected with many Gram-positive bacilli, including *Clostridium tetani, Bacillus anthracis*, and *Listeria monocytogenes*, as well as some *Actinomyces* and *Nocardia* species.

Resistance to tetracyclines has emerged for many Gram-negative aerobic pathogens. This is particularly true for *N. gonorrhoeae*, for which tetracycline monotherapy is no longer considered adequate. *N. meningitidis* is sensitive to selected tetracyclines (e.g., minocycline), but because they are bacteriostatic, not bactericidal, these agents have likewise been judged incomplete therapy for meningococcal infections.

The activity of tetracyclines is also variable against many enteric Gram-negative species. Many strains of *E. coli, Klebsiella, Enterobacter, Proteus*, and *Serratia* are resistant and almost all *Pseudomonas aeruginosa* and many *Acinetobacter* species are resistant. The tetracyclines are also less than completely effective against Gram-negative anaerobic pathogens, since resistance is common among many *Bacteroides* strains as well as *Fusobacterium.*

Tetracyclines are, however, among the agents of choice in treating infections caused by certain Gram-negative bacilli. These include, among others, *H. pylori, Vibrio cholerae, Brucella, Yersinia enterocolitica, Bordetella pertussis*, and many strains of *Hemophilus influenzae*. Both tetracycline and doxycycline are active against *Legionella pneumophilia*; however, combination treatment employing erythromycin plus rifampin remains the therapy of choice for this microorganism. Tetracyclines are also among the preferred therapy for infections caused by *M. pneumoniae*, *Chlamydia trachomatis*, *C. pneumoniae*, many *Rickettsia* species, *Borrelia burgdorferi* (the Lyme disease pathogen), *Treponema pallidum, Leptospira,* and, in high concentrations, the following protozoal infestations: *Plasmodium falciparum* (selected strains) and *Entamoeba histolytica*, among others.

Resistance to the tetracyclines is attributed to one of two primary mechanisms: (1) plasmid-mediated interference with the ability of a tetracycline to accumulate within the bacterial cell often seen in the *Enterobacteriaceae* and (2) ribosomal protection, which prevents effective binding of the tetracyclines to bacterial ribosomes, common in a variety of Gram-positive and Gram-negative bacteria, among them *Neisseria* species.

All the tetracyclines can be administered orally and are absorbed with bioavailabilities ranging from 58% (oxytetracycline) to 95% (minocycline). The oral absorption of the short- and intermediate-acting drugs is diminished in the presence of food, but food appears to have little influence on the bioavailability of the long-acting tetracyclines. As a group, the tetracyclines form insoluble chelates with a variety of bivalent and trivalent cations which are found in the diet or in other medications. These include calcium, magnesium, and aluminum, which are found in over-the-counter antacids and laxatives, and zinc and iron, which are components of multivitamins, among other dietary supplements. Since the elderly frequently use these products they must be instructed to avoid them during concomitant therapy with the tetracyclines. Interestingly, dairy products, although they contain calcium, have been reported to influence absorption of minocycline and doxycycline only minimally.

Although available for parenteral administration as well as oral dosing, rapid intravenous injection of doxycycline and minocycline should be avoided. Oxytetracycline can be administered by intramuscular injection, but the route is painful, poorly bioavailable, and is therefore not recommended. Plasma protein binding, although variable, appears to be less for the short-acting tetracyclines, greater for the long- and intermediate-acting agents. The volumes of distribution are, conversely, lowest for the long-acting tetracyclines. Tissue penetration can generally be predicted on the basis of the lipid to water partition coefficient of the tetracyclines. Doxycycline and minocycline, for example, the most lipid-soluble tetracyclines, penetrate into tissues (renal, prostatic, endometrial, etc.) and secretions (cerebrospinal fluid, saliva, tears, etc.) more readily than the short-acting agents. This phenomenon has been implicated in the vestibular toxicity associated with minocycline, since the cells of the vestibular apparatus have a high lipid content. Tetracyclines preferentially distribute into rapidly metabolizing and growing tissues, including bone, teeth (in the fetus and neonate), and hepatic tissue.

Renal clearance is not the exclusive route of tetracycline elimination, but is the most important factor in determining the durations of action of the tetracyclines. The short-acting agents have high renal clearance and the intermediate-acting agents moderate renal clearance. The half-lives of all these agents are significantly prolonged in renal insufficiency. The long-acting tetracyclines depend much less upon renal clearance for their elimination. Minocycline may undergo considerable biotransformation and enterohepatic recirculation. The pharmacokinetics of doxycycline are likewise apparently not influenced by renal function or, for that matter, hepatic function. Excretion is by fecal elimination of an inactive chelate, which does not modify the colonic microflora. These pharmacokinetic attributes, among others, present certain advantages in the use of doxycycline over other drugs in this class, particularly in patients with renal insufficiency, including the elderly. No other dose adjustment recommendations have appeared in the literature regarding the use of the tetracyclines in the elderly, nor do the manufacturers of these agents offer any specific advice about their use in this population.

GI complaints are among the most common adverse reactions associated with the tetracyclines. These include epigastric discomfort, nausea, vomiting, and diarrhea which are attributed to the direct local irritation of the GI tract. After several days of oral administration, all the tetracyclines (with the exception of doxycycline) alter the balance of the intestinal microflora. Although this rarely results in *Clostridium difficile*-mediated colitis, *Pseudomonas, Proteus,* staphylococci, resistant coliforms, and *Candida* can become prominent. When pseudomembranous colitis associated with *Clostridium difficile* does emerge it must be treated promptly with oral vancomycin.

High-dose intravenous therapy with tetracyclines has been associated with impaired hepatic function. This is especially likely when these drugs are used in pregnant patients or those with existing hepatic insufficiency. Intravenous administration of 4 g/d or more has been reported to cause hepatic necrosis in some cases. Pre-existing renal insufficiency can likewise be exacerbated by all the tetracyclines except doxycycline. This has been attributed to an inhibition of protein synthesis and resultant azotemia. Renal tubular acidosis and other renal injury resulting from nitrogen retention has been associated with the use of outdated tetracyclines.

The above-mentioned vestibular toxicity, associated particularly with minocycline, is manifested by dizziness, tinnitus, vertigo, ataxia, nausea, and vomiting. Fortunately, this symptom complex which usually appears after several days of therapy is reversible after discontinuation of the drug. Because of the risk of hip fractures and other injuries which may result in the elderly, use of minocycline in this population requires careful monitoring and may not present sufficient benefit to offset these potential problems.

True drug allergy to one tetracycline implies a class allergy for the affected patient. Allergic reaction associated with tetracycline, including skin rashes and drug fever, are uncommon. Systemic administration of the tetracyclines, particularly demeclocycline, can induce sensitivity to sunlight and ultraviolet light, especially in fair-skinned individuals. Patients often confuse GI intolerance, common to the tetracyclines, with drug allergy and must be questioned carefully to distinguish between these types of adverse experiences.

Tetracyclines are widely used for many types of infections. They were the first broad-spectrum antibiotics developed and their effectiveness against a wide variety of microorganisms has resulted, unfortunately, in their indiscriminate administration. This had led to the emergence of bacterial resistance and the advent of superinfecting, tetracycline-resistant organisms in the hospital setting. Earlier indiscriminate use of these agents in the livestock industry has also led to the spread of tetracycline-resistant bacteria among those working in this field and the public at large.

On the positive side, tetracyclines are among the agents of choice for treating infections attributed to *M. pneumonia*, *Chlamydia, Rickettsia*, and some *Spirochetes*. They are also among the preferred agents for ehrlichiosis, a tick-borne Rickettsial infection caused by *Ehrlichia chaffeensis*, as well as brucellosis, cholera, melodiosis, leiptospirosis, relapsing fever, and *V. vulnificus* infections. They are used successfully in respiratory tract mixed-bacterial infections including sinusitis and bronchitis, as well as other mixed Gram-positive and Gram-negative infections, provided resistance is not present. In early Lyme disease (stage I) a 3-week course of oral tetracycline or doxycycline is the preferred therapy for adults (not pregnant women, however) and children ages 8 and older. A 30-day course of therapy with these agents may also be useful in the treatment of stage II and/or stage III Lyme disease when accompanied by mild neurologic or cardiac findings and arthritis, respectively.

The tetracyclines are accepted second-line therapy in the treatment of syphilis, *Y. enterocolitica* gastroenteritis, tularemia, and actinomycosis. In brucellosis, tularemia and plague, tetracyclines are often combined with an aminoglycoside. Protozoal infections including chloroquine-resistant *P. falciparum* and *Entamoeba histolytica* can be treated with tetracyclines as alternate therapy.

Although at one time tetracycline was used inappropriately for the systemic treatment of mild acne, these agents do have a recognized role as the therapy of choice in the treatment of severe chronic inflammatory lesions attributable to *Acne vulgaris* which are unresponsive to topical therapy alone.

Finally, tetracyclines combined with metronidazole and bismuth subsalicylate constitutes the preferred "triple therapy" of *Helicobacter pylori*-mediated peptic ulcer disease, including those patients with complications and/or those who would otherwise be considered for surgery.

Besides the above-mentioned interference with tetracycline absorption caused by certain cations, these agents participate in several important drug-drug interactions which must be considered in any multiple-drug therapeutic regimen that includes the tetracyclines.

Pharmacokinetic drug interactions which involve tetracyclines are caused by concomitant administration of agents which enhance hepatic biotransformation, among them phenytoin, carbamazapine, barbiturates, and chronic ethanol ingestion. These agents accelerate the cytochrome P450-dependent metabolism of the tetracyclines and produce lower antibiotic plasma levels. Bismuth subsalicylate has been reported to decrease the absorption of doxycycline and other tetracyclines when they are used as combination therapy for travelers' diarrhea. The use of an alternating administration regimen for the bismuth salt and antibiotic can prevent this problem.

Alteration of the gut microflora by the tetracyclines (all except doxycycline) can prevent inactivation of digoxin by these microorganisms, significantly raising serum digoxin levels and the risk of toxicity. Because the impact of most of the tetracyclines on bowel microflora is persistent, clinical and laboratory monitoring for digoxin toxicity is recommended and may be of particular value in elderly patients taking cardiac glycosides regularly. The same mechanism may be responsible for the decrease of vitamin K-dependent clotting factors and a prolongation of the prothrombin time of patients receiving coumarin-type anticoagulants. Monitoring of the prothrombin status in these patients, many of whom are elderly, may likewise be valuable. Tetracyclines have also been reported to elevate serum lithium concentrations, but the mechanism is unknown.

Other drug interactions include serious renal toxicity and deaths reported following the concomitant use of tetracyclines and the gaseous anesthetic methoxyflurane. Concurrent use of tetracyclines and diuretics has been reported to increase the blood urea nitrogen concentration, suggesting that caution be exercised in patients with pre-existing renal insufficiency, including the elderly, who may be receiving both these classes of drugs. Since tetracyclines are frequently used in combination with other antimicrobials there have been reports of their interference with the bactericidal effect of some other agents, particularly penicillin. Tetracyclines have also been reported to increase the effect of oral hypoglycemic agents (tolbutamide) and insulin in some patients.

E. NITROMIDAZOLES

- Metronidazole

This synthetic antimicrobial was developed to treat protozoal infections, and first saw clinical use in the early 1960s as oral therapy for urogenital (vaginal) trichomoniasis. Since that time, however, metronidazole has been proven an effective bactericidal agent against obligate anaerobic Gram-negative bacteria, including *Bacteroides* species. It is less effective against Gram-positive anaerobes such as *Peptococcus*, *Peptostreptococcus*, and *Clostridium* species. It is also effective against anaerobic protozoa including *Enamoeba histolytica*, *Giardia lamblia*, and *Balantidium coli*. Except for *Gardnerella vaginalis* and *Campylobacter fetus*, metronidazole is not effective against obligate aerobic microorganisms, facultative aerobes, or microaerophiles. Acquired resistance to metronidazole is rare and the precise mechanism of resistance, when it does emerge, is not understood. Cross resistance does not develop, probably because metronidazole is chemically and structurally different from other agents used in the therapy of anaerobic bacterial infections.

Metronidazole can be administered parenterally, orally, or rectally. Oral bioavailability is approximately 80 to 85%, which is unaffected by food. Food, however, does prolong the time required to achieve peak plasma concentrations. Rectal absorption is variable. Metronidazole is widely distributed to all tissues, including the CNS, the cerebrospinal fluid, and even penetrates into abscesses. Metronidazole is only 10 to 20% bound to plasma proteins.

Less than 20% of an administered dose is excreted unchanged in the urine. The majority of its clearance is attributed to hepatic biotransformation with the metabolites excreted primarily in the urine and to a lesser extent in the bile. In patients with normal hepatic and renal function, metronidazole has an elimination half-life which ranges from 4 to 7 hours. In patients with renal failure, half-life is prolonged to approximately 10 hours.

Metronidazole dosage should be adjusted in patients with severe hepatic insufficiency. While renal insufficiency does not impair clearance to the point at which dose adjustment is necessary, renal failure can lead to the accumulation of the biotransformation products of metronidazole which may be associated with neurotoxicity. In such cases dosage adjustment may also be warranted. In clinical trials elderly patients have demonstrated reduced renal excretion of both the parent drug and hydroxy metabolite of metronidazole. Interestingly, this appears to influence the clearance of the metabolite, but not the metronidazole itself. In general, the ability to eliminate metronidazole appears to be preserved in old age, and consequently age-related dose adjustments are usually not needed.[36,37] However, because the pharmacokinetics of metronidazole may be altered in the elderly, according to the manufacturer, the monitoring of serum drug levels may be necessary to adjust the dosage accordingly.

Few side effects are associated with metronidazole therapy. Mild GI symptoms including xerostomia, anorexia, nausea, vomiting, and a bitter metallic taste are among the most frequent complaints associated with its use. Other effects include headache, confusion, dizziness, rash, urticaria, vaginal and urethral burning, and darkening of the urine. The most serious adverse experiences affect the CNS, including peripheral neuropathy and convulsions. For these reasons the drug should be used cautiously in patients with a history of seizures. Reversible neutropenia occurs rarely during metronidazole therapy, and leukocyte counts (total and differential) are recommended before, during, and after therapy for this reason.

Several drugs interact with metronidazole. Concurrent alcohol use causes a disulfuram-like reaction including headache, facial flushing, nausea, vomiting, and abdominal cramps. Clearly, metronidazole should never be combined with disulfuram itself. Inhibitors of the cytochrome P450-dependent biotransformation of metronidazole by cimetidine and stimulation of its biotransformation by phenobarbital may cause toxicity or therapeutic failure, respectively.

Metronidazole itself interferes with the biotransformation of the oral anticoagulants coumarin and warfarin and, consequently, increases their anticoagulant activity. Metronidazole also interferes with serum chemistry assays for aspartate aminotransferase, alanine aminotransferase, lactic dehydrogenase, and triglycerides, among other things.

Metronidazole is useful in the therapy of infections caused by obligate anaerobic bacteria. However, because many such infections are mixed involving both anaerobic and aerobic pathogens, metronidazole is often combined with another drug which is effective against aerobic bacteria.

Metronidazole is a therapy of choice for endocarditis caused in rare circumstances by *Bacteroides fragilis* or other *Bacteroides* species and is also effective against intra-abdominal soft tissue and pelvic infections caused by susceptible microorganisms. Its reliable bactericidal activity and penetration into the CNS have made metronidazole a mainstay in the therapy of brain abscesses caused by Gram-negative anaerobes.

Because of recently emerged drug resistance on the part of someGram-positive aerobic bacteria to vancomycin, metronidazole is now the drug of choice to treat other clinical uses include the therapy of bacterial vaginosis (applied as a local cream), antibiotic-induced *Clostridium difficile* colitis, and as a component of the three-part therapy of susceptible *H. pylori* gastritis (together with either amoxicillin or tetracycline and bismuth salts).

Finally, metronidazole is the therapy of choice for various parasitic infestations including amebiasis, giardiasis, and trichomoniasis.

F. QUINOLONES

- Ciprofloxacin
- Norfloxacin
- Ofloxacin
- Enoxacin
- Lomefloxacin

The fluorinated piperazinyl quinolones are potent, broad-spectrum antimicrobial agents which interfere with the repair, replication, transposition, and transcription of bacterial DNA. These agents are effective against Gram-negative aerobic bacteria including *Pseudomonas aeruginosa* as well as many Gram-positive aerobic species. Because of bacterial resistance, which is either chromosomally mediated or due to reduced drug permeability, quinolones are ineffective against anaerobic bacteria including *B. fragilis* and *C. difficile*. Five fluorinated quinolones, ciprofloxacin, norfloxacin, ofloxacin, enoxacin, and lomefloxacin, are available commercially. With few exceptions, the spectrum of antibiotic activity is similar for all the fluoroquinolones. Ciprofloxacin is the most potent agent in treating infections caused by the Gram-negative bacteria including *P. aeruginosa*, against which most other quinolones are less effective. Among Gram-positive bacteria most fluoroquinolones generally have poor activity against *Streptococcus* species; otherwise, ciprofloxacin and ofloxacin are the quinolone antibiotics most effective in treating Gram-positive bacterial infections as well as *Mycobacterium tuberculosis* and several other mycobacterial species.

Oral bioavailability of the quinolones varies from a low of 40% (norfloxacin) to over 90% (ofloxacin, lomefloxacin, and enoxacin). The bioavailability of ciprofloxacin (75%) falls between these two extremes. Absorption of lomefloxacin is unchanged in the elderly.

Orally administered quinolones can form insoluble chelates when they are given with foods, drugs, or vitamins containing metals such as calcium, iron, magnesium, zinc, and aluminum. Examples of such ingested substances include dairy products (calcium), antacids (calcium, magnesium, aluminum), iron supplements, and multivitamins (zinc and iron). To avoid reduced bioavailability, ingestion of these substances should be separate from dosing with quinolones by 2 to 3 hours.

The fluoroquinolones are well distributed throughout the body, achieving high intracellular concentrations in neutrophils and monocytes. These agents demonstrate poor distribution into the cerebrospinal fluid in most cases. Although inflammation of the meninges improves this, even low concentrations of these agents in the cerebrospinal fluid (10% of serum levels) provide activity against CNS infections, including meningitis attributable to Gram-negative rods. Plasma protein binding varies from 10 to 40%.

Glomerular filtration and, to a lesser extent, tubular secretion are the primary excretory pathways for most of the fluoroquinolones. All fluoroquinolones except ofloxacin, which is cleared renally essentially unchanged, are also biotransformed in the liver through a combination of cleavage (oxidation, hydroxylation) and conjugation (glucuronidation) reactions. Consequently, the elimination half-life of ofloxacin is significantly prolonged (500% increase) in renal failure compared to the other fluoroquinolones. In healthy elderly volunteers with normal renal function based upon their age, but reduced compared to young adults, norfloxacin is cleared more slowly and has a slightly longer elimination half-life. Mean peak plasma enoxacin concentrations were 50% higher in elderly patients vs. young adults reflecting their age-related reduction in renal function. Plasma clearance of lomefloxacin is reduced, however, by about 25% and the AUC increased by approximately 32% in elderly patients reflecting age-related decreases in renal function. Some investigators have suggested that ofloxacin, lomefloxacin, and enoxacin, which have higher 24-h urinary excretion rates, should be administered at lower doses according to the age of the patient, in order to prevent adverse reactions.[38] It has also been suggested that the dose of ofloxacin be reduced in patients more than 75 years old, to at least to one half of that given to younger patients.[39] However, the reports are contradictory. Other studies have concluded that dosage adjustments should not be necessary in elderly patients with only minor reductions in renal function caused by age-related changes.[40–42] It appears that no consistent conclusions can be made regarding the necessity of dose reductions from a pharmacokinetic point of view. However, reports of adverse reactions to quinolones in the elderly, especially concentration-dependent CNS symptoms, and the risk of interaction with other drugs, suggest the need for caution in determining dosages of all of these compounds in elderly subjects.[43] Despite these pharmacokinetic differences, the safety and efficacy of this drug in elderly patients was the same as in younger patients. Renal and hepatic insufficiency both variably prolong the elimination half-lives of these drugs.

The fluoroquinolones are generally well tolerated. The most commonly reported adverse experiences are GI symptoms (nausea, vomiting, and abdominal pain), and these are noted by fewer than 5% of the patients using these agents. Rarely, *C. difficile* has been implicated in the diarrhea sometimes observed during fluoroquinolone therapy. Mild CNS findings including headache, blurred vision, anxiety, restlessness, insomnia, and confusion have been reported following fluoroquinolone use. More serious CNS findings including seizures and convulsions, however, have been reported to occur with all these agents, especially in elderly patients. In multiple-dose clinical studies in elderly patients the elderly experienced significantly more adverse reactions than individuals under age 65, although the incidence of reactions judged to be drug related was comparable across age groups.[43]

Allergic reactions including rashes, photosensitivity, and acute anaphylaxis have also been reported. Because of cartilage damage observed in animal studies, fluoroquinolones are not recommended for use in pregnant women or children, but cartilage damage has not been observed as a problem in elderly patients using these antibiotics. However, arthritis symptoms have been reported following the intravenous use of ofloxacin.

The fluoroquinolones have been demonstrated to interfere with the hepatic clearance of a variety of drugs which are biotransformed by cytochrome P450-mediated mixed-function oxidation reactions. Examples include theophylline, warfarin, and caffeine. This inhibition varies among the fluoroquinolones, being highest for enoxacin, lower for ciprofloxacin and norfloxacin, and minimal for the other fluoroquinolones. Because of this interaction, fluoroquinolones should be cautiously used with narrow therapeutic window drugs like theophylline, which rely on hepatic P450-mediated oxidation for their clearance. When administered concomitantly, blood levels, for example, serum theophylline concentrations, should be monitored frequently to assess the impact of this interaction on the pharmacokinetics of such narrow therapeutic window agents.

Clinically, the fluoroquinolones are useful in the treatment of infections caused by multidrug-resistant Gram-negative aerobic bacteria including *P. aeruginosa*. The fluoroquinolones have been used successfully in the treatment of genitourinary infections including complicated infections of the urinary tract, gonococcal urethritis, cervicitis, and bacterial prostatitis. They are also indicated for Gram-negative bacillary infections of the respiratory tract and for osteomyelitis and septic arthritis caused by susceptible Gram-negative organisms. Other indications for the fluoroquinolones include skin and soft tissue infections, bacterial gastroenteritis, fever, and Gram-negative bacteremia. Ciprofloxacin has been used interchangeably with ofloxacin in the therapy of multidrug-resistant tuberculosis. Data from one clinical trial indicate that ciprofloxacin and rifampin may be given concomitantly in standard clinical dosing regimens. The combination results in therapeutic levels of both drugs and appears to be safe for administration to elderly nursing home patients.[44]

G. VANCOMYCIN

Vancomycin, introduced in 1956, is a narrow-spectrum polypeptide antibiotic which is effective against Gram-positive aerobic bacteria including methicillin-resistant staphylococci, enterococci, and anaerobic bacteria including *C. difficile*. While most enterococci are sensitive to vancomycin, this drug administered alone is only bacteriostatic against these organisms and must be combined with an aminoglycoside to achieve a bactericidal effect. Vancomycin has no activity against Gram-negative bacteria.

Vancomycin inhibits bacterial cell wall synthesis at a different location than the β-lactam antibiotics. Both plasmid- and chromosomal-mediated bacterial resistance to this drug on the part of some Gram-positive organisms has emerged as a limiting factor in vancomycin therapy. In fact, many hospitals now restrict vancomycin use to infectious disease specialists and to cases of life threatening infections in which a failure to respond to metronidozale therapy has been documented.

Vancomycin is not absorbed orally, and since intramuscular injections are quite painful this drug is exclusively administered by the intravenous route, except when used orally for *C. difficile* colitis. It is well distributed to most tissues; however, penetration into the cerebrospinal fluid is poor. Clearance is predominantly renal via glomerular filtration of the unchanged drug. In normal individuals the elimination half-life ranges from 4 to 6 hours; this increases to up to 7 days in renal failure patients. The drug is not dialyzable. Dosage reduction is therefore required in patients with compromised renal function. Therapy in such cases must be monitored by routine plasma vancomycin assays for peak and trough levels. The total systemic and renal clearance of vancomycin may be reduced in elderly patients. Results of one clinical trial suggest that elderly patients exhibit significant differences in vancomycin pharmacokinetic parameters compared with young patients, and the investigator recommends individualized vancomycin dosing in the elderly.[45]

Once a problem for earlier dosage forms, nephrotoxicity is now uncommon with vancomycin except when it is given in combination with an aminoglycoside. The same holds true for ototoxicity. Because of the risks for both ototoxicity and nephrotoxicity, vancomycin should be used cautiously in the elderly, for whom a decrease in kidney function and hearing are common occurrences. Vancomycin is associated with common hypersensitivity reactions including fevers and rashes and an unusual response to rapid intravenous infusion called the "red man syndrome". This reaction, which results from histamine release, is not immunologic in nature, but is related to the rate of infusion of the drug. The reaction produces a characteristic erythema of the head, neck, and torso, and this cutaneous manifestation of histamine release is often accompanied by hypertension. All symptoms usually resolve quickly after the vancomycin infusion is stopped, and the syndrome can be avoided by slow infusion of this drug.

H. CLINDAMYCIN

Clindamycin, a lincosamide antibiotic which inhibits bacterial protein synthesis, is bacteriostatic against anaerobic bacteria and Gram-positive aerobic bacteria. Clindamycin is active against most *Streptococcus* and many *Staphylococcus* species. *Enterococci* are always resistant to clindamycin, as are Gram-negative aerobic bacteria. Methicillin-resistant staphylococcal strains are usually resistant to clindamycin.

Clindamycin is available in two different oral formulations, both of which are well absorbed, and one parenteral dosage form. It is well distributed to most tissues except cerebrospinal fluid. It also achieves high intracellular concentrations in monocytes and neutrophils. Clearance is primarily via hepatic biotransformation and renal excretion, with a small amount excreted in the bile. Only approximately 10% of an administered dose is excreted unchanged in the urine, and dosage adjustment is unnecessary in renal failure patients with normal hepatic function. The normal elimination half-life is 2.5 hours.

GI complaints including epigastric distress, nausea, vomiting, and diarrhea are frequently associated with clindamycin administration. The diarrhea, which more often accompanies oral administration of the antibiotic, is sometimes attributed to the cytotoxin of *C. difficile* and is more common in the elderly than in younger patients.

Clindamycin is indicated for the treatment of staphylococcal and anaerobic infections including female pelvic infections and intra-abdominal infections. In penicillin-allergic patients it can be used in the treatment of a variety of anaerobic infections normally treated with β-lactam antibiotics, including lung abscess and aspiration pneumonia, a common infection of the debilitated elderly patient.

I. TRIMETHOPRIM-SULFAMETHOXAZOLE COMBINATION THERAPY

Trimethoprim combined with sulfamethoxazole in a 5:1 ratio is one of the most commonly used fixed antibiotic combinations. Both agents individually interfere with bacterial folate synthesis, ultimately inhibiting bacterial DNA synthesis and reproduction. The individual components are only bacteriostatic, whereas the combination product is bactericidal due to the synergism achieved by the co-administration of these two drugs. The combination of trimethoprim and sulfamethoxazole is active against *Streptococcus pneumoniae*, *Hemophilus influenzae*, *Escherichia coli*, *Proteus mirabilis*, *P. vulgaris*, *Morganella morganii*, *Klebsiella* species, and *Enterobacter* species. This combination is also active against susceptible strains of *Shigella*, *Salmonella*, several species of enterotoxigenic *Escherichia coli*, and protozoa including *Pneumocystis*.

Trimethoprim and sulfamethoxazole are both absorbed well following oral administration. Neither component influences the oral absorption of the other, nor of the combination. Trimethoprim is lipid soluble and is consequently more widely distributed than sulfamethoxazole. Trimethoprim distributes well into the cerebrospinal fluid, as does sulfamethoxazole. Distribution into the cerebrospinal fluid approximately doubles for both agents when the meninges are inflamed. Following distribution the active forms of these agents achieve an optimal ratio of approximately 20 to 1 in the blood and tissues.

Approximately 80% of trimethoprim and 30% of sulfamethoxazole are excreted unchanged in the urine. In both cases the remaining percentages of each drug are cleared by hepatic biotransformation into metabolites which are subsequently excreted in the urine. The normal elimination half-lives of both components are about 10 hours, and this increases approximately 2.5 to 3.0 times in renal failure patients. Consequently, dosage adjustment in patients with renal insufficiency is necessary.

A variety of adverse experiences are associated with the sulfonamides (skin rashes, febrile mucocutaneous syndromes), some of the them serious, including Stevens-Johnson syndrome, toxic epidermal necrolysis, fulminant hepatic necrosis, agranulocytosis, aplastic anemia, and other blood dyscrasias. Nausea, diarrhea, and hypersensitivity reactions are the adverse experiences most often associated with trimethoprim. The combination of trimethoprim and sulfamethoxazole is frequently associated with severe, sometimes fatal, hematologic reactions including neutropenia, thrombocytopenia, pancytopenia, and hemolytic and megaloblastic anemia. These adverse experiences are especially common in older patients who have been administered high doses of the combination over ten or more days and in patients with depleted folate stores, including chronic alcoholics, the malnourished, and those receiving chronic anticonvulsant therapy. Not surprisingly, the elderly may experience an increased risk of severe adverse reactions when other conditions, for example, impaired kidney or liver function or concomitant drug use, are present. The adverse experiences most frequently reported in elderly patients include severe skin reactions, generalized bone marrow suppression, and thrombocytopenia.

The combination of trimethoprim and sulfamethoxazole should be used cautiously in patients with renal dysfunction because of the risk of crystalluria. Dosage adjustment should be made in renal insufficiency as noted above, and the use of this combination is not recommended when creatinine clearance is below 15 mL/min. Trimethoprim combined with sulfamethoxazole has also been reported to interact with and potentiate the action of several other medications (phenytoin, tolbutamide, coumarin anticoagulants, chlorpropamide) and cause erroneous results in some laboratory tests (methotrexate assay).

This combination has been employed in the treatment and prophylaxis of urinary tract infections and in the acute exacerbations of chronic bronchitis in adults. Trimethoprim and sulfamethoxazole are also indicated in traveler's diarrhea caused by susceptible strains of *E. coli* and in the treatment of various genitourinary infections including bacterial epididymitis, prostatitis, pyelonephritis, and cystitis. It is also a drug of choice for the treatment of *Pneumocystis carinii* infections in immunocompromised patients, among them, HIV-infected individuals. Trimethoprim alone can be used for urinary tract infections in patients who cannot tolerate sulfonamides.

J. ANTITUBERCULOSIS DRUGS

- Isoniazid
- Ethambutol
- Pyrazinamide
- Rifampin

Tuberculosis is reemerging as a public health concern in the general population. The elderly who as a group have diminished immunologic function are at particular risk, especially those who reside in nursing homes, in whom reactivation of an earlier infection and new active cases of tuberculosis are more frequently encountered.[46] Primary therapy for tuberculosis and other mycobacterial infections consists of isoniazid, also known as isonicotinic acid hydrazide, rifampin, pyrazinamide, and ethambutol. Streptomycin, the first clinically effective agent to be made commercially available for the treatment of tuberculosis, is now often included in this group. Most patients with tuberculosis can be treated effectively with a combination of these medications. For those who cannot, therapy with alternate medications, including para-amino salicylic acid, kanamycin, and amikacin, among other drugs, may be employed. This discussion will focus on the drugs considered primary therapy for tuberculosis, with the exception of streptomycin. In general, it has been suggested that for some antituberculosis agents, specifically isoniazid, pyrazinamide, and rifampin, dose modification (i.e., reduction) should be considered for elderly patients because of the sensitivity which they have demonstrated to the adverse effects of these agents.[47]

1. Isoniazid

Isoniazid is a bactericidal agent; the mechanism of its antimycobacterial activity, which is limited to *Mycobacterium tuberculosis* and *M. bovis*, is related to its inhibition of mycolic acid synthesis. Mycolic acid, which is a unique and important component of mycobacterial cell walls, has no counterpart in mammalian cell metabolism, and this difference confers effectiveness and selective toxicity to isoniazid. When used alone, resistance develops to isoniazid within a few weeks. Consequently, in the treatment of active tuberculosis it is always combined with other antimycobacterial agents. Isoniazid used alone, however, is the drug of choice for the prophylaxis of uninfected patients who are at risk for developing tuberculosis by virtue of close contact with an infected individual or those with positive tuberculosis skin tests in whom prophylaxis is indicated.

Isoniazid is available for both oral and parenteral administration. It is well absorbed after oral dosing, and is well distributed to all tissues including the CNS where it penetrates into the cerebrospinal fluid. Isoniazid is biotransformed in the liver by acetylation, a reaction which is subject to genetic variation. About half of the Caucasian population of the U.S., for example, are slow acetylators while approximately 80% of Asians are rapid acetylators. Both isoniazid and its biotransformation products are cleared renally.

Isoniazid therapy is associated with two major adverse experiences, both of which have important implications for elderly patients. Peripheral neuropathy, a frequent complication of high-dose therapy with isoniazid, results from depletion of pyridoxine (vitamin B_6). This is a particular problem with diabetic patients and the malnourished, and for this reason patients at risk for this toxicity, include many of the elderly. Other at-risk groups are alcoholics and those with chronic renal insufficiency. All patients at risk should receive regular pyridoxine supplementation to avoid this toxicity, which manifests itself as paresthesias and neuritis in individuals receiving isoniazid without such supplementation.

The most serious adverse experience associated with isoniazid therapy is hepatic toxicity caused by acetyl hydrazine, a toxic product of isoniazid biotransformation. Patients over the age of 50 have been identified as having an increased risk (approximately 3%) for such hepatotoxicity by the U.S. Department of Public Health, prompting concern about the safe use of isoniazid in the elderly. Other risk factors for hepatic toxicity include rapid acetylation of isoniazid, which predisposes a patient to produce the toxic metabolite, and alcohol consumption. The hepatotoxicity is more common during continuous, as compared to intermittent, isoniazid therapy.

Isoniazid interacts with antacids which are reported to decrease its absorption. Other drug interactions include alteration of the metabolism of carbamazepine, which increases the toxicity of both drugs, the reduction in blood levels and effect of ketoconazole as well as increased phenytoin toxicity due to decreased biotransformation.

2. Rifampin

Rifampin, which is also called rifampicin, was first used clinically in 1968. It inhibits DNA-dependent RNA polymerase, and consequently RNA synthesis, in a number of aerobic bacteria including the mycobacteria and many strains of methicillin-resistant *staphylococci*. Rifampin is bactericidal against *M. tuberculosis* and a variety of atypical mycobacteria. Bacterial resistance to rifampin develops rapidly as a result of bacterial mutation and can be avoided by combining rifampin with another effective therapeutic agent.

Rifampin is available for both oral and parenteral administration. It is highly lipid soluble and quickly absorbed and distributed widely to tissues, including the CNS and cerebrospinal fluid after oral dosing. It also penetrates well into neutrophils, monocytes, and peripheral nerves. Rifampin is cleared primarily by hepatic biotransformation, specifically by deacetylation to desacetyl rifampin, which is an active metabolite. Both the parent compound and this biotransformation product are excreted via the bile into the feces. The extensive hepatic clearance of rifampin requires dose reduction in patients with hepatic disease, but no reduction is required in renal failure patients. A small percentage of the metabolites of rifampin are cleared by the kidneys.

Minor adverse experiences associated with rifampin use include orange discoloration of the urine, saliva, and other secretions; allergic reactions, nausea, vomiting, abdominal distress, and flu-like symptoms. Other rare, but more serious adverse reactions include acute renal failure, hemolytic anemia, thrombocytopenia, and neutropenia. Elevated serum transaminase levels have been reported without and with overt hepatitis, which is reported to occur in about 1% of all treated patients. Rifampin accelerates the hepatic biotransformation of a variety of drugs including chloramphenicol, chlorpropamide, coumarin anticoagulants, cyclosporin, dapsone, diazepam, digitoxin, disopyramide, estrogens, glucocorticoids, methodone, metoprolol, mexiletine, phenytoin, propranolol, quinidine, sulfasalazine, sulfonylureas, theophylline, and verapamil. It also increases its own biotransformation.

Because of rapid resistance rifampin is never employed as single-drug therapy in the treatment of tuberculosis. Rifampin combined with either nafcillin or vancomycin plus gentamicin is the therapy of choice for prosthetic heart valve infections caused by coagulase negative staphylococci and is also used in combination to treat some cases of bacterial meningitis. Rifampin and ciprofloxacin may be given concomitantly to treat methicillin-resistant *Staphylococcus aureus* in nasal carriers and other nonlife-threatening infections using standard clinical dosing regimens. The combination results in therapeutic levels of both drugs and appears to be safe for administration to elderly nursing home patients.[40]

3. Ethambutol

Ethambutol inhibits *M. tuberculosis* and *M. bovis* by a mechanism which is not completely understood. It is not bactericidal, and is always combined with other antituberculosis drugs to provide effective therapy. Its primary role in such combination therapy is to slow the development of mycobacterial resistance to the agent with which it is combined. Ethambutol has no activity against other bacteria.

Ethambutol is available only for oral use and is approximately 80% bioavailable when administered by this route. It is widely distributed to tissues, including the lung parenchyma and cerebrospinal fluid, and is approximately 30% bound to plasma proteins. Ethambutol is cleared primarily via the renal route with about 65% of an oral dose excreted unchanged in the urine. Hepatic biotransformation is minimal. The normal elimination half-life of about 4 hours is prolonged to about 16 hours in renal failure, and dosage must be adjusted in patients with reduced renal function.

Optic neuritis, which is manifest by blurred vision, red-green color blindness, and central scotoma, unilaterally or bilaterally, is the most serious adverse experience associated with ethambutol use. While reversible if the drug is promptly discontinued, this ocular toxicity can produce permanent visual impairment if ethambutol is continued after these symptoms occur. For this reason patients using ethambutol should receive regular vision evaluations.

Ethambutol is used clinically in the combination therapy of both tuberculosis and in *M. avium* infections in AIDS patients.

4. Pyrazinamide

Pyrazinamide, a derivative of nicotinamide, was introduced as an antituberculosis drug in 1952. Although an effective bactericidal agent against *M. tuberculosis* in an acidic environment and against intracellular tuberculosis bacilli which have been phagocytized, it has no activity at neutral pH or against extracellular tuberculosis lesions.

Pyrazinamide is well absorbed and widely distributed after oral administration. Less than 10% of pyrazinamide is excreted unchanged by the kidneys. It is cleared primarily by hepatic biotransformation to metabolites which are then excreted in the urine. Renal clearance of the parent drug and metabolites is via glomerular filtration. However, about 98% of filtered pyrazinamide is subsequently reabsorbed. The elimination half-life is about 9 hours.

Insufficient numbers of elderly patients were studied in clinical trials of pyrazinamide to detect any differences from younger individuals. In general, doses for the elderly should be carefully selected, based upon their higher likelihood of concomitant disease, their other medications, and the competence of their organs of clearance.

Clinical use of pyrazinamide is limited by its hepatic toxicity, which is dose related and occurs in 1 to 5% of patients treated with doses of up to 30 mg/kg/d. Pyrazinamide metabolites interfere with the tubular secretion of uric acid, causing hyperuricemia, which sometimes advances to overt gout.

The role of pyrazinamide in the therapy of tuberculosis is the eradication of intracellular mycobacteria which is essential to avoid recrudescence of clinical disease after completion of drug therapy. This role is limited, however, to the early part of treatment (up to 2 months), after which pyrazinamide does not appear to provide any additional clinical benefit.

REFERENCES

1. **Lamy, P.,** Pharmacotherapeutics in the elderly, *Md. Med. J.*, 38, 144–148, 1989.
2. **Burns, E. A. and Goodwin, J. S.,** Immunology and infectious disease, in *Geriatric Medicine*, 2nd ed., K. Casel, Riesenberg, Sorensen, Walsh, Eds., Springer-Verlag, New York, 1990, 312–329.

3. **Bryan, C. S. and Reynolds, K. L.,** Community-acquired bacteremic urinary tract infections, *J. Urol.*, 132(3), 490–493, 1984.
4. **Bryan, C. S., and Reynolds, K. L.,** Hospital-acquired bacteremic urinary tract infections. *J. Urol.*, 132(3), 494-498, 1984.
5. **Kaye, D.,** Urinary tract infections in the elderly, *Bull. N.Y. Acad. Med.*, 56, 209, 1980.
6. **Esposito, A. L. et al.,** Community-acquired bacteremia in the elderly: analysis of one hundred consecutive episodes, *J. Am. Geriatr. Soc.*, 28(7), 315–319, 1980.
7. **Gleckman, R. A.,** The chronically catheterized elderly patient: a selective review. *J. Am. Geriatr. Soc.*, 33(7), 489–491, 1985.
8. **Yoshikawa, T. T. and Norman, D. C.,** Ageing and infectious diseases, in *Principles and Practice of Geriatric Medicine*, 2nd ed., Pathy, M. S. J., Ed., John Wiley & Sons, New York, 1991.
9. **Setia, U. et al.,** Bacteremia in a long term care facility, spectrum and mortality, *Arch. Intern. Med.*, 144, 1633–1635, 1984.
10. **Barrons, R. W., Murray, K. M. et al.,** Populations at risk for penicillin-induced seizures, *Ann. Pharmacother.*, 26(1), 26–9, 1992.
11. **Gleckman, R. A.,** Reviewing the safe use of antibiotics in the elderly, *Geriatrics*, 44(7), 1989.
12. **Raveendran, R., Adithan, C. et al.,** Ampicillin pharmacokinetics in Indian geriatric subjects, *Ind. J. Med. Sci.*, 44(3), 61–4, 1990.
13. **Janknegt, R., Boogaard-Van den Born, J. et al.,** Pharmacokinetics of amoxycillin in elderly in-patients, *Pharm. Weekbl. Sci. Ed.*, 14(1), 27–9, 1992.
14. **Meyers, B. R., Wilkinson, P. et al.,** Pharmacokinetics of ampicillin-sulbactam in healthy elderly and young volunteers, *Antimicrob. Agents Chemother.*, 35(10), 2098–101, 1991.
15. **Santoro, J., Agarwal, B. N., Martinelli, R., Wenger, N., and Levison, M. E.,** Pharmacology of Cefaclor in Normal Volunteers and Patients with Renal Failure, Antimicrob. *Agents Chemother.*, 13(6), 951–954, 1978.
16. **Satterwhite, J. H., Cerimele, B. J. et al.,** Pharmacokinetics of cefaclor AF: effects of age, antacids and H2-receptor antagonists, *Postgrad. Med. J.*, 68 (Suppl. 3), S3–9, 1992.
17. **Karki, S. D., Bentley, D. W. et al.,** Disposition of intramuscular cefonicid in elderly patients, *JAGS*, 41(8), 808–10, 1993.
18. **Barriere, S. L.,** Pharmacology and pharmacokinetics of cefprozil, *Clin. Infect. Dis.*, 14 (Suppl. 2), S184–8, discussion S195–6, 1992.
19. **Ridgway, E., Stewart, K. et al.,** The pharmacokinetics of cefuroxime axetil in the sick elderly patient, *J. Antimicrob. Ther.*, 27(5), 663–8, 1991.
20. **Borin, M. T., Peters, G. R., and Smith, T. C.,** Pharmacokinetics and dose proportionality of cefmetazole in healthy young and elderly volunteers, *Antimicrob. Agents Chemother.*, 34(10), 1944–8, 1990.
21. **Backhouse, C., Wade, A. et al.,** Multiple dose pharmacokinetics of cefpodoxime in young adult and elderly patients, *J. Antimicrob. Ther.*, 26 (Suppl. E), 29–34, 1990.
22. **Tremblay, D., Dupront, A. et al.,** Pharmacokinetics of cefpodoxime in young and elderly volunteers after single doses, *J. Antimicrob. Ther.*, 26 (Suppl. E), 21–8, 1990.
23. **Sirgo, M. A. and Norris, S.,** Ceftazidime in the elderly: appropriateness of twice-daily dosing, *DICP*, 25(3), 284–8, 1991.
24. **Slaker, R. A. and Danielson, B.,** Neurotoxicity associated with ceftazidime therapy in geriatric patients with renal dysfunction, *Pharmacotherapy*, 11(4), 351–2, 1991.
25. **Vlasses, P. H., Bastion, W. A. et al.,** Ceftazidime dosing in the elderly: economic implications, *Ann. Pharmacother.*, 27(7–8), 967–71, 1993.
26. **Barbhaiya, R. H., Knupp, C. A. et al.,** Effects of age and gender on pharmacokinetics of cefepime, *Antimicrob. Agents Chemother.*, 36(6), 1181–5, 1992.
27. **Kovarik, J. M. et al.,** Pharmacokinetics of cefepime in patients with respiratory tract infections, *Antimicrob. Agents Chemother.*, 34(10), 1885–8, 1990.
28. **Deeter, R. G., Weinstein, M. P. et al.,** Crossover assessment of serum bactericidal activity and pharmacokinetics of five broad-spectrum cephalosporins in the elderly, *Antimicrob. Agents Chemother.*, 34(6), 1007-13, 1990.
29. **Meyers, B. R., Wilkinson, P. et al.,** Pharmacokinetics of aztreonam in healthy elderly and young adult volunteers, *J. Clin. Pharm.*, 33(5), 470–4, 1993.
30. **Van der Auwera, P.,** Pharmacokinetic evaluation of single daily dose amikacin, *J. Antimicrob. Chemother.*, 27 (Suppl. C), 63–71, 1991.
31. **Maller, R., Emanuelsson, B. M. et al.,** Amikacin once daily: a new dosing regimen based on drug pharmacokinetics, *Scand. J. Infect. Dis.*, 22(5), 575–9, 1990.
32. **Miglioli, P. A., Pivetta, P. et al.,** Effect of age on single- and multiple-dose pharmacokinetics of erythromycin, *Eur. J. Clin. Pharmacol.*, 39(2), 161–4, 1990.
33. **Coates, P., Daniel, R. et al.,** An open study to compare the pharmacokinetics, safety and tolerability of a multiple-dose regimen of azithromycin in young and elderly volunteers, *Eur. J. Clin. Microb. Infect. Dis.*, 10(10), 850–2, 1991.

34. **Chu, S. Y., Wilson, D. S. et al.,** Clarithromycin pharmacokinetics in healthy young and elderly volunteers, *J. Clin. Pharmacol.*, 32(11), 1045–9, 1992.
35. **Wallace, R. J., Jr., Brown, B. A. et al.,** Drug intolerance to high-dose clarithromycin among elderly patients, *Diag. Microb. Infect. Dis.*, 16(3), 215–21, 1993.
36. **Lau, A. H., Lam, N. P. et al.,** Clinical pharmacokinetics of metronidazole and other nitromidazole anti-infectives, *Clin. Pharmacokinetics*, 23(5), 328–64, 1992.
37. **Loft, S., Egsmose, C. et al.,** Metronidazole elimination is preserved in the elderly, *Hum. Exp. Toxicol.*, 9(3), 155–9, 1990.
38. **Morita, M., Hasuda, A. et al.,** Accumulation of new quinolones in the blood of elderly patients, *J. Int. Med. Res.*, 21(6), 334–41, 1993.
39. **Molinaro, M., Villani, P. et al.**, Pharmacokinetics of ofloxacin in elderly patients and in healthy young subjects, *Eur. J. Clin. Pharmacol.*, 43(1), 105–7, 1992.
40. **Schentag, J. J. and Goss, T. F.,** Quinolone pharmacokinetics in the elderly, *Am. J. Med.*, 92(4A), 33S–37S, 1992.
41. **Cowling, P., Rogers, S. et al.,** The pharmacokinetics of lomefloxacin in elderly patients with urinary tract infection following daily dosing with 400 mg, *J. Antimicrob. Chemother.*, 28(1), 101–7, 1991.
42. **Lepage, J. Y., Caillon, J. et al.,** Pharmacokinetics of norfloxacin in the elderly, *Fundam. Clin. Pharmacol.*, 5(3), 203–8, 1991.
43. **Nilsson-Ehle, I. and Ljungberg, B.,** Quinolone disposition in the elderly. Practical implications, *Drugs Aging*, 1(4), 279–88, 1991.
44. **Chandler, M. H., Toler, S. M. et al.,** Multiple-dose pharmacokinetics of concurrent oral ciprofloxacin and rifampin therapy in elderly patients, *Antimicrob. Agents Chemother.*, 34(3), 442–7, 1990.
45. **Guay, D. R., Vance-Bryan, K. et al.,** Comparison of vancomycin pharmacokinetics in hospitalized elderly and young patients using a Bayesian forecaster, *J. Clin. Pharmacol.*, 33(10), 918–22, 1993.
46. **Garibaldi, R. A., Neuhaus, E. G., and Nurse, B. A.,** Infections in the elderly, *Am. J. Med.*, 81 (Suppl. 1A), 53–58, 1986.
47. **Walubo, A. and Chan, K., et al.,** The disposition of antituberculous drugs in plasma of elderly patients. II. Isoniazid, rifampicin and pyrazinamide, *Methods Findings Exp. Clin. Pharmacol.*, 13(8), 551–6, 1991.

Chapter 17

PHARMACOLOGY OF CANCER CHEMOTHERAPEUTIC AND IMMUNOTHERAPEUTIC AGENTS WITH COMMENTS ON THE EFFECTS OF AGE

Ti Li Loo, Emil J. Freireich, and H. George Mandel

CONTENTS

0-8493-8306-4/96/$0.00+$.50

I. INTRODUCTION

A. TUMOR CHEMOTHERAPY

Modern rational chemotherapy was born in 1942 when the clinical trial of nitrogen mustards was initiated, because these compounds had shown selective toxicity to lymphoid tissues.[1–5] Since then, cancer chemotherapy has advanced to become one of the most important and exciting modalities for treating certain kinds of cancer today. The chemotherapy of cancer differs basically from that of infectious parasitic diseases in that the agents used are seldom specific against the malignant cell alone, in sharp contrast to those of infectious diseases that are selectively toxic to the invading organism. Obviously, a degree of specificity does exist or cancer chemotherapy would not be effective at all. Toxicity is usually expressed in rapidly growing normal cells such as bone marrow stem cells, gastrointestinal mucosa cells, and hair follicles. However, contrary to the popular misconception, not all malignant cells proliferate faster (namely, having a shorter cycle time) than normal cells. Indeed, the doubling time of some tumors, including those of the colon, breast, and lung, is very long. In addition, the invasiveness, metastatic potential, and degree of differentiation vary appreciably from one kind of malignancy to another; human tumor cells are highly heterogeneous, varying widely in growth rate, cell kinetics, and metastatic potential. Taking all of these variables into consideration, one must conclude that cancer chemotherapy is indeed an exacting challenge.

B. ANTITUMOR AGENTS

Anticancer agents can be of natural or synthetic origin. Almost all naturally occurring anticancer agents were discovered by chance or through initially random, but later systematic, screening. Examples of natural compounds include the vinca alkaloids and the anthracycline antibiotics. Synthetic antineoplastic agents were discovered by "enlightened empiricism", since a first principle to guide their synthesis was obviously nonexistent. A number of clinically important antimetabolites such as cytarabine, mercaptopurine (6-MP), and fluorouracil (FU) are synthetic products derived by structural modifications of their natural counterparts. Another major group of synthetic antitumor drugs consists of alkylating agents, such as nitrogen mustard, which form covalent linkages to vital cellular components. Tumors of endocrine origin frequently respond to hormonal treatment. More recently, immunotherapy has provided innovative approaches to controlling tumor growth.

C. TUMOR CELL KINETICS

Studies on the kinetics of tumor cells growing in culture or in animal models have provided critical information on the mechanisms by which tumors replicate. At early stages of tumor development cancer cells duplicate at logarithmic rates. As tumors grow in size, limitations due to nutrient and oxygen availability to tumor cells slow, but do not stop, cancer growth. Eventually, tumors reach a critical size or tumor cell number which is fatal to the host.

Drugs which destroy tumor cells will kill a given percentage of these cells, depending on the dose and other determinants. Low drug concentrations will reduce the tumor cell population minimally because of a low "logarithmic cell kill", but higher doses with a higher logarithmic cell kill may produce serious host toxicity. The drugs thus reduce the tumor burden, but once the drug action has terminated, tumor growth resumes at its previous rate. The drug-induced delay results in the increase in host survival until the lethal tumor number is reached and accounts for the palliation produced by chemotherapy. Drugs usually do not permit sufficient tumor cell kill for immunological or other body defenses to complete tumor destruction, and thereby to allow for patient survival.

The relative selectivity of antitumor agents rests in part on the comparatively high "growth fraction" of tumor cells (the fraction in mitotic cycle) compared with susceptible normal host cells. Since most antitumor drugs produce their cytotoxicity during the mitotic cycle, a significant portion of normal cells, not being in mitotic cycle, may be spared from the killing effects of the drug.

D. DRUG RESISTANCE

A serious shortcoming of most clinically useful anticancer agents is their limited spectrum of activity. Unfortunately, those tumors responsible for most human deaths (e.g., lung, colon, breast) are frequently insensitive to chemotherapy, i.e., they exhibit primary or intrinsic resistance. In addition, tumors initially responsive to an anticancer agent often acquire resistance by a number of mechanisms so that they become refractory to subsequent treatment with the same agent. A newly recognized type of resistance, multiple (or pleiotropic) drug resistance, pertains to the phenomenon exhibited by certain malignant cell lines that although initially made resistant to only a single chemotherapeutic agent (usually a natural product), later become cross resistant to multiple, structurally unrelated cytotoxic drugs.

E. OTHER DETRIMENTS TO SUCCESSFUL CHEMOTHERAPY

The lack of high specificity against tumor cells as compared with normal cells, leading to serious toxicity, is another shortcoming of cancer chemotherapeutic agents. Moreover, many anticancer agents fail to penetrate into the anatomical sanctuaries where malignant cells are often sequestered. Obviously, therefore, an ideal anticancer agent, in addition to lacking serious systemic toxicity, should be able to induce long and complete remissions in a large population of patients with a variety of neoplastic diseases, especially those highly fatal.

F. DRUG DEVELOPMENT

In drug development, before clinical trials, screening of the candidate drug usually uses an animal model,[7] frequently a rodent, and toxicological evaluations are then carried out in other experimental animals also. The model systems have had some predictive value, although, regrettably, drugs active against animal tumor systems that later demonstrated useful clinical activities are few. More recently, screening has extended to cultured cells,[8] but such drug evaluation bypasses all of the *in vivo* pharmacokinetic barriers such as drug absorption, compartmentalization, excretion, and especially *in vivo* metabolic activation. The use of short-term *in vitro* assays with cultured human tumor cells taken from patients as a means of individualizing therapy also has not lived up to its initial promise thus far.

All anticancer agents are cytotoxic; unless they display some selectivity and specificity against human malignancies, they have no significant lasting clinical value. The clinical efficacy of an antitumor agent, representing the sum total expression of its toxicity, selectivity, specificity, pharmacokinetic and pharmacodynamic properties in humans, is often exquisitely sensitive to manipulations of dose, schedule, and route of its administration. Consequently, the increase in effectiveness of a new agent necessarily depends on the availability of pertinent pharmacologic information derived from experiments with the agent initially in laboratory animals, but eventually also in humans.

G. PRESENT STATUS OF CANCER CHEMOTHERAPY

In spite of an incomplete understanding of tumor biology, the lack of exploitable differences between malignant and normal cells, and the inadequate specificity of drugs against tumors, cancer chemotherapy has scored some remarkable successes. Most of these breakthroughs, usually involving combinations of antitumor drugs, have occurred against more rapidly growing neoplasms where cures now can be frequently expected from tumor chemotherapy. The list includes acute lymphocytic leukemia, Wilms' tumor, and neuroblastoma in children; Hodgkin's disease; choriocarcinoma; and testicular tumors.

Only the major cancer chemotherapeutic agents selected on the strength of their clinical usefulness will be discussed in this chapter; however, hormonal and immunotherapeutic agents are also included. Table 17.1 represents a summary of the principal anticancer agents described, together with the major clinical indications and the most common and often dose-limiting toxicities. Figure 17.1 is a representation of the sites of action of most of the drugs believed to be responsible for their antitumor effects. The last section briefly reviews the relevance of pharmacologic studies of cancer chemotherapeutic agents in relation to elderly patients. A broader and more in-depth perspective of cancer chemotherapy can be found in the more specialized literature.[1–5]

II. CYTOTOXIC CHEMOTHERAPY

A. ALKYLATING AGENTS[9]

These are compounds that cause cytotoxicity by interacting with cellular macromolecular nucleophilic centers.

1. Nitrogen Mustards, $R\text{-}N(CH_2CH_2Cl)_2$

Modern rational cancer chemotherapy was ushered in some 50 years ago when mechlorethamine (HN2) was first used to treat Hodgkin's disease and other lymphomas.[3] It soon became apparent that at physiologic pH one of the 2-chloroethyl moieties of HN2 is converted to an aziridinium cation that readily reacts with ("alkylates") cellular nucleophiles; these include most frequently the N-7 position, and to a lesser extent, the O-6 positions of guanine, as well as other sites on purines, pyrimidines, phosphates of nucleic acids, and proteins. Moreover, the second 2-chloroethyl moiety in turn reacts similarly with these nucleophiles (Figure 17.2). The alkylation results in DNA base mispairing and subsequent miscoding and

TABLE 17.1.
Survey of Major Clinical Indications and Toxicities of Anticancer Agents

Drug	Major indications	Dose-limiting toxicities
	Alkylating agents	
Mechlorethamine	Lymphomas, especially Hodgkin's disease, mycosis fungoides	Nausea, vomiting, and myelosuppression
Melphalan	Myeloma, acute leukemias, lymphomas, ovarian cancer	Myelosuppression
Chlorambucil	Chronic lymphocytic leukemia	Myelosuppression, nausea, and vomiting
Cyclophosphamide	Breast cancer, Ewing's sarcoma, small cell lung cancer, lymphomas (especially Burkitt's), neuroblastoma, acute lymphocyte leukemia	Myelosuppression, nausea, vomiting, alopecia, and hemorrhagic cystitis
Ifosfamide	Small cell lung cancer, testicular tumors, sarcomas, breast cancer, cervical cancer, lymphomas	Myelosuppression, nausea, vomiting, and hemorrhagic cystitis
Busulfan	Chronic myelocytic leukemia not in blastic crisis	Myelosuppression, fibrosis of the lung
Carmustine, lomustine, semustine	Brain tumors, Hodgkin's disease, myeloma	Delayed and cumulative myelosuppression, nausea, and vomiting
Thio-TEPA	Intravesical bladder carcinoma	Myelosuppression, nausea, and vomiting
	Antimetabolites	
Methotrexate	Pediatric acute lymphocytic leukemia, lymphomas, choriocarcinoma, breast cancer, and other solid tumors	Myelosuppression, nausea and vomiting, gastrointestinal disturbances, stomatitis, pulmonary infiltrates, and fibrosis
Mercaptopurine	Acute lymphocytic leukemia	Myelosuppression, nausea, and vomiting
Thioguanine	Acute leukemia (other than lymphocytic)	Myelosuppression, nausea, and vomiting
Cytarabine	Acute myelocytic leukemia	Myelosuppression, nausea, and vomiting
Fluorouracil, floxuridine	Colorectal carcinoma, breast, gastric, head, and neck cancers	Oral and gastrointestinal ulcers, myelosuppression
	Natural products	
Vinblastine	Hodgkin's disease, testicular tumor, breast cancer, choriocarcinoma	Nausea, vomiting, and myelosuppression
Vincristine	Acute lymphocytic leukemia, lymphomas, pediatric solid tumors	Peripheral neuropathy, alopecia
Etoposide	Lung and testicular cancers	Myelosuppression, nausea, and vomiting
Teniposide	Hematologic malignancies	Myelosuppression, nausea, and vomiting
Daunorubicin	Acute leukemias	Cardiomyopathy, myelosuppression
Doxorubicin	Breast, endometrial, liver, small cell lung cancer, osteogenic sarcoma, lymphomas	Cardiomyopathy, myelosuppression
Bleomycin	Testicular cancer, lymphomas, and squamous cell carcinomas	Pneumonitis, pulmonary fibrosis
Dactinomycin	Choriocarcinoma	Myelosuppression, stomatitis
Mitomycin C	Breast and gastric cancers	Myelosuppression
L-Asparaginase	Acute lymphocytic leukemia	Allergic reactions
Taxol	Breast and ovarian cancer, nonsmall cell lung cancer	Hypersensitivity, myelosuppression, mucositis, peripheral neuropathy
	Miscellaneous agents	
Cisplatin	Small cell, squamous cell, and adenocarcinomas of the lung, breast, ovary, and testicular cancers	Nephrotoxicity, ototoxicity, myelosuppression
Carboplatin	Similar to cisplatin	Myelosuppression

TABLE 17.1. (Continued)
Survey of Major Clinical Indications and Toxicities of Anticancer Agents

Drug	Major indications	Dose-limiting toxicities
Dacarbazine	Melanoma	Nausea and vomiting, myelosuppression
Hydroxyurea	Chronic myelocytic leukemia, melanoma, ovarian cancer	Myelosuppression, nausea, and vomiting
Mitoxantrone	Acute myelocytic leukemia, lymphomas, breast cancer	Myelosuppression, cardiomyopathy, alopecia
	Hormonal agents	
Prednisone, prednisolone	Acute lymphocytic leukemia, lymphoma	Cushingoid syndrome
Diethylstilbestrol, ethinyl estradiol	Prostatic carcinoma	Tumor flare, skeletal pain, hypercalcemia
Leuprolide	Prostatic carcinoma	Impotence, testicular dystrophy
Flutamide	Prostatic carcinoma	Nausea, diarrhea, gynecomastia
Tamoxifen	Breast cancer	Hot flashes, nausea and vomiting, vaginal bleeding, tumor flare
Aminoglutethimide	Breast cancer, prostatic carcinoma	Drowsiness, nausea, myelosuppression, masculinization
Medroxyprogestrone, megestrol	Endometrial carcinoma	Hot flashes, fluid retention, hypercalcemia, vaginal bleeding
Testosterone	Breast cancer	Masculinization
Fluoxymesterone	Breast cancer	Masculinization, cholestatic hepatitis, hepatoma
	Immunotherapeutic agents	
Levamisole	Colorectal cancer (with fluorouracil)	Agranulocytosis, myalgias, arthralgias, flu-like symptoms
Interferon-α	Lymphoreticular tumors, renal cell carcinoma, hairy cell leukemia	Flu-like symptoms, myelosuppression
Interleukin-2	Renal cell carcinoma	Fever, fluid retention, hypotension, respiratory difficulties

mutation, while bialkylation gives rise to DNA strand cross linking. The bifunctional alkylating agent can additionally link a DNA strand to proteins. Also, depurination of DNA may lead to DNA strand breakage. Such damage is especially lethal to dividing cells in late G and S phases of the mitotic cycle, although alkylating agents are not cell cycle specific and may exert deleterious effects on cells in any phase of the cycle. It is quite likely that the alkylation of DNA by these drugs may be responsible for their observed carcinogenicity.

All nitrogen mustards are derivatives of bis(2-chloroethyl)amine. To improve the selectivity of HN2, numerous nitrogen mustards have been synthesized with various R groups as the prosthetic carrier molecule. However, disappointingly, no significant improvement in selectivity has been observed, and currently only a few alkylating agents are used clinically. As briefly outlined above, they presumably share the same cytotoxic mechanism.

a. *Mechlorethamine (HN2, Nitrogen Mustard; R = CH_3)*

This prototype nitrogen mustard has enjoyed early prominence as the first rationally developed cancer chemotherapeutic agent. HN2 itself is unstable, and for parenteral administration HN2 solution must be prepared freshly and used immediately. Its chemical and biological half-life is less than 10 min. Care must be taken to prevent necrotic extravasation and direct vesicant tissue injury.

Alkylation of various cellular macromolecular nucleophiles by HN2 undoubtedly accounts for its cytotoxicity, directed particularly to the rapidly proliferating cells in the bone marrow,

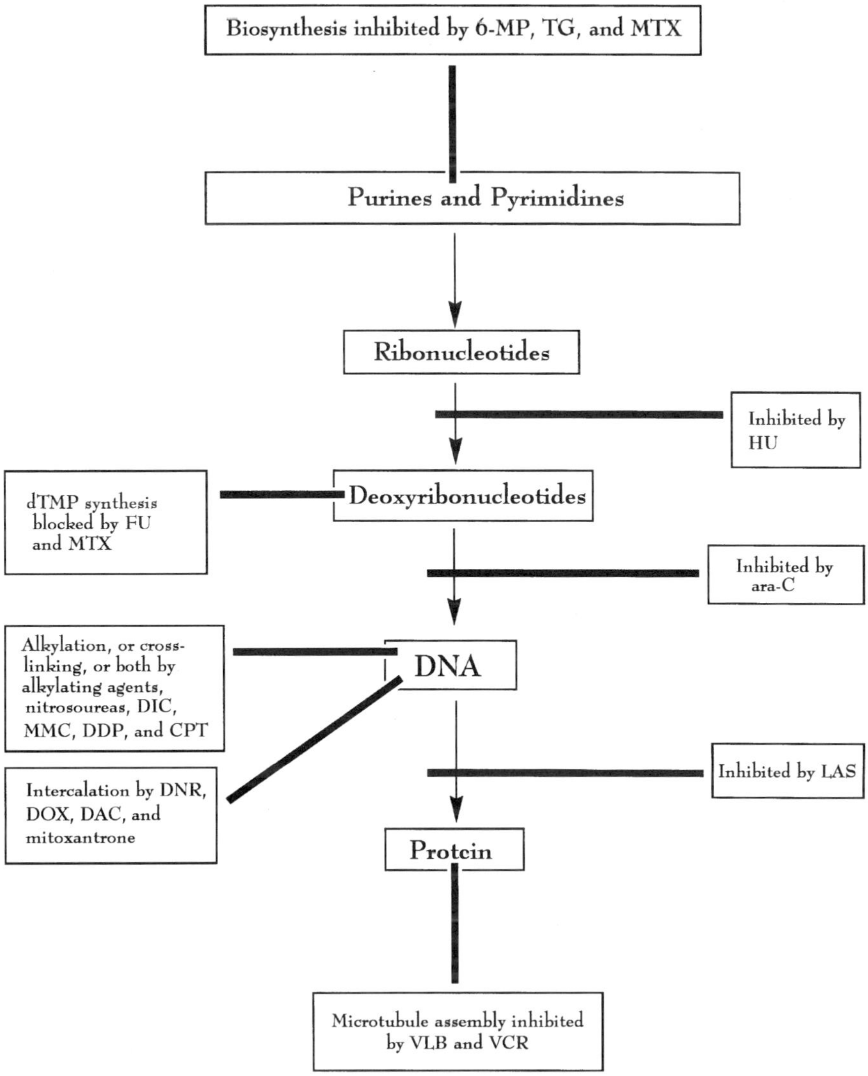

Figure 17.1. Overall scheme of cellular biosynthesis, with indication of sites of action or anticancer agents. Abbreviations: 6-MP, mercaptopurine; TG, thioguanine; MTX, methotrexate; HU, hydroxyurea; ara-C, cytarabine; LAS, L-asparaginase; dTMP, thymidylate; FU, 5-fluorouracil; DIC, dacarbazine; MMC, mitomycin C; DDP, cisplatin; CPT, carboplatin; DNR, daunorubicin; DOX, doxorubicin; DAC, dactinomycin; VLB, vinblastine; VCR, vincristine.

gastrointestinal tract, gonads, and hair follicles. Major clinical toxicity of HN2 manifests itself in myelosuppression, nausea, and vomiting. The latter can be alleviated by pretreatment with antiemetics.

Cellular resistance to HN2 in part seems to be attributable to impaired uptake of the agent, but increased DNA repair of lesions caused by HN2 alkylation, and enhanced trapping of HN2 by thiols and other competing nucleophiles, have also been reported.

HN2 is useful in treating Hodgkin's disease and other lymphomas, especially mycosis fungoides where it is applied topically. It is rapidly degraded *in vivo*; owing to its short half-life, in patients with severe organ failure, such as that of liver or kidney secondary to rapidly advancing lymphoma or other malignancies, HN2 can be used in full dosage without further aggravating the existing organ dysfunction. It is usually used in combination with other agents,

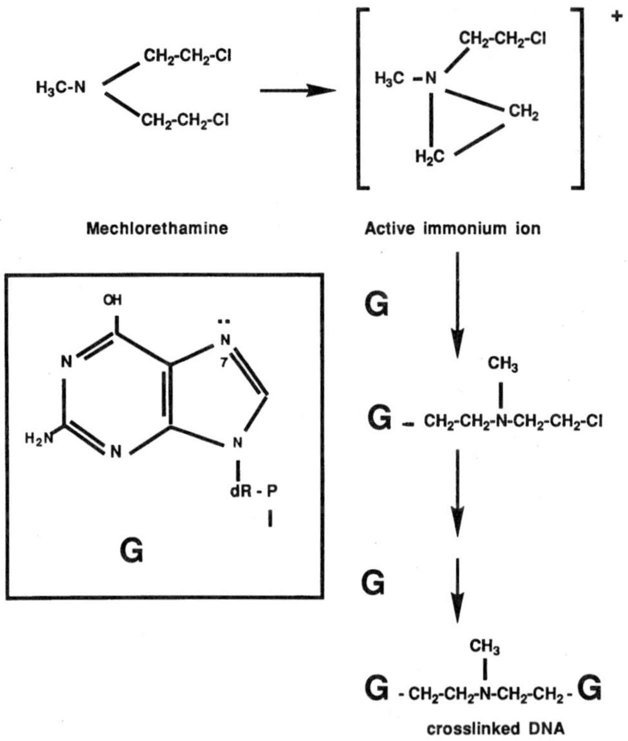

Figure 17.2. Activation of the alkylating agent mechlorethamine (nitrogen mustard), [R-N $(CH_2CH_2Cl)_2$, where R is CH_3] and interaction with guanine moieties (G) of DNA strands to form cross-linked DNA.

as, for instance, with vincristine (Oncovin), prednisone, and procarbazine in the MOPP regimen for treating Hodgkin's disease.

b. Melphalan (Alkeran)

Melphalan, an arylnitrogen mustard (R = L-phenylalanine, Figure 17.2), was originally synthesized in the hope of achieving selectivity against malignant melanomas, since L-phenylalanine is a precursor of melanin; however, its actions differed from those as originally intended. Because of its slower reactivity compared with HN2, and its greater infiltration into tissues, the drug may be administered orally. Melphalan undergoes spontaneous chemical degradation and *in vivo* metabolism.

Considerably less effective than cyclophosphamide (see below) in acute leukemia, lymphomas, and other solid tumors, melphalan is nevertheless the agent of choice for the treatment of multiple myeloma. Also, it has been used for the management of ovarian cancer. Myelosuppression is its major clinical toxicity; other organ toxicities are rare.

c. Chlorambucil (Leukeran)

Originally synthesized as a soluble aryl nitrogen mustard for parenteral administration, chlorambucil (R = phenylbutyric acid, in Figure 17.2) is also effective orally. Compared with other chemotherapeutic agents, chlorambucil is much better tolerated. Its chief toxicity is reversible myelosuppression; nausea is relatively mild. Chlorambucil is used principally in the treatment of chronic lymphocytic leukemia, other low-grade lymphoid malignancies, and ovarian carcinoma. However, because of increasing frequencies of secondary malignancies following therapy with alkylating agents and because of the discovery of more effective treatment for those tumors, the clinical application of chlorambucil has decreased.

d. Cyclophosphamide (CPA, Cytoxan)

An important and extensively used anticancer agent with a broad spectrum of clinical activities, CPA was initially conceived as a transport or latent form of *nor*-nitrogen mustard that remains inactive until putatively cleaved intracellularly by phosphoramidase found in relative abundance in a number of tumor cells. However, CPA is not cytotoxic until metabolically activated, but its activation is an oxidative process involving the P450 hepatic microsomal mixed-function oxidases. The metabolism of CPA is outlined in Figure 17.3.

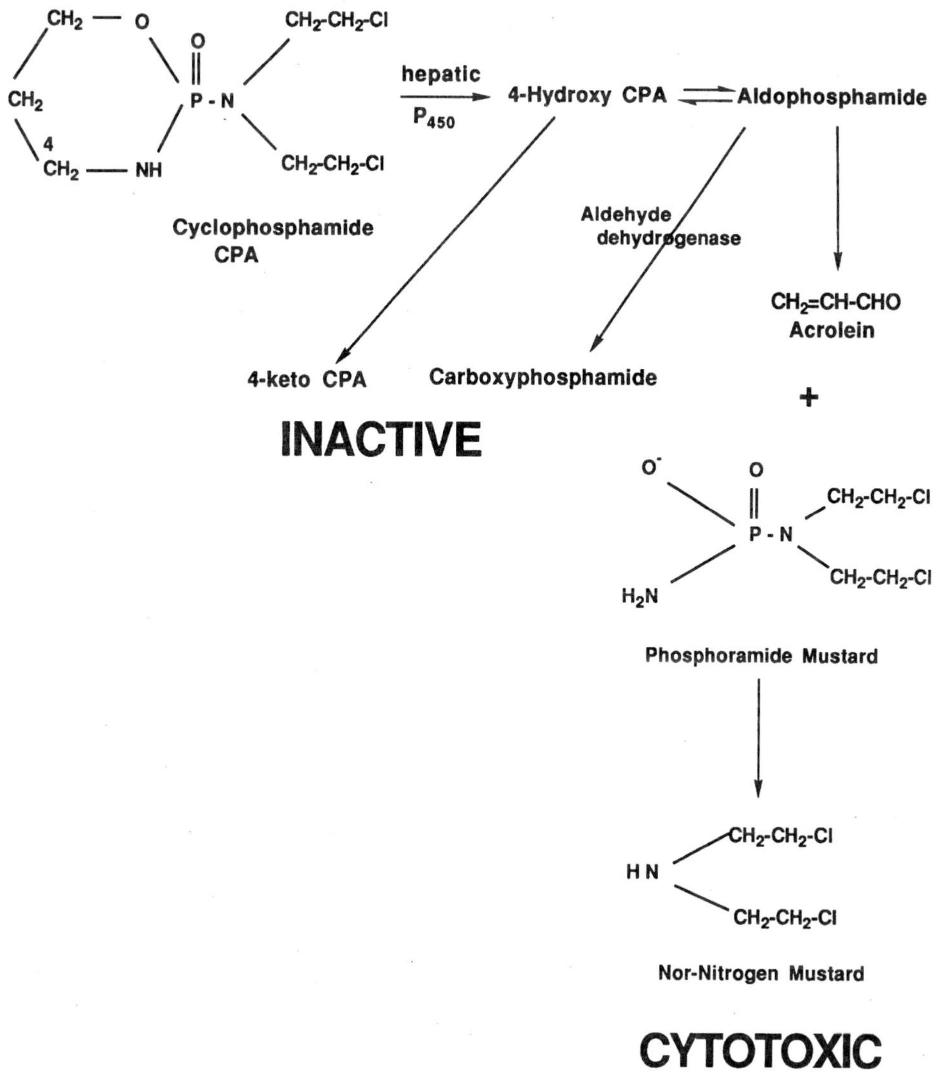

Figure 17.3. Activation of cyclophosphamide (CPA) leading to formation of inactive metabolites 4-keto CPA and carboxyphosphamide; cytotoxic products are acrolein, phosphoramide mustard, and *nor*-nitrogen mustard. The latter two are associated with antitumor activity.

As discussed above, oxidation of CPA is mediated by hepatic microsomal oxidases to form 4-hydroxy-CPA and 4-aldo-CPA. Most of an administered dose of CPA is biotransformed to the inactive 4-keto- and 4-carboxy-CPA. Spontaneous decomposition produces acrolein and phosphoramide mustard. The unstable phosphoramide mustard may decompose to cytotoxic *nor*-nitrogen mustard. However, most investigators believe that phosphoramide mustard is principally responsible for DNA cross linking by CPA, which then results in the antitumor effect, but also toxicity.

CPA is completely bioavailable after oral administration. In patients with low creatinine clearance, or in severe liver failure, normal clearance is reduced and plasma CPA half-life is progressively lengthened.

As a single agent administered orally or intravenously, CPA is often curative in patients with Burkitt's lymphoma. The drug is also incorporated in a large number of regimens for the treatment of lymphomas, other solid tumors, and leukemias. In combination with anthracycline antibiotics, apparent clinical synergism has been observed; thus the CHOP (CPA, doxorubicin, vincristine, and prednisone) regimen is one of the most effective for lymphoma treatment. Another important use of CPA is as a conditioning agent for allogeneic bone marrow transplantation, especially in high dose coupled with total body radiation. This regimen has been successful in patients with acute myeloblastic leukemia, chronic granulocytic leukemia, or myelodysplastic syndromes.

The major clinical toxicities are myelosuppression with infrequent thrombocytopenia, reversible alopecia, nausea and vomiting, and occasionally hemorrhagic cystitis probably due to acrolein. The latter toxicity may be reduced or prevented by hydration, bladder irrigation with N-acetylcysteine, and frequent voiding.

e. Ifosfamide (IFA)

Though a structural analog of CPA, IFA differs noticeably from CPA in clinical activity, pharmacology, and toxicology. Like CPA, IFA is metabolically activated *in vivo* by hepatic microsomal enzymes resulting in the generation of alkylating species. Clinically, the antitumor action and toxicity are probably associated with the production of IFA-mustard, [*N,N′*-2-di(2-chloroethyl)]phosphorodiamidic acid, and other alkylating entities. In contrast to CPA, a large percentage of unchanged IFA is excreted in the urine, consistent with a slow rate of *in vitro* metabolic activation of this agent. To some extent IFA can cross the blood-brain barrier.

The major toxic effects of IFA are dose-limiting hematuria and dose-dependent leukopenia; other toxicities are alopecia, nausea, and vomiting. Central nervous system (CNS) toxicities such as lethargy and confusion after high doses of the drug have been attributed to 2-chloroacetaldehyde generated from the oxidative cleavage of the 2-chloroethyl side chain. The hemorrhagic cystitis caused by the cytotoxic IFA metabolites excreted in the urine is ameliorated by hydration and particularly the systemic administration of Mesna (sodium 2-mercaptoethanesulfonate).

IFA has shown activities against a wide spectrum of malignant diseases, including small cell lung cancer, testicular tumors of all histologic types, soft tissue sarcoma, mammary carcinoma, cervical carcinoma, hypernephroma, pancreatic tumor, and lymphomas. Moreover, IFA has demonstrated activity in the therapy of patients with testicular tumors and soft tissue sarcomas previously treated with CPA. It is also useful in combination regimens with anthracycline antibiotics and etoposide because of its mild myelosuppressive toxicity at full doses.

2. Alkyl Sulfonates

a. Busulfan (Myleran)

This compound differs chemically from the nitrogen mustards, but is still considered to be an alkylating agent. Alkylation of proteins rather than nucleic acid may be the predominant lesion caused by busulfan. It is rapidly metabolized.

Busulfan is highly selective against chronic myelocytic leukemia except in patients in blastic crisis. Myelosuppression is the dose-limiting toxicity, including thrombocytopenia and anemia, but little lymphocytopenia. However, busulfan elicits interstitial fibrosis of the lung, as well as bone marrow and other organ toxicities after prolonged use at low doses, and therefore is increasingly being replaced by hydroxyurea (HV) and interferon (IFN) as initial treatment for this disease. Clinically, busulfan and CPA are apparently synergistic, and this combination is an effective conditioning regimen for allogeneic and autologous bone marrow transplantation.

3. Nitrosoureas

The observation that analogs of 1-methyl-3-nitro-1-nitrosoguanidine, a precursor of the simple alkylating agent, diazomethane, have exhibited activity against leukemias in experimental systems has led to the development of nitrosoureas as cancer chemotherapeutic agents with improved efficacy. Carmustine (BCNU), lomustine (CCNU), and semustine (MeCCNU) currently have clinical applications. As a group the unusually high lipid solubility makes the nitrosoureas the drugs of choice in the therapy of diseases such as CNS malignancies.

An early suggestion that BCNU decomposes *in vitro* to both alkylating and carbamoylating entities may explain the *in vivo* mechanisms of its anticancer actions. It is now commonly accepted that alkylation of nucleic acids by the nitrosoureas is responsible for their antitumor activity, whereas carbamoylation of proteins causes their host toxicity. Alkylation results in DNA interstrand and DNA-protein cross links. The nitrosoureas are unstable and highly reactive. They undergo denitrosation, apparently mediated by hepatic microsomal enzymes to produce nitric oxide, a biochemically and pharmacologically highly active neurohormone. Conceivably, this oxidative cleavage may also occur *in vivo*. If this intermediary is indeed produced in man, the therapeutic pharmacology and toxicologic consequences of such a denitrosation clearly deserve future investigation.

a. Carmustine (BCNU)

BCNU is the most investigated of this group of agents. It is unstable in human plasma with an *in vitro* half-life of 17 min. The major indications of BCNU are in the treatment of brain tumors, Hodgkin's disease, and multiple myeloma. Its characteristic clinical toxicity is delayed and cumulative myelosuppression; nausea and vomiting also occur. Because of its distinctive mechanism of interaction with DNA, BCNU has been used in combination with other alkylating agents, particularly CPA.

b. Lomustine (CCNU) and Semustine (MeCCNU)

CCNU, after oral administration, is useful for treating brain tumors and lymphomas, especially Hodgkin's disease. Delayed myelosuppression, nausea, and vomiting are the major clinical toxicities. Clinical applications and toxicities of semustine are similar to those of CCNU.

4. Ethylenimines

a. Triethyline Thiophosphoramide (Thio-TEPA)

Thio-TEPA is an older and almost abandoned agent, but doses higher than those employed previously are now possible when followed by reinfusion of cryopreserved autologous bone marrow. Interest in thio-TEPA has recently been revived because of its activity against intravesical bladder carcinoma.

B. ANTIMETABOLITES

Synthetic structural analogs of natural precursors in biosynthetic pathways of nucleic acids are of considerable importance in cancer chemotherapy. Since they inhibit cell proliferation by interfering with cellular intermediary metabolism, they are grouped together under "antimetabolites". In general, they may be incorporated into nucleic acids as a fraudulent constituent, or compete with their natural counterparts in binding to the active or regulatory site of a critical enzyme, or allosterically inhibit a feedback control process. Usually they require prior metabolic activation before exerting their inhibitory effects. Many antimetabolites have been synthesized and evaluated as cancer chemotherapeutic agents, but only a few have proven clinically valuable because of lack of selectivity.

1. Folate Antagonists[10,11]

Folate in its reduced form, tetrahydrofolate (FH_4), serves as a vital coenzyme in microorganisms as well as mammalian species, acting as a carrier of one-carbon units in the biosynthesis of a large variety of essential cellular constituents including thymidylate, purines, glycine, serine, and methionine. By interfering with these vital functions, mainly of thymidylate and purines, folate antagonists exert cytotoxic actions. Not all folate antagonists are useful cancer chemotherapeutic agents; methotrexate (MTX) is the major folate antagonist applied in tumor therapy.

a. Methotrexate (MTX)

To function as a cofactor in numerous normal biochemical reactions, folate (F) must first be reduced to FH_4, via dihydrofolate, FH_2, both reactions being mediated by dihydrofolate reductase (DHFR), but FH_2 is a far better substrate. With a high affinity for DHFR, MTX, a structural analog of folate, acts as a potent inhibitor of FH_4 formation. Thus, it interferes with many biosynthetic processes requiring FH_4, so that the folate coenzymes are trapped as the metabolically ineffective FH_2 polyglutamates. MTX is also converted to polyglutamates, especially in tumor cells. These polyglutamates bind to DHFR and are retained in the cells where they then produce cytotoxicity.

The biosynthetic pathway most sensitive to MTX inhibition is the conversion of 2′-deoxyuridylate (dUMP) to thymidylate (dTMP), that requires the donation of a methyl group from 5-10-methylene FH_4 to the uracil moiety of dUMP (Figure 17.4). Since exogenous thymidine is readily phosphorylated by thymidine kinase to dTMP independent of the supply of FH_4, it can circumvent the MTX inhibition. Therapeutically, however, leucovorin (folinic acid, citrovorum factor, 5-formyl FH_4) is the agent widely used to "rescue" patients from toxicities at some time after high-dose MTX treatment. This is because leucovorin, a fully reduced FH_4 derivative, does not need DHFR for its reductive activation, and can be directly and efficiently utilized for the biosyntheses of other FH_4 cofactors.

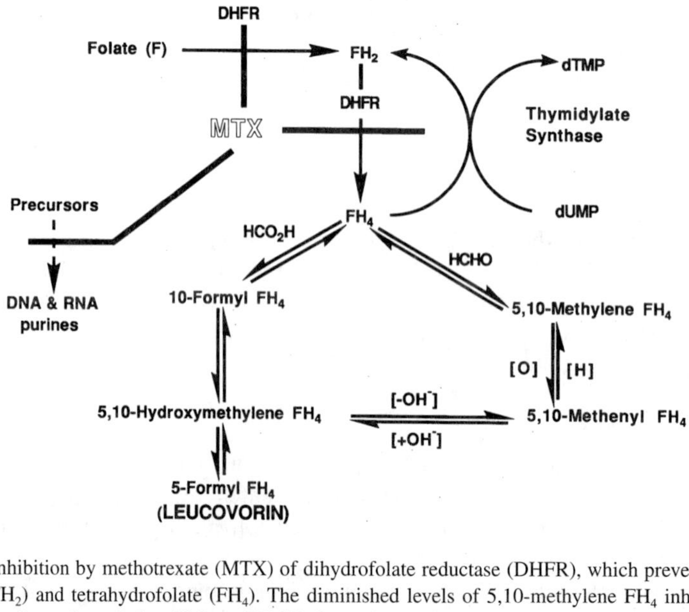

Figure 17.4. Inhibition by methotrexate (MTX) of dihydrofolate reductase (DHFR), which prevents formation of dihydrofolate (FH_2) and tetrahydrofolate (FH_4). The diminished levels of 5,10-methylene FH_4 inhibit thymidylate synthase and the formation of thymidylate (dTMP) from deoxyuridylate (dUMP). The reduced levels of 5,10-methenyl-FH_4 and 10-formyl-FH_4 prevent RNA and DNA purine formation from *de novo* precursors. Leucovorin rescues from MTX toxicity by resupplying a source of FH_4.

Possible cellular resistance mechanisms to MTX are (1) increased production of DHFR through gene amplification; (2) altered DHFR with lowered affinity for MTX; (3) impaired MTX transport; and (4) defective conversion of MTX to its polyglutamate derivatives. Following administration of MTX intramuscularly or by mouth, wide variability in MTX pharmacokinetics has been the rule rather than the exception, with somewhat better absorption by the intramuscular route. A high percentage of MTX is excreted in the urine. With MTX at high doses given by slow intravenous infusion, urinary excretion is accelerated when the patient is hydrated and the urine alkalinized. In humans, serum MTX half-life seems to vary directly with age and inversely with endogenous creatinine clearance. To initiate the "rescue" with leucoverin during high-dose MTX therapy, pharmacokinetic monitoring is essential. MTX does not readily penetrate into the CNS. There is no evidence that MTX is metabolized in man after conventional low doses. However, in patients receiving high-dose MTX, 7-hydroxymethotrexate has been found in the urine.

MTX is an important chemotherapeutic agent with a broad spectrum of clinical anticancer properties. It is curative against childhood acute lymphocytic leukemia, lymphomas other than Hodgkin's disease, choriocarcinoma, and head and neck epithelial as well as squamous cell carcinoma. In combination with other agents it frequently induces remissions in breast cancer and other solid tumors. Major clinical toxicities include myelosuppression, gastrointestinal disturbances, stomatitis, and alopecia. At very high doses followed by leucovorin rescue, MTX has shown substantial antitumor activity against many common malignancies such as lung cancer and breast cancer. In this regimen the dose-limiting nephrotoxicity that is frequently encountered can be avoided by careful monitoring plasma MTX concentrations. Another important use of MTX pertains to the control of diffuse leptomeningeal infiltration in lymphoblastic leukemia and other types of malignancies. Direct administration of MTX into the cerebrospinal fluid, sufficient to produce adequate CNS drug concentrations, has proven effective and even curative.

2. Purine Analogs[12]

Of the purine antimetabolites, initially only 6-MP plays a role in cancer chemotherapy; however, other purine analogs, such as thioguanine (6-TG), cladribine, fludarabine, and pentostatin are gradually gaining clinical importance.

Both 6-MP and 6-TG are readily converted by hypoxanthine-guanine phosphoribosyltransferase (HGPRT) to the respective sulfur analogs of inosinate and guanylate. Thus, thioinosinate (TIMP) and thioguanylate (TGMP) are potent inhibitors of several vital biochemical reactions. In a pseudo-feedback fashion, both TIMP and TGMP interfere with the first step of purine *de novo* biosynthesis, i.e., the reaction of phosphoribosyl pyrophosphate with glutamine to form ribosylamine-5′-phosphate, catalyzed by amidophosphoribosyltransferase. In addition, TIMP inhibits the purine interconversions to GMP and AMP. Probably even more important, the incorporation of TGMP directly and TIMP indirectly as fraudulent nucleotides into cellular DNA has also been implicated in thiopurine cytotoxicity.

a. Mercaptopurine (6-MP, Purinethol)

Although 6-MP is often administered by mouth, its gastrointestinal absorption is erratic and incomplete. The drug is extensively anabolized *in vivo* to biologically active nucleotide analogs. Catabolic oxidation to 6-thiouric acid is mediated by xanthine oxidase. Bioavailability is increased fivefold in patients pretreated with allopurinol, a xanthine oxidase inhibitor, which, because it diminishes first-pass metabolism of orally administered 6-MP to inactive products, can cause major toxicity. Several mechanisms of resistance to 6-MP, such as the loss of HGPRT or decreased affinity for 6-MP by this enzyme, have been demonstrated.

6-MP is used mostly for treating acute leukemia, usually in combination with agents such as MTX, prednisolone, or cytarabine. The chief clinical toxicities are myelosuppression, stomatitis, nausea, and vomiting. It has been reported that parenteral administration of 6-MP can avoid its hepatoxicity and results in enhanced tolerance of the agent by the patient. In the POMP regimen, 6-MP is combined with vincristine, MTX, and prednisone.

b. Thioguanine (TG)

TG is readily converted to its 5′-monophosphate or TGMP, a reaction catalyzed by HGPRT. TGMP is slowly converted stepwise to the diphosphate, TGDP, and triphosphate, TGTP, and ultimately incorporated into cellular DNA where it produces chromosomal abnormalities. Cellular resistance to TG can be caused by either the depletion of HGPRT, or a reduction of its affinity for substrates, or an increase in alkaline phosphatase activity.

TG is usually used in combination with cytarabine in the treatment of acute leukemias other than the lymphocytic variety. Its dose-limiting clinical toxicity is granulocytopenia; other toxicities include emesis and alopecia. Because it does not require xanthine oxidase for catabolism, TG has been frequently used in high-dose regimens such as cytarabine-TG combinations for acute myeloblastic leukemia therapy. This is an important advantage particularly in patients with very large tumor burdens; uric acid nephropathy can be prevented by combining TG with allopurinol, which does not produce the toxicity of the 6-MP-allopurinol combination.

3. Pyrimidine Analogs

Analogs of the pyrimidine bases, cytosine, thymine, and uracil, which mimic certain vital biochemical functions of the natural metabolites, also exhibit antineoplastic properties. Cytarabine, fluorouracil (FU), and floxuridine are currently clinically useful cancer chemotherapeutic agents.

a. Cytarabine [Ara-C, 1-β-D-Arabinofuranosylcytosine][13]

Ara-C differs from the natural metabolite cytidine in having an arabinose sugar in place of the ribose; it is a deoxycytidine and not a cytidine analog. To exert its cytotoxicity, ara-C must first be converted to the 5′-monophosphate, ara-CMP, by deoxycytidine kinase; ara-CMP is ultimately phosphorylated to the triphosphate, ara-CTP, catalyzed by deoxycytidylate kinase. After incorporation into DNA, ara-CTP blocks initiation and elongation of the growing DNA strand. It also interrupts cell replication by inhibiting DNA polymerase α responsible for *de novo* DNA synthesis, and DNA polymerase β responsible for DNA repair. Ara-C undergoes rapid *in vivo* detoxication by deamination to arabinosyluridine (ara-U), a reaction catalyzed by deoxycytidine deaminase; ara-U is relatively innocuous, at least when produced from low doses of ara-C.

High intracellular ara-CTP concentrations appear to be closely linked to ara-C cytotoxicity. A correlation seems to exist between remission duration and intracellular ara-CTP levels, as well as ara-CTP retention *in vitro* by cells from patients with acute myelocytic leukemia.

The plasma elimination half-life of ara-C is relatively short, and gastrointestinal absorption of ara-C is unreliable. Ara-C elimination from the CNS is slower than that from the plasma so that the drug concentration in the cerebrospinal fluid during the terminal phase may exceed that in the concurrent plasma.

Several possible mechanisms for natural and acquired clinical resistance to this agent have been reported. The deletion of the activating anabolic enzyme deoxycytidine kinase, or the overproduction of the inactivating catabolic enzyme deoxycytidine deaminase, reduce the intracellular ara-CTP concentration, leading to resistance. Alternatively, expansion of the cellular dCTP pool which counteracts the damaging effect of ara-C, impairment of ara-C transport into the tumor cell, and DNA polymerase with diminished affinity for ara-CTP have all been demonstrated in resistant cells.

Particularly useful in treating acute leukemia, ara-C is the single most effective agent for cures in adult acute myelocytic leukemia; in fact, the disease of approximately 15% of these patients is controlled by ara-C. Ara-C is usually administered in combination with a

DNA-binding drug such as an anthracycline antibiotic, or TG, or etoposide, all of which may improve the effectiveness of ara-C. The dose-limiting toxicity of ara-C is myelosuppression. Other toxicities include gastrointestinal disturbances and stomatis. High-dose ara-C may overcome resistance to conventional doses of ara-C. When ara-C is given at high doses, substantial drug concentrations are achieved in cerebrospinal and other body fluids. This has become an important strategy for the treatment of diffuse subarachnoid leukemic infiltration and intracerebral leukemic deposits such as those observed in association with the inversion of chromosome 16.

b. Fluorouracil (FU, 5-Fluorouracil)[14]

As a cancer chemotherapeutic agent FU, with the replacement of the hydrogen by fluorine in the 5 position of uracil, is one of the first drugs rationally designed based on the original observation that in the rat the utilization of endogenous uracil for nucleic acid biosynthesis by chemically induced hepatoma is more avid than by normal tissues; however, this now appears to be a general phenomenon in growing vs. nonproliferating tissues. The stability of the C–F bond precludes the replacement of the fluorine by a methyl group, analogous to the conversion of dUMP to dTMP, in which the 5-H in dUMP is replaced with a methyl group. These and other biochemical differences between FU and uracil ultimately manifest themselves as FU participates in critical steps in a replicating cell.

FU exerts its cytotoxic action indirectly after intracellular metabolism to 5-fluorouridine 5′-monophosphate, FUMP, and its deoxy derivative, FdUMP (Figure 17.5). Ultimately, as a fraudulent substrate, FUMP is phosphorylated to FUTP which is incorporated into RNA where it replaces the natural substrate UTP. FdUMP competes with the natural substrate dUMP for the catalytic sites of thymidylate synthase, a key enzyme in DNA synthesis. Inactivation of this important enzyme is due to the formation of a stable, covalently bonded ternary complex consisting of thymidylate synthase, 5,10-methylenetetrahydrofolate, and FdUMP. With RNA and protein syntheses continually proceeding, FdUMP inhibition of DNA synthesis causes the sensitive cell to die a thymineless death. FU is catabolized *in vivo* to the 5,6-dihydro derivative and other inactive breakdown products. Mechanisms of resistance to FU include the deletion of FU-activation enzymes and the induction of thymidylate synthase refractory to the action of FdUMP.

FU is widely used in the treatment of many solid tumors, particularly in colorectal carcinoma and breast cancer. In combination with levamisole it is effective in the adjuvant treatment of advanced primary colon cancer that has been resected. The major clinical toxicities are mucositis and gastrointestinal disturbances. In addition, severe myelosuppression has been observed after continuous FU infusion.

c. Floxuridine (2′-deoxy-5-fluorouridine, FdUrd)[14]

Because FdUrd is more soluble than FU, by the continuous intra-arterial infusion of FdUrd a much higher concentration of FU is achievable than when FU is given, resulting in enhanced anabolism to FdUMP. Since this metabolite is considered to be closely associated with the antitumor action of FU, it may have more selective benefits in cancer chemotherapy.

C. NATURAL PRODUCTS

As an alternative to rationally designed synthetic antitumor agents, attention has also focused on natural products.

1. Vinca Alkaloids[15,16]

a. Vinblastine (VLB) and Vincristine (VCR)

In the search for hypoglycemic plant medicines, crude extracts of the periwinkle plant were found to cause granulocytopenia and myelosuppression in the rat, and to exhibit antileukemic activity. At least two isolated components of these extracts, VLB and VCR, have

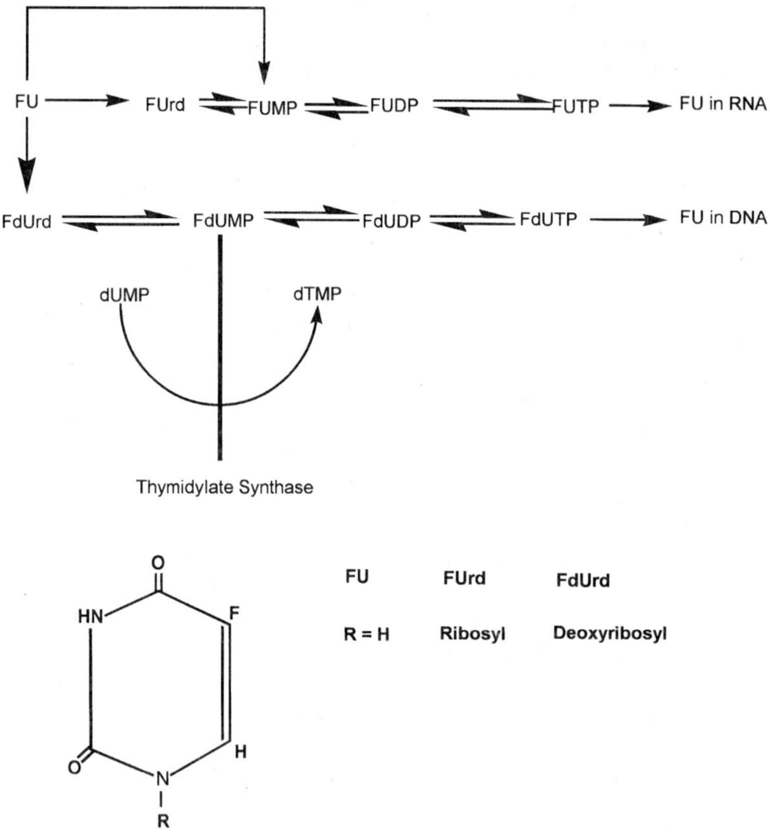

Figure 17.5. Conversion of 5-fluorouracil (FU) to the ribosyl conjugate (FUrd), ribosylmonophosphate (FUMP), diphosphate (FUDT), and triphosphate (FUTP) which allows FU to be incorporated into RNA. Attachment of FU to deoxyribose produces corresponding deoxyribosyl compounds which lead to incorporation of FU into DNA. Fluorodeoxyuridylate (FdUMP) inhibits thymidylate synthase, which blocks formation of thymidylate (dTMP) and DNA synthesis. 5,10-Methylene FH_4 is a cofactor for this enzyme.

important anticancer activity. Both drugs are capable of specific binding to tubulin, the precursor of microtubules responsible for mitosis and other vital cellular functions such as substrate transport, cell motility, and structural integrity. The inhibition of mitotic spindle formation leads to arrest of cells in metaphase of the mitotic cycle. However, cultured cells are susceptible to the cytotoxic actions of the vinca alkaloids during all phases of the cell cycle, especially late S phase, implying additional mechanisms of cytotoxicity. Although structural differences between VLB and VCR appear to be minor, the drugs exhibit significantly different pharmacological, toxicological, and therapeutic features. Cross resistance among them has not been reported. The vinca alkaloids have often been implicated in eliciting multiple drug resistance, presumably because they share a common cellular transport mechanism with a number of other structurally unrelated cytotoxic agents to which cell lines have become resistant.

While neurotoxicity, manifested chiefly as peripheral neuropathy, is rare with VLB, it is dose limiting with VCR. In contrast, VLB is myelosuppressive. Because of its lack of myelosuppressive toxicity, VCR has found broad application in combination with other antitumor drugs since it can be used in full doses together with other myelosuppressive agents. However, VCR can cause cumulative neurotoxicity which is only slowly reversible. The absence of significant neurotoxicity makes VLB much more generally useful in combinations where myelosuppression is not a major problem.

The very long plasma half-life of VCR suggests increasing drug deposition and cumulative toxicity if administered more often than once weekly; neither VLB nor VCR crosses the blood-brain barrier readily. The principal route of excretion of the vinca alkaloids is through the bile, and renal elimination plays only a minor part. Both undergo extensive metabolic degradation; VLB is apparently deacetylated to a more active metabolite. In the few patients studied, favorable antitumor response was associated with slow clearance of the alkaloid. In spite of the very long plasma half-life of VCR, infusion with the agent may lead to improved therapeutic efficacy.

VLB is usually administered intravenously, care being taken to avoid extravasation. Oral dosing is not recommended owing to incomplete and erratic gastrointestinal absorption. In combination with agents such as doxorubicin (DOX), bleomycin (BLM), and dacarbazine (DIC) it is effective for treating advanced Hodgkin's disease. It is also useful for chemotherapy of other solid tumors, including testicular tumor, breast carcinoma, and choriocarcinoma. High-dose VLB combined with BLM was the first regimen to cure a substantial fraction of patients with testicular cancers. The dose-limiting toxicity is leukopenia; thrombocytopenia and anemia are less frequent.

VCR, with a broad spectrum of antitumor activity which may actually be curative, is effective against acute lymphocytic leukemia, lymphomas including Hodgkin's disease, and childhood solid tumors. Its usefulness is limited by neurotoxicity, while hematologic toxicity is uncommon. Alopecia occurs quite regularly with VCR usage.

2. Podophyllotoxins[16,17]

Podophyllum peltatum L., also known as American mandrake or May apple, occupies a notable niche in American folk medicine; early settlers used its root and rhizome as a cathartic, emetic, and cholagogue. Alcohol extraction of the dried roots and rhizomes of the *Podophyllum* species affords a resinous product, podophyllin. The antimitotic and antitumor constituents of podophyllin are podophyllotoxins; they are lignans and not alkaloids. Podophyllotoxins are effective topically against warts; however, they are very toxic. Semisynthetic analogs were therefore developed, culminating in the discovery of etoposide (VP) and teniposide (VM). DNA breakage correlates with cytotoxicity of these compounds. The current consensus is that topoisomerase II is the most likely intracellular target of the epipodophyllotoxins. Those congeners active in inducing protein-associated DNA breaks are also potent inhibitors of the catenation, i.e., the double-stranded breaking and resealing activity of mammalian DNA topoisomerase II, while topoisomerase I that catalyzes the breaking of one strand of DNA remains unaffected.

a. *Etoposide (VP, VP-16)*

The principal route of excretion of etoposide is renal. Over a wide range of concentrations VP is more than 94% bound to serum albumin; this is one of the reasons why VP penetrates the blood-brain barrier poorly. Hepatic impairment seems not to affect VP pharmacokinetics; however, renal dysfunction greatly decreases VP total clearance so that dose reduction in these patients is indicated. An oxidation product of VP may be responsible for the cytotoxic actions that damage DNA.

Etoposide is assuming an increasingly significant role in cancer chemotherapy, especially in combination with other agents. Combined with cisplatin, VP is highly effective in small cell lung cancer as well as squamous carcinoma and adenocarcinomas of the lung. It is curative in the salvage treatment for testicular cancers that have failed primary treatment with VLB, BLM, and cisplatin. Recent studies have indicated that prolonged and repeated dosing schedules increase the effectiveness of VP. Its dose-limiting toxicity is leukopenia; thrombocytopenia is less frequent. Nausea and vomiting are encountered occasionally, particularly with the oral preparation. The availability of the oral preparation has greatly extended the potential range of its therapeutic applications.

b. Teniposide (VM, VM-26)

In general, VM seems to be biologically more active than VP. Like VP, VM shows wide interpatient variations in its pharmacokinetics. In patients with leukemia, those with higher steady-state plasma VM concentrations and slower drug clearance were more likely to respond. Virtually completely bound to serum albumin, VM does not penetrate the blood-brain barrier well. Teniposide is a clinically useful agent, especially in combination with other agents in treating hematologic malignancies.

3. Anthracycline Antibiotics[18]

Isolated from cultures of various species of *Streptomyces*, the anthracycline antibiotics, including daunorubicin (DNR) and DOX, and several of their semisynthetic analogs, are an important class of anticancer agents with a broad spectrum of clinical activity.

The linear planar tetrahydrotetracene ring system incorporating quinone and hydroquinone moieties together with an unusual amino-sugar, daunosamine, is responsible for a variety of pharmacologic consequences: (1) chelation with divalent cations, (2) biological redox reactions, (3) the *in vivo* generation of free radicals, (4) intercalation between DNA base pairs followed by interaction of the amino group of daunosamine with the sugar-phosphate backbone of the DNA helix, and (5) inhibition of DNA topoisomerase II. Any and all of these events can ultimately be detrimental to cell replication and survival. For instance, intercalation can cause DNA strand breaks and sister chromatid exchange, and the eventual inhibition of nucleic acid synthesis. Free radicals originating from these drugs can lead to the subsequent formation of not only highly toxic intermediates such as superoxide anion and hydroxyl radicals, but other reactive radicals with alkylating properties. In fact, the deleterious myocardiac toxicity of these antibiotics has been attributed to myocardiac mitochondrial and cell membrane damage caused by these radicals. Continuing efforts are being expended at structural modifications of the anthracycline antibiotics to improve their clinical efficacy and selective toxicity to tumors.

a. Daunorubicin (Daunomycin, DNR)

DNR has a plasma half-life of 20 hr, is highly protein bound, and is extensively metabolized in the body. In combination with other agents, DNR is effective in the treatment of acute leukemias. It is also used in treating certain solid tumors; however, in this regard, it is much less efficacious than DOX. Its dose-limiting toxicity is leukopenia; nausea and vomiting are relatively mild. Cardiomyopathy is the most serious and dose-limiting side effect. However, its 4-demethoxy derivative, or idarubicin, is less cardiotoxic, and gaining clinical application.

b. Doxorubicin (Adriamycin, DOX)

It is surprising that the spectrum of anticancer activity of DOX is so much wider than that of DNR, given the apparently minor difference in structure. The early DOX clearance during the distribution phase seems to correlate with patient age. DOX is extensively metabolized in the body, and the predominant route of elimination is through the bile. A major product of DOX metabolism mediated by cytoplasmic aldoketoreductases is its reduced 13-hydroxy metabolite, doxorubicinol (DOX-ol), which has cytotoxic properties. The plasma half-life of DOX-ol, 30 hr, is approximately the same as that of DOX. It has been suggested that DOX cardiomyopathy may be related to the formation of another metabolite, deoxydoxorubicinone.

DOX has an impressive spectrum of anticancer activity, being effective against a variety of hematologic malignancies and solid tumors. It is the single most effective agent against metastatic breast cancer and soft tissue sarcomas. Significant clinical synergism has been observed when given with either CPA or FU and CPA. Like DNR, its dose-limiting toxicity is also hematologic, primarily leukopenia. Serious cardiomyopathy often occurs after chronic treatment with DOX and appears to be related to the total dose administered. Dose reduction is advocated in patients with liver disease or hyperbilirubinemia.

4. Bleomycins (BLM)[19]

A group of cytotoxic glycopeptide antibiotics, isolated from a culture filtrate of a strain of the microorganism *Streptomyces verticillus*, are collectively known as the bleomycins. They share a complex common structure. The clinical preparation of BLM is a mixture of analogs, mostly A_2 (70%) and B_2 (28%). BLM chelates with metal ions such as those of copper and iron and binds to DNA through intercalation. In the presence of ferrous ions and oxygen it generates free radicals that induce single- as well as double-strand breaks in DNA, but not RNA. These breaks are manifested in chromosomal aberrations and fragmentations, as seen in cultured cells in the G_2 phase of the cell cycle. Also, in the presence of not only oxygen, but also a reducing agent such as dithiothreitol, the Cu·BLM chelate is capable of behaving like a minienzyme, a monooxygenase, to degrade DNA.

Approximately 60% of the administered dose is slowly excreted in the urine. In patients with renal failure the plasma half-life of BLM is considerably increased with decreasing creatinine clearance. Although all tissues contain a BLM-degrading enzyme, BLM hydrolase, levels of this enzyme are low in skin and lung where significant toxicity has been reported.

The absence of myleosuppressive toxicity in BLM makes it a valuable member in various combinations with other anticancer agents in curative regimens for treating testicular cancer, squamous cell carcinomas, and lymphomas. Its most serious toxicity is a unique form of pulmonary fibrosis in the subpleural areas; this peculiar toxicity is related to the total dose and the risk increases with advancing age.

5. Dactinomycin (DAC, Actinomycin D)[18,20]

DAC, first introduced into the clinic in 1954, is the oldest antineoplastic antibiotic. A model RNA synthesis inhibitor, DAC forms a complex with DNA and then selectively interferes with DNA-dependent RNA synthesis, specifically that of ribosomal RNA. The planar phenoxazone ring intercalates between adjacent G-C base-pairs of DNA, and the cyclic peptides interact with the amino groups of G through hydrogen bonding.

The plasma half-life of the antibiotic is estimated to be 36 hr; in 7 d on average 20% of the dose is excreted in the urine and a lesser amount in the feces. The drug is minimally metabolized and does not penetrate readily into the CNS. However, it is selectively concentrated in the nucleated blood elements. In general, the response of tumors to the drug is related to the intratumoral drug concentration and the retention of this antibiotic in the tumor. Myelosuppression is its dose-limiting toxicity.

As a single agent DAC is effective in choriocarcinoma. In combination regimens it is used for the treatment of solid tumors such as Ewing's sarcoma, Wilms' tumor, and rhabdomyosarcoma.

6. Mitomycin C (MMC)[20]

The presence of the quinoid moiety in MMC may facilitate its participation in biological redox reactions to generate highly reactive and cytotoxic free radicals, and that of the aziridine ring may further confer alkylating properties on the agent, probably after *in vivo* reductive activation. In short, MMC is expected potentially to alkylate, cross link, cleave, and depurinate DNA after forming various intermediates in cyclic redox reactions, thus leading to inhibition of cell replication. Its dose-limiting toxicity is myelosuppression. MMC is active against a number of solid tumors. In combination with other agents it is useful for treating stomach and breast cancers.

7. L-Asparaginase (LAS, L-Asparagine Amidohydrolase)[21]

LAS, the only enzyme of some application in clinical cancer chemotherapy, mediates the cleavage of the generally considered nonessential amino acid L-asparagine to aspartate and ammonia; the reverse reaction, on the other hand, is catalyzed by asparagine synthetase. The identification of LAS in guinea pig serum as the inhibitory factor of rodent tumors has been initially hailed as a major breakthrough in cancer biochemistry: the first definitive demonstration of a unique, distinct metabolic difference between normal and cancer cells. It was hoped that this difference could form the basis for specific chemotherapy, at least of lymphoid malignancies, since human lymphoid tissues are particularly deficient in asparagine synthetase so that the depletion of L-asparagine would be selectively deleterious. Depletion of L-asparagine is the prelude to inhibition of protein synthesis and ultimately cell death. Unfortunately, the cellular difference in sensitivity to the action of LAS is only quantitative.

For clinical use the enzyme is prepared from *Escherichia coli* or *Erwinia carotovora.* It is an agent with a narrow spectrum of anticancer activity, particularly useful for remission induction in pediatric patients with acute lymphocytic leukemia. In adults with acute lymphoblastic leukemia its role is limited when used alone. However, it is used widely in combination with MTX for the treatment of adult acute lymphoblastic leukemia because of its ability to modulate side effects of MTX. However, in adults it elicits a variety of toxicities including hyperglycemia, lowering of plasma proteins (particularly fibrinogen), severe anorexia, and weight loss, and in very high doses CNS depression. LAS has similarly been reported to modulate the toxic side effects of ara-C; for this reason it is used for remission induction in acute myeloblastic leukemia. LAS is prone to induce allergic reactions. Patients becoming allergic to *Escherichia coli* preparation have been found to tolerate the *Erwinia* preparation and thus allowed continuing LAS therapy. Resistance to LAS therapy develops readily and rapidly. To reduce LAS immunogenicity and to prolong its plasma half-life, LAS from *Escherichia coli* covalently linked to polyethylene glycol, PEG-LAS, has been developed. In humans, the plasma half-life of PEG-LAS is several times longer than that of native LAS, thus permitting less frequent administration. Moreover, in pediatric patients it is less immunogenic. Currently it is in clinical trial.

8. Taxol[15] (Paclitaxel)

A complex diterpene extracted from the bark of the Pacific yew, *Taxus brevifolia*, taxol promotes microtubule assembly *in vitro* at concentrations attainable clinically during prolonged infusions; it produces abnormal morphological effects on these cellular structures, a unique mechanism of cytotoxicity. Recent clinical trials have shown that taxol is active against drug-resistant ovarian cancer, breast cancer, and nonsmall cell lung cancer. Major toxicities include acute hypersensitivity reactions, neutropenia, mucositis, and peripheral neuropathy; cardiac rhythm disturbances have also been observed.

D. MISCELLANEOUS AGENTS

1. Platinum Coordination Compounds[9]

The inorganic antitumor agent cis-diamminedichloroplatinum (II) (cisplatin) was discovered serendipitously when, upon electrolysis, cultured bacteria were killed by platinum salts emanating from the electrodes. Its establishment as an important anticancer agent has prompted the synthesis and development of a host of coordination compounds of platinum and other metals in the hope of finding more efficacious agents. But thus far, in addition to cisplatin, carboplatin is the only member of the family of platinum coordination compounds that has been accepted clinically.

For these coordination compounds to show antitumor activity, first, the two ammine groups (ammonia ligands) must be in a *cis*-configuration. Second, the compounds must have suitable leaving groups such as chloride and carboxylate anions; other anions such as iodide, nitrate, nitrite, and perchlorate render the compounds inactive. Third, the platinum-bound nitrogen must contain a hydrogen donor, that is, at least one NH group. Lastly, tetravalent platinum compounds are seldom active per se; the platinum must first undergo reduction to the square planar divalent state.

a. Cisplatin (DDP)

DDP exists in cis and trans isomeric forms; however, only the *cis*-isomer is active. It has long been recognized that DDP reacts with pyrimidines and nucleic acids to produce "platinum blues" of undefined structures. Since DDP is an active antitumor agent while the *trans*-isomer is markedly less active or totally inactive, it suggests that the interaction between DDP and DNA, the likely target molecule, is stereospecific. At concentrations barely cytotoxic to HeLa cells, DDP indeed inhibits DNA, but not RNA or protein synthesis. Apparently this inhibition is the consequence of both intrastrand and interstrand DNA cross linking. Therefore, it is currently believed that inhibition of DNA synthesis constitutes the mechanism of cytotoxicity of DDP. However, it must be reiterated that DDP is a reactive molecule that generates a number of products *in vivo*. The contributions of these products to the selective cytotoxicity of DDP to cancer cells remain to be elucidated. A significant proportion of DDP is excreted in the urine. Repeated courses of DDP lead to a reduction in the renal elimination of platinum, probably through a decrease in tubular secretion of DDP.

Its most serious side effect is nephrotoxicity. Severe debilitating nausea and vomiting are common. Ototoxicity such as tinnitus and hearing loss, even deafness, may also occur. The infusion of DDP over periods as long as 5 d attenuates many of the acute side effects, such as nausea and vomiting. All of the DDP toxicities are strongly dose related and can be largely avoided at lower dosages. Hydration and diuresis ameliorate the nephrotoxicity, but not the ototoxicity.

DDP is now widely used for the treatment of a variety of solid tumors. It is an important component of the combination regimens that are curative for testicular cancer. It is also effective against gynecologic malignancies, particularly ovarian cancer. DDP is highly effective in metatastic breast cancer, and very useful for the treatment of both small cell lung cancer as well as squamous carcinoma and adenocarcinomas of the lung.

b. Carboplatin (CPT)[9]

CPT is a platinum coordination compound with antitumor activity, but with less nephrotoxicity, ototoxicity, and neurotoxicity than DDP. However, it is myelosuppressive. CPT is active against a variety of solid tumors, especially ovarian cancer; its spectrum of antitumor activity is similar to that of DDP except that its therapeutic index seems to be significantly better. Its dose-limiting toxicity is hematologic, mostly leukopenia. Nausea and vomiting are mild; ototoxicity, neuropathy, and nephrotoxicity are rare. In patients with ovarian cancer who fail or relapse after standard conventional cisplatin-containing therapy, significant responses including complete remissions have been elicited; however, marked cross resistance between CPT and DDP has been observed.

2. Dacarbazine (DIC, DTIC)[22]

Although derived from the purine precursor, 5-aminoimidazole-4-carboxamide, DIC apparently is not an antimetabolite, but rather an alkylating agent. *In vivo* it undergoes N-demethylation mediated by the hepatic microsomal mixed function oxidase to give the N-monomethyl metabolite that ultimately generates the active antitumor methylating species. Because of poor oral absorption the drug is given intravenously. Excretion is mainly by the kidney and may be delayed with renal impairment. It is extremely emetic, and mild myelosuppression has been reported.

DIC currently is the most active single agent against malignant melanoma, although the response rate is only 20%. It is also effective in Hodgkin's disease and soft tissue sarcomas in combination regimens.

3. Hydroxyurea (Hydrea, HU)[23]

The simplest one-carbon organic antitumor agent, HU, has been known for more than a century; however, its anticancer activity has been demonstrated only relatively recently. There is ample evidence that, at noncytotoxic doses, HU *in vitro* and *in vivo* blocks DNA, but not RNA and protein syntheses by inhibiting ribonucleoside diphosphate reductase. Cells in S phase are killed while those in other phases are allowed to progress to the G_1-S junction where they are synchronized.

After oral administration of large doses, HU is rapidly and completely absorbed and penetrates readily into the cerebrospinal and ascites fluids. The plasma half-life is approximately 4 hr, and most of the drug is eliminated by urinary excretion. Unlike urea, HU does not diffuse freely through all body tissues.

HU is an effective oral agent for treating chronic myelogenous leukemia and some solid tumors. Its dose-limiting toxicity is leukopenia. At high doses nausea, vomiting, and stomatitis have been reported. Since, unlike busulfan, HU produces no delayed toxicity after chronic administration in patients with chronic myeloblastic leukemia, it has become the primary agent of choice for the benign phase of the disease. HU can additionally rapidly reduce circulating blasts in patients with acute leukemia, and is therefore used in the short term for this purpose.

4. Mitoxantrone[18]

Although not exactly an analog of the anthracycline antibiotics, conceptually mitoxantrone (first termed DHQ by its discoverer) may be considered a derivative of DOX following removal of its amino sugar. This chemical modification was believed to lessen the myocardiac toxicity of this family of compounds.

Mitoxantrone intercalates into DNA, causes intra- and interstrand cross linkings with G-C pairs preferred, induces single- and double-strand breaks, and finally inhibits both DNA and RNA syntheses; however, it apparently does not generate cytotoxic free radicals. Moreover, it elicits nuclear aberrations and chromosomal scattering. It is not cell cycle phase-specific with regard to cell killing, but it blocks cells at the G_2 phase to result in an increase of cellular RNA content and polypoidy. Cellular resistance to mitoxantrone is attributed to impaired transport of the agent. The intercalation may impair DNA transcription and RNA processing; however, that effect is not believed to kill cancer cells. In human autopsy specimens, the highest mitoxantrone concentration is in the thyroid and liver, followed by heart. Myelosuppression, especially granulocytopenia, is dose limiting. Other occasional toxic manifestations include cardiomyopathy, thrombocytopenia, nausea and vomiting, mucositis, and alopecia.

Mitoxantrone is an active agent against breast cancer, hepatocellular carcinoma, lymphoma, and acute leukemia. In combination with ara-C it is effective and well tolerated and produces high remission rates in elderly patients with acute myelocytic leukemia. Compared with DOX, it is perhaps not as effective against breast cancer, but certainly less prone to elicit myocardiac toxicity.

III. HORMONE THERAPY[24]

The growth of certain tumors such as those of the breast, endometrium, and prostate frequently depends on stimulation by sex hormones. Such tumors therefore can be inhibited by surgical ablation of hormone-producing tissues, biochemical blockade of hormone synthesis, or the application of hormone antagonists. Unfortunately, however, hormonal treatment is only palliative.

Androgens have long been known to maintain prostate size and function, whereas castration or estrogen treatment shrinks prostate tumors. More recently, prostate tumors have been controlled with synthetic luteinizing hormone release hormone (LHRH) agonists such as leuprolide, which, when given clinically, reduces plasma testosterone levels through inhibition of gonadotropin secretion.

Since the growth of normal breast tissue is exquisitely dependent upon endocrinal stimulation and control, it is not surprising that the growth of breast cancer is similarly sensitive to hormonal manipulations. As will be discussed later, both pre- and postmenopausal metastatic breast cancers are treated with tamoxifen, an antiestrogen with relatively little toxicity. Also the aromatase inhibitor, aminoglutethimide, which prevents the production of estrogens from fat tissue, is effective in treating breast cancer. Formerly, hypophysectomy or ovariectomy served a similar purpose of reducing estrogen activity. Endometrial cancer frequently responds to progestins, which apparently antagonize the estrogen dependence of the tumor. The use of glucocorticoids against lymphomas and leukemias probably rests on the lympholytic action of these hormones.

Sex and adrenocorticoid hormones react via specific receptors located in certain neoplastic cells. The binding of the hormones to a cytoplasmic or nuclear protein receptor then leads to interaction with genomic DNA which, following transcription of mRNA and translation, produces proteins that mediate the actions of the hormones.

The receptor status of the tumor determines its response to the specific hormone. This aspect has been studied intensively in the case of the estrogen receptor for breast cancer. Whereas about 60% of patients whose breast cancer is estrogen receptor positive respond to endocrine treatment (ablation, antiestrogen, or aromatase inhibitors), only about 10% of estrogen receptor-negative tumors have similarly responded. Since the progesterone receptor is induced by estrogens and thus reflects estrogen function, the tumor response to estrogens is increased to about 75% in tumors which are both estrogen and progesterone receptor positive. With endometrial cancer, the tumor response to progestin treatment is close to 90% in progesterone receptor-positive tumors, but only 17% in progesterone receptor-deficient neoplasms. A relationship between androgen receptor presence and response to endocrine therapy of prostate tumors has also been observed. Usually well differentiated tumors have high receptor levels, but when such tumors become less hormone dependent the cells become dedifferentiated and receptors are lost. Such cells usually show a high rate of DNA synthesis, and may become susceptible to cytotoxic chemotherapy.

A. GLUCOCORTICOIDS

These drugs are lympholytic agents, especially against T-cells. They produce fragmentation of DNA, and are useful in the treatment of lymphocytic leukemia and lymphomas. Their use in breast cancer may be due to some additional direct growth-inhibitory action against tumor cells. They are also used as supportive therapy in managing hypercalcemia in cancer. Prednisone, a glucocorticoid that differs from the naturally occurring cortisone in having an extra double bond linking C1 and C2, is most frequently selected. It is converted to the active form of the steroid, prednisolone, by reduction of the ketone at carbon 11. Prednisolone has a half-life of about 3 hr and is further metabolized by the liver. Cushingoid syndrome, manifested by hypertension, fluid retention, and moon face, as well as hirsutism, hyperglycemia, osteoporosis, euphoria, glaucoma, and skin abnormalities, are side effects. Withdrawal from prednisone treatment should be gradual to permit return of normal adrenal function. Resistance to glucocorticoid therapy has been associated with a decrease in receptor binding to the steroid or a mutation of the receptor.

B. ESTROGENS

Diethylstilbestrol (DES) and ethinyl estradiol are used in the treatment of prostate carcinomas. These compounds are far more potent than the natural estrogen, estradiol. The exact mechanism of anticancer action of these agents is unknown. By inhibiting LH production, testosterone synthesis is decreased, thereby reducing the stimulus to prostate tumor growth. Also, they cause disturbances in mitosis, induce chromosomal nondisjunction, and possibly inhibit estrogen receptor resynthesis. Both drugs are largely inactivated by hepatic metabolism. The initial plasma half-life of DES is 80 min, followed by a slow second phase, and that of ethinyl estradiol is 28 hr.

Typical toxicities of estrogens include a transient exacerbation of various symptoms termed the tumor flare, which involves an increase in swelling of tumor metastases, skeletal pain, and hypercalcemia. Treatment should be stopped until normal calcium levels have been restored. Hypertension, congestive heart failure, thromboembolism, vaginal bleeding, breast and bone pain, gynecomastia, corneal alterations, and rashes have been reported, together with nausea, vomiting, and diarrhea. Long-term use of estrogens has resulted in endometrial and breast carcinoma. *In utero* exposure to DES increases alarmingly the risk of developing vaginal clear cell adenocarcinoma in young women, probably due to the action of an oxidative metabolite of DES in the fetal genital tract.

C. GONDADOTROPIN (GnRH) OR LUTEINIZING HORMONE-RELEASING HORMONES (LHRH)

This hormone stimulates anterior pituitary cells to release LH after binding to LHRH receptors, culminating in down-regulation of the receptor. Chronic exposure to LHRH agonists or intermittent exposure to high doses reduces LH release, and plasma concentrations of testosterone and related steroids decline, producing a reversible pharmacological orchiectomy. The synthetic polypeptides leuprolide and goserelin are LHRH agonists, used mainly in the therapy of prostate cancer, usually in combination with the antiandrogen, flutamide (see below). This treatment produces a profound and protracted reduction in testosterone levels. Most common side effects of LHRH agonists are hot flashes, decreased libido, and impotence.

D. ANTIANDROGEN

Flutamide is a nonsteroidal antiandrogen; it and its α-hydroxy metabolite compete with dihydrotestosterone for binding to the androgen receptor. To protect against a transient rise in plasma testosterone levels, flutamide is co-administered with an LHRH agonist in the therapy of prostate cancer. The drug is activated by hydroxylation to hydroxyflutamide, which is the actual competitor. Side effects include gynecomastia, nausea, diarrhea, and dizziness.

E. ANTIESTROGEN

Tamoxifen is the therapeutic estrogen antagonist of choice. By binding to estrogen receptors it competes with endogenous estradiol, and therefore inhibits breast cancer cells dependent on estrogen stimulation. It also possesses some estrogen agonist properties.

Its major action is in estrogen receptor-positive postmenopausal women with breast cancer, but it also has anticancer efficacy in estrogen receptor-negative and premenopausal patients, suggesting additional mechanisms of action. It is used in hormonal therapy for breast cancer in postmenopausal women, in advanced disease in premenopausal patients, and as an adjuvant in postmenopausal disease. Currently it is being tested as a prophylactic agent against breast cancer in tumor-free women with a high risk of that disease. The drug is metabolized to 4-hydroxy-tamoxifen, N-desmethyl-tamoxifen, and other products, some of which have long half-lives and themselves bind to the estrogen receptor. It is excreted largely in the feces, and renal impairment does not result in elevated drug concentration in plasma.

Toxicity is usually minimal, including hot flashes, nausea, a transient tumor flare, and occasional thrombocytopenia. Chronic administration enhances the risk of endometrial carcinomas.

F. AROMATASE INHIBITORS

Whereas in premenopausal women most of the estrogen is synthesized in the ovary, in postmenopausal women it is derived from extraglandular tissues. The conversion of androstenedione to estrone and ultimately to estradiol is mediated by an enzyme system collectively known as aromatase located largely in adipose tissue. Aminoglutethimide, originally studied because of its anticonvulsive properties, inhibits aromatase. It is useful in treating breast cancer in estrogen or progesterone receptor-positive postmenopausal women or ovariectomized premenopausal women. Because hydrocortisone synthesis is also blocked by aminoglutethimide, hydrocortisone is usually co-administered with the aromatase inhibitor.

The drug has an average plasma half-life of 13 hr that declines to about half that value upon chronic use, probably because of hepatic microsomal enzyme induction. Aminoglutethimide is more toxic than tamoxifen, producing CNS depression, ataxia, skin rashes, and nausea.

G. PROGESTINS

Exactly how progestins exert their antitumor effects is not known. Medroxyprogesterone and megestrol are synthetic progestins that can be given orally. Both are extensively metabolized. Principal toxicities include hot flashes, fluid retention, vaginal bleeding, and hypercalcemia. There is a risk of thrombophlebitis, thromboembolism, and lowering of plasma HDL, leading to increased incidence of atherosclerosis. The drugs are used mainly against advanced, inoperable, or recurrent endometrial carcinoma and occasionally in metastic breast cancer.

H. ANDROGENS

These hormones nowadays are used infrequently against metastic breast cancer where they probably act indirectly to reduce endogenous estrogen synthesis by suppressing LH production. Testosterone is activated by reduction to dihydrotestosterone which then binds to the androgen receptor. Now fluoxymesterone is used and has a longer plasma half-life than does testosterone. Major side effects involve masculinization, including facial growth, baldness, water retention, occasional hypercalcemia, and, for fluoxymesterone, cholestatic hepatitis and hepatic adenocarcinoma after prolonged exposure.

IV. IMMUNOTHERAPY OF CANCER[26]

While chemotherapy has established itself as one of the generally accepted modalities of cancer treatment, immunotherapy is still under development, sometimes with tantalizingly encouraging results. Early observations in animal models that tumor-associated antigens (TAA) could evoke host immunity in carcinogen- and virus-induced tumors (as contrasted with spontaneous tumors), have lent considerable impetus to experimental cancer immunotherapy. Immunotherapy promises to offer at least one definitive advantage over cytotoxic chemotherapy, namely, exquisite selectivity.

The development of cancer immunotherapy has largely been following the traditional two-pronged approach, active immunization and passive immunization. In the former, humoral or cellular immunity is provoked by administration of, or exposure to, appropriate antigen, whereas in the latter, antibodies produced in another person or species are utilized to confer immunity on the recipient.

Active immunization with autochthonous tumors after attenuation by irradiation, or neuraminidase treatment to unmask TAA on cell surface, or hybridization with cultured cells, or admixing with viral, bacterial, or other adjuvant to enhance tumor immunogenicity, has been tried with minor successes in a variety of cancers such as malignant melanoma, renal cell carcinoma, and acute myelogenous leukemia. However, these malignancies are known to undergo spontaneous remission. To prolong remissions or to increase remission reinduction rates in acute leukemias when the patients are already in remission after intensive chemotherapy and radiotherapy, irradiated allogenic tumor cells have been administered with bacterial or other adjuvants with limited success. Clinical improvement has also been reported by reinfusion of autologous lymphocytes activated *in vitro* with either tumor cells or mitogens such as phytohemagglutinin, leading to recent research with lymphocyte-activated killer (LAK, see below) cells. The use of immunostimulants has opened another avenue to active immunization; for instance, bacterial and chemical contact allergens have been reported to produce regression of cutaneous basal cell and squamous cell carcinomas, and metastatic melanoma lesions. Similarly, direct intralesional administration of viable *Bacillus Calmette-Guérin* has caused up to 60% regression of cutaneous metastases in patients with malignant melanoma. Although its tumor inhibitory effects are not consistent, heat-inactivated *Corynebacterium parvum* administered intraperitoneally has produced regression of metastatic lesions in 30% of patients with epithelial ovarian carcinoma. Taken together, these observations suggest that in immunocompetent patients these bacterial adjuvants are effective against small tumor volumes if direct contact with tumor cells is possible. Immunorestorative agents including certain traditional Chinese herbal medicines and the veterinary anthelmintic levamisole, a relatively simple organic compound, have also shown promise. Levamisole exerts an effect on macrophage and T-cell function; in combination with 5-FU it is significantly more effective than the latter alone in prolonging the survival of patients with Dukes stage C colorectal carcinoma.

Interferons (IFN) are glycoproteins elaborated by host cells in response to exogenous harmful stimuli. They were noted first for their antiviral, but later for their antiproliferative and differentiative properties as well as their effects on the immune system. The three major kinds of IFNs are classified according to their cellular sources: IFN-α from leukocytes and macrophages, IFN-β from fibroblasts and epithelial cells, and IFN-γ from T-cells and large granular lymphocytes. Highly homogeneous IFN preparations are now available from recombinant DNA technology. Many lymphoreticular tumors are sensitive to IFN-α therapy, in particular hairy cell leukemia, chronic myelogenous leukemia, and nodular lymphoma. Occasionally patients with chronic lymphocytic leukemia and multiple myeloma also respond. IFN-α therapy is also effective in some patients with glioblastoma, Kaposi's sarcoma, carcinoids, malignant melanoma, and renal cell carcinoma. By regional or intralesional administration it is impressively active against basal cell, ovarian, and bladder carcinomas. It rarely produces any serious side effects, but often elicits an influenza-like syndrome. IFNs exert their antitumor effects directly by interacting with tumor cells and indirectly through immunomodulation. Combination chemo- and immunotherapy is currently under investigation; promising results have already been reported by combining 5-FU with recombinant IFN-α-2a against advanced colorectal carcinoma. Interleukin-2 (IL-2) is another cytokine intensively studied as an immunotherapeutic agent; it has recently been approved by the FDA for the treatment of renal cell carcinoma; however, IL-2 exerts no direct effect on malignant cells.

Attempts to develop specific antitumor vaccines have been mostly unsuccessful. Recently it has been reported that a small fraction, 8 to 16%, of metastases regressed in melanoma patients inoculated with an autologous tumor-cell vaccine. IL-2 may augment the tumor response to vaccines containing TAA. Clearly, further investigations in anticancer vaccines are warranted.

Passive immunization remains an attractive and promising approach to cancer immunotherapy. Recent progress in this field has been encouraging; for example, temporary reduction in lymphocyte counts has been achieved in patients with chronic lymphocytic leukemia and in T- and B-cell lymphomas. The availability of monoclonal antibodies against TAA has greatly enhanced interest in passive immunization, but few TAAs have actually been identified. Moreover, they are not really exclusively associated with tumors, but generally are expressed by one or more normal cell types. This may not be as detrimental as it appears to be because, as an example, most lymphomas are monoclonal, and antibodies against human B-cell lymphoma react at most with only a small fraction of the patient's normal B-cells. In addition, although some TAA may be expressed by a large number of host cells, the quantitative difference in expression may still be therapeutically exploitable. To produce large amounts of human monoclonal antibodies that recognize TAA is technically difficult. Even if available in sufficient amounts for clinical applications, the efficacy of monoclonal antibodies may be impeded by free antigen, failure to penetrate tumor tissues, and absence of antigen expression by some tumor cells. Nevertheless, significant objective response rates lasting 29 to 72 months have been observed in patients with B-cell lymphoma treated with anti-idiotypic antibodies. Also, regression of metastatic melanoma has been reported after systemic administration of monoclonal antibodies against the tumor-associated antigenic ganglioside GD_3 and intralesional administration of monoclonal antibodies against the ganglioside GD_2. Most recently, a sizable number of patients with colorectal cancer of Dukes stage C were randomly assigned to either an observational regimen or postoperational monoclonal antibody therapy; they were followed up for 5 years. The overall death rate of the antibody-treated patients was reduced by 30%, and recurrence rate by 27%. Conjugation of antibodies with cytotoxic agents to target the latter for tumor cells is another interesting approach. In fact, similar conjugation with radionuclides has also shown activity in lymphomas and ovarian carcinoma; myelotoxicity is dose limiting. In general, unconjugated monoclonal antibodies are well tolerated, however. A number of the unconjugated antibodies are currently in clinical trial.

The availability of cytokines produced by recombinant DNA technology has similarly significantly facilitated clinical evaluations of adoptive immunotherapy. Administration of autologous LAK cells with IL-2 has elicited significant objective response in patients with renal cell carcinoma, melanoma, and colorectal carcinoma, including some long-lasting complete remissions; however, IL-2 alone without LAK is also active against renal cell carcinoma and melanoma. High-dose IL-2 with LAK produces fever, nausea and vomiting, diarrhea, erythema, fluid shifts, weight gain, increase in serum creatinine, hyperbilirubinemia, hypotension, supraventricular arrythmia, and pulmonary edema; all these are reversible. Tumor infiltrating lymphocytes (TIL) from tumors with specific antitumor reactivity and cultured with low concentrations of IL-2 are more potent than LAK in animal models. TIL produced regression in 11 of 20 patients with metastatic melanoma. Compared with LAK cells, TIL may localize at tumor sites more effectively.

V. AGING AND PHARMACOLOGY OF ANTICANCER AGENTS[27,28]

In the U.S., though only approximately 20% of the population is 55 years of age or older, 80% of malignancies occurs in this ever-increasing group. As chemotherapy has now established itself as one of the modalities of cancer treatment, an understanding of the effects of aging on the pharmacology of antitumor agents has become a prerequisite for the efficacious use of therapeutic drugs. Unfortunately, difficulties of collecting data on this subject have impaired the attainment of such a goal. There are only a few studies on younger patients to provide a reference standard. In clinical trials, selection bias prevails because most investigators are reluctant to enter elderly patients into developmental therapeutic protocols. Traditional classification of elderly patients on the basis of chronological rather than biological age is arbitrary and a poor predictor of pharmacological changes related to the aging process. The elderly population is vastly heterogeneous, and the interpatient variability can be staggering. In addition, comorbid diseases frequently accompany older age, and patients must be considered on an individual basis. Nonetheless, certain generalizations have been reached regarding the effects of aging on the pharmacology of cancer chemotherapeutic agents.

Aging sets in motion a number of irreversible physical and biological changes, many of which can only be demonstrated by careful laboratory tests; we list a few such alterations. Total body water and lean body mass decrease, with a concomitant increase in body fat. There is a shift in drug partition so that the apparent volume of distribution of lipophilic drugs is enlarged while that of hydrophilic drugs is diminished. The liver decreases in size and weight, especially in women; its blood flow and extraction capacity fall off, and, in general, all hepatobiliary functions decline. The combined outcome is a lessening of the first-pass effect, and the bioavailability of a drug is thus enhanced. Bioavailability of highly protein-bound drugs is also increased by age-associated hypoalbuminemia. Although phase II reactions (conjugation reactions) do not appear to be affected, phase I biotransformations (conversion of parent drug to a more polar metabolite) in the elderly are reduced. Therefore, drug deactivation or activation is lessened. The kidney becomes smaller in size, its blood flow decreases, and creatinine clearance usually declines with age. As a result, drug elimination is less effective in the elderly, particularly if hepatic function is impaired at the same time. When coupled with an expanded volume of distribution, the slowed clearance will significantly lengthen the plasma half-life of the drug. These age-related physiological alterations, especially if they occur in combination, will lead to far-reaching pharmacokinetic, pharmacodynamic, and toxicological consequences.

There are a few examples where age has appeared to influence the pharmacological action of anticancer agents. Although the absorption of orally administered anticancer agents does not seem to be influenced by aging, age-related alterations in toxicity secondary to changes in drug distribution have been reported. For example, in the elderly the more severe myelotoxicity of lipid-soluble drugs such as semustine (methyl-CCNU) and other nitrosoureas may be attributable to their partition in favor of adipose tissue, which is increased relative to lean body mass in the elderly. During the early distribution phase, DOX clearance is inversely related to the age of the patient, being slower in the elderly. To avoid the observed increased risk of DOX-induced cardiotoxicity in this population of patients, dose modulation is mandatory. Although there is no evidence so far that metabolism of anticancer agents is altered in any fashion in these patients, renal function such as the glomerular filtration rate, tubular reabsorption and secretion, is diminished in most (70%) of the elderly. In these patients, to avoid serious toxicity caused by chemotherapeutic agents such as BLM, cisplatin, CPA, melphalan, and MTX, that are eliminated primarily by urinary excretion, dosage should be based on creatinine clearance rather than body surface. Such a rational therapeutic approach in treating elderly women with advanced breast cancer with the cyclophosphamide-methotrexate-5-fluorouracil combination, when the initial CPA and MTX doses were calculated as a linear function of creatinine clearance, reduced both the incidence and severity of myelotoxicity. Finally, older women are more likely to be estrogen-receptor positive; when age and menopausal status of the patients are analyzed together, age turns out to be the primary determinant of the increased estrogen receptor concentration.

Some investigators believe that older patients with malignancies should be treated as aggressively as younger ones to receive the necessary chemotherapeutic benefits. However, exceptions should be based on physiological functional parameters and performance status instead of chronological age. Myelotoxicity following very aggressive chemotherapy in patients with leukemia and lymphoma other than Hodgkin's disease seems more severe and prolonged in patients over 65. As already mentioned, aging increases the risk of DOX-induced cardiotoxicity. In general, an increase in clinical bleeding and infection in cancer patients may occur in the elderly patient given chemotherapy. Repair of mucosal damage by anticancer agents is frequently slow and inadequate in older patients, which aggravates chemotherapy-induced mucositis. Moreover, the elderly are at higher risk of cisplatin-caused ototoxicity as well as peripheral neurotoxicity from VCR.

In summary, aging exerts definite effects on the pharmacology and toxicology of cancer chemotherapeutic agents. Whether or not an elderly patient should receive aggressive chemotherapy must be decided judiciously on an individual basis, taking into consideration the individual's physiological and not chronological age.

REFERENCES

1. **Holland, J. F., Frei, E. III, Bast, R. C., Jr., Kufe, D. W., Moreton, D. L., and Weichselbaum, R. R.,** *Cancer Medicine*, Lea & Febinger, Philadelphia, 1993, Sec. XVI.
2. **Chabner, B. A. and Longo, D. L., Eds.,** *Cancer Chemotherapy*, Lippincott-Raven, Philadelphia, 1990.
3. **Calabresi, P. and Chabner, B. A.,** *Chemotherapy of Neoplastic Diseases*, Sec. X in *The Pharmacological Basis of Therapeutics*, 9th ed., Hardman, J. G., Limbird, L. E., Molinoff, P. B., Ruddon, R. W., and Gilman, A. G., Eds., McGraw-Hill, Columbus, OH, 1996.
4. **Pratt, W. B., Ruddon, R. W., Ensminger, W. D., and Maybaum, J.,** *The Anticancer Drugs*, 2nd ed., Oxford University Press, New York, 1994.
5. **DeVita, V. T., Jr., Hellman, S., and Rosenberg, S. A.,** *Cancer, Principles and Practice of Oncology*, 4th ed., J. B. Lippincott, Philadelphia, 1993.
6. **Morrow, C. S. and Cowan, K. H.,** *Drug resistance and its clinical circumvention*, chap. XV-2 in Ref. 1.
7. **Khleif, S. N. and Curt, G A.,** *Animal models in drug development*, chap. XV-5 in Ref. 1
8. **Hanauske, A.-R. and von Hoff, D. D.,** *In vitro and in vivo predictive tests*, chap. XV-6 in Ref. 1.
9. **Colvin, M.,** *Alkylating agents and platinum antitumor compounds*, chap. XVI-3 in Ref. 1.
10. **Bertino, J. R.,** *Folate antagonists*, chap. XVI-1 in Ref. 1.
11. **Allegra, C. J.,** *Antifolates*, chap. 5 in Ref. 2.
12. **McCormack, J. J. and Johns, D. G.,** *Purine and purine nucleoside antimetabolites*, chap. 9 in Ref. 2.
13. **Chabner, B. A.,** *Cytidine analogues*, chap. 6 in Ref. 2.
14. **Grem, J. L.,** *Fluorinated pyrimidines*, chap. 7 in Ref. 2.
15. **Beck, W. T., Cass, C. E., and Houghton, P. J.,** *Anticancer drugs from plants: vinca alkaloids and taxol*, chap. XVI-8 in Ref. 1.
16. **Bender, R. A., Hamel, E., and Hande, K. R.,** *Plant alkaloids*, chap. 10 in Ref. 2.
17. **Wozniak, A. and Ross, W. E.,** *Epipodophyllotoxins*, chap. XVI-6 in Ref. 1.
18. **Myers, C.,** *Anthracyclines and DNA intercalators*, chap. XVI-5 in Ref. 1.
19. **Chabner, B. A.,** *Bleomycin*, chap. 13 in Ref. 2.
20. **Verweij, J., Hartigh, J. D., and Pinedo, H. M.,** *Antitumor antibiotics*, chap. 15 in Ref. 2.
21. **Chabner, B. A.,** *Enzyme therapy*: L-asparaginase, chap. 16 in Ref. 2.
22. **Averbuch, S.D.,** *Dacarbazine, procarbazine, hexamethyl-melamine*, chap. XVI-4 in Ref. 1.
23. **Donehower, R. C.,** *Hydroxyurea*, chap. 8 in Ref. 2.
24. Ref. 1, Sec XVII, *Principles of endocrine therapy*.
25. **Swain, S. M. and Lippman, M. E.,** *Endocrine therapy of cancer*, chap. 4 in Ref. 2.
26. Ref. 1, Sec. XVIII, *Principles of biotherapeutics*.
27. **Kerr, I. G. and DeAngelis, C.,** Cancer chemotherapy in the elderly — clinical pharmacologic considerations, chap. 9 in Zenser, T. V. and Coe, R. M., Eds., *Cancer and Aging, Progr. Res. Treat.*, Springer-Verlag, New York, 1989.
28. **Egorin, M. J.,** Cancer pharmacology in the elderly, *Semin. Oncol.*, 20, 43, 1993.

Chapter 18

NONSTEROIDAL ANTI-INFLAMMATORY DRUGS

James D. Winkler

CONTENTS

1. NONSTEROIDAL ANTI-INFLAMMATORY DRUGS

A. INTRODUCTION

The nonsteroidal anti-inflammatory drugs (NSAIDs) are a collection of drugs of several different structural classes that share in common both a therapeutic profile and a mechanism of action. The major activity in the therapeutic profile of these compounds is implied from the name anti-inflammatory, and most of the compounds in this collection possess moderate anti-inflammatory activity. This anti-inflammatory activity is observed against inflammation resulting from a number of pathological settings, such as musculoskeletal disorders, rheumatoid conditions, and infections. Other activities contributing to the therapeutic profile of these compounds are efficacy against pain and fever and the ability to block aggregation of platelets. The prototypical compound in this collection is aspirin, whose therapeutic profile has been

0-8493-8306-4/96/$0.00+$.50

known for over 100 years. Within the last several decades, aspirin has been joined by dozens of structurally different compounds, all of which have activities comparable to aspirin.

The unifying mechanism of action of these different compounds is their ability to inhibit the enzyme cyclooxygenase (COX). COX (prostaglandin [PG] H syntase) is an enzyme responsible for the conversion of arachidonic acid into PG H_2, the first step in the formation of a series of different prostaglandins and thromboxane (TX). These prostanoids, under the right conditions, can mediate or promote inflammatory responses, pain, fever, and platelet aggregation. Thus, inhibition of COX by NSAIDs leads to a predictable therapeutic outcome.

The NSAIDs can be divided into several groups based on structural similarities. The groups of NSAIDs (and examples of compounds) include the salicylates (aspirin), pyrazoles (phenylbutazone), para-aminophenols (acetaminophen), indols (indomethacin), fenamates (meclofenamate), propionic acids (ibuprofen), benzothiazine carboxamides (piroxicam), and phenylacetic acids (diclofenac).

In any discussion of NSAIDs, there are many issues where the drugs can be treated as one group and issues where there will be important differences between individual drugs. Generally speaking, the NSAIDs can be considered as one group when discussing issues that concern the effects of inhibition of COX, a property shared by all NSAIDs. In contrast, the NSAIDs must be discussed as individual agents when issues such as pharmacokinetics are examined, due to differences in metabolism caused by different chemical structures. In this chapter, we will be discussing the NSAIDs as one group, unless the particular issue requires separation of individual agents.

B. QUESTIONS ABOUT NSAID AND THE AGING POPULATION

A discussion of the use of NSAIDs in the aging population is important for several reasons. There is a real need for more frequent therapy with NSAIDs with aging. As a person gets older, there is an increased incidence of rheumatoid diseases, neuromuscular disorders, and other disorders in which the patient will benefit from the use of NSAIDs.[1] It is estimated that almost half of people over 65 have rheumatic disease to some degree, and these rheumatic symptoms account for a third of doctor visits.[2] Overlaying on this real increase in disease incidence is an increase in daily aches and pains, a "getting older" feeling of decreased mobility, and increased muscle pains, which lead to large increases in NSAID use, of both over-the-counter and prescription forms. For these reasons, the elderly are the largest consumers of NSAIDs. For males and females, respectively, the percent of people taking NSAIDs during a 12-month period is 3 and 6% for ages 17 to 44, 20 and 31% for ages 45 to 64, and 34 and 51% for ages 65 and older.[3] In fact, women over 65 are more likely than not to have taken NSAIDs.[4] Because of this tremendous increase in NSAIDs use with age, the therapeutic and toxic effects of these drugs in the elderly are a major concern.

To help focus the discussion of aging and NSAIDs, there are several types of questions that can be raised. The first type of question concerns the aging process and the system that NSAIDs interact with in the aging human. Specifically, what are the changes that occur with aging in the inflammatory response that may alter the use of anti-inflammatory agents? What are the changes that occur in the specific inflammatory system that NSAIDs act upon, including changes in COX activity and the ability of the aged person to form and catabolize PG?

The second type of question concerns the aging process and NSAIDs themselves. Specifically, are there changes that occur with aging that alter the ability of a person to metaboline NSAIDs and are there changes that occur in the ability of an older person to respond to NSAIDs? Are there differences in older people in the ability of NSAIDs to cause therapeutic or adverse affects?

The third type of question concerns a summation of the previous two questions. Specifically, what can we learn about the aging process from an examination of changes that occur in the PG inflammatory system? What can we learn about therapy in the elderly, using information about the therapeutic use of NSAIDs in the elderly as a guide?

II. EFFECT OF AGE ON INFLAMMATORY AND IMMUNE SYSTEMS

Taken as a total population, the elderly have a clear increase in morbidity and mortality from infections compared to a younger population. The simple conclusion from such data is that there are decreases in the ability of older people to mount immune and inflammatory responses to infectious organisms, demonstrating an overall decreased function with aging. However, this simple picture may not be correct. The elderly can be divided into two general populations, one elderly, but generally in good health and the other elderly with underlying disease(s). Now it is important to re-examine the question of altered immune and inflammatory function in aging, looking at the two populations separately. In fact, a review of studies of hospitalizations due to infection reveals that infection and ensuing complications are much more common in the elderly with underlying disease than in healthy, age-matched controls.[5] Thus, in a population of "healthy" older people, it is not clear if alterations in immune and inflammatory function have indeed occurred.

A more detailed examination of the immune system indicates a depressed response in the elderly. There is a decrease in the magnitude of the immune response with aging.[6] There is a decrease in the proliferative capacity of lymphocytes in older animals.[7] The number of cells that can respond to antigen or mitogens in *in vitro* assays is reduced, and there is increased activity of suppressor T-cells.[5] Part of the decreased ability of lymphocytes to respond to stimulation may be due to the modulatory effects of PG. Treatment with PGE_2 reduces the ability of lymphocytes to respond to mitogens, and lymphocytes from older people appear to be more responsive to PGE_2 than those from younger people.[8,9] The largest changes in the immune system with aging appear to be at the level of T-cells and their function. Some authors have suggested that this decrease in T-cells function does not in fact represent a diminution in immune function, but rather is a display of a very mature immune system that has already responded to a broad range of environmental pathogens and that T-cells have in general already served their function and are now naturally quiescent.[6]

In contrast to decreases in the function of immune-responsive cells documented in the elderly, there are data to indicate that there is no major defect in the inflammatory response in the elderly.[5] For example, there was no significant difference between young and old subjects in their inflammatory response to urate crystals, measured by both *in vitro* and *in vivo* tests.[10] Inflammatory cells from older individuals are present in normal numbers and have undiminished capacity to adhere, respond to chemotactic stimuli, and to kill infectious organisms.[5]

In addition to using inflammatory cells, increased body temperature is used as a mechanism to fight infection. Elderly patients have been reported to have a decreased febrile response to infection.[11] While the mechanism of this decreased response with age is not clear, PGs have an important role to play in regulation of elevated body temperature. Grahn et al.[12] studied PGE_2 release from brains from young and old mice in response to endotoxin challenge. They found that some older mice fail to produce PGE_2 when challenged, and they hypothesize that this lack of PGE_2 could translate into a lack of ability to produce fever in older patients with infection.

The picture that is developing of the older person is one in which there may be small reductions in the immune response and ability to produce fever. Some of these reductions may in fact be appropriate reductions due to increased efficiency of their immune systems. In contrast, there is no strong evidence for reductions in the inflammatory response of these people.

III. EFFECT OF AGE ON CYCLOOXYGENASE

Decades after the discovery of the therapeutic actions of aspirin, the discovery was made that NSAIDs act by inhibition of COX activity. Within the last several years this information has been extended by the discovery that there are two forms of COX.[13,14] These two forms, designated COX-1 and COX-2, are different at the genetic, messenger RNA and enzymatic levels. There is approximately 60 to 70% homology between the two forms of COX,[13] but there are also some very important differences, as will be discussed presently.

The enzyme COX-1 appears to be widely distributed in many tissues of the body and may provide a low, constitutive level of PG production.[15] In contrast, COX-2 appears to be induced by a variety of inflammatory stimuli[16-18] and to be present in high levels in inflammatory tissues, such as rheumatoid synovial tissue.[19] The discovery of two forms of COX opens the possibility that they can be differentially inhibited.[20–22] It may be possible in the future with isozyme-selective COX inhibitors to have compounds with different therapeutic and side effect profiles from those of the current NSAIDs.

Studies in which there is a direct comparison of COX levels between younger and older human populations have not been reported, and few studies exist in which a comparison has been performed in animals. In the rat, COX content in aortic smooth muscle and kidney has been examined in young and old animals, and no significant differences were uncovered.[23,24] More recently, human umbilical vein endothelial cells taken from young and senescent populations were studied *in vitro* and expression of COX-2 mRNA was evaluated. COX-2 was elevated in cells from the senescent population,[25] suggesting that cells from older people have the ability to express ample amount of COX. Although no sequence work has been reported, presumably the COX produced in elderly people is identical to that produced in younger people in terms of sequence, function, and ability of inhibitors to block its activity. This assumption is supported both by reports that tissues from elderly people have unchanged responses to COX inhibitors[26] and by the reported clinical efficacy of NSAIDs in the elderly.[2]

At this juncture, there is no evidence to conclude that there are any differences in COX content, character, or function between young and old people. Clearly, more studies need to be performed to examine this issue. In addition, there is no information at this time comparing the ability of young and old people to increase the content of COX-2 in response to various inflammatory or pathological stimuli. This is an important question, not only in terms of understanding the differential regulation of COX in different aged populations, but also in comprehending the potential benefit of selective inhibition of COX isoforms.

IV. EFFECT OF AGE ON THE FUNCTION OF THE PROSTAGLANDIN SYSTEM

COX is a key enzyme mediating the production of PG and TX inflammatory lipid mediators. However, COX is only one part of a complex system that exists to regulate the levels of these mediators. This system includes: (1) processes involved in the storage of arachidonate, the form of arachidonic acid contained within cellular phospholipids used for PG formation; (2) enzymes involved in the production of specific PG products; and (3) enzymes involved in the catabolism or removal of PG. These systems act in concert to produce specific concentrations of lipid mediators. In addition, these mediators act through specific and selective receptors on the effector cells. Certainly, alterations in any of these enzymes or receptors will change the function of the PG system. We will briefly review studies on the effects of aging on these parameters of the PG system.

A. ARACHIDONATE METABOLISM

Arachidonic acid is handled in special ways by inflammatory cells, with specific enzymes involved in the activation of arachidonic acid into arachidonoyl-CoA, in the incorporation of arachidonoyl-CoA into phospholipids, in the movement of arachidonate between phospholipids into potential releasable pools and in the release of arachidonate to provide substrate for COX.[27–30] Few studies have been done to compare the activity of this complex system in young and old animals. The uptake and incorporation of arachidonic acid into cellular phospholipids has been examined in brains from young and old rats. Terracina et al.[31] found a 50% increase in the content of arachidonoyl-CoA in brains from aged rats. However, there was a significant decrease in the incorporation of arachidonic acid into brain phospholipids. This decreased incorporation can account for the 20% decrease in rat brain arachidonate content, as reported by Gaiti.[32] In aging rats, the ability of the liver to incorporate arachidonic acid into phospholipids remains steady for 50 weeks, then increases over the final 40 weeks of life.[33] Human lung fibroblasts have been aged in culture and arachidonic acid release examined. In such studies, there is reported to be an increased release of arachidonic acid,[34] although whether or not this phenomenon is observed in *ex vivo* tissues from older humans is not clear.

B. PROSTAGLANDIN PRODUCTION

Changes with aging on the production of PG have been studied in a variety of species and cellular models. Looking first at cellular models of aging, decreases in PG production have been reported in human lung fibroblasts (6-keto-$PGF_{1\alpha}$, $PGF_{2\alpha}$),[35] in rat vascular smooth muscle cells,[36] and in human endothelial cells (6-keto-$PGF_{1\alpha}$).[37] However, these studies in cellular models of aging, in which PG production decreased, are not always in agreement with studies from whole tissues taken from young and old animals. For example, increases during aging in PG production have been reported in skeletal muscle from Rhesus monkeys,[38] rat kidney (6-keto-$PGF_{1\alpha}$, PGE_2, TXB_2),[39,40] and rat aorta.[41] In another study of rat kidney, there was no change reported in the production of TXB_2, while decreases in PGI_2 production were apparent.[24] 6-Keto-$PGF_{1\alpha}$, PGE_2, and $PGF_{2\alpha}$ production by homogenates of human aorta was unaffected by age or sex.[42] In livers from aging rats, however, there is a decline in the production of PGE_2 and $PGF_{2\alpha}$ with age.[33] Clearly, the effects of aging on PG production may vary with the specific eicosanoid and tissue examined.[37] However, there is no evidence for an overly striking deficit in the ability of older animals to produce PG.

C. PROSTAGLANDIN ELIMINATION

There are few reports on the effects of aging on the elimination of PG. Chang and Tai[24] looked directly at an enzyme involved in PG catabolism, NAD^+-dependent PG dehydrogenase, and found that there was a decrease with age in the activity of this enzyme in rat kidney. Studies of excretion of PG into the urine of human subjects have demonstrated mixed effects of aging. For example, there is a report that aging decreases the excretion of 6-keto-$PGF_{1\alpha}$ while increasing the excretion of TXB_2.[43] Similarly, excretion of PGE_2 is reduced while there is no change in PGF_2.[44] Again, the effects of aging on PG elimination may vary with the specific eicosanoid examined.

D. PROSTAGLANDIN CONCENTRATIONS

There are various reports that have examined the effects of aging on PG concentrations in various tissues. Here, the authors are not looking at production or elimination, but at the net concentration resulting from the summation of these processes. An examination of human plasma has revealed either no change (6-keto-$PGF_{1\alpha}$, PGE_2) or slight increases ($PGF_{2\alpha}$, TXB_2) in eicosanoid levels with aging.[44] Aorta tissue from young and old humans showed no significant difference with respect to 6-keto-$PGF_{1\alpha}$, PGE_2, or $PGF_{2\alpha}$ concentrations.[42] Several investigators have examined the PG content of human gastrointestinal mucosal tissue. Whereas Moore et al.[45,46] found no change with age in 6-keto-$PGF_{1\alpha}$ content, other reports document decreases with age in PGE_2 and $PGF_{2\alpha}$ concentrations.[47,48] These decreases in PG content with age appear to correlate with increases in acid secretion,[49] suggesting that these changes may have an important functional consequence. In studies in mice, there were declines in serum PGE_2 in the plasma from male mice, but not female mice, while in both sexes $PGF_{2\alpha}$ was unchanged.[50] These results suggest that there may be changes in PG content, depending on the tissue or PG examined, as well as possible differences due to the sex of the animal studied. There is some evidence to suggest that these differences may result in altered physiology with aging.

E. PROSTAGLANDIN RECEPTOR RESPONSES

PG cause their physiological and pathological effects by stimulation of specific receptors on effector cells. Any alteration in the number, affinity, or second messenger generation capacity of these receptors will change the response of the animal to a given concentration of PG. This is an area that has been little studied. In rats, the vasoconstriction response to the TX mimic U46619 was not altered during aging, suggesting the receptor/response mechanism in those tissues was not changed.[51] In contrast, the vascular response curves to PGI_2 and PGE_2 showed a rightward shift with aging,[52] suggesting that aging decreased the responsiveness of this tissue. In guinea pig trachea preparations, PGE_2 responses were unchanged with aging, whereas the response of the taenia caeci increased with age.[53] PGE_1 is more efficacious in inhibiting lipolysis in adipocytes from older rats.[54,55]

V. EFFECT OF AGING ON THE PHARMACOKINETICS OF NSAIDs

Some of the changes that occur in the interaction of aging people with NSAIDs may be due to alterations in the ability of older people to absorb, distribute, metabolize, and excrete these drugs. This section will briefly review some of the important differences in the pharmacokinetic handling of NSAIDs that occur with aging.

A. PHYSIOLOGICAL CHANGES WITH AGING

There are clear and consistent differences in general physiology that occur with aging (see review by Tümer et al.).[56] In general, in people with intact gastrointestinal tracts, there is little change with age in the ability to absorb drugs.[57] Naturally, this generalization does not hold in people with reduced gastrointestinal function due to surgery, disease, or drugs that modify gastrointestinal performance. In contrast to the lack of changes that occur in absorption, clear differences are observed in distribution of drugs in the elderly. These differences are due, in large part, to decreased serum protein concentrations, increased effective volume of distribution, and alterations in percentage of body fat and lean mass.[57,58] In general, liver weight and blood flow decline with age.[59] In spite of this decline, hepatic metabolism of most drugs is not greatly affected by aging, with the exception of the ability of the liver to perform oxidative metabolism, which may decrease metabolism of some drugs with aging.[59] The lack of change of metabolism of most drugs may be due to a broad excess in metabolic capacity of the liver. Decreases in renal blood flow, glomerular filtration, and tubular secretion have been observed to occur with aging, and these changes can result in decreases in drug clearance for drugs cleared primarily by the renal route.[58]

B. PATHOLOGICAL DIFFERENCES WITH AGING

Regardless of the age of a person, disease processes can have a dramatic effect on drug pharmacokinetics. In this regard, the elderly are special in that they have a higher incidence of ongoing or underlying diseases than a younger population. A number of studies have been made of the effect of disease on the pharmacokinetics of NSAIDs in the elderly. Liver impairment diseases or conditions have the largest effect on NSAIDs metabolism, as most of these drugs are eliminated by action of the liver.[60] In general, in the presence of decreased liver function in the elderly, the dose of NSAIDs must be reduced, often to half of the normal dose, although solid pharmacokinetic data in elderly patients with liver dysfunction are only available for a limited number of compounds.[60] In a similar manner, renal impairment due to disease could decrease the clearance of NSAIDs, as has been reported for diflunisal.[61] However, many NSAIDs are not dependent on renal clearance, and their kinetics is not altered in people with slight to moderate renal impairment.[62]

By far the most common disease states in the elderly for which NSAIDs are used are arthritic diseases. Studies in elderly patients with arthritis have disclosed no changes in the pharmacokinetics of sulindac[63] or diflunisal,[61] and only slight decreases in area under the concentration-time curve for nabumatone.[64]

C. PHARMACOKINETIC DIFFERENCES IN NSAIDS WITH AGING

A number of reports exist on the pharmacokinetics of NSAIDs in the aging population. In general, these studies are performed on patients with no major known disease conditions that would alter their pharmacokinetic response to NSAIDs. The findings of these studies are summarized in Table 18.1. Of the drugs that have been studied, about half show important reductions in the ability of older people to metabolize, distribute, and/or eliminate them. Other drugs that have been studied show no pronounced changes in pharmacokinetics with age.

TABLE 18.1.
The Effects of Age on Pharmacokinetics of Some NSAIDs

Class	Drug	Comment	Ref.
Salicylates	Salicylate	No change in PK	86
		No change in AUC	87
	Diflunisol	Little change in PK	61
Pyrazoles	Phenylbutazone	No change $T_{1/2}$	88
Indols	Indomethacin	Decreased clear.	89
	Sulindac	No change in PK	63
Propionic acids	Ibuprofen	Decreased clear.	90
	Indoprofen	Increased $T_{1/2}$	91
	Naproxen	Decreased clear.	92–94
Benzothiazine carbox	Piroxicam	No change in PK	95–97
Phenylacetic acids	Diclofenac	No change AUC	98

Note: The abbreviations used in the Table are AUC, area under the concentration-time curve; clear., clearance; PK, pharmacokinetics; $T_{1/2}$, half-life.

In general, there are important differences between individual drugs, due to differences in pharmacokinetics caused by different chemical structures and different properties of each drug. For example, although decreases in serum albumin occur with aging, this may only have an important effect on a drug that is normally highly bound, such as salicylic acid.[65,66] Another general consideration is that for many NSAIDs there are no major changes in pharmacokinetics with aging. However, this point must be tempered with a last general observation that for several of the NSAIDs there is insufficient information of the effects of aging on their pharmacokinetics.[60]

D. DRUG-DRUG INTERACTIONS

The major drug-drug interactions of NSAIDs involve competition for drug binding sites on serum proteins and for renal secretion of organic acids.[60] Due to general decreases in serum protein and renal function observed with age, as described above, as well as to the increase in overall drug use in the elderly, there is an increase with age in the incidence of drug-drug interactions involving NSAIDs.[56]

VI. EFFECT OF AGING ON THE PHARMACODYNAMICS OF NSAIDs

This section is a summation of the previous sections in the following sense: given that there may or may not be changes with age in the inflammation system, in COX, in the PG system, and in the pharmacokinetics of individual NSAIDs, in a global way, how do these drugs act in elderly patients? Are there changes in their ability to be effective anti-inflammatory agents? Are there changes in their ability to produce a range of adverse effects? These questions will now be addressed.

A. THERAPEUTIC EFFECTS

The therapeutic effectiveness of NSAIDs does not appear to diminish with age. In general, the doses of NSAIDs that produce anti-inflammatory effects in younger patients will produce equal efficacy in older patients. This is especially true if the effective free plasma drug concentration is used for the comparison, eliminating any differences due to changes with age in the pharmacokinetics of the drugs.[60] The fact that NSAIDs are so widely used by the elderly is a testimony to their effectiveness in that population.

B. ADVERSE EFFECTS

There is a common belief that older people are more sensitive to NSAIDs and suffer from a higher incidence of adverse effects. Among the questions to be addressed are, is there truly an increased incidence of adverse effects in the elderly? Is the increased incidence of adverse effects due to changes in pharmacokinetics (more drug getting to the site of the effect)? Is the increased incidence of adverse effects due to changes in pharmacodynamics (more activity per unit of drug at the site of the effect)?

The most common adverse effects of NSAIDs are gastrointestinal effects. Numerous studies have reported that gastrointestinal side effects are positively correlated with the use of NSAIDs and that there is an increased risk of adverse effects with age.[67–73] While this is the general consensus of the reports, there is one report that fails to show changes with age in the frequency of gastric lesions.[45] In addition, a study of NSAID-induced decreases in gastric mucosal blood flow failed to show any changes with age.[74]

Other adverse effects that are said to be associated with NSAID use are hepatic, renal, hematological, and hypersensitivity. For hepatic effects, there are actually no strong data to link NSAIDs with hepatic adverse effects and no effect of age can be detected.[69,75] In a study of the effects of NSAIDs on renal function, Allred et al.[76] could not show any effect of these drugs in an elderly population. There is a belief that renal function is affected by PG production and the NSAIDs, by their blockade of renal PG production, can alter renal function, renal blood flow, and produce renal side effects, including necrosis, nephrotic syndrome, and electrolyte disturbances.[75,77] Older patients may be at greater risk for renal side effects, especially NSAID-induced acute interstitial nephritis.[78] Concerning hematological adverse effects, there is a report of a slight increased risk with aging in NSAID-induced neutropenia.[69] Hypersensitivity reactions, while very serious, are too rare and too little data exist to determine if their incidence increases with age.[69]

In general, there is evidence to suggest that there is an increase in adverse effects of NSAIDs with age.[79] However, this view is not universally held[58] and some reports examined numbers of adverse effect reports, not the incidence of adverse effects. To alleviate this problem, Bollini et al.[80] examined the role of quality and study design on the results of epidemiological studies of the effects of NSAIDs on gastrointestinal adverse effects. They found that increased risks of adverse effects were found in the more poorly designed and executed studies. Conversely, satisfactory studies that controlled for major confounding variables were associated with lower risk estimates. Using their conservative analysis, there still remained an age-associated risk factor in NSAID-induced gastrointestinal adverse effects, with the relative risk index increasing from 3.2 in people less than 60 to 7.1 in people over 60 years of age.[80] It appears that by the best estimates that NSAID-induced gastrointestinal adverse effects increase with age.

The mechanism of this increase in adverse effects is not clear, and several possible explanations can be proposed. One possibility is that the differences observed in gastrointestinal adverse effects are due to differences in the "baseline". That is, older patients may start with a higher level of pre-existing gastrointestinal damage before starting NSAID therapy. In support of this notion is the observation that the elderly are less able to recover from an episode of ulcer bleeding than is a younger patient.[81] Another factor is that older people may take more frequent courses of NSAID therapy. In an interesting study, Hutchinson et al.[82] showed that total drug adverse effects appeared to increase with age when examined as a percent of the number of patients reporting effects, yet the same data showed no increase with age when expressed as the percent of adverse effects per course of therapy. A strong possibility for the increased incidence of adverse effects among the elderly is the alteration in pharmacokinetics that occurs with aging, as described above. In most, if not all, of the studies of the effects of NSAIDs on gastrointestinal effects in the elderly, no evaluation was made of age-associated differences in effective dosage of the drugs.[83] Finally, it is possible that the elderly have an increased response to a given concentration of NSAID, a pharmacodynamic alteration. In support of this idea is a report that older people are more sensitive to central nervous system effects of NSAIDs than younger people.[84] The hypothesis was made that older people are more sensitive to PG and NSAIDs,[8] yet to date little evidence exists to support this idea.

VII. CONCLUSIONS AND FUTURE QUESTIONS

In conclusion, there are few minor or no demonstrated changes in the ability of the elderly to mount an inflammatory response, including their ability to manufacture COX and regulate PG concentrations. Whereas there is little evidence for changes in the therapeutic efficacy of NSAIDs in the elderly, there is ample evidence for significant changes in pharmacokinetics of some NSAIDs and for an increased incidence of adverse effects in the older population.

Important questions remain for future investigation. The discovery of two forms of COX has raised many questions about the regulation of these enzymes by disease and age. The possible therapeutic potential of isotype-selective COX inhibitors in the elderly needs to be explored. We need to know more about the regulation and responsiveness of PG receptors in different tissues from older people, to explore the possibility that altered sensitivity of these receptors with age may alter the ability of NSAIDs to produce therapeutic or adverse effects. Finally, the mechanism that accounts for the increased incidence of adverse effects of NSAIDs in the elderly must be inspected. Do changes in the pharmacokinetics of NSAIDs explain the increases in adverse effects, and are there changes in receptor sensitivity or is the increase in adverse effects due to a yet to be defined change that occurs with aging? Answers to these questions, as well as judicious use of current information,[85] can result in an increase in the safe use of this important class of therapeutic agents.

REFERENCES

1. **Hodinka, L.**, Improving the risk-benefit ratio of nsaid therapy in the elderly, *Scand. J. Rheumatol. Suppl.*, 20, 3, 1991.
2. **Nuki, G.**, Pain control and the use of non-steroidal analgesic anti-inflammatory, *Br. Med. Bull.*, 46, 262, 1990.
3. **Bulpitt, C. J.**, Risks and benefits of drug treatment of hypertension in the elderly, *J. R. Soc. Med. Suppl.*, 87, 16, 1994.
4. **Hughes, G. R. V.**, The problems of using NSAIDs in the elderly, *Scand. J. Rheumatol. Suppl.*, 91, 19, 1991.
5. **Phair, J. P., Hsu, C. S., and Hsu, Y. L.**, Ageing and infection, *Ciba. Found. Symp.*, 134, 143, 1988.
6. **Siskind, G. W.**, Aging and the immune system, in *Modern Biological Theories of Aging*, Warner, H. R., Ed., Raven Press, New York, 1987, 235.
7. **Licastro, F. and Walford, R. L.**, Effects exerted by prostaglandins and indomethacin on the immuneresponse during aging, *Gerontology*, 32,1, 1986.
8. **Goodwin, J. S. and Messner, R. P.**, Sensitivity of lymphocytes to prostaglandin E2 increases in subjects over age 70, *J. Clin. Invest.*, 64, 434, 1979.
9. **Goodwin, J. S.**, Changes in lymphocyte sensitivity to prostaglandin E, histamine, hydrocortisone, and X irradiation with age: studies in a healthy elderly population, *Clin. Immunol. Immunopathol.*, 25, 243, 1982.
10. **McGill, N. W., Dieppe, P. A., and Swan, A.**, The effect of age on the inflammatory response to arthritis-associated crystals, *Aust. N.Z. J. Med.*, 22, 458, 1992.
11. **Gleckman, R. and Hibert, D.**, Afebrile bacteremia. A phenomenon in geriatric patients, *J. Am. Med. Assoc.*, 248, 1478, 1982.
12. **Grahn, D., Norman, D. C., and Yoshikawa, T. T.**, Fever and aging: central nervous system prostaglandin E2 in response to endotoxin, *Exp. Gerontol.*, 22, 249, 1987.
13. **Kujubu, D. A., Fletcher, B. S., Varnum, B. C., Lim, R. W., and Herschman, H. R.**, TIS10, a phorbol ester tumor promoter-inducible mRNA from Swiss 3T3 cells, encodes a novel prostaglandin synthase/cyclooxygenase homologue, *J. Biol. Chem.*, 266, 12866, 1991.
14. **O'Banion, M. K., Sadowski, H. B., Winn, V., and Young, D. A.**, A serum- and glucocorticoid-regulated 4-kilobase mRNA encodes a cyclooxygenase-related protein, *J. Biol. Chem.*, 266, 23261, 1991.
15. **O'Neill, G. P. and Ford-Hutchinson, A. W.**, Expression of mRNA for cyclooxygenase-1 and cyclooxygenase-2 in human tissues, *FEBS Lett.*, 330, 156, 1993.
16. **O'Sullivan, M. G., Chilton, F. H., Huggins, E. M., Jr., and McCall, C. E.**, Lipopolysaccharide priming of alveolar macrophages for enhanced synthesis of prostanoids involves induction of a novel prostaglandin H synthase, *J. Biol. Chem.*, 267, 14547, 1992.
17. **Lyons-Giordano, B., Pratta, M. A., Galbraith, W., Davis, G. L., and Arner, E. C.**, Interleukin-1 differentially modulates chondrocyte expression of cyclooxygenase-2 and phospholipase A_2, *Exp. Cell Res.*, 206, 58, 1993.
18. **Jackson, B. A., Goldstein, R. H., Roy, R., Cozzani, M., Taylor, L., and Polgar, P.**, Effects of transforming growth factor b and interleukin-1b on expression of cyclooxygenase 1 and 2 and phospholipase A_2 mRNA in lung fibroblasts and endothelial cells in culture, *Biochem. Biophys. Res. Commun.*, 197, 1465, 1993.
19. **Crofford, L. J., Wilder, R. L., Ristimäki, A. P., Sano, H., Remmers, E. F., Epps, H. R., and Hla, T.**, Cyclooxygenase-1 and -2 expression in rheumatoid synovial tissues. Effects of interleukin-1b, phorbol ester, and corticosteroids, *J. Clin. Invest.*, 93, 1095, 1994.
20. **Meade, E. A., Smith, W. L., and DeWitt, D. L.**, Differential inhibition of prostaglandin endoperoxide synthase (cyclooxygenase) isozymes by aspirin and other non-steroidal anti-inflammatory drugs, *J. Biol. Chem.*, 268, 6610, 1993.
21. **Futaki, N., Takahashi, S., Yokoyama, M., Arai, I., Higuchi, S., and Otomo, S.**, NS-398, a new anti-inflammatory agent, selectively inhibits prostaglandin G/H synthase/cyclooxygenase (COX-2) activity in vitro, Prostaglandins, 47, 55, 1994.
22. **Mitchell, J. A., Akarasereenont, P., Thiemermann, C., Flower, R. J., and Vane, J. R.**, Selectivity of nonsteroidal antiinflammatory drugs as inhibitors of constitutive and inducible cyclooxygenase, *Proc. Natl. Acad. Sci. U.S.A.*, 90, 11693, 1993.
23. **Chang, W. C., Murota, S. I., Nakao, J., and Orimo, H.**, Age-related decrease in prostacyclin biosynthetic activity in rat aortic smooth muscle cells, *Biochim. Biophys. Acta*, 620, 159, 1980.
24. **Chang, W. C. and Tai, H. H.**, Changes in prostacyclin and thromboxane biosynthesis and their catabolic enzyme activity in kidneys of aging rats, *Life Sci.*, 34, 1269, 1984.
25. **Garfinkel, S., Brown, S., Wessendorf, J. H. M., and Maciag, T.**, Post-transcriptional regulation of interleukin 1a in various strains of young and senescent human umbilical vein endothelial cells, *Proc. Natl. Acad. Sci. U.S.A.*, 91, 1559, 1994.
26. **Schoeffter, P. and Godfraind, T.**, Spontaneous rhythmic contractions of human saphenous veins isolated from old subjects are sensitive to cyclooxygenase inhibitors, *Experientia*, 45, 459, 1989.
27. **MacDonald, J. I. S. and Sprecher, H.**, Phospholipid fatty acid remodeling in mammalian cells, *Biochim. Biophys. Acta*, 1084, 105, 1991.

28. **Snyder, F., Lee, T.-C., and Blank, M. L.,** The role of transacylases in the metabolism of arachidonate and platelet-activating factor, *Prog. Lipid Res.*, 31, 65, 1992.
29. **Winkler, J. D. and Chilton, F. H.,** The role of CoA-independent transacylases in the production of platelet-activating factor and the metabolism of arachidonate, *Drug News Perspec.*, 6, 133, 1993.
30. **Mayer, R. J. and Marshall, L. A.,** New insights on mammalian phospholipase A_2(s); comparison of arachidonoyl-selective and -nonselective enzymes, *FASEB J.*, 7, 339, 1993.
31. **Terracina, L., Brunetti, M., Avellini, L., DeMedio, G. E., Trovarelli, G., and Gaiti, A.,** Arachidonic and palmitic acid utilization in aged rat brain areas, *Mol. Cell. Biochem.*, 115, 35, 1992.
32. **Gaiti, A.,** The aging brain. A normal phenomenon with not-so-normal arachidonic acid metabolism, *Ann. N.Y. Acad. Sci.*, 559, 365, 1989.
33. **Morita, I. and Murota, S.,** Effect of aging on the prostaglandin-synthesizing system in rat liver, *Prostaglandins Med.*, 4, 45, 1980.
34. **Huang, N. N., Wang, D. J., and Heppel, L. A.,** Stimulation of aged human lung fibroblasts by extracellular ATP via suppression of arachidonate metabolism, *J. Biol. Chem.*, 268, 10789, 1993.
35. **Taylor, L., Schneider, E., Smith, J., and Polgar, P.,** Prostaglandin production and cellular aging, *Mech. Ageing Dev.*, 16, 311, 1981.
36. **Takeuchi, K., Abe, K., Sato, M., Yasujima, M., Hagino, T., Fang, S., and Yoshinaga, K.,** Effect of in vitro aging on prostaglandin synthesis in cultured rat vascular smooth muscle cells, *Agents Actions Suppl.*, 22, 49, 1987.
37. **Lennon, E. A. and Poyser, N. L.,** Effect of age on vascular prostaglandin production in male and female rats, *Prostaglandins Leukot. Med.*, 25, 1, 1986.
38. **Young, M. K., Bocek, R. M., Herrington, P. T., and Beatty, C. H.,** Aging: effects on the prostaglandin production by skeletal muscle of male rhesus monkeys (Macaca mulatta), *Mech. Ageing Dev.*, 16, 345, 1981.
39. **Rathaus, M., Greenfeld, Z., Podjarny, E., Brezis, M., Green, J., and Bernheim, J.,** Altered prostaglandin synthesis and impaired sodium conservation in the kidneys of old rats, *Clin. Sci. (Colch).*, 83, 301, 1992.
40. **Rathaus, M., Greenfeld, Z., Podjarny, E., Brezis, M., and Bernheim, J.,** Sodium loading and renal prostaglandins in old rats, *Prostaglandins Leukot. Essent. Fatty Acids,* 49, 815, 1993.
41. **Markov, KhM., Ivanova, I. A., and Zadkova, G. F.,** Vozrastnye osobennosti prostaglandinovoi sistemy vnekotorykh organakh, *Fiziol. Zh. S.S.S.R.*, 69, 832, 1983.
42. **Lennon, E. A., Ansell, I., Davies, G. C., and Poyser, N. L.,** The effect of age and smoking on vascular prostaglandin production in men and women, *Prostaglandins Leukot. Essent. Fatty Acids,* 32, 15, 1988.
43. **Hornych, A., Forette, F., Bariety, J., Krief, C., Aumont, J., and Paris, M.,** The influence of age on renal prostaglandin synthesis in man, *Prostaglandins Leukot. Essent. Fatty Acids,* 43, 191, 1991.
44. **Tokar, A. V. and Negarae, A. I.,** Prostaglandins in elderly humans with normal and high arterial pressure, *Gerontology,* 34, 82, 1988.
45. **Moore, J. G., Bjorkman, D. J., Mitchell, M. D., and Avots-Avotins, A.,** Age does not influence acute aspirin-induced gastric mucosal damage, *Gastroenterology,* 100, 1626, 1991.
46. **Moore, J. G. and Bjorkman, D. J.,** NSAID-induced gastropathy in the elderly: understanding and avoidance, *Geriatrics,* 44, 51, 1989.
47. **Cryer, B., Lee, E., and Feldman, M.,** Factors influencing gastroduodenal mucosal prostaglandin concentrations: roles of smoking and aging, *Ann. Intern. Med.*, 116, 636, 1992.
48. **Goto, H., Sugiyama, S., Ohara, A., Hoshino, H., Hamajima, E., Kanamori, S., and Ozawa, T.,** Age-associated decreases in prostaglandin contents in human gastric mucosa, *Biochem. Biophys. Res. Commun.*, 186, 1443, 1992.
49. **Cryer, B., Redfern, J. S., Goldschmiedt, M., Lee, E., and Feldman, M.,** Effect of aging on gastric and duodenal mucosal prostaglandin concentrations in humans, *Gastroenterology,* 102, 1118, 1992.
50. **Parkening, T. A., LaGrone, L. F., and Brouhard, B. H.,** Concentrations of prostaglandins in plasma, seminal vesicles, and ovaries of aging C57BL/6NNia mice, *Exp. Gerontol.*, 20, 291, 1985.
51. **Mayhan, W. G., Faraci, F. M., Baumbach, G. L., and Heistad, D. D.,** Effects of aging on responses of cerebral arterioles, *Am. J. Physiol.*, 258, H1138, 1990.
52. **Jackson, E. K., Herzer, W. A., and Lawson, J. A.,** Defective modulation of noradrenergic neurotransmission by exogenous prostaglandins in aging spontaneously hypertensive rats, *J. Pharmacol. Exp. Ther.,* 251, 858, 1989.
53. **Vermue, N. A. and Den Hertog, A.,** The prostaglandin response in guinea-pig taenia caeci and trachea smooth muscle of different ages, *Eur. J. Pharmacol.,* 147, 273, 1988.
54. **Hoffman, B. B., Chang, H., and Reaven, G. M.,** Stimulation and inhibition of lipolysis in isolated rat adipocytes: evidence for age-related changes in responses to forskolin and PGE1, *Horm. Metab. Res.*, 19, 358, 1987.
55. **Chang, W. C. and Roth, G. S.,** Changes in prostaglandin E1 stimulation of glucose oxidation in rat adipocytes during maturation and aging, *Life Sci.*, 28, 623, 1981.
56. **Tumer, N., Scarpace, P. J., and Lowenthal, D. T.,** Geriatric pharmacology: basic and clinical considerations, *Annu. Rev. Pharmacol. Toxicol.*, 32, 271, 1992.

57. **Hernadi, F.**, Pharmacodynamic and pharmacokinetic relations of aging, *Int. J. Clin. Pharmacol. Ther. Toxicol.*, 30, 545, 1992.
58. **Buchanan, W. W.**, Implications of NSAID therapy in elderly patients, *J. Rheumatol. Suppl.*, 20, 29, 1990.
59. **Woodhouse, K. W. and Wynne, H.**, The pharmacokinetics of non-steroidal anti-inflammatory drugs in the elderly, *Clin. Pharmacokinet.*, 12, 111, 1987.
60. **Brater, D. C.**, Drug-drug and drug-disease interactions with nonsteroidal anti-inflammatory drugs, *Am. J. Med.*, 80, 62, 1986.
61. **Erikson, L. O., Wahlin-Boll, E., Odar-Cederlof, I., Lindholm, L., and Melander, A.**, Influence of renal failure, rheumatoid arthritis and old age on the pharmacokinetics of diflunisal, *Eur. J. Clin. Pharmacol.*, 36, 165, 1989.
62. **Hyneck, M. L.**, An overview of the clinical pharmacokinetics of nabumetone, *J. Rheumatol.*, 19 (Suppl. 36), 20, 1992.
63. **Sitar, D. S., Owen, J. A., MacDougall, B., Hunter, T., and Mitenko, P. A.**, Effects of age and disease on the pharmacokinetics and pharmacodynamics of sulindac, *Clin. Pharmacol. Ther.*, 38, 228, 1985.
64. **Kendall, M. J., Chellingsworth, M. C., Jubb, R., Thawley, A. R., Undre, N. A., and Kill, D. C.**, A pharmacokinetic study of the active metabolite of nabumetone in young healthy subjects and older arthritis patients, *Eur. J. Clin. Pharmacol.*, 36, 299, 1989.
65. **Viani, A., Rizzo, G., Carrai, M., and Pacifici, G. M.**, The effect of ageing on plasma albumin and plasma protein binding of, *Br. J. Clin. Pharmacol.*, 33, 299, 1992.
66. **Viani, A., Rizzo, G., Carrai, M., and Pacifici, G. M.**, Differential effect of aging on albumin and plasma protein binding of, *Pharmacol. Res.*, 25, 43, 1992.
67. **Fries, J. F.**, Assessing and understanding patient risk, *Scand. J. Rheumatol. Suppl.*, 92, 21, 1992.
68. **Llewellyn, J. G. and Pritchard, M. H.**, Influence of age and disease state in nonsteroidal antiinflammatory drug associated gastric bleeding, *J. Rheumatol.*, 15, 691, 1988.
69. **Carson, J. L. and Rees Willett, L.**, Toxicity of nonsteroidal anti-inflammatory drugs: an overview of the, *Drugs*, 46, 243, 1993.
70. **Schubert, T. T., Bologna, S. D., Nensey, Y., Schubert, A. B., Mascha, E. J., and Ma, C. K.**, Ulcer risk factors: interactions between helicobacter pylori infection, *Am. J. Med.*, 94, 413, 1993.
71. **Guess, H. A., West, R., and Strand, L. M.**, Fatal upper gastrointestinal hemorrhage or perforation among users and nonusers of nonsteroidal anti-inflammatory drugs in Saskatchewan, Canada, *J. Clin. Epidemiol.*, 41, 35, 1988.
72. **Collier, D. S. and Pain, J. A.**, Nonsteroidal anti-inflammatory drugs and peptic ulcer perforation, *Gut*, 26, 359, 1985.
73. **Griffin, M. R., Ray, W. A., and Schaffner, W.**, Nonsteroidal anti-inflammatory drug use and death from peptic ulcer in elderly persons, *Ann. Intern. Med.*, 109, 359, 1988.
74. **Taha, A. S., Angerson, W., Nakshabendi, I., Beekman, H., Morran, C., Sturrock, R. D., and Russell, R. I.**, Gastric and duodenal mucosal blood flow in patients receiving non-steroidal anti-inflammatory drugs. Influence of age, smoking, ulceration and Helicobacter pylori, *Aliment. Pharmacol. Ther.*, 7, 41, 1993.
75. **Weinblatt, M. E.**, Nonsteroidal anti-inflammatory drug toxicity: increased risk in the elderly, *Scand. J. Rheumatol. Suppl.*, 91, 9, 1991.
76. **Allred, J., Wong, W., and Kafetz, K.**, Elderly people taking non-steroidal anti-inflammatory drugs are unlikely to have excess renal impairment, *Postgrad. Med. J.*, 65, 735, 1989.
77. **Menkes, C. J.**, Renal and hepatic effects of NSAIDs in the elderly, *Scand. J. Rheumatol. Suppl.*, 83, 11, 1989.
78. **Garella, S. and Matarese, R. A.**, Renal effects of prostaglandins and clinical adverse effects of nonsteroidal anti-inflammatory agents, *Medicine*, 63, 165, 1984.
79. **Clark, D. W. and Ghose, K.**, Neuropsychiatric reactions to nonsteroidal anti-inflammatory drugs (NSAIDs). The New Zealand experience, *Drug. Saf.*, 7, 460, 1992.
80. **Bollini, P., Garcia Rodriguez, L. A., Gutthann, S. P., and Walker, A. M.**, The impact of research quality and study design on epidemiologic, *Arch. Intern. Med.*, 152, 1289, 1992.
81. **Irvin, T. T.**, Mortality and perforated peptic ulcer: a case of risk stratification in elderly patients, *Br. J. Surg.*, 76, 215, 1989.
82. **Hutchinson, T. A., Flegel, K. M., Kramer, M. S., Leduc, D. G., and Kong, H. H.**, Frequency, severity and risk factors for adverse drug reactions in adult out-patients: a prospective study, *J. Chronic Dis.*, 39, 533, 1986.
83. **Gurwitz, J. H. and Avorn, J.**, The ambiguous relation between aging and adverse drug reactions, *Ann. Intern. Med.*, 114, 956, 1991.
84. **Johnson, A. G. and Day, R. O.**, The problems and pitfalls of NSAID therapy in the elderly (Part I), *Drugs Aging*, 1, 130, 1991.
85. **Girgis, L. and Brooks, P.**, Nonsteroidal anti-inflammatory drugs. Differential use in older patients, *Drug Ther.*, 4, 101, 1994.
86. **Needs, C. J. and Brooks, P. M.**, Clinical pharmacokinetics of the salicylates, *Clin. Pharmacokinet.*, 10, 164, 1985.

87. **Netter, P., Faure, G., Regent, M. C., Procknal, J. A., and Levy, G.,** Salicylate kinetics in old age, *Clin. Pharmacol. Ther.*, 38, 6, 1985.
88. **Triggs, E. J., Nation, R. L., Long, A., and Ashley, J. J.,** Pharmacokinetics in the elderly, *Eur. J. Clin. Pharmacol.*, 8, 55, 1975.
89. **Oberbauer, R., Krivanek, P., and Tunheim, K.,** Pharmacokinetics of indomethacin in the elderly, *Clin. Pharmacokinet.*, 24, 428, 1993.
90. **Greenblatt, D. J., Abernethy, D. R., Methis, R., Marmatz, J. S., and Shader, R. I.,** Absorption and disposition of ibuprofen in the elderly, *Arthritis Rheum.*, 27, 1066, 1984.
91. **Lund, B., Egsmose, C., Knudsen, O., and Andersen, R. B.,** Pharmacokinetic profile of indoprofen in elderly subjects, *Br. J. Clin. Pharmacol.*, 22, 721, 1986.
92. **Upton, R. A., Williams, R. L., Kelly, J., and Jones, R. M.,** Naproxen pharmacokinetics in the elderly, *Br. J. Clin. Pharmacol.*, 18, 207, 1984.
93. **Van den Ouweland, F. A., Jansen, P. A., Tan, Y., Van de Putte, L. B., Van Ginneken, C. A., and Gribnau, F. W.,** Pharmacokinetics of high-dosage naproxen in elderly patients, *Int. J. Clin. Pharmacol. Ther. Toxicol.*, 26, 143, 1988.
94. **McVerry, R. M., Lethbridge, J., Martin, N., Mukerjee, S. K., Littler, T., Tallis, R., Sibeon, R., and Orme, M. L.,** Pharmacokinetics of naproxen in elderly patients, *Eur. J. Clin. Pharmacol.*, 31, 463, 1986.
95. **Olkkola, K. T., Brunetto, A. V., and Mattila, M. J.,** Pharmacokinetics of oxicam nonsteroidal anti-inflammatory agents, *Clin. Pharmacokinet.*, 26, 107, 1994.
96. **Rudy, A. C., Figueroa, N. L., Hall, S. D., and Brater, D. C.,** The pharmacokinetics of piroxicam in elderly persons with and without renal impairment, *Br. J. Clin. Pharmacol.*, 37, 1, 1994.
97. **Hundal, O., Rugstad, H. E., and Husby, G.,** Naproxen free plasma concentrations and unbound fractions in patients with osteoarthritis: relation to age, sex, efficacy, and adverse events, *Ther. Drug. Monit.*, 13, 478, 1991.
98. **Kendall, M. J., Thornhill, D. P., and Willis, J. V.,** Factors affecting the pharmacokinetics of diclofenac sodium, *Rheumatology*, Suppl. 2, 38, 1979.

INDEX

A

B

C

D

I

O

P

Q

R

S

U

V

W

X

Y

Z